# PEDIATRIC HYPERTENSION

# Clinical Hypertension and Vascular Diseases

William B. White, MD
*Series Editor*

---

***Pediatric Hypertension,*** edited by *Ronald J. Portman, MD, Jonathan M. Sorof, MD, and Julie R. Ingelfinger, MD, 2004*

***Secondary Hypertension:*** *Clinical Presentation, Diagnosis, and Treatment,* edited by *George A. Mansoor, MD, 2004*

# PEDIATRIC HYPERTENSION

*Edited by*

RONALD J. PORTMAN, MD

*Division of Pediatric Nephrology and Hypertension,*
*University of Texas-Houston, Medical School, Houston, TX*

JONATHAN M. SOROF, MD

*Division of Pediatric Nephrology and Hypertension,*
*University of Texas-Houston, Medical School, Houston TX*

JULIE R. INGELFINGER, MD

*Department of Pediatrics, Harvard Medical School,*
*and Division of Pediatric Nephrology, Massachusetts General Hospital,*
*Boston, MA*

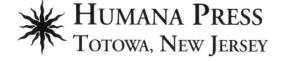

HUMANA PRESS
TOTOWA, NEW JERSEY

999 Riverview Drive, Suite 208
Totowa, New Jersey 07512

**www.humanapress.com**



Production Editor: Tracy Catanese
Cover design by Patricia F. Cleary.

For additional copies, pricing for bulk purchases, and/or information about other Humana titles, contact Humana at the above address or at any of the following numbers: Tel.: 973-256-1699; Fax: 973-256-8341, E-mail: humana@humanapr.com; or visit our Website: www.humanapress.com

This publication is printed on acid-free paper. ∞
ANSI Z39.48-1984 (American National Standards Institute) Permanence of Paper for Printed Library Materials.



Printed in the United States of America. 10 9 8 7 6 5 4 3 2 1

1-59259-797-1 (e-book)

Library of Congress Cataloging-in-Publication Data

Pediatric hypertension / edited by Ronald J. Portman, Jonathan M. Sorof, Julie R. Ingelfinger.
p. ; cm. -- (Clinical hyptertension and vascular diseases)
Includes bibliographical references and index.
ISBN 1-58829-385-8 (alk. paper)
1. Hypertension in children.
[DNLM: 1. Hypertension--diagnosis--Child. 2. Hypertension--diagnosis--Infant. 3. Hypertension--etiology--Child. 4. Hypertension--etiology--Infant. 5. Hypertension--therapy--Child. 6. Hypertension--therapy--Infant. WG 340 P3725 2004] I. Portman, Ronald J. II. Sorof, Jonathan M. III. Ingelfinger, Julie R. IV. Series.
RJ426.H9P435 2004
618.92'132--dc22

200327615

# Foreword

The importance of hypertension in children and adolescents is becoming increasingly recognized by physicians and scientists in the 21st century. However, in contrast to the attention that hypertension has received in the adult population for the past three decades since the first Joint National Committee (JNC) report, research and clinical knowledge that involves hypertension in children is still very much in its own childhood. *Pediatric Hypertension*, edited by Drs. Portman, Sorof, and Ingelfinger, is undoubtedly the most up-to-date and clinically relevant contribution to the field of hypertension in children available because it brings together the numerous pathophysiologic, diagnostic, and therapeutic advances in the evaluation of high blood pressure in infants, children, and adolescents.

The editors have carefully organized their volume into sections that cover blood pressure regulation in infants and children, blood pressure measurement issues, pathophysiology and clinical assessment for essential and secondary forms of hypertension during childhood, and nonpharmacologic and pharmacologic approaches to the treatment of hypertension in children.

In Chapters 12 through 19 of the volume, substantial coverage has appropriately been given to the impact of genomics and the environment as they contribute to the development of hypertension in childhood. These sections do contribute to the novelty of this book because the chapters are grounded in basic, translational, and clinical investigations that have led to enhanced understanding of the development of hypertension during youth. The clinical management chapters outline the complications of hypertension in children, which have been underestimated and consequently call for much more thoughtful consideration to intervention.

The chapters in *Pediatric Hypertension* are superbly written by contributors who have provided comprehensive, scientifically sound, and clinically appropriate information. As series editor of *Clinical Hypertension and Vascular Diseases*, I am quite impressed by this timely and excellent book and know that *Pediatric Hypertension* will certainly become a standard textbook for all hypertension specialists as well as all physicians who take care of children and adolescents.

***William B. White,*** MD
*Professor of Medicine*
*University of Connecticut School of Medicine, Farmington*
*Series Editor,* Clinical Hypertension and Vascular Diseases

# Preface

More than a quarter of a century has elapsed since the first Task Force on Blood Pressure Control in Children was published in 1977. Since that seminal publication, normative data have been obtained for both casual and ambulatory children's blood pressure. Blood pressure measurement in infants, children, and adolescents, once an afterthought, has become routine. *Pediatric Hypertension* discusses the many aspects of pediatric hypertension—a multidisciplinary subspecialty that is comprised of pediatric nephrologists, cardiologists, endocrinologists, pharmacologists, and epidemiologists. Although some areas of our discipline have become well established, others, such as routine use of ambulatory blood pressure recording and well-designed trials in pediatric hypertension, are still emerging. Accordingly, we have included chapters that focus on aspects of blood pressure control and hypertension in the very young that are particularly relevant to those caring for infants, children, and adolescents.

*Pediatric Hypertension* opens with chapters concerning blood pressure regulation in the very young: the transition from fetal life to infant circulation, the factors that regulate blood pressure in early childhood, and the chronobiology of pediatric blood pressure. We then move on to the assessment of blood pressure in children. The book addresses both casual and ambulatory blood pressure measurement methodologies and norms, as well as the epidemiology of hypertension in children.

Definitions of hypertension in children, predictors of future hypertension, risk factors, and special populations are discussed at length. Comprehensive chapters on both primary and secondary hypertension in children point out differences in presentation of hypertension in the pediatric, in comparison to the adult, population. The contributions of genetics to the understanding of hypertension are presented, as well as those events during gestation and perinatal life that may influence the development of later hypertension. Risk factors that are discussed include the influences of race and ethnicity, diet, obesity, and society. Special populations, including the neonate with hypertension and the child with chronic renal failure or end-stage renal disease, are each discussed in a separate chapter. In those chapters, the pathophysiology insofar as it is known is also considered.

This text concludes with a section that focuses on the evaluation and management of pediatric hypertension. Suggestions for evaluation are presented, and both nonpharmacologic and pharmacologic therapy are discussed at length. The 1997 Food and Drug Administration Modernization Act, which offers extension of market exclusivity in return for approved clinical trials of medications with pediatric indication, has had a major impact on the conduct of pediatric antihypertensive medication trials. The current status of such pediatric antihypertensive trials is presented. In the appendix, the reader will find the latest tables for the definition of hypertension in children from the Fourth Report on the Diagnosis, Evaluation, and Treatment of High Blood Pressure in Children and Adolescents, to be published in *Pediatrics* in the summer of 2004.

We hope that *Pediatric Hypertension* provides a catalyst for more interest in pediatric hypertension as well as a guide for the interested clinician or clinical researcher already active in this discipline. Very shortly, the results of additional trials concerning new antihypertensive agents in children will be available with the mandate that new antihypertensive medications be evaluated in children. An update by the Task Force on Blood Pressure Control in Children will also be completed in 2004. A number of groups that have a special interest in blood pressure and its control in the very young will continue to contribute to the field, among them, most notably, the International Pediatric Hypertension Association; the National Heart, Lung, and Blood Institute; the American Society of Hypertension; and the American Society of Pediatric Nephrology. These initiatives will lead to a better understanding of the definition, causes, consequences, prevention, and treatment of pediatric hypertension. In addition to advances in molecular and genetics laboratories, new technologies in assessment of human cardiac and vascular anatomy and physiology will help to elucidate the pathophysiology of hypertension and its response to management. In so doing, our hope is that the trend towards reduction in cardiovascular morbidity and mortality will continue for the current generation of children.

Finally, we wish to acknowledge the pioneering work of so many in the field of pediatric hypertension that has given us the foundation and tools to advance our field.

***Ronald J. Portman,*** MD
***Jonathan M. Sorof,*** MD
***Julie R. Ingelfinger,*** MD

*International Pediatric Hypertension Association*

# CONTENTS

# Contributors

RAYMOND D. ADELMAN, MD • *Division of Nephrology, Phoenix Children's Hospital, Phoenix, AZ*

BRUCE S. ALPERT, MD • *Professor of Pediatrics, Division of Pediatric Cardiology, University of Tennessee Medical Center, Memphis, TN*

GERALD S. BERENSON, MD • *Departments of Epidemiology, Medicine, Pediatrics, and Biochemistry, Tulane Center for Cardiovascular Health, Tulane University Health Sciences Center, New Orleans, LA*

DOUGLAS L. BLOWEY, MD • *Associate Professor, Divisions of Nephrology and Pediatric Pharmacology and Toxicology, Departments of Pediatrics and Pharmacology, University of Missouri-Kansas City, Children's Mercy Hospitals and Clinics, Kansas City, MO*

LAVJAY BUTANI, MD • *Assistant Professor of Pediatrics, University of California Davis Medical Center, Sacramento, CA*

STEPHEN R. DANIELS, MD, PhD • *Professor and Associate Chairman, Division of Cardiology, Department of Pediatrics, Children's Hospital Medical Center, Cincinnati, OH*

MICHAEL J. DILLON, MD • *Professor of Paediatric Nephrology, Nephro-Urology Unit, Institute of Child Health, University College London, and Consultant Physician and Senior Clinical Nephrologist, Renal Unit, Great Ormond Street Hospital for Children, London, UK*

CRAIG K. EWART, PhD • *Professor of Psychology, Department of Psychology, Syracuse University, Syracuse, NY*

BONITA FALKNER, MD • *Professor of Medicine and Pediatrics, Department of Medicine, Thomas Jefferson University, Philadelphia, PA*

JOSEPH T. FLYNN, MD, MS • *Associate Professor of Pediatrics and Director, Pediatric Hypertension Program, Division of Pediatric Nephrology, Montefiore Medical Center, Albert Einstein College of Medicine, Bronx, NY*

ALAN B. GRUSKIN, MD (DECEASED) • *Professor and Chairman, Department of Pediatrics, Children's Hospital of Michigan, Wayne State University School of Medicine, Detroit, MI*

GREGORY A. HARSHFIELD, PhD • *Georgia Prevention Institute, Department of Pediatrics, Medical College of Georgia, Augusta, GA*

MICHAEL HASSELLE, BS • *Division of Pediatric Cardiology, University of Tennessee Medical Center, Memphis, TN*

ERHARD HAUS, MD, PhD • *Professor, Department of Laboratory Medicine and Pathology, University of Minnesota/HealthPartners Medical Group, St. Paul, MN*

JULIE R. INGELFINGER, MD • *Liaison, Executive Committee, International Pediatric Hypertension Association, Professor of Pediatrics, Harvard Medical School, Senior Consultant in Pediatric Nephrology, Massachusetts General Hospital, Boston, MA*

JOHN E. JONES, PhD • *Assistant Professor of Pediatrics, Division of Pediatric Nephrology, Georgetown University School of Medicine, Washington, DC*

PEDRO A. JOSE, MD, PhD • *Professor of Pediatrics and Physiology and Biophysics, Georgetown University School of Medicine, Washington, DC*

EMPAR LURBE, MD • *Pediatric Nephrology, University of Valencia, Hospital General, Valencia, Spain*

TEJ K. MATTOO, MD, DCH, FRCP (UK) • *Professor of Pediatrics and Director of Pediatric Nephrology, Children's Hospital of Michigan, Wayne State University School of Medicine, Detroit, MI*

OTTO MEHLS, MD • *Professor of Pediatrics and Director, Division of Pediatric Nephrology, University Children's Hospital, University of Heidelberg, Heidelberg, Germany*

BRUCE Z. MORGENSTERN, MD • *Associate Professor of Pediatrics, Chair, Division of Pediatric Nephrology; Vice-Chair for Education, Department of Pediatric and Adolescent Medicine, Mayo Clinic, Rochester, MN*

ARUNA R. NATARAJAN, MBBS, DCh • *Assistant Professor, Department of Pediatrics, Division of Critical Care, Georgetown University Hospital, Washington, DC*

SIDNEY ORNDUFF, PhD • *Associate Professor of Psychiatry, University of Tennessee Medical Center, Memphis, TN*

RONALD J. PORTMAN, MD • *Chairman, Executive Committee, International Pediatric Hypertension Association, and Professor and Director, Division of Pediatric Nephrology and Hypertension, University of Texas-Houston Medical School, Houston, TX*

JOSEP REDON, MD, FAHA • *Hypertension Clinic, Hospital Clinico, University of Valencia, Valencia, Spain*

JEAN E. ROBILLARD, MD • *Professor of Pediatrics, and Dean, Roy J. and Lucille A. Carver College of Medicine, University of Iowa, Iowa City, IA*

ALBERT P. ROCCHINI, MD • *Professor of Pediatrics, Division of Pediatric Cardiology, C. S. Mott Hospital, University of Michigan School of Medicine, Ann Arbor, MI*

FRANZ SCHAEFER, MD, PhD • *Professor of Pediatrics, Division of Pediatric Nephrology, University Children's Hospital, University of Heidelberg, Heidelberg, Germany*

KARL SCHÄRER, MD • *Professor of Pediatrics, Division of Pediatric Nephrology, University Children's Hospital, University of Heidelberg, Heidelberg, Germany*

JEFFREY L. SEGAR, MD • *Associate Professor of Pediatrics, Roy J. and Lucille A. Carver College of Medicine, University of Iowa, Iowa City, IA*

MICHAEL H. SMOLENSKY, PhD • *Professor of Environmental Physiology, School of Public Health, University of Texas-Houston Health Science Center, Houston, TX*

HAROLD SNIEDER, PhD • *Associate Professor of Pediatrics, Georgia Prevention Institute, Department of Pediatrics, Medical College of Georgia, Augusta, GA*

JONATHAN M. SOROF, MD • *Vice Chairman, Executive Committee, International Pediatric Hypertension Association, and Associate Professor, Department of Pediatric Nephrology and Hypertension, University of Texas-Houston Medical School, Houston, TX*

SATHANUR R. SRINIVASAN, PhD • *Tulane Center for Cardiovascular Health, Tulane University Health Sciences Center, New Orleans, LA*

RITA D. SWINFORD, MD • *Associate Professor of Pediatrics, Division of Pediatric Nephrology and Hypertension, University of Texas-Houston Medical School, Houston, TX*

Frank A. Treiber, PhD • *Director, Georgia Prevention Institute, Regents Professor of Pediatrics and Psychiatry, Medical College of Georgia, Augusta, GA*
Elaine M. Urbina, MD • *Tulane Center for Cardiovascular Health, Tulane University Health Sciences Center, New Orleans, LA*
Thomas G. Wells, MD • *Associate Professor of Pediatrics, University of Arkansas for Medical Sciences, Little Rock, AR*
Dawn K. Wilson, PhD • *Research Associate Professor, Arnold School of Public Health and Prevention Research Center, University of South Carolina, Columbia, SC*
Martha E. Wilson, MA • *Georgia Prevention Institute, Medical College of Georgia, Augusta, GA*

# I

# Regulation of Blood Pressure in Children

# 1 Neurohumoral Regulation of Blood Pressure in Early Development

*Jeffrey L. Segar,* MD *and Jean E. Robillard,* MD

**CONTENTS**



## INTRODUCTION

Circulatory function is mediated through interacting neural, hormonal, and metabolic mechanisms acting at both central and local levels. The central nervous system (CNS) in particular is critical for cardiovascular homeostasis *(1,2)*. Autonomic tone to the heart and vasculature is continuously modulated by an array of peripheral sensors, including arterial baroreceptors and chemoreceptors *(3)*. Brain cardiovascular centers located between afferent and efferent pathways of the reflex arc integrate a variety of visceral and behavioral sensations, allowing for a wide range of modulation of specific autonomic, cardiovascular, and endocrine responses. Although these basic mechanisms exist in the fetus and newborn, different rates of maturation of these systems influence the ability of the developing animal to maintain blood pressure (BP) and organ blood flow.

The contribution of the autonomic nervous system to cardiovascular homeostasis changes during development. Both α-adrenergic blockade and ganglionic blockade produce greater decreases in BP in term fetal sheep than in preterm fetal sheep or newborn lambs, suggesting that sympathetic tone is high late in fetal life *(4,5)*. The influence of the parasympathetic system on resting heart rate (HR) appears to increase with maturation *(6)*. Cholinergic blockade produces no consistent effect on HR in premature fetal sheep, a slight increase in HR in term fetuses and the greatest effect in lambs beyond the first week of life *(4,7,8)*.

Arterial pressure displays natural oscillation within a physiological range, the degree of which is similar in fetal and postnatal life *(9–12)*. In the adult, ganglionic blockade increases

From: *Clinical Hypertension and Vascular Disease: Pediatric Hypertension*
Edited by: R. J. Portman, J. M. Sorof, and J. R. Ingelfinger © Humana Press Inc., Totowa, NJ

arterial pressure variability *(11,13)*, suggesting that a component of arterial pressure lability is peripheral or humoral in origin and is buffered by autonomic functions. In contrast, ganglionic blockade in term fetal sheep significantly attenuates HR and arterial pressure variability *(10)*. Changes in sympathetic tone, as recorded from the renal sympathetic nerves, have been shown to correlate positively with fluctuations in HR and arterial pressure *(10)*. Oscillations in basal sympathetic tone appear to be related to changes in the behavioral state of the fetus *(14–16)*. Although fetal electrocortical and sympathetic activity have not been recorded simultaneously, HR, arterial pressure, and catecholamine levels are highest during periods of high voltage, low frequency electrocortical activity *(14,17–19)*. Other physiologic parameters, including organ blood flows, regional vascular resistances and cerebral oxygen consumption are also dependent on electrocortical state and likely reflect changes in autonomic activity *(18,20,21)*.

## THE ARTERIAL BAROREFLEX

Arterial baroreceptors are major sensing elements of the cardiovascular regulatory system *(1,2)*. Arterial baroreceptors in the carotid sinus and aortic arch are stimulated by changes in vascular stretch related to increases in BP *(1)*. This increase in nerve activity, transmitted to the brain, results in alterations in parasympathetic and sympathetic nerve activities that influence HR and peripheral vascular resistance, and buffer changes in arterial pressure *(22,23)*. Studies in sheep, which to date have served as the most common model for studying integrative developmental cardiovascular physiology, demonstrate that the arterial baroreflex is functional during fetal and postnatal life *(6,9,24,25)*. Investigators disagree, however, on the influence of these reflexes in controlling HR and arterial pressure. Early studies indicate that the threshold for baroreceptor activity is above the normal range of arterial pressure during fetal and neonatal life, and that baroreceptors may not be loaded during fetal life *(26,27)*. However, studies demonstrating that sinoaortic denervation produces marked fluctuations in fetal arterial pressure and HR *(9,24)* suggest that the arterial baroreflex contributes to cardiovascular homeostasis. Single fiber recordings of baroreceptor afferents *(28–32)* in fetal and newborn animals demonstrate that carotid sinus nerve activity is phasic and pulse synchronous, and that activity increases with a rise in arterial or carotid sinus pressure *(28,30,32)*. Basal discharge of baroreceptor afferents does not change during fetal and postnatal maturation, despite a considerable increase in mean arterial pressure during this time, indicating that baroreceptors reset during development, continuing to function within the physiologic range for arterial pressure *(28,29)*. The sensitivity of carotid baroreceptors to increases in carotid sinus pressure is greater in fetal than in newborn and 1-mo-old lambs *(28)*, and in newborn compared to adult rabbits *(29)*. These findings suggest that reduced HR responses to changes in arterial pressure during fetal life are not owing to underdeveloped afferent activity of baroreceptors but to differences in central integration and efferent parasympathetic nerve activity. The mechanisms that regulate the changes in sensitivity of the baroreceptors early in development have not been investigated, but may be related to changes in the degree of mechanical deformation of nerve endings and thus to strain sensitivity, ionic mechanisms that operate at the receptor membrane to cause hyperpolarization, or substances released from the endothelium, including prostacyclin and nitric oxide, that modulate baroreceptor activity *(33–38)*.

Baroreflex control of fetal HR is dominated by changes in cardiac vagal tone, although integrity of the reflex is dependent upon both sympathetic and parasympathetic pathways *(39)*.

A number of studies describe a relatively reduced HR response to alterations in arterial pressure in fetal and newborn animals, and in human infants *(27,40–42)*. Using reflex bradycardia in response to increased BP by balloon inflation, Shinebourne et al. *(40)* found that baroreflex activity is present as early as 0.6 gestation in fetal lambs, and that the sensitivity of the reflex increased up to term. Additional studies in sheep *(41)* and other species *(43,44)* have similarly found increasing baroreflex sensitivity with postnatal age. Reflex bradycardia in response to carotid sinus stimulation is absent in the newborn piglet, although vagal efferents exert a tonic action on the heart at this stage of development *(44)*. Age-related changes in HR in response to phenylephrine are also greater in 2-mo-old piglets than in 1-d-old animals *(43)*.

Other studies suggest that the sensitivity of the arterial baroreflex is in fact greater in the fetus than in the newborn and decreases with maturation *(45,46)*. Recordings of HR and efferent renal sympathetic nerve activity (RSNA) in response to increases and decreases in BP in fetal, newborn, and 4–6-wk-old sheep demonstrate that: baroreceptor activity regulates sympathetic outflow as well as HR during fetal life; that functional baroreflex control of RSNA and HR shifts toward higher pressures during development; and that the sensitivity of the RSNA baroreflex function curve is greater early in development and decreases following the transition from fetal to newborn life (Fig. 1) *(47)*. Interestingly, studies during postnatal life have shown that baroreflex control of HR and sympathetic nerve activity is impaired with senescence *(48)*, an effect that may contribute to the development of hypertension.

### *Resetting of the Arterial Baroreflex*

Resetting of the arterial baroreflex is defined as a change in the relation between arterial pressure and HR, or between pressure and sympathetic and parasympathetic nerve activities *(33,34)*. A number of studies demonstrate that the sensitivity of the baroreflex changes with maturation, and shifts or resets toward higher pressures *(47–49)*. This shift occurs during fetal life, is present immediately after birth, and continues with postnatal maturation, paralleling the naturally occurring increase in BP *(50)*. The mechanisms that regulate developmental changes in baroreflex sensitivity and control the resetting of the baroreflex are poorly understood. Changes in the relationship between arterial pressure and sympathetic activity, or HR, occur at the level of the baroreceptor itself (peripheral resetting), and from altered coupling of afferent impulses, from baroreceptors to efferent sympathetic or parasympathetic activities within the CNS (central resetting) *(33)*.

Changes in the levels of locally produced factors, such as nitric oxide, and circulating hormones and neuropeptides, such as angiotensin II (ANG II) and vasopressin (AVP), activate additional neural reflex pathways that may modulate the changes in arterial baroreflex during development *(33,51,52)*.

### *Baroreflex Function in the Human Neonate*

In the human infant, neural control of the circulation has been assessed most often by recording alterations in the HR in response to postural changes. Several studies have demonstrated in healthy term and preterm infants that unloading arterial baroreceptor by head-up tilting produces a significant HR response *(53,54)*. In contrast, other investigators have been unable to demonstrate a consistent response of HR to tilting, and concluded that the HR component of the baroreflex is poorly developed during the neonatal period *(55)*. Using venous occlusion plethsmography, Waldman et al. *(55)* found in healthy preterm and term infants that 45° head-up tilting produced on average a 25% decrease in limb blood flow, suggestive of an increase in peripheral vascular resistance, although no significant tachycardia was observed.

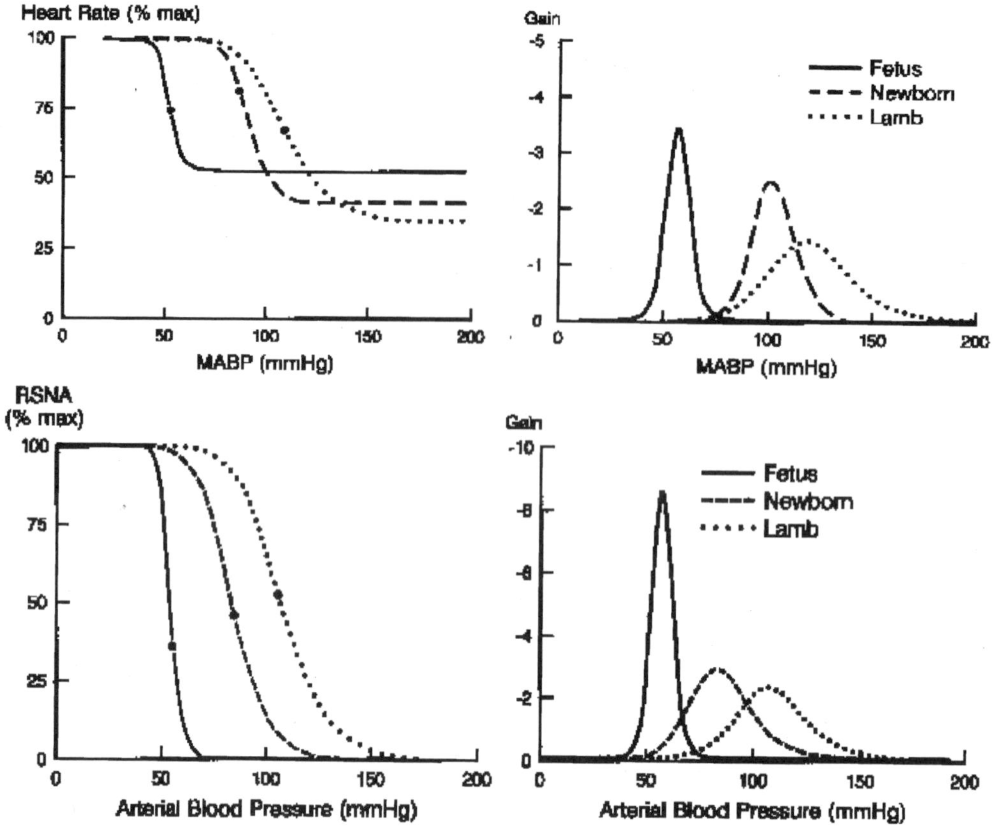


Fig. 1. Baroreflex function relating heart rate (top) or renal sympathetic nerve activity (RSNA) (bottom) and mean arterial blood pressure (MABP) in near-term fetal, newborn (7-d-old), and 4- to 6-wk-old lambs. RSNA and heart rate are expressed as % of maximum response. •, point on curves representing resting values. The gains of the reflexes (right hand panels) represent the slopes of the curves are obtained using the first derivatives of the baroreflex curves. (Reproduced from Segar JL et al. *[47]*.)

Power spectral analysis, a computer technique of quantifying the small spontaneous beat-by-beat variations in HR has been used in human adults *(56)*, infants *(57, 58)*, and fetuses *(59)* to evaluate the contribution of the autonomic nervous system in maintaining cardiovascular homeostasis. Fetal electrocardiogram tracings have shown that younger fetuses have a greater total energy of the power spectrum compared with more mature fetuses, consistent with the evolution of a stable and mature autonomic nervous system *(59)*. Maturational changes in the power spectra of HR variability have also been shown by comparing preterm to term infants *(57,58)*. There is a progressive decline in the low frequency/high frequency (LF/HF) power ratio associated with both increasing postnatal and gestational age, indicating an increase in parasympathetic contribution to control of resting HR with maturation. Clairembault et al. *(58)* found that changes in the HF component of the spectrum were greater at 37–38 wk, suggesting a steep increase in vagal tone at this age.

Power spectral analysis has also been used to characterize developmental changes in sympathovagal balance in response to arterial baroreceptor unloading in preterm infants beginning at 28–30 wk postconceptional age *(60)*. Longitudinal examination of HR power *(60)* found that infants at 28–30 wk the LF/HF ratio did not change with head-up postural change, whereas with increasing postnatal age the LF component of the spectrum increases with head-up tilt. These findings suggest that neural regulation of cardiac function undergoes changes with maturation, becoming more functional with postnatal development.

## CARDIOPULMONARY REFLEXES

Cardiopulmonary receptors are sensory endings located in the four cardiac chambers, in the great veins, and in the lungs *(61)*. In the adult, the volume sensors mediating reflex changes in cardiovascular and renal function are believed to be primarily those residing in the atria *(62,63)* and the ventricles *(61)*, with the ventricular receptors being of utmost importance during decreases in cardiopulmonary pressures *(61,64,65)*. The majority of ventricular receptor vagal afferents are unmyelinated C-fibers that can be activated by exposure to chemical irritants (chemosensitive) and changes in pressure or stretch (mechanosensitive receptors) *(66,67)*. These receptors have a low basal discharge rate, which exerts a tonic inhibitory influence on sympathetic outflow and vascular resistance *(61)*, and regulates plasma AVP concentration *(68)*. Interruption of this basal activity results in increases in HR, BP, and sympathetic nerve activity, whereas activation of cardiopulmonary receptors results in reflex bradycardia, vasodilation, and sympathoinhibition *(61)*.

Characterization of the cardiopulmonary reflex during the perinatal and neonatal periods was initially performed by stimulation of chemosensitive cardiopulmonary receptors *(43,69,70)*. These studies *(69,70)* demonstrated that the HR, BP, and regional blood flow responses to stimulation of chemosensitive cardiac receptors were smaller during early development than later in life, and absent in premature fetal lambs *(70)* and piglets under 1 wk old *(69)*. Stimulation of cardiopulmonary receptors with volume expansion had no effect on basal renal nerve activity in the fetus, but significantly reduced RSNA in newborn and 8-wk-old sheep *(71,72)*. However, the decrease in RSNA in response to volume expansion was totally abolished in sinoaortic denervated (SAD) newborn lambs but was not affected by sinoaortic denervation in 6–8-wk-old sheep *(73)*. These results indicate that cardiopulmonary reflexes are not fully mature early in life, and that stimulation of sinoaortic baroreceptors plays a greater role than cardiopulmonary mechanoreceptors in regulating changes in sympathetic activity in response to expansion of vascular volume early during development.

During development, cardiopulmonary mechanoreceptors also respond to reductions in blood volume by eliciting reflexes that influence systemic hemodynamics. Hemorrhage produces a significant decrease in arterial BP without accompanying changes in HR in fetal sheep less than 120 d gestation, whereas BP remains stable and HR increases in near-term fetuses *(74)*. However, other investigators *(75,76)* found the hemodynamic response to hemorrhage to be similar in immature and near-term fetuses, with reductions in both HR and BP. Inhibition of vagal afferents during slow and nonhypotensive hemorrhage blocks the normal rise in plasma vasopressin but does not alter the rise in plasma renin activity in near-term fetal sheep *(75)*.

When input from cardiopulmonary receptors is removed by section of the cervical vagosympathetic trunks, the decrease in fetal BP in response to hemorrhage is similar to that in intact fetuses *(77)*, whereas vagotomy with sinoaortic denervation enhances the decrease in BP *(75)*. Therefore, it is likely that activation of fibers from the carotid sinus (arterial baroreceptors and chemoreceptors) but not vagal afferents (cardiopulmonary baroreceptors and chemoreceptors) are involved in the maintenance of BP homeostasis during fetal hemorrhage.

Cardiopulmonary receptors also appear to have a diminished role in early postnatal life, as reflex changes in newborn lamb RSNA during nonhypotensive and hypotensive hemorrhage are dependent upon the integrity of arterial baroreceptors, but not cardiopulmonary receptors *(78)*. In addition, the cardiovascular responses to hemorrhage in newborn lambs are dependent upon intact renal nerves that in turn modulate release of AVP *(79)*.

The RSNA responses to vagal afferent nerve stimulation are similar in sinoaortic denervated fetal and postnatal lambs *(80)*, suggesting that delayed maturation of the cardiopulmonary reflex is not secondary to incomplete central integration of vagal afferent input. On the other hand, the decreased sensitivity of the cardiopulmonary reflex early in development in the face of a sensitive arterial baroreflex response (as outlined above) is intriguing. One may suggest that there is an occlusive interaction between these two reflexes during development. In support of this hypothesis, studies in adults *(81,82)* have shown that activation of arterial baroreceptors may impair the reflex responses to activation of cardiopulmonary receptors.

## PERIPHERAL CHEMOREFLEX RESPONSES

Peripheral chemoreceptors located in the aortic arch and carotid bodies are functional during fetal life and participate in cardiovascular regulation *(83–85)*. Acute hypoxemia evokes integrated cardiovascular, metabolic, and endocrine responses. The fetal cardiovascular responses to acute hypoxemia include transient bradycardia, an increase in arterial BP, and an increase in peripheral vascular resistance *(84,86)*. The bradycardia is mediated by parasympathetic efferents while the initial vasoconstriction results from increased sympathetic tone *(85,87)*. The release of circulating factors such as AVP and catecholamines serve to maintain peripheral vasoconstriction while the HR returns toward basal levels. In fetal lambs, the cardiovascular response to acute hypoxemia is eliminated by carotid but not aortic chemodenervation *(88)*. Although chemoreceptors are active and responsive in the fetus and newborn, studies in sheep and human infants suggest that chemoreceptor sensitivity and activity is reduced immediately after birth *(89,90)*. This decreased sensitivity persists for several days until the chemoreceptors adapt and reset their sensitivity from the low oxygen tension of the fetus to the higher levels seen postnatally *(90,91)*. The mechanisms involved with this resetting are not known, although the postnatal rise in $PaO_2$ appears to be crucial; raising fetal $PaO_2$ produces a rightward shift in the response curve of carotid baroreceptors to differing oxygen tension *(92)*. Holgert et al. *(93)* hypothesized that developmental changes in dopamine turnover within the carotid body contribute the postnatal resetting of the arterial chemoreceptors, whereas others suggest differences in intracellular calcium mobilization during hypoxia may be an important component of chemoreceptor maturation *(94)*.

The purine nucleoside adenosine appears to play an important role in chemoreceptor mediated responses as adenosine receptor blockade abolishes hypoxia-induced bradycardia and hypertension in fetal sheep *(95,96)*. Treatment with an adenosine receptor antagonist, or with carotid sinus denervation, before acute fetal hypoxemia, also prevents an increase in plasma epinephrine, and markedly reduces the increase in plasma norepinephrine *(97,98)*. Thus, adenosine receptor blockade may act, via chemoreceptor-dependent mechanisms, to abolish circulatory and adrenergic responses to acute hypoxemia in fetal sheep, although chemoreflex-independent mechanisms likely also exist. In postnatal animals adenosine increases carotid body afferent discharge, whereas hypoxia-induced increases in afferent activity are attenuated by adenosine receptor antagonists *(99)*.

The cardiovascular response to acute fetal hypoxemia depends on the prevailing intrauterine condition *(86,100)*. Gardner et al. *(86)* studied chronically instrumented fetal sheep grouped according to $PaO_2$. Chronically hypoxic fetuses (baseline $PaO_2$ 17.3 ± 0.5 mm Hg) displayed greater increases in arterial BP and femoral vascular resistance than control fetuses (baseline $PaO_2$ 22.9 ± 1.0 mm Hg) in response to acute hypoxia. Functional chemoreflex analysis during early hypoxemia, performed by plotting the change in $PaO_2$ against the change in HR and femoral vascular resistance, demonstrated that the slopes of the cardiac and vasoconstrictor chemoreflex curves were enhanced in hypoxic fetuses relative to control. Additional evidence suggests that exposure to hypoxia for a limited period of time (hours to days) has a sensitizing effect on the chemoreflex, whereas sustained hypoxia (days to weeks) may have a desensitizing effect *(100)*. The mechanisms regulating this alteration in response are unclear. In the chick embryo, hypoxia increases sympathetic nerve fiber density and neuronal capacity for norepinephrine synthesis *(101)*. Thus, augmented efferent pathways may contribute to the enhanced responses. On the other hand, recordings from carotid chemoreceptors in chronically hypoxic kittens demonstrate blunted responses to acute decreases in $PaO_2$ relative to control animals *(102)*. It is therefore possible that, with prolonged hypoxia, blunting of the chemoreflex responses may be related to afferent mechanisms.

## SYMPATHETIC ACTIVITY AT BIRTH

The transition from fetal to newborn life is associated with numerous hemodynamic adjustments, including changes in HR and peripheral vascular resistance and redistribution of blood flow *(103,104)*. Activation of the sympathetic nervous system appears to be an important part of this adaptive process. Marked increases in circulating catecholamine levels occur with birth *(105,106)*. while arterial pressure and cardiac function, including HR and cardiac output, are depressed by ganglionic blockade in newborn (1–3 d), but not in older lambs *(107)*. In direct support of the hypothesis that sympathetic tone is high during the immediate postnatal period, renal sympathetic nerve activity increases nearly 250% following delivery of term fetal sheep by cesarean section, and parallels the rise in arterial pressure and HR *(50)*. Delivery appears to produce near-maximal stimulation of renal sympathetic outflow, because further increases cannot be elicited by unloading of arterial baroreceptors *(50)*. Furthermore, reflex inhibition of this increase in RSNA could not be achieved by arterial baroreceptor stimulation, as seen in fetal and 3–7-d-old lambs *(47)*, suggesting that central influences exist which override the arterial baroreflex and that the maintenance of a high sympathetic tone is vital during this transition period. A similar pattern of baroreceptor reflex inhibition has been well described in adult animals as part of the defense reaction *(108)*.

The factors mediating the large increase in sympathetic outflow at birth are unclear. *In utero* ventilation studies of fetal sheep have shown that rhythmic lung inflation increases plasma catecholamine concentrations, although there are no consistent effects on BP or HR *(109,110)*. Fetal RSNA increases only 50% during *in utero* ventilation, while oxygenation and removal of the placental circulation by umbilical cord occlusion produces no additional effect *(111)*. Such studies demonstrate that lung inflation and an increase in arterial oxygen tension contribute little to the sympathoexcitation process at birth. The increases in HR, mean arterial BP, and RSNA following delivery are similar in intact and sinoaortic denervated and vagotomized fetal lambs *(112)*, suggesting that afferent input from peripheral chemoreceptors and mechanoreceptors also contribute little to the hemodynamic and sympathetic responses at delivery.

The change in environmental temperature at birth may play an important role in the sympathoexcitatory response at birth. Cooling of the near-term fetus both *in utero* and in exteriorized preparations results in an increase in HR, BP, and norepinephrine concentrations, which is consistent with sympathoexcitation *(113,114)*. In contrast, exteriorization of the near-term lamb fetus into a warm water bath does not produce the alterations in systemic hemodynamics or catecholamine values typically seen at birth *(113)*. Fetal cooling, but not ventilation or umbilical cord occlusion, also initiates nonshivering thermogenesis via neurally mediated sympathetic stimulation of brown adipose tissue *(115)*. In utero cooling of fetal lambs also produces an increase in RSNA of similar magnitude to that seen at delivery by cesarean section *(55)*, suggesting that cold-stress plays a role in the activation of the sympathetic nervous system at birth. These changes occur before a decrease in core temperature, and are reversible with rewarming, suggesting that sensory input from cutaneous cold-sensitive thermoreceptors rather than a response to a change in core temperature is mediating the response.

Studies in adults suggest that multiple brain centers are involved in autonomic control of the systemic circulation. Sympathetic outflow is controlled not only by the medulla oblongata *(116)*, as well described, but also by higher centers, especially the hypothalamus *(117,118)*, allowing for a wide range of modulation. In fetal sheep, electrical stimulation of the hypothalamus evokes tachycardia and a pressor response which are attenuated by α-adrenoreceptor blockade *(119)*. Stimulation of the dorsolateral medulla and lateral hypothalamus in the newborn piglet similarly increases BP and femoral blood flow *(43)*. Because the responses to hypothalamic stimulation are lost during stress (hypoxia, hypercapnia, hemorrhage) whereas those elicited from the medulla are not, some investigators have proposed that the hypothalamus exerts little influence of cardiovascular function until later in postnatal development *(43)*. However, other studies suggest forebrain structures are vital for normal physiological adaptation following the transition from fetal to newborn life *(111)*. The increases in HR, mean arterial BP, and RSNA which normally occur at birth are absent in animals subjected to transection of the brain stem at the level of the rostral pons prior to delivery. These data suggest that supramedullary structures are involved in mediating the sympathoexcitation seen at birth. Ablation of the paraventricular nucleus of the hypothalamus attenuates the postnatal increase in sympathetic outflow and alters baroreflex function *(120)*. Consequently, this structure appears to be intimately involved in the regulation of circulatory and autonomic functions during the transition from fetal to newborn life.

The hemodynamic and sympathetic responses at birth are markedly different in prematurely delivered lambs (0.85 of gestation) compared to those delivered at term *(121)*. Postnatal increases in HR and BP are attenuated, and the sympathoexcitatory response, as measured by RSNA, is absent *(121)*. This impaired response occurs despite the fact that the descending pathways of the sympathetic nervous system are intact and functional at this stage of development, as demonstrated by a large pressor and sympathoexcitatory response to *in utero* cooling *(121)*. Antenatal administration of glucocorticoids, which has been shown to improve postnatal cardiovascular as well as pulmonary function, augments sympathetic activity at birth in premature lambs and decreases the sensitivity of the cardiac baroreflex *(121)*. The mechanisms for antenatal glucocorticoid administration augmenting cardiovascular and sympathetic responses at birth are unclear, although stimulation of the peripheral renin-angiotensin system (RAS) and activation of systemically accessible $AT_1$ receptors are not involved *(122)*.

## HUMORAL FACTORS

### *Renin-Angiotensin System (RAS)*

The RAS is active in the fetal and perinatal periods *(123–125)*. During embryonic and early fetal life, the primary function of the RAS may be to regulate organ growth and development as ANG II stimulates cell growth and replication and regulates vascular proliferation *(126)*. Only later during fetal development does the RAS become involved in modulating cardiovascular function and renal hemodynamics. In sheep, fetal plasma levels of renin are elevated when compared with adults *(127)*. In normal children, plasma renin activity is elevated during the newborn period, declines rapidly in the first year of life, and then continues with a gradual decline until adulthood *(128,129)*. In preterm infants, plasma renin activity is markedly elevated and has close inverse relationship to postconceptual age *(130)*. A large number of studies also report that administration of inhibitors of ANG II, including angiotensin converting enzyme inhibitors and ANG II subtype 1 receptor blockers, decreases fetal and newborn arterial BP *(125,131–133)*.

Fetal plasma renin activity and plasma ANG II concentration increase after aortic constriction, hypotension, and blood volume reduction *(123)*. Conversely, a rise in arterial BP and volume expansion reduces plasma renin activity in fetal and newborn animals *(134)*. The vasopressor response, and renal vascular reactivity to exogenous ANG II, are less pronounced in fetal lambs than in adult sheep *(135)*. Factors explaining the higher activity of the RAS and decreased sensitivity to ANG II early in development have not been explored in detail. One may speculate that differences in localization and expression of the ANG II receptor subtypes contribute to this effect.

Baroreceptors and chemoreceptors regulate the release of vasoactive hormones, such as ANG II *(52,136)*. Changes in the levels of circulating hormones in turn influence neural regulation of cardiovascular function. For example, in the sheep fetus, a rise in arterial BP produced by ANG II administration produces little or no cardiac slowing *(135,137)*, although others have reported dose-dependent decreases in HR *(46,138)*. The bradycardic and sympathoinhibitory responses to a given increase in BP is less for ANG II than for other vasoconstrictor agents *(51)*. In the adult, ANG II facilitates activation of sympathetic ganglia and enhances the release of norepinephrine at the neuroeffector junction *(139)*. Within the CNS, ANG II stimulates sympathetic outflow and alters baroreceptor reflexes by acting on ANG II type 1 ($AT_1$) receptors located within the hypothalamus, medulla, and circumventricular organs *(140,142)*. The site of action of ANG II in regulating baroreflex function in the fetus is not known.

Endogenous ANG II participates in regulating arterial baroreflex responses early during development. The absence of rebound tachycardia after reduction in BP by angiotensin converting enzyme (ACE) inhibitors is well described in fetal and postnatal animals *(131)*, as well as in human adults and infants *(57)*. In the newborn lamb, ACE inhibition or $AT_1$ receptor blockade decreases RSNA and HR, and resets the baroreflex toward lower pressure *(51,143)*. Resetting of the reflex is independent of changes in prevailing BP. Lateral ventricle administration of an $AT_1$, but not an $AT_2$, receptor antagonist also lowers BP. Additionally, it resets the baroreflex toward lower pressure in newborn and 8-wk-old sheep at doses that have no effect when given systemically *(143)*.

## *Arginine Vasopressin*

Several lines of evidence suggest that arginine vasopressin (AVP) plays an important role in maintaining cardiovascular homeostasis during fetal and postnatal development. Graded infusions of AVP increase fetal BP and decrease fetal HR in a dose-dependent manner *(144,145)*. Plasma AVP concentrations in the fetus are increased by multiple stimuli, including hypotension, hemorrhage, hypoxemia, acidemia, and hyperosmolality *(136,146–148)*. Vasopressin responses to hypotension are partially mediated by arterial baroreceptors, whereas the contribution of carotid or aortic chemoreceptors appears to play little role in the AVP response to hypoxia *(149,150)*. While AVP appears to provide an important component of the cardiovascular response to acute stress, vasopressin appears to have little impact on basal fetal circulatory regulation. Blockade of AVP receptors in fetal sheep has no measurable effects on arterial BP, HR, or renal sympathetic nerve activity in fetal sheep or newborn lambs *(151,152)*. However, AVP receptor inhibition impairs the ability of the fetus to maintain BP during hypotensive hemorrhage and reduces the catecholamine response *(153)*.

In several adult species, vasopressin modulates parasympathetic and sympathetic tone and baroreflex function *(52,141,154)*. Administration of AVP evokes a greater sympathoinhibition and bradycardia than other vasoconstrictors, resulting in a comparable increase in BP *(52,155)*. This modulation of the baroreflex has been attributed to AVP enhancing the gain of the reflex, as well as resetting the reflex to a lower pressure *(52,155)*. Studies during fetal and newborn life demonstrate that AVP secretory mechanisms are well-developed early in life, and that AVP increases fetal arterial pressure and decreases HR in a dose-dependent manner *(145,156)*. However, sequential increases in plasma AVP in fetal and newborn sheep do not alter baroreflex control of RSNA and HR in response to acute changes in BP *(151)*.

Circulating endogenous AVP also appears to have little effect on baroreflex function in early stages of development. Peripheral administration of a $V_1$-receptor antagonist has no measurable effects on resting hemodynamics in fetal sheep or on basal arterial BP *(152)*, HR, RSNA, or baroreflex response in newborn lambs *(151)*. This lack of baroreflex modulation by AVP may facilitate the pressor response to AVP in fetuses and newborns during stressful situations such as hypoxia and hemorrhage. In this way, AVP could play a particularly important role in maintaining arterial pressures during these states early in development.

The role of central vasopressin in maintaining hemodynamic homeostasis in the developing animal has not been extensively studied. Under basal conditions fetal AVP levels are ten-fold higher in the cerebrospinal fluid than in plasma, suggesting that AVP contributes to central regulation of autonomic function *(157)*. Intracerebroventricular infusion of AVP produces significant decreases in mean arterial BP and HR in newborn lambs, although no reflex changes in RSNA have been seen *(158)*. Interestingly, intracerebroventricular administration of AVP increases RSNA in 8-wk-old sheep, demonstrating that the role of AVP receptors within the CNS in regulation autonomic function is developmentally regulated *(158)*. The changes in BP and HR are completely inhibited by administration of a $V_1$ antagonist, demonstrating that the central cardiovascular effects of AVP are mediated by $V_1$ receptors, as it has been reported in mature animals *(159)*.

## *Corticosteroids*

Adrenal steroids are vital for normal physiological development. Fetal adrenalectomy attenuates the normal gestational age-dependent increase in BP that occurs in late gestation, while cortisol replacement produces a sustained increase in fetal BP *(160,161)*. Antenatal exposure to exogenous glucocorticoids increases fetal postnatal arterial BP by enhancing peripheral vascular resistance and cardiac output without altering HR *(162–164)*. The mechanisms accounting for the increase in fetal vascular resistance are not clear. In the adult, administration of hydrocortisone or dexamethasone suppresses resting and stimulated muscle sympathetic nerve activity, suggesting little role for augmented sympathetic tone *(165,168)*. On the other hand, glucocorticoids enhance pressor responsiveness and vascular reactivity to norepinephrine and ANG II *(167,168)*, in part by increasing $\alpha_1$-adrenergic and $AT_1$ receptor levels and potentiating ANG II and vasopressin-induced inosital triphosphate production *(169,170)*. Glucocorticoids also reduce the activity of depressor systems, including vasodilator prostaglandins and nitric oxide (NO), and have been shown to decrease serum $NO2^-/NO3^-$, endothelial nitric oxide synthase mRNA stability and protein levels *(171)*.

In the sheep fetus, cortisol infusion increases BP as well as the hypertensive response to intravenous ANG II, but not to norepinephrine *(161)*. However, infusions of synthetic glucocorticoids, which also increase arterial BP, do not alter the pressor response to phenylephrine, ANG II, or vasopressin *(172)*. Furthermore, the increase in BP is not inhibited by blockade of the RAS *(122)*. In vitro studies demonstrate fetal treatment with betamethasone enhances the contractile response of femoral arteries to depolarizing potassium solutions, supporting a role for enhanced calcium channel activation *(173)*. Glucocorticoid exposure enhances in vitro responses of peripheral arteries to vascontrictors, including norepinephrine and endothelin 1, while attenuating vasodilator effects of forskolin and bradykinin and nitric oxide production *(173–176)*.

In addition to peripheral effects on vascular reactivity, antenatal glucocorticoids also modify autonomic and endocrine functions. Increases in fetal BP and vascular resistance following betamethasone treatment occur despite marked suppression of circulating vasoconstrictors, including catecholamines, ANG II, and AVP *(121,164,177)*. Circulating neuropeptide Y concentration, which may provide an index of peripheral sympathetic activity, is increased following fetal exposure to dexamethasone *(178)*. Glucocorticoid treatment accelerates postnatal maturation of brain catecholaminergic signaling pathways in rats, and enhances renal sympathetic nerve activity in prematurely delivered lambs *(179–181)*.

Endogenous production of cortisol is important for normal maturational changes in autonomic and baroreflex function. Adrenalectomized sheep fail to display the normal postnatal increase in RSNA, while the response is restored by cortisol replacement *(182)*. Restoring circulating cortisol levels to the prepartum physiological range shifts the fetal and immediate postnatal HR and RSNA baroreflex curves toward higher pressure without altering the slope of the curves *(182)*. In a similar manner, elevation of corticosterone levels in adult rats resets baroreflex control of HR and RSNA, and reduces the gain of the responses *(183,184)*. Antenatal administration of betamethasone decreases the sensitivity of baroreflex mediated changes in HR in preterm fetuses and premature lambs *(121)*. Antenatal glucocorticoid exposure also alters baroreflex and chemoreflex function in fetal and newborn animals *(172,179)*. Baroreflex control of HR and RSNA are reset towards higher pressures in steroid-exposed animals. In response to acute hypoxia, fetuses exposed to glucocorticoids display prolonged bradycardia and attenuated plasma catecholamine and vasopressin responses *(178)*. Taken together, these findings indicate that glucocorticoids modify autonomic and endocrine control of cardiovascular function during development. These effects may even persist well after cessation of exposure *(178)*.

### *Nitric Oxide (NO)*

A role for NO in the control of systemic hemodynamics is suggested by a number of studies. Nitric oxide normally contributes to regulation of fetal BP and organ-specific vascular resistance as acute blockade of NO production causes an immediate rise in BP and umbilicoplacental resistance, and decreases in HR, renal blood flow velocity, and plasma renin concentration *(185,186)*. These cardiovascular effects are significantly attenuated by prolonged or repeated exposure to NO synthesis inhibition, indicating that other vasodilatory regulatory mechanisms are functioning during fetal life *(186)*. Nitric oxide also functions as a neurotransmitter and acts centrally to regulate fetal arterial BP. Administration of the NO donor nitroglycerin into the fourth cerebral ventricle of the ovine fetus decreases mean arterial pressure, whereas blocking NO synthase in the 4th ventricle increases fetal BP *(187)*. Inhibition of endogenously produced NO also increases BP in 1- and 6-wk-old lambs to similar extents although the concomitant decreases in HR are greater in the young lamb *(188)*. Endogenous nitric oxide regulates arterial baroreflex control of HR in 1- but not 6-wk-old lambs, and may contribute to developmental changes in baroreflex function during this period *(188)*.

## CONCLUSION

Understanding the mechanisms regulating cardiovascular function in the fetal and postnatal periods, particularly as they relate to the physiological adaptations occurring with the transition from fetal to newborn life, is of great importance. Failure to regulate arterial pressure, peripheral resistance, and blood volume may lead to significant variations in organ blood flow and substrate delivery, resulting in ischemic or hemorrhagic injury. There is abundant evidence to suggest that autonomic regulatory mechanisms, including baroreceptors and chemoreceptors, are important modulators of BP and circulatory function in the developing fetus and newborn. Additional humoral and endocrine factors act directly and indirectly to regulate vascular tone and cardiac function. A large number of cardiovascular regulatory factors, including opioids, natriuretic peptides, and prostanoids act centrally and peripherally to regulate systemic hemodynamics, and have not been addressed. Further work is needed to determine the role of these factors and their interactions during relevant pathophysiological conditions. A more complete understanding of neurohumoral control of cardiovascular function early in life could potentially result in the development of new therapeutic strategies to prevent complications during the perinatal period.

## REFERENCES

1. Persson P. Cardiopulmonary receptors and "neurogenic hypertension." Acta Physiol Scand 1988;570:1–53.
2. Kirscheim HR. Systemic arterial baroreceptor reflexes. Physiol Rev 1976;56:100–177.
3. Spyer KM. Central nervous mechanisms contributing to cardiovascular control. J Physiol 1994;474:1–19.
4. Vapaavouri EK, Shinebourne EA, Williams RL, Heymann MA, Rudolph AM. Development of cardiovascular responses to autonomic blockade in intact fetal and neonatal lambs. Biol Neonate 1973;22:177–188.
5. Tabsh K, Nuwayhid B, Murad S, et al. Circulatory effects of chemical sympathectomy in fetal, neonatal and adult sheep. Am J Physiol 1982;243:H113–H122.
6. Walker AM, Cannata J, Dowling MH, Ritchie B, Maloney J. Sympathetic and parasympathetic control of heart rate in unanaesthetized fetal and newborn lambs. Biol Neonate 1978;33:1350–1143.
7. Woods JR, Dandavino A, Murayama K, Brinkman CR, Assali NS. Autonomic control of cardiovascular functions during neonatal development and in adult sheep. Circ Res 1977;40:401–407.
8. Nuwayhid B, Brinkman CR, Bevan JA, Assali NS. Development of autonomic control of fetal circulation. Am J Physiol 1975;228:237–344.

9. Yardly RW, Bowes G, Wilkinson M, et al. Increased arterial pressure variability after arterial barorecptor denervation in fetal lambs. Circ Res 1983;52:580–588.
10. Segar JL, Merrill DC, Smith BA, Robillard JE. Role of sympathetic activity in the generation of heart rate and arterial pressure variability in fetal sheep. Pediatr Res 1994;35:250–254.
11. Alper RH, Jacob JH, Brody MJ. Regulation of arterial pressure lability in rats with chronic sinoaortic deafferentation. Am J Physiol 1987;253:H466–H474.
12. Barres C, Lewis SJ, Jacob HJ, Brody MJ. Arterial pressure lability and renal sympathetic nerve activity are disassociated in SAD rats. Am J Physiol 1992;263:R639–R646.
13. Robillard JE, Nakamura KT, DiBona GF. Effects of renal denervation on renal responses to hypoxemia in fetal lambs. Am J Physiol 1986;250:F294–F301.
14. Mann LI, Duchin S, Weiss RR. Fetal EEG sleep stages and physiologic variability. Am J Obstet Gynecol 1974;119:533–538.
15. Zhu Y, Szeto HH. Cyclic variation in fetal heart rate and sympathetic activity. Am J Obstet Gynecol 1987;156:1001–1005.
16. Davidson SR, Rankin JHG, Martin CB, Reid DL. Fetal heart rate variability and behavioral state: analysis by power spectrum. Am J Obstet Gynecol 1992;167:712–717.
17. Wakatsuki A, Murata Y, Ninomoya Y, Masaoka N, Tyner JG, Kutty KK. Physiologic baroreceptor activity in the fetal lamb. Am J Obstet Gynecol 1992;167:820–827.
18. Clapp JF, Szeto HH, Abrams R, Mann LI. Physiologic variability and fetal electrocortical activity. Am J Obstet Gynecol 1980;136:1045–1050.
19. Reid DL, Jensen A, Phernetton TM, Rankin JHG. Relationship between plasma catecholamine levels and electrocortical state in the mature fetal lamb. J Dev Physiol 1990;13:75–79.
20. Jensen A, Bamford OS, Dawes GS, Hofmeyr G, Parkes MJ. Changes in organ blood flow between high and low voltage electrocortical activity in fetal sheep. J Dev Physiol 1986;8:187–194.
21. Richardson BS, Patrick JE, Abduljabbar H. Cerebral oxidative metabolism in the fetal lamb: relationship to electrocortical state. Am J Obstet Gynecol 1985;153:426–431.
22. Abboud F, Thames M. Interaction of cardiovascular reflexes in circulatory control. In: Shepherd JT, Abboud FM, eds. Handbook of Physiology, Section 2, Vol III, Part 2. Bethesda, MD: American Physiological Society, 1983:675–753.
23. Persson PB, Ehmke H, Kirchheim HR. Cardiopulmonary-arterial baroreceptor interaction in control of blood pressure. News in Physiol Sci 1989;4:56–59.
24. Itskovitz J, LaGamma EF, Rudolph AM. Baroreflex control of the circulation in chronically instrumented fetal lambs. Circ Res 1983;52:589–596.
25. Brinkman CRI, Ladner C, Weston P, Assali NS. Baroreceptor functions in the fetal lamb. Am J Physiol 1969;217:1346–1351.
26. Bauer DJ. Vagal reflexes appearing in the rabbit at different ages. J Physiol 1939;95:187–202.
27. Dawes GS, Johnston BM, Walker DW. Relationship of arterial pressure and heart rate in fetal, new-born and adult sheep. J Physiol 1980;309:405–417.
28. Blanco CE, Dawes GS, Hanson MA, McCooke HB. Carotid baroreceptors in fetal and newborn sheep. Pediatr Res 1988;24:342–346.
29. Tomomatsu E, Nishi K. Comparison of carotid sinus baroreceptor sensitivity in newborn and adult rabbits. Am J Physiol 1982;243:H546–H550.
30. Downing SE. Baroreceptor reflexes in new-born rabbits. J Physiol 1960;150:201–213.
31. Biscoe TJ, Purves MJ, Sampson SR. Types of nervous activity which may be recorded from the carotid sinus nerve in the sheep foetus. J Physiol 1969;202:1–23.
32. Ponte J, Purves MJ. Types of afferent nervous activity which may be measured in the vagus nerve of the sheep foetus. J Physiol 1973;229:51–76.
33. Chapleau MW, Hajduczok G, Abboud FM. Mechanisms of resetting of arterial baroreceptors: an overview. Am J Med Sci 1988;295:327–334.
34. Chapleau MW, Hajduczok G, Abboud FM. Resetting of the arterial baroreflex: peripheral and central mechanisms. In: Zucker IH, Gilmore JP, eds. Reflex Control of the Circulation. Boca Raton, FL: CRC, 1991:165–194.
35. Andresen MC. Short and long-term determinants of baroreceptor function in aged normotensive and spontaneously hypertensive rats. Circ Res 1984;54:750–759.
36. Heesch CM, Abboud FM, Thames MD. Acute resetting of carotid sinus baroreceptors. II. Possible involvement of electrogenic Na+ pump. Am J Physiol 1984;247:H833–H839.

37. Matsuda T, Bates JN, Lewis SJ, Abboud FM, Chapleau MW. Modulation of baroreceptor activity by nitric oxide and S-nitrocysteine. Circ Res 1995;76:426–433.
38. Jimbo M, Suzuki H, Ichikawa M, Kumagai K, Nishizawa M, Saruta T. Role of nitric oxide in regulation of baroreceptor reflex. J Auton Nerv Syst 1994;50:209–219.
39. Yu ZY, Lumbers ER. Measurement of baroreceptor-mediated effects on heart rate variability in fetal sheep. Pediatr Res 2000;47:233–239.
40. Shinebourne EA, Vapaavuori EK, Williams RL, Heymann MA, Rudolph AM. Development of baroreflex activity in unanesthetized fetal and neonatal lambs. Circ Res 1972;31:710–718.
41. Vatner SF, Manders WT. Depressed responsiveness of the carotid sinus reflex in conscious newborn animals. Am J Physiol 1979;237:H40–H43.
42. Young M. Responses of the systemic circulation of the new-born infant. Br Med Bull 1966;22:70–72.
43. Gootman PM. Developmental aspects of reflex control of the circulation. In: Zucker IH, Gilmore JP, eds. Reflex Control of the Circulation. Boca Raton, FL: CRC,1991:965–1027.
44. Buckley NM, Gootman PM, Gootman GD, Reddy LC, Weaver LC, Crane LA. Age-dependent cardiovascular effects of afferent stimulation in neonatal pigs. Biol Neonate 1976;30:268–279.
45. Maloney JE, Cannata JP, Dowling MH, Else W, Ritchie B. Baroreflex activity in conscious fetal and newborn lambs. Biol Neonate 1977;31:340–350.
46. Scroop GC, Marker JD, Stankewytsch B, Seamark R. Angiotensin I and II in the assessment of baroreceptor function in fetal and neonatal sheep. J Dev Physiol 1986;8:123–137.
47. Segar JL, Hajduczok G, Smith BA, Robillard J. Ontogeny of baroreflex control of renal sympathetic nerve activity and heart rate. Am J Physiol 1992;263:H1819–H1826.
48. Hajduczok G, Chapleau MW, Johnson SL, Abboud FM. Increase in sympathetic activity with age. I. Role of impairment of arterial baroreflexes. Am J Physiol 1991;260:H1113–H1120.
49. Palmisano BW, Clifford PS, Coon RL, Seagard JL, Hoffmann RG, Kampine JP. Development of baroreflex control of heart rate in swine. Pediatr Res 1989;27:148–152.
50. Segar JL, Mazursky JE, Robillard JE. Changes in ovine renal sympathetic nerve activity and baroreflex function at birth. Am J Physiol 1994;267:H1824–H1832.
51. Segar JL, Merrill DC, Smith BA, Robillard JE. Role of endogenous angiotensin II on resetting of the arterial baroreflex during development. Am J Physiol 1994;266:H52–H59.
52. Bishop VS, Haywood JR. Hormonal control of cardiovascular reflexes. In: Zucker IH, Gilmore JP, eds. Reflex Control of the Circulation. Boca Raton, FL: CRC, 1991:253–271.
53. Picton-Warlow CG, Mayer FE. Cardiovascular responses to postural changes in the neonate. Arch Dis Child 1970;45:354–359.
54. Thoresen M, Cowan F, Walløe L. Cardiovascular responses to tilting in healthy newborn babies. Early Human Dev 1991;26:213–222.
55. Waldman S, Krauss AN, Auld PAM. Baroreceptors in preterm infants: their relationship to maturity and disease. Dev Med Child Neurol 1979;21:714–722.
56. Malliani A, Pagani M, Lombardi F. Clinical and experimental evaluation of sympatho-vagal interaction: power spectral analysis of heart rate and arterial pressure variabilities. In: Zucker IH, Gilmore JP, eds. Reflex Control of the Circulation. Boca Raton, FL: CRC, 1991:937–964.
57. Chatow U, Davidson S, Reichman BL, Akselrod S. Development and maturation of the autonomic nervous system in premature and full-term infants using spectral analysis of heart rate fluctuations. Pediatr Res 1995;37:294–302.
58. Clairambault J, Curzi-Dascalova L, Kauffmann F, Médigue C, Leffler C. Heart rate variability in normal sleeping full-term and preterm neonates. Early Human Dev 1992;28:169–183.
59. Karin J, Hirsch M, Akselrod S. An estimate of fetal autonomic state by spectral analysis of fetal heart rate fluctuations. Pediatr Res 1993;34:134–138.
60. Mazursky JE, Birkett CL, Bedell KA, Ben-Haim SA, Segar JL. Development of baroreflex influences on heart rate variability in preterm infants. Early Hum Dev 1998;53:37–52.
61. Minisi AJ, Thames MD. Reflexes from ventricular receptors with vagal afferents. In: Zucker IH, Gilmore JP, eds. Reflex Control of the Circulation. Boca Raton: CRC, 1991:359.
62. Goetz KL, Madwed JB, Leadley RJ Jr. Atrial receptors: reflex effects in quadripeds. In: Zucker IH, Gilmore JP, eds. Reflex Control of the Circulation. Boca Raton: CRC, 1991:291.
63. Hainsworth R. Reflexes from the heart. Physiol Rev 1991;71:617–658.

64. Victor RG, Thoren PN, Morgan DA, Mark AL. Differential control of adrenal and renal sympathetic nerve activity during hemorrhagic hypertension in rats. Circ Res 1989;64:686–694.
65. Togashi H, Yoshioka M, Tochihara M, Matsumoto M, Saito H. Differential effects of hemorrhage on adrenal and renal nerve activity in anesthetized rats. Am J Physiol 1990;259:H1134–H1141.
66. Baker DG, Coleridge HM, Coleridge JCG. Vagal afferent C fibers from the ventricle. In: Hainsworth R, Kidd C, Linden RJ, eds. Cardiac Receptors. Cambridge University Press, Cambridge: 1979:117.
67. Gupta BN, Thames MD. Behavior of left ventricular mechanoreceptors with myelinated and nonmyelinated afferent vagal fibers in cats. Circ Res 1983;52:291–301.
68. Thames MD, Donald SE, Shepherd JT. Stimulation of cardiac receptors with Veratrum alkaloids inhibits ADH secretion. Am J Physiol 1980;239:H784–H788.
69. Gootman PM, Buckley BJ, DiRusso SM, et al. Age-related responses to stimulation of cardiopulmonary receptors in swine. Am J Physiol 1986;251:H748–H755.
70. Assali NS, Brinkman CR, Wood R Jr, Danavino A, Nuwayhid B. Ontogenesis of the autonomic control of cardiovascular function in the sheep. In: Longo LD, Reneau DD, eds. Fetal and Newborn Cardiovascular Physiology.Garland STPM, New York: 1978:47–91.
71. Smith F, Klinkefus J, Robillard J. Effects on volume expansion on renal sympathetic nerve activity and cardiovascular and renal function in lambs. Am J Physiol 1992;262:R651–R658.
72. Merrill DC, Segar JL, McWeeny OJ, Smith BA, Robillard JE. Cardiopulmonary and arterial baroreflex responses to acute volume expansion during fetal and postnatal development. Am J Physiol 1994;267:H1467–H1475.
73. Merrill DC, McWeeny OJ, Segar JL, Robillard JE. Impairment of cardiopulmonary baroreflexes during the newborn period. Am J Physiol 1995;268:H134–H1351.
74. Gomez RA, Meernik JG, Kuehl WD, Robillard JE. Developmental aspects of the renal response to hemorrhage during fetal life. Pediatr Res 1984;18:40–46.
75. Chen HG, Wood CE. Reflex control of fetal arterial pressure and hormonal responses to slow hemorrhage. Am J Physiol 1992;262:H225–H233.
76. Toubas PL, Silverman NH, Heymann MA, Rudolph AM. Cardiovascular effects of acute hemorrhage in fetal lambs. Am J Physiol 1981;240:H45–H48.
77. Wood CE, Chen H-G, Bell ME. Role of vagosympathetic fibers in the control of adrenocorticotropic hormone, vasopressin, and renin responses to hemorrhage in fetal sheep. Circ Res 1989;64:515–523.
78. O'Mara MS, Merrill DC, McWeeny OJ, Robillard JE. Ontogeny and regulation of arterial and cardiopulmonary baroreflex control of renal sympathetic nerve activity (RSNA) in response to hypotensive (NH) and hypotensive hemorrhage (HH) postnatally. Pediatr Res 1995;37:31A.
79. Smith FG, Abu-Amarah I. Renal denervation alters cardiovascular and endocrine responses to hemorrhage in conscious newborn lambs. Am J Physiol 1998;275:H285–H291.
80. Merrill DC, Segar JL, McWeeny OJ, Robillard JE. Sympathetic responses to cardiopulmonary vagal afferent stimulation during development. Am J Physiol 1999;277:H1311–H1316.
81. Cornish KG, Barazanji MW, Yong T, Gilmore JP. Volume expansion attenuates baroreflex sensitivity in the conscious nonhuman primate. Am J Physiol 1989;257:R595–R598.
82. Hajduczok G, Chapleau MW, Abboud FM. Increase in sympathetic activity with age: II. Role of impairment of cardiopulmonary baroreflexes. Am J Physiol 1991;260:H1121–H1127.
83. Bishop VS, Hasser EM, Nair UC. Baroreflex control of renal nerve activity in conscious animals. Circ Res 1987;61:I76–I81.
84. Cohn EH, Sacks EJ, Heymann MA, Rudolph AM. Cardiovascular responses to hypoxemia and acidemia in fetal lambs. Am J Ob Gyn 1974;120:817–824.
85. Giussani DA, Spencer JAD, Moore PJ, Bennet L, Hanson MA. Afferent and efferent components of the cardiovascular reflex responses to acute hypoxia in term fetal sheep. J Physiol 1993;461:431–449.
86. Gardner DS, Fletcher JW, Bloomfield MR, Fowden AL, Giussani DA. Effects of prevailing hypoxaemia, acidaemia or hypoglycaemia upon the cardiovascular, endocrine and metabolic responses to acute hypoxaemia in the ovine fetus. J Physiol 2002;540:351–366.
87. Iwamota HS, Rudolph AM, Mirkin BL, Keil LE. Circulatory and humoral responses of sympathectomized fetal sheep to hypoxemia. Am J Physiol 1983;245:H267–H772.
88. Bartelds B, Van Bel F, Teitel DF, Rudolph AM. Carotid, not aortic, chemoreceptors mediate the fetal cardiovascular response to acute hypoxemia in lambs. Pediatr Res 1993;34:51–55.

89. Blanco CE, Dawes GS, Hanson MA, McCooke HB. The response to hypoxia of arterial chemoreceptors in fetal sheep and newborn lambs. J Physiol 1984;351:25–37.
90. Hertzberg T, Lagercrantz H. Postnatal sensitivity of the peripheral chemoreceptors in newborn infants. Arch Dis Child 1987;62:1238–1241.
91. Kumar P, Hanson MA. Re-setting of the hypoxic sensitivity of aortic chemoreceptors in the new-born lamb. J Dev Physiol 1989;11:199–206.
92. Blanco CE, Hanson MA, McCooke HB. Effects on carotid chemoreceptor resetting of pulmonary ventilation in the fetal lamb in utero. J Dev Physiol 1988;10:167–174.
93. Hertzberg T, Hellstrom S, Holgert H, Lagererantz H, Pequignot JM. Ventilatory response to hyperoxia in newborn rats born in hypoxia—possible relationship to carotid body dopamine. J Physiol 1992;456:645–654.
94. Sterni LM, Bamford OS, Tomares SM, Montrose MH, Carroll JL. Developmental changes in intracellular $Ca^{2+}$ response of carotid chemoreceptor cells to hypoxia. Am J Physiol 1995;268:L801–L808.
95. Koos BJ, Chau A, Ogunyemi D. Adenosine mediates metabolic and cardiovascular responses to hypoxia in fetal sheep. J Physiol (Lond) 1995;488:761–766.
96. Koos BJ, Maeda T. Adenosine $A_{2A}$ receptors mediate cardiovascular responses to hypoxia in fetal sheep. Am J Physiol 2001;280:H83–H89.
97. Giussani DA, Gardner DS, Cox DT, Fletcher AJW. Purinergic contribution to circulatory, metabolic, and adrenergic responses to acute hypoxemia in fetal sheep. Am J Physiol 2001;280:R678–R685.
98. Jensen A, Hanson MA. Circulatory response to acute asphyxia in intact and chemodenervated fetal sheep near term. Reprod Fert Develop 1995;7:1351–1359.
99. McQueen DS, Ribeiro JA. Pharmacological characterization of the receptor involved in chemoexcitation induced by adenosine. Br J Pharmacol 1986;88:615–620.
100. Hanson MA. Role of chemoreceptors in effects of chronic hypoxia. Comp Biochem Physiol 1997;119A:695–703.
101. Ruijtenbeek K, LeNoble FA, Janssen GM, et al. Chronic hypoxia stimulates periarterial sympathetic nerve development in chicken embryo. Circulation 2000;102:2892–2897.
102. Hanson MA, Kumar P, Williams BA. The effect of chronic hypoxia upon the development of respiratory chemoreflexes in the newborn kitten. J Physiol 1989;411:563–574.
103. Dawes GS. Changes in the circulation at birth. Br Med Bull 1961;17:148–153.
104. Padbury JF, Martinez AM. Sympathoadrenal system activity at birth: integration of postnatal adaptation. Sem Perinatal 1988;12:163–172.
105. Lagercrantz H, Bistoletti P. Catecholamine release in the newborn at birth. Pediatr Res 1973;11:889–893.
106. Padbury JF, Diakomanolis ES, Hobel CJ, Perlman A, Fisher DA. Neonatal adaptation: sympatho-adrenal response to umbilical cord cutting. Pediatr Res 1981;15:1483–1487.
107. Minoura S, Gilbert RD. Postnatal changes of cardiac function in lambs: effects of ganglionic block and afterload. J Dev Physiol 1986;9:123–135.
108. Hilton SM. The defense-arousal system and its relevance for circulatory and respiratory control. J Exp Biol 1982;100:159–174.
109. Ogundipe OA, Kullama LK, Stein H, Nijland MJ, Ervin G, Padbury J, Ross MG. Fetal endocrine and renal responses to in utero ventilation and umbilical cord occlusion. Am J Obstet Gynecol 1993;169:1479–1486.
110. Smith FG, Smith BA, Segar JL, Robillard JE. Endocrine effects of ventilation, oxygenation and cord occlusion in near-term fetal sheep. J Dev Physiol 1991;15:133–138.
111. Mazursky JE, Segar JL, Nuyt A-M, Smith BA, Robillard JE. Regulation of renal sympathetic nerve activity at birth. Am J Physiol 1996;270:R86–R93.
112. Segar JL, Smith OJ, Holley AT. Mechano- and chemoreceptor modulation of renal sympathetic nerve activity at birth in fetal sheep. Am J Physiol 1999;276:R1295–R1301.
113. Van Bel F, Roman C, Iwamoto HS, Rudolph AM. Sympathoadrenal, metabolic, and regional blood flow responses to cold in fetal sheep. Pediatr Res 1993;34:47–50.
114. Gunn TR, Johnston BM, Iwamoto HS, Fraser M, Nicholls MG, Gluckman PD. Haemodynamic and catecholamine responses to hypothermia in the fetal sheep in utero. J Dev Physiol 1985;7:241–249.
115. Gunn TR, Ball KT, Power GG, Gluckman PD. Factors influencing the initiation of nonshivering thermogenesis. Am J Obstet Gynecol 1991;164:210–217.
116. Calaresu FR, Yardley CP. Medullary basal sympathetic tone. Ann Rev Physiol 1988;50:511–524.
117. Gebber GL. Central determinants of sympathetic nerve discharge. In: Loewy AD, Spyer KM, eds. Central Regulation of Autonomic Function. New York, NY: Oxford University Press, 1990:126–144.

118. Loewy AD. Central autonomic pathways. In: Loewy AD, Spyer KM, eds. Central Regulation of Autonomic Functions. New York, NY: Oxford University Press, 1990:88–103.
119. Williams RL, Hof RP, Heymann MA, Rudolph AM. Cardiovascular effects of electrical stimulation of the forebrain in the fetal lamb. Pediatr Res 1976;10:40–45.
120. Segar JL, Ellsbury DL, Smith OM. Inhibition of sympathetic responses at birth in sheep by lesion of the paraventricular nucleus. Am J Physiol 2002;283:R1395–R1403.
121. Segar JL, Lumbers ER, Nuyt AM, Smith OJ, Robillard JE. Effect of antenatal glucocorticoids on sympathetic nerve activity at birth in preterm sheep. Am J Physiol 1998;274:R160–R167.
122. Segar JL, Bedell KA, Smith OJ. Glucocorticoid modulation of cardiovascular and autonomic function in preterm lambs: role of ANG II. Am J Physiol 2001;280:R646–R654.
123. Guillery EN, Robillard JE. The renin-angiotensin system and blood pressure regulation during infancy and childhood. In: Rocchini AP, ed. The Pediatric Clinics of North America: Childhood Hypertension. Philadelphia: W.B. Saunders, 1993:61–77.
124. Lumbers ER. Functions of the renin-angiotensin system during development. Clin Exp Phamarcol Physiol 1995;22:499–505.
125. Iwamota HS, Rudolph AM. Effects of endogenous angiotensin II on the fetal circulation. J Dev Physiol 1979;1:283–293.
126. Kim S, Iwao H. Molecular and cellular mechanisms of angiotensin II-mediated cardiovascular and renal diseases. Pharmacol Rev 2001;52:11–34.
127. Broughton-Pipkin F, Kirkpatrick SM, Lumbers ER, Mott JE. Renin and angiotensin-like levels in foetal, newborn and adult sheep. J Physiol (London) 1974;241:575–588.
128. Bartunek J, Weinberg EO, Tajima M, Rohrbach S, Lorell BH. Angiotensin II type 2 receptor blockade amplifies the early signals of cardiac growth response to angiotensin II in hypertrophied hearts. Circulation 1999;99:22–25.
129. Stalker HB, Holland NH, Kotchen JM, Kotchen TA. Plasma renin activity in healthy children. J Pediatr 1976;89:256–258.
130. Richer C, Hornych H, Amiel-Tison C, Relier JP, Giudicelli JF. Plasma renin activity and its postnatal development in preterm infants. Preliminary report. Biol Neonate 1977;31:301–304.
131. Robillard JE, Weismann DN, Gomez RA, Ayres NA, Lawton WJ, VanOrden DE. Renal and adrenal responses to converting-enzyme inhibition in fetal and newborn life. Am J Physiol 1983;244:R249–R256.
132. Scroop GC, Stankewytsch-Janusch B, Marker JD. Renin-angiotensin and automatic mechanisms in cardiovascular homeostasis during hemorrhage in fetal and neonatal sheep. J Dev Physiol 1992;18:25–33.
133. Weismann DN, Herrig JE, McWeeny OJ, Ayres NA, Robillard JE. Renal and adrenal responses to hypoxemia during angiotensin-converting enzyme inhibition in lambs. Circ Res 1983;52:179–187.
134. Robillard JE, Weitzman RE. Developmental aspects of the fetal renal response to exogenous arginine vasopressin. Am J Physiol 1980;238:F407–F414.
135. Robillard JE, Gomez RA, VanOrden D, Smith FGJ. Comparison of the adrenal and renal responses to angiotensin II in fetal lambs and adult sheep. Circ Res 1982;50:140–147.
136. Wood CE. Baroreflex and chemoreflex control of fetal hormone secretion. Reprod Fert Develop 1995;7:479–489.
137. Jones III OW, Cheung CY, Brace RA. Dose-dependent effects of angiotensin II on the ovine fetal cardiovascular system. Am J Obstet Gynecol 1991;165:1524–1533.
138. Ismay MJ, Lumbers ER, Stevens AD. The action of angiotensin II on the baroreflex response of the conscious ewe and the conscious fetus. J Physiol 1979;288:467–479.
139. Reid IA. Interactions between ANG II, sympathetic nervous system and baroreceptor reflex in regulation of blood pressure. Am J Physiol 1992;262:E763–E778.
140. Bunnemann B, Fuxe K, Ganten D. The renin-angiotensin system in the brain: an update 1993. Reg Peptides 1993;46:487–509.
141. Toney GM, Porter JP. Effects of blockade of $AT_1$ and $AT_2$ receptors in brain on the central angiotensin II pressor response in conscious spontaneously hypertensive rats. Neuropharmacol 1993;32:581–589.
142. Head GA, Mayorov DN. Central angiotensin and baroreceptor control of circulation. Ann NY Acad Sci 2001;940:361–379.
143. Segar JL, Minnick A, Nuyt AM, Robillard JE. Role of endogenous ANG II and $AT_1$ receptors in regulating arterial baroreflex responses in newborn lambs. Am J Physiol 1997;272:R1862–R1873.

144. Irion GL, Mack CE, Clark KE. Fetal hemodynamic and fetoplacental vasopressin response to exogenous arginine vasopressin. Am J Obstet Gynecol 1990;162:115–120.
145. Tomita H, Brace RA, Cheung CY, Longo LD. Vasopressin dose-response effects on fetal vascular pressures, heart rate, and blood volume. Am J Physiol 1985;249:H974–H980.
146. Weitzman RE, Fisher DA, Robillard J, Erenberg A, Kennedy R, Smith F. Arginine vasopressin response to an osmotic stimulus in the fetal sheep. Pediatr Res 1978;12:35–38.
147. Robillard JE, Weitzman RE, Fisher DA, Smith FGJ. The dynamics of vasopressin release and blood volume regulation during fetal hemorrhage in the lamb fetus. Pediatr Res 1979;13:606–610.
148. Wood CE, Chen HG. Acidemia stimulates ACTH, vasopressin, and heart rate responses in fetal sheep. Am J Physiol 1989;257:R344–R349.
149. Raff H, Kane CW, Wood CE. Arginine vasopressin responses to hypoxia and hypercapnia in late-gestation fetal sheep. Am J Physiol 1991;260:R1077–R1081.
150. Giussani DA, McGarrigle HHG, Spencer JAD, Moore PJ, Bennet L, Hanson MA. Effect of carotid denervation on plasma vasopressin levels during acute hypoxia in the late-gestation sheep fetus. J Physiol 1994;477: 81–87.
151. Nuyt A-M, Segar JL, Holley AT, O'Mara MS, Chapleau MW, Robillard JE. Arginine vasopressin modulation of arterial baroreflex responses in fetal and newborn sheep. Am J Physiol 1996;271:R1643–R1653.
152. Ervin MG, Ross MG, Leake RD, Fisher DA. $V_1$ and $V_2$-receptor contributions to ovine fetal renal and cardiovascular responses to vasopressin. Am J Physiol 1992;262:R636–R643.
153. Kelly RT, Rose JC, Meis PJ, Hargrave BY, Morris M. Vasopressin is important for restoring cardiovascular homeostasis in fetal lambs subjected to hemorrhage. Am J Obstet Gynecol 1983;146:807–812.
154. Berecek KH, Swords BH. Central role for vasopressin in cardiovascular regulation and the pathogenesis of hypertension. Hypertension 1990;16:213–224.
155. Luk J, Ajaelo I, Wong V, et al. Role of $V_1$ receptors in the action of vasopressin on the baroreflex control of heart rate. Am J Physiol 1993;265:R524–R529.
156. Miyake Y, Murata Y, Hesser J, Tyner J. Cardiovascular responses to norepinephrine and arginine vasopressin infusion in chronically catheterized fetal lambs. J Reproduct Med 1991;36:735–740.
157. Stark RI, Daniel SS, Husain MK, Tropper PJ, James LS. Cerebrospinal fluid and plasma vasopressin in the fetal lamb: basal concentration and the effect of hypoxia. Endocrinol 1985;116:65–72.
158. Segar JL, Minnick A, Nuyt A-M, Robillard JE. Developmental changes in central vasopressin regulation of cardiovascular function. Pediatr Res 1995;37:34A.
159. Unger T, Rohmeiss P, Demmert G, Ganton D, Lang RE, Luft F. Opposing cardiovascular effects of brain and plasma AVP: role of $V_1$- and $V_2$-AVP receptors. In: Buckley JP, Ferrario CM, eds.. Brain Peptides and Catecholamines in Cardiovascular Regulation. New York: Raven, 1987:393–401.
160. Unno N, Wong CH, Jenkins SL, et al. Blood pressure and heart rate in the ovine fetus: ontogenic changes and effects of fetal adrenalectomy. Am J Physiol 1999;276:H248–H256.
161. Tangalakis T, Lumbers ER, Moritz KM, Towstoless MK, Wintour EM. Effect of cortisol on blood pressure and vascular reactivity in the ovine fetus. Exp Physiol 1992;77:709–717.
162. Stein HM, Oyama K, Martinez A, et al. Effects of corticosteroids in preterm sheep on adaptation and sympathoadrenal mechanisms at birth. Am J Physiol 1993;264:E763–E769.
163. Padbury JF, Polk DH, Ervin G, Bery LM, Ikegami M, Jobe AH. Postnatal cardiovascular and metabolic responses to a single intramuscular dose of betamethasone in fetal sheep born prematurely by cesarean section. Pediatr Res 1995;38:709–715.
164. Derks JB, Giussani DA, Jenkins SL, et al. A comparative study of cardiovascular, endocrine and behavioural effects of betamethasone and dexamethasone administration to fetal sheep. J Physiol 1997;499:217–226.
165. Dodt C, Keyser B, Molle M, Fehm HL, Elam M. Acute suppression of muscle sympathetic nerve activity by hydrocortisone in humans. Hypertension 2000;35:758–763.
166. Macefield VG, Williamson PM, Wilson LR, Kelly JJ, Gandevia SC, Whitworth JA. Muscle sympathetic vasoconstrictor activity in hydrocortisone-induced hypertension in humans. Blood Press 1998;7:215–222.
167. Grünfeld JP, Eloy L. Glucocorticoids modulate vascular reactivity in the rat. Hypertension 1987;10:608–618.
168. Grünfled JP. Glucocorticoids in blood pressure regulation. Horm Res 1990;34:111–113.
169. Provencher PH, Saltis J, Funder JW. Glucocorticoids but not mineralocorticoids modulate endothelin-1 and angiotensin II binding in SHR vascular smooth muscle cells. J Steroid Biochem Mol Biol 1995;52:219–225.
170. Sato A, Suzuki H, Iwaita Y, Nakazato Y, Kato H, Saruta T. Potentiation of inositol trisphosphate production by dexamethasone. Hypertension 1992;19:109–115.

171. Wallerath T, Witte K, Schäfer SC, et al. Down-regulation of the expression of endothelial NO synthase is likely to contribute to glucocorticoid-mediated hypertension. Proc Natl Acad Sci 1999;96:13357–13362.
172. Fletcher AJW, McGarrigle HHG, Edwards CMB, Fowden AL. Effects of low dose dexamethasone treatment on basal cardiovascular and endocrine function in fetal sheep during late gestation. J Physiol 2002;545:649–660.
173. Anwar MA, Schwab M, Poston L, Nathanielsz PW. Betamethasone-mediated vascular dysfunction and changes in hematological profile in the ovine fetus. Am J Physiol 1999;276:H1137–H1143.
174. Docherty CC, Kalmar-Nagy J. Development of fetal vascular responses to endothelin-1 and acetycholine in the sheep. Am J Physiol 2001;280:R554–R562.
175. Docherty CC, Kalmar-Nagy J, Engelen M, et al. Effect of in vivo fetal infusion of dexamethasone at 0.75 GA on fetal ovine resistance artery responses to ET-1. Am J Physiol 2001;281:R261–R268.
176. Molnar J, Nijland M, Howe DC, Nathanielsz PW. Evidence for microvascular dysfunction after prenatal dexamethasone at 0.7, 0.75, and 0.8 gestation in sheep. Am J Physiol 2002;283:R561–R567.
177. Ervin MG, Padbury JF, Polk DH, Ikegami M, Berry LM, Jobe AH. Antenatal glucocorticoids alter premature newborn lamb neuroendocrine and endocrine responses to hypoxia. Am J Physiol 2000;279:R830–R838.
178. Fletcher AJW, Gardner DG, Edwards CMB, Fowden AL, Giussani DA Cardiovascular and endocrine responses to acute hypoxaemia during and following dexamethasone infusion in the ovine fetus. J Physiol 2003;549:271–287.
179. Semenza GL. HIF-1: mediator of physiological and pathophysiological responses to hypoxia. J Appl Physiol 2000;88:1474–1480.
180. Slotkin TA, Lappi SE, Tayyeb MI, Seidler FJ. Dose-dependent glucocorticoid effects on noradrenergic synaptogenesis in rat brain: ontogeny of [$^3$H]desmethylimipramine binding sites after fetal exposure to dexamethasone. Res Commun Chem Pathol Pharmacol 1991;73:3–19.
181. Slotkin TA, Lappi SE, McCook EC, Tayyeb MI, Eylers JP, Seidler FJ. Glucocorticoids and the development of neuronal function: effects of prenatal dexamethasone exposure on central noradrenergic activity. Biol Neonate 1992;61:326–336.
182. Segar JL, Van Natta T, Smith OJ. Effects of fetal ovine adrenalectomy on sympathetic and baroreflex responses at birth. Am J Physiol 2002;283:R460–R467.
183. Scheuer DA, Bechtold AG. Glucocorticoids modulate baroreflex control of heart rate in conscious normotensive rats. Am J Physiol 2001;282:R475–R483.
184. Scheuer DA, Mifflin SW. Glucocorticoids modulate baroreflex control of renal sympathetic nerve activity. Am J Physiol 2001;280:R1440–R1449.
185. Yu ZY, Lumbers ER, Simonetta G. The cardiovascular and renal effects of acute and chronic inhibition of nitric oxide production in fetal sheep. Exp Physiol 2002;87:343–351.
186. Chlorakos A, Langille BL, Adamson SL. Cardiovascular responses attenuate with repeated NO synthesis inhibition in conscious fetal sheep. Am J Physiol 1998;274:H1472–H1480.
187. Sheng-Xing M, Fang Q, Morgan B, Ross MG, Chao CR. Cardiovascular regulation and expressions of NO synthase-tyrosine hydroxylase in nucleus tractus solitarius of ovine fetus. Am J Physiol 2003;284:H1057–H1063.
188. McDonald TJ, Le WW, Hoffman GE. Brainstem catecholaminergic neurons activated by hypoxemia express GR and are coordinately activated with fetal sheep hypothalamic paraventricular CRH neurons. Brain Res 2000;885:70–78.

# 2 Cardiovascular and Autonomic Influences on Blood Pressure

*John E. Jones,* PhD, *Aruna R. Natarajan,* MBBS, DCh, *and Pedro A. Jose,* MD, PhD

*CONTENTS*



## INTRODUCTION

The cardiovascular system provides appropriate organ and tissue perfusion at rest and at times of stress by regulation of blood pressure (BP). The arterial pressure level at any given time reflects the composite activities of the heart and the peripheral circulation.

## CONTROL OF BLOOD PRESSURE

Although the relationship between pressure and flow through the vascular tree is not linear, BP can be expressed as the product of cardiac output (CO) and peripheral resistance *(1)* (Table 1). These variables are closely intertwined, and the control mechanisms for pressure regulation involve more than simply a direct change in either CO or peripheral resistance *(2)*. The major determinant of BP at rest is arteriolar resistance; during exercise, CO assumes a more important role.

### *Cardiac Output*

CO is defined as the volume of blood pumped by the left ventricle of the heart into the aorta and, subsequently, to the circulation. In general, CO is expressed in L/min. It represents the circulatory status of the organism and plays a critical role in maintenance of BP in health and disease. BP is determined by the product of CO and systemic vascular resistance.

From: *Clinical Hypertension and Vascular Disease: Pediatric Hypertension*
Edited by: R. J. Portman, J. M. Sorof, and J. R. Ingelfinger © Humana Press Inc., Totowa, NJ

Table 1
Factors Influencing Arterial Pressure as the Product of Cardiac Output and Peripheral Resistance

*Cardiac output*
Heart rate
Stroke volume
  Venous return
  Myocardial contractility
Blood volume
*Peripheral resistance*
Adrenergic nerves
Circulating catecholamines
Other vasoactive substances
    Acetylcholine
    Angiotensin II
    Endothelium-derived contracting factor
    Kinins
    Neuropeptides (neurotensin, NPY, substance P)
    Nitric oxide
    Oxytocin
    Prostanoids (prostaglandins, HETEs, leukotrienes, thromboxanes)
    Serotonin
    Vasopressin (antidiuretic hormone)
Ions and cellular regulators (e.g., calcium, sodium, chloride, potassium, magnesium, manganese, and trace metals, pH, etc.)
Hematocrit (viscosity)
Reactive oxygen species

Reproduced from ref. *85*, with permission.

CO varies widely depending on metabolic and physical activity, age, and size of the body. For healthy young males, resting CO is 5.6 L/min. The value is 20% less in females. As this value varies consistently with the surface area of the body, it is also expressed as cardiac index, which is the CO per square meter of body surface area. This value is about 3 L/min/$m^2$. Babies have a higher cardiac index at 5.5 L/min/$m^2$, and this value is even higher in preterm babies.

Control of CO is governed by two kinds of mechanisms: primary mechanisms, which operate quickly for acute regulation, and secondary mechanisms, which have a slower onset and regulate long-term aspects of cardiac function. CO is derived from the product of stroke volume (volume represented by the volume of blood pumped by the heart in one beat) and the heart rate (HR) per minute. In infancy and early childhood, CO is increased mainly by an increase in HR because the capacity of the cardiac muscle to increase stroke volume during this period is limited.

### *Stroke Volume*

Stroke volume depends on three primary factors, all of which are interrelated and not mutually exclusive. These factors are preload, afterload, and myocardial contractility. Preload is determined by venous filling of the right ventricle and, subsequently, the left ventricle, determining the volume of blood available to be pumped. Preload is classically compromised in dehydration and hemorrhage. Afterload is determined by peripheral arterial resistance and intrinsic ventricular wall stress. Afterload determines diastolic pressure and, by extension, mean arterial pressure and tissue perfusion. Afterload is reduced in septic shock with profound vasodilatation, and it is increased in hypothermia. Myocardial contractility is defined as the inherent ability of cardiac muscle to pump blood. This function is compromised in myocarditis and some forms of cardiomyopathy. These primary factors could be altered by secondary factors in response to the physiological state of the individual.

### *Preload*

CO is determined primarily by preload, that volume of venous blood that fills the ventricle during diastole. This is also called venous return or end diastolic volume. The adult heart is capable of pumping up to 15 L/min, but the usual resting CO is only 5.6 L/min. The Frank-Starling law describes the inherent ability of the heart to regulate its output despite a rapidly varying venous return. Increasing venous return increases end-diastolic volume resulting in the stretch of the muscle fibers. Consequently, increased volume at the end of diastole leads to immediate, increased, and effective ejection during systole, which is defined as increased stroke volume. This ensures that even when end-diastolic volume or filling is increased, the end-systolic volume, or the volume of blood left in the ventricle does not increase, as all the extra volume is pumped out. The energy output of a heart muscle fiber increases with increasing fiber length up to a point, beyond which further extension of the fiber results in a decrease in its contractile force, which then causes a reduction in stroke volume. An important aspect of the Frank-Starling law is that a change in the afterload (or outflow resistance) has almost no influence on cardiac output. Preload-dependent regulation of stroke volume is also called *heterometric regulation*. Stretching of the ventricle stretches the sinus node in the wall of the right atrium, which increases its rate of firing, and increases the HR by 10–15%. The stretched right atrium also initiates a reflex called the Bainbridge reflex, which increases HR. In summary, increasing preload increases stroke volume and HR. Therefore, preload is a major factor in the enhancing of CO.

### *Afterload*

Afterload is the force that opposes or resists ventricular emptying. After the ventricle has ejected its contents, the rise in aortic pressure closes the aortic valve and maintains a back pressure that the next cycle of systole has to overcome. Components of the aortic back pressure include the tension developed in the aortic walls, peripheral vascular resistance, the reflected pressure waves within the ventricle, and its distribution throughout the ventricular wall. Ventricular pressure, myocardial thickness, and peripheral resistance all contribute to systolic wall stress, which signifies afterload. Mean arterial pressure (calculated as 2× diastolic plus 1× systolic BP divided by 3), which is related to CO and peripheral resistance, gives an indication of afterload. Mean afterload is normally kept constant by central cardiovascular and autonomic control.

Because the afterload does not allow the ventricle to empty completely, a percentage of the original venous return remains in the heart. The term *ejection fraction* (EF) describes the amount of blood ejected from the ventricle during one systolic wave (stroke volume [SV]) divided by the amount of blood in the ventricle at the end of diastole (left ventricular end-diastolic volume [LVEDV]).

$$EF = SV/LVEDV$$

This can be quantified with echocardiography by measuring the shortening fraction of the muscle fiber, which correlates directly with contractility. Typically, the EF for a normal adult is 0.50–0.75. This fraction does not change with gestational or postnatal age. Left and right ventricular diastolic volumes, however, increase with gestational and postnatal age *(3)*.

### *Myocardial Contractility*

Myocardial contractility accounts for the increases in contractile force of a muscle fiber, with no accompanying change in fiber length. This capacity of cardiac muscle is called *homeotropic regulation*. The heart is richly supplied with both sympathetic and parasympathetic nerves that have profound effects on heart rate and contractility. The resting normal sympathetic tone maintains cardiac contractility at 20% greater than in the denervated heart. Increased sympathetic input to the heart can significantly increase both HR and contractile force up to 100%. Parasympathetic innervation, on the other hand, reduces HR and contractile force through nerve fibers predominantly supplying the atria. However, contractility can only be decreased to about 20%. Sympathetic enhancement of cardiac contractility is mediated by norepinephrine from the cardiac sympathetic nerves. Norepinephrine causes an increase in the shortening of the muscle fiber with a constant preload and total load, resulting in increased stroke volume. This effect is mediated by the stimulation of β-adrenergic receptors, mainly of the $\beta_1$ subtype (*see* Table 2) on the cardiac membranes, leading to an increase in cyclic AMP (cAMP). cAMP increases phosphorylase B activity, stimulating glycogen metabolism, and increasing energy supply for enhanced contractility. Combined with its effect on increasing HR, sympathetic stimulation can cause a two- to threefold increase in CO.

Calcium is necessary for effective contraction of cardiac muscle. Action potential causes release of calcium into the sarcoplasm of the muscle. Instantaneously, calcium ions diffuse into the myofibrils and catalyze the chemical reactions that promote sliding of actin and myosin filaments along one another, producing muscle contraction. Because muscle sarcoplasm does not have a large store of calcium, large amounts of extracellular calcium are needed to diffuse into the T-tubules, where they are bound to glycoproteins, and released as needed, to enhance contractility.

### *Heart Rate and Rhythm*

Factors affecting HR do so by altering the electric properties of the cardiac pacemaker cells, which have an intrinsic rate and are age-dependent, being higher in infancy and diminishing with age. The autonomic nervous system has the most profound influence on HR. The sympathetic and parasympathetic systems act by changing the rate of spontaneous depolarization of the resting potential in the cardiac pacemaker cells. While sympathetic stimulation causes the HR to increase, parasympathetic stimulation causes it to fall. These reflexes are immediate and represent critical survival mechanisms. During periods of tachycardia, peak ejection velocity is increased. The net effect of the tachycardia is an increased CO. However, outside the normal adult physiologic range, large increases or decreases in HR result in a decrease in the net CO. In the adult, tachycardia of 170 bpm or greater allows too little time for ventricular filling. The small ejection volume cannot be overcome by the increased HR. Lower than normal HR, or bradycardia, causes a decreased CO because of a reduced stroke volume relative to the requirements of the individual. In the case of reduced HR below 40 bpm (in the adult), the increase in preload owing to increased filling time is limited because major ventricular filling, which occurs early in diastole, is not maintained for the duration of the diastolic period. CO decreases because stroke volume does not increase sufficiently.

Table 2
Some Drugs Showing Selectivity for Adrenergic and Dopamine Receptor Subtypes *(19)*

| *Drug name* | *Agonists* | *Antagonists* |
|---|---|---|
| Nonselective | Norepinephrine | Phentolamine |
| $\alpha_1$ | Cirazoline | Prazosin |
| $\alpha_{1A}$ | A61603 Oxmetazoline | (+) Niguldipine, 5-methyl urapidil, KMD-3213 |
| $\alpha_{1B}$ | | (+) -Cyclazosin |
| $\alpha_{1D}$ | BMY 7378 | BMY-7378 |
| $\alpha_2$ | UK14304 | Idazoxan<br>Rauwolscine<br>Yohimbine |
| $\alpha_{2A/D}$ | Oxymetazoline | BRL 44408 |
| $\alpha_{2B}$ | Guanfacine | Imiloxan |
| $\alpha_{2C}$ | | ARC 239 |
| β-Adrenoceptor | | |
| Nonselective | Isoproterenol | Propranolol |
| $\beta_1$ | Xamoterol | Betaxolol<br>Atenolol |
| $\beta_2$ | Salmeterol<br>Terbutaline | Butoxamine<br>ICI 118,551 |
| $\beta_3$ | BR 37344<br>CL 316243 | SR-59230A<br>SR 58894 |
| Dopamine receptor | | |
| Nonselective | Dopamine | |
| $D_1$-like | Fenoldopam[a] | R(+)-SCH 23390[a] |
| $D_1$ | | |
| $D_5$ | | |
| $D_2$-like | LY 171555<br>SKF103376 | YM 09151<br>Domperidone |
| $D_2$ | U91356A | L741,626 |
| $D_3$ | PD128907<br>R(+)-7-hydroxyPIPAT | S(–)-Nafadotride<br>U-99,194A |
| $D_4$ | PD168077 | L-745, 870 |

[a] Selective for $D_1$-like receptors but cannot distinguish between $D_1$ and $D_5$ receptors.
Reproduced from ref. *85*, with permission.

HR is one of the most important determinants of myocardial energy consumption. Generally it is more energy efficient to increase CO by increasing stroke volume, rather than by increasing HR. Infants and children are more likely to increase their HR, and thus expend more energy in increasing their CO during stress.

### *Primary Regulation of Cardiac Output During Development*

Effective circulation is necessary in very early embryonic development, and parallels structural development of the heart *(4)*. As early as 5 wk postconception in humans, the basic circulatory parameter, HR, is present at about 100 bpm. CO is very dependent on HR and also on atrioventricular synchrony after formation of the four-chambered heart. Systolic function of the heart and, consequently CO, increases with gestational age. The EF of the embryonic ventricle is roughly 30–50%. The fetal heart has a limited ability to increase work following stretch, so the Frank-Starling curve is limited compared to adults. The lower wall stress in the embryo, owing to a smaller ventricular size and lower pressures, reduces the total afterload and enhances CO in the face of a high peripheral resistance. Afterload owing to wall stress increases as gestation progresses, reflecting the increase in ventricular size and transmural pressures while peripheral vascular resistance decreases.

### *Secondary Regulation of Cardiac Output*

A variety of factors operate in the normal person to regulate CO over the long-term. These secondary control mechanisms do not have as great an influence on the heart as the components previously described. Secondary controls include cardiovascular reflexes and hormonal influences. Cardiopulmonary receptors, which are sensory nerve endings in the atria, ventricles, coronary vessels, and lungs, have chemo- and mechano-sensitive properties. The activity of these receptors is relayed to the nucleus of the tractus solitarius, via vagal afferents and spinal sympathetic afferent fibers. Stimulation of these receptors evokes responses similar to those noted with arterial baroreceptors. Thus, an increase in distension of the atria results in a decrease in circulating levels of vasopressin, aldosterone, and renin, among other hormones, but causes an increase in the natriuretic factors synthesized by the atrium and the ventricles (atrial natriuretic peptide, brain natriuretic peptide, C-type natriuretic peptide). Circulating atrial natriuretic peptide decreases with gestational and postnatal age *(5)*. Depressor reflexes in the heart originating mainly from the inferoposterior wall of the left ventricle promote bradycardia, vasodilatation, and hypotension (Bezold–Jarisch reflex) *(6)*. These are mediated by increased parasympathetic and decreased sympathetic activity. Left ventricular mechanoreceptor stimulation can also attenuate arterial baroreflex control of HR. Decreased activity of cardiac vagal afferents results in enhanced sympathetic activity and increased vascular resistance, renin release, and vasopressin secretion. Alterations in extracellular fluid volume influence CO via changes in venous return and BP. In fetal and newborn animals, however, cardiopulmonary receptors have minimal influence in the regulation of cardiovascular and autonomic responses to changes in BP or blood volume *(7)*.

### *Peripheral Resistance*

Blood flow through a vessel is determined by two primary factors: the amount of pressure forcing the blood through the vessel, and the resistance to flow. The resistance to flow in a blood vessel is best described as impedance because this takes into account inertial properties and viscosity of blood, elastic properties of blood vessels, and the variable geometries of blood vessels during phasic flow. One of the most important factors influencing the flow through the arteries is the vessel diameter, since the conductance is proportional to the fourth power of the diameter. Therefore, flow is influenced more by changes in vascular resistance than by pressure changes. The variables influencing peripheral resistance are listed in Table 1.

### *Control Mechanisms for Blood Pressure Regulation*

The short-term adjustment and long-term control of BP are supplied by a hierarchy of pressure controls *(2)*. The cardiovascular reflexes are the most rapidly acting pressure control mechanisms. They are activated within seconds and the effects may last a few minutes to a few days. The pressure controls acting with intermediate rapidity include capillary fluid shifts, stress relaxation, and hormonal control that includes the angiotensin and vasopressin systems. These systems, like the cardiovascular reflexes, function to buffer acute changes in pressure. Long-term control is afforded by long-term regulation of body fluids *(2)*.

### *Arterial Baroreceptors*

The degree of arteriolar constriction is determined by a balance between tonic output from the pressor areas of the cardiovascular center and the degree of inhibition from the baroreceptors. The arterial baroreceptors are the major fast-reacting, slowly adapting feedback elements to the central-neural cardiovascular regulatory system. Their function is to limit sudden changes in BP. Their mechano-sensitive nerve endings are located at the medial-adventitial border of blood vessels with elastic structure, mainly at the aortic arch and carotid sinuses. The receptors respond to deformation of the vessel in any direction, i.e., circumferential and longitudinal stretch. This results in the stimulation of mechano-sensitive channels that contain degenerative/epithelial sodium channel (DEG/ENaC) *(8,9)*. The pressure diameter relationship is concave with the greatest distensibility at about 120–140 mmHg. There are two types of receptors in the carotid sinus: type I receptors are thin myelinated fibers; type II receptors are thick myelinated fibers with fine end branches terminating in neurofibrillar end plates. The latter receptors are also seen in the aortic arch.

An increase in BP stimulates the mechanosensitive receptors in the baroreceptors, inhibits the sympathetic nervous system, and activates the parasympathetic nervous system. This results in a decrease in HR, myocardial contractility, peripheral vascular resistance, and venous return. A decrease in BP decreases mechanosensitive stimulation of the baroreceptors, inhibits the parasympathetic nervous system, and activates the sympathetic nervous system. This results in an increase in HR, myocardial contractility, peripheral vascular resistance, and venous return *(10)*. A second system, endogenous nitric oxide (NO), is involved in the short-term regulation of BP; increased arterial pressure increases shear stress, which leads to the generation of NO opposing the rise in BP by vasodilatation.

Sensory innervation of the aortic arch is derived from the vagus, while the carotid sinus nerve originates from the glossopharyngeal nerve. The majority of afferent nerves are myelinated type A fibers. These fibers have large and intermediate spikes of 40–120 μV corresponding to the high distensibility region. At normal pressure levels, these fibers primarily transmit the dynamic components of BP, pulse pressure *(dp/dt)*, and pulse frequency. The receptor sensitivity is highest at the lower end (60–100 mmHg) of the high distensibility region of the blood vessel. There are a few nonmyelinated type C fibers, located mainly in the carotid sinus nerve. The spikes are small (5–10 μV), have a higher static threshold (120–150 mmHg), correspond to the low distensibility region, and mainly transmit mean pressure. The type C fibers can be activated independently by sympathetic stimuli.

The arterial baroreceptors are more effective in compensating for a fall rather than a rise in mean arterial pressure. The interaction between mean and pulsatile components can be of considerable importance in the hemodynamic response to hemorrhage. For example, the initial response to moderate hemorrhage results in a decrease in pulse pressure with maintenance of mean arterial pressure. Decreasing pulse pressure results in a redistribution of CO to the mesenteric and cardiac circulations, with no effect on the renal circulation.

Information carried by the afferent limb of the reflex arc from the baroreceptors is relayed to the lower brainstem via the vagus and glossopharyngeal nerves. Most secondary neurons are located at the nucleus of the tractus solitarius, and projections are directed to various regions of the brainstem. The effectors of the baroreceptors include systems that have an immediate, but short-term, effect on circulatory function, and those that have delayed, but long-term effects. Examples of the former are resistance vessels, arterioles throughout the systemic circulation, the capacitance vessels, veins and arteries, and the heart. An example of a system with a long-term effect is the kidney. In addition, neural reflexes may influence circulating levels of several hormones (e.g., renin, vasopressin) with short- and long-term effects on cardiovascular regulation. The effect of neural reflexes on the kidneys may be direct, through renal sympathetic nerve activity, or indirect, through circulating catecholamines.

Nerve endings containing norepinephrine are found in the carotid sinus and aortic arch, and may influence the sensitivity of the sinus reflex. Norepinephrine given intravenously decreases distensibility of the sinus at low pressures, but increases distensibility at high pressure. In the conscious dog, sinus hypotension induces a reflex tachycardia and sympathetic vasoconstriction of the skeletal resistance vessels. The changes in the renal and mesenteric beds (45% of total peripheral resistance) seem to owe solely to autoregulation. In the anesthetized dog, sinus hypotension induces a greater magnitude and a more generalized pattern of sympathetic vasoconstriction, and may include both resistance and capacitance vessels. Several paracrine factors that affect the sensitivity of arterial baroreceptors have been reported, including prostanoids and NO. In general, vasoconstrictors decrease baroreceptor sensitivity while vasodilators increase baroreceptor sensitivity. However, NO decreases baroreceptor sensitivity independent of its vasodilator action. Reactive oxygen species (ROS) also decrease baroreceptor sensitivity, a mechanism that may contribute to the increase in systemic BP caused by ROS *(11)*.

### *Adaptation of the Baroreceptors*

The baroreceptors exert a tonic inhibitory influence on peripheral sympathetic activity. Baroreceptor nerves interact by mutual inhibitory addition; with a decrease in pressure, there is less reflex inhibition and a resultant increase in sympathetic outflow. While transient baroreceptor-induced changes in HR are primarily mediated by the parasympathetic nervous system, steady-state responses are owing to a greater involvement of the sympathetic nervous system. A sudden increase in pressure (with resultant stretching of the receptors) causes an immediate increase in baroreceptor firing rate. With continued elevation of the pressure, however, there is a decrease in the rate of baroreceptor firing. Initially the decrease is rapid, and during the succeeding hours and days it slows down. This adaptation, or resetting, in response to a lower or higher pressure seems to be complete in 2 d. This adaptation can occur at the receptor and nervous signal pathway *(2)*. The resetting of the baroreflex is much more rapid in adults than in infants *(12)*.

### *Arterial Baroreceptors During Development*

Studies in humans and experimental animals suggest that arterial baroreceptors are present in the fetus and undergo postnatal maturation *(12)*. There is an enhanced sensitivity of the efferent limb of the baroreflex in fetal life *(12)*. In adults with intact arterial baroreceptors, a rapid head-up tilt is accompanied by an immediate increase in HR, and peripheral vascular resistance with maintenance of mean arterial pressure in the upper body. Several studies have suggested that in healthy preterm and term human infants, head-up tilting also increases HR in proportion to the degree of tilting. However, other studies have shown that in healthy preterm infants with a postconceptional age of 28–32 wk, a 45° head-up tilt results in an increase in peripheral resistance without any significant changes in HR *(7)*. The increase in HR with a 45° head-up tilt increases with postconceptional age. In the conscious newborn dog, the magnitude of the increase in mean arterial pressure and peripheral resistance following bilateral carotid occlusion is less than in the adult. In addition, these changes occur without alterations in HR, similar to the effects noted in infants. In fetal sheep, only the increase in HR with a decrease in BP is noted. There is no relationship of arterial pressure and HR variability immediately after birth, but the fetal pattern resumes a few hours later *(13)*.

Newborn lambs exhibit the classic inverse relationship between HR and BP, but the sensitivity is only about 50% that of an adult. The responses to small changes in BP is similar in fetal and newborn lambs. However, when the change in BP is greater than 15% the responses are different. In newborn lambs, a progressive tachycardia accompanies the increasing hypotension, owing to a combination of increased sympathetic outflow and parasympathetic withdrawal. There is no progressive tachycardia in the fetus; in fact, when the BP change is greater than 50%, bradycardia occurs, apparently due to augmentation of vagal parasympathetic tone.

There are age-dependent differences in the ability of the piglet to compensate for hemorrhage and hypoxia *(14)*. Neonatal swine are better able to compensate for venous hemorrhage than for arterial hemorrhage *(15)*. Volume expansion inhibits the sympathetic nervous system to a greater extent in older than in newborn lambs. Increasing arterial pressure by intravenous administration of vasoconstrictor agents results in smaller changes in HR in the newborn animal as well. Completion of sympathetic efferent pathways occurs before baroreceptor reflex activity is capable of modulating cardiac sympathetic activity. Therefore, maturation of baroreceptor reflex activity may be dependent on development of baroreceptor function, or of connections between baroreceptor and sympathetic efferents *(12)*. The changes in baroreflexes during development are thought to be caused by afferent, central integration, and efferent pathways. The maturation of receptors for various humoral and hormonal agents (e.g., angiotensin II [ANG II], glucocorticoids, prostanoids, vasopressin) has been shown to affect baroreflex function.

### *Autonomic Regulation of Blood Pressure*

Regulation of the distribution of CO and maintenance of BP are major functions of the autonomic nervous system. The arterioles are normally in a continuous state of partial constriction, largely determined by an equilibrium between vasoconstrictor influences from the cardiovascular centers and the inhibitory input from the peripheral baroreceptors. The veins also receive autonomic innervation. Adrenergic nerves induce venous constriction with a resultant decrease in capacitance which increases venous return and CO. The effects of the adrenergic nervous system are conveyed by the neurotransmitters norepinephrine, epinephrine, and dopamine.

### Catecholamines

Epinephrine is released mainly from the adrenal medulla, while norepinephrine is released mainly in terminal nerve endings. In organs with dopaminergic nerves, a greater proportion of catecholamine released is dopamine. Norepinephrine synthesized at peripheral nerve endings is stored in subcellular granules. After a specific stimulus it is released into the synaptic cleft, where it interacts with specific receptors presynaptically and at the effector cell. The neurotransmitter is inactivated to a large extent by reuptake into the storage granules. This reuptake process (reuptake-1) is stereoselective, sodium-dependent, and of high affinity. A presynaptic reuptake that is of low affinity and nonsodium-dependent has been termed reuptake-2. There are specific amine transporters. Although the enzymatic degradation of the neurotransmitter by monoamine oxidase and catechol-*O*-methyl transferase is much less important in termination of neurotransmitter action in nervous tissue, this metabolism plays an important role in vascular smooth muscles *(16)*. The remainder of the neurotransmitter which escapes reuptake-1 and -2 is released into the circulation. Since only about 20% of the total appears in the circulating pool, the plasma levels of catecholamines are merely a rough index of adrenergic activity.

### Adrenergic and Dopaminergic Receptors

For the neurotransmitter to exert its specific effect, it must occupy a specific receptor on the cell surface. Catecholamines can occupy specific pre- and postsynaptic receptors. Each receptor has different subtypes *(17–19)*. Table 2 lists some drugs that have relative selectivity for each particular receptor subtype in the peripheral vascular bed. Occupation of presynaptic $\alpha_2$-adrenergic and $S_2$-like dopamine receptors inhibits norepinephrine release. Occupation of presynaptic $\beta_2$-receptors enhances norepinephrine release. At low levels of nerve stimulation, norepinephrine release is increased; at high levels of stimulation, the inhibitory effects of presynaptic $\alpha_2$-adrenergic receptors predominate, acting as a short-loop feedback. The antihypertensive effects of dopamine agonists and ($\beta$-adrenergic antagonists) may owe in part to their ability to decrease release of norepinephrine at the terminal nerve endings.

### $\alpha_1$-Adrenergic Receptors

Three $\alpha_1$-adrenergic receptors are expressed in mammals, $\alpha_{1A}$ (originally designated as the $\alpha_{1C}$ when cloned), $\alpha_{1B}$, and $\alpha_{1D}$. Vascular bed may impart receptor subtype specificity. Thus, $\alpha_{1A}$ may mediate contraction of renal and caudal arteries, whereas $\alpha_{1D}$-adrenergic receptors may regulate the contraction of the aorta, femoral, iliac, and superior mesenteric arteries. Mice deficient for the $\alpha_{1A}$-adrenergic receptor have decreased BP, as do mice deficient for the $\alpha_{1D}$-adrenergic receptor *(20)*. The $\alpha_{1D}$-receptor-deficient mice are resistant to the hypertensive effects of sodium chloride. In contrast, $\alpha_{1B}$-adrenergic receptors may not regulate vascular smooth muscle contraction. Mice deficient for these receptors have normal BP in the basal state. Pharmacological evidence for this has been shown in studies of mice deficient for a specific $\alpha_1$-adrenergic receptor subtype *(21,22)*. Hypertrophy in neonatal cardiac myocytes is mediated primarily by the $\alpha_{1A}$- and $\alpha_{1B}$-adrenergic receptors. Aortic hypertrophy, on the other hand, is primarily owing to the actions of the $\alpha_{1D}$-adrenergic receptors.

### $\alpha_2$-Adrenergic Receptors

There are three $\alpha_2$-adrenergic receptor subtypes, $\alpha_{2A/D}$, $\alpha_{2B}$, and $\alpha_{2C}$. The $\alpha_{2A}$ class predominates, and these receptors decrease BP and mediate most of the classical effects of $\alpha_2$-adrenergic stimulation. In contrast, $\alpha_B$-adrenergic receptors, predominantly found outside of the central nervous system at extrajunctional or postsynaptic sites, produce vasoconstriction and thus counteract the hypotensive effects of $\alpha_{2A}$-adrenergic receptor stimulation. $\alpha_{2C}$-adrenergic receptors do not have cardiovascular effects but may mediate the hypothermic response *(23)*.

### β-Adrenergic Receptors

Disruption of either the $\beta_1$, $\beta_2$-adrenergic receptor, or both, does not affect HR or resting BP in mice. Mice lacking the $\beta_1$-adrenergic receptor are unresponsive to cardiac β-adrenergic receptor stimulation, suggesting that neither $\beta_2$- nor $\beta_3$-adrenergic receptors play a role in the inotropic or chronotropic responses in the mouse *(24)*, and indeed, the effect of the non-β-adrenergic subtype receptor agonist isoproterenol is not altered in $\beta_2$-adrenergic-receptor null mice. However, the hypotensive response to isoproterenol is impaired in both $\beta_1$ or $\beta_2$-adrenergic null mice *(25,26)*. $\beta_3$-adrenergic receptors do not have major effects on the cardiovascular system *(27)*.

### Dopamine Receptors

Dopamine is an important regulator of BP. Presynaptic/junctional and postsynaptic/junctional, or extrasynaptic dopamine receptors, are found in many organs and vascular beds. Dopamine receptors have also been described in the heart, but their function remains to be determined *(28,29)*. Dopamine's actions on renal hemodynamics, epithelial transport, and humoral agents such as aldosterone, catecholamines, endothelin, prolactin, pro-opiomelanocortin, renin, and vasopressin place it in a central homeostatic position for the regulation of extracellular fluid volume and BP. Dopamine also modulates fluid and sodium intake via its actions in the central nervous system (CNS) and gastrointestinal (GI) tract, and by regulation of cardiovascular centers that control the functions of the heart, arteries, and veins. Abnormalities in dopamine production and receptor function accompany a high percentage of human essential hypertension and several forms of rodent genetic hypertension. Dopamine receptor genes, as well as genes encoding their regulators, are in loci that have been linked to hypertension in humans and in rodents. Moreover, allelic variants (single nucleotide polymorphisms [SNPs]) of genes that encode the regulators of the dopamine receptors, alone or in combination with variants of genes that encode proteins that regulate the renin-angiotensin system (RAS), are associated with human essential hypertension.

Each of the five dopamine receptor subtypes ($D_1$, $D_2$, $D_3$, $D_4$, and $D_5$) participates in the regulation of blood pressure by mechanisms specific to the subtype. Some receptors ($D_2$ and $D_5$) influence the central and/or peripheral nervous system; others influence epithelial transport *(30–33)*. Both the $D_1$-like dopamine receptors ($D_1$ and $D_5$) and the $D_3$ receptor decrease epithelial sodium transport *(30,31)*. $D_4$ receptors inhibit the effects of aldosterone and vasopressin in the renal cortical collecting duct *(32,33)*. $D_2$-like receptors, under certain circumstances, may increase sodium transport *(34,35)*. Dopamine can regulate the secretion and receptors of several humoral agents (e.g., the $D_1$, $D_3$, and $D_4$ receptors interact with the RAS). The $D_1$-like receptors are vasodilatory while the $D_2$-like receptors can mediate vasodilation or vasoconstriction depending upon the starting vascular resistance. When vascular resistance is high, $D_2$-like receptors are vasodilatory by inhibition of norepinephrine release. However, when vascular resistance is low, $D_2$-like receptors mediate vasoconstriction probably via the $D_3$ receptor *(34)*. Modifications of the usual actions of the receptor can produce blood pressure changes. In addition, abnormal functioning of these dopamine receptor subtypes impairs their antioxidant function *(36)*.

### Signal Transduction

The signal resulting from occupation of cell membrane receptors is amplified by the intervention of other agents called second messengers. Occupation of either β-adrenergic receptor subtype or the $D_1$-like class of dopamine receptor by agonists stimulates adenylyl cyclases; agonist occupancy of $\alpha_2$-adrenergic receptors, or dopamine $D_2$ receptors, leads to inhibition of adenylyl cyclases. The changes in intracellular cyclic adenosine monophosphate levels alter the activities of certain enzymes, e.g., protein kinase A, and mediate the eventual response of the effector cell. Certain drugs (e.g., nitrites) exert their vasodilatory effect by stimulation of guanylate cyclase activity *(37)*. Another second messenger is associated with the phosphoinositide system. The $\alpha_1$-adrenergic and the $D_1$ dopamine receptors are linked to phospholipase C; stimulation leads to an increase in formation of inositol phosphates and diacylglycerol. Inositol phosphates increase intracellular calcium, whereas diacylglycerol stimulates protein kinase C. Occupation of $\alpha_1$-adrenergic and $D_1$ dopamine receptors may also result in the activation of phospholipase $A_2$, increasing the formation of biologically active arachidonate metabolites by the action of cyclooxygenases (prostaglandins, thromboxanes), lipoxygenases (leukotrienes), and cytochrome p450 monooxygenase (e.g., 20 hydroxyeicosanotetraenoic acid).

### Receptor Regulation

Signal transduction involves "on" and "off" pathways to ensure that signaling is achieved in a precisely regulated manner *(38–40)*. One "off" pathway is receptor desensitization, or loss of receptor responsiveness. Receptor desensitization is a mechanism to dampen short-term agonist effects following repeated agonist exposure. Desensitization involves several processes, including phosphorylation, sequestration/internalization, and degradation of receptor protein *(38–40)*. An initial step in the desensitization process is the phosphorylation of the receptor by a member or members of the G protein-coupled receptor kinases (GRKs) family. GRKs are serine and threonine kinases that phosphorylate G protein-coupled receptors (GPCRs) in response to agonist stimulation. The phosphorylation of GPCRs, including $D_1$ receptors, leads to the binding of a member or members of the arrestin family, an uncoupling of the receptor from its G protein complex, and a decrease in functional response *(38–41)*. The phosphorylated GPCR and arrestin complex undergo internalization via clathrin-coated pits into an endosome where the GPCR is dephosphorylated *(38–40)*, facilitated by protein phosphatases *(42)*, and recycled back to the plasma membrane, or degraded by lysosomes and/or proteasomes. These processes may be specific to a particular receptor.

### Development of Receptor Regulation

There are developmental changes in the desensitization process. The neonatal rat heart is resistant to β-adrenergic receptor desensitization *(43)*. Rather, β-adrenergic agonists produce sensitization caused by the induction of adenylyl cyclase activity, as a consequence of loss of $G\alpha_i$ protein and function, enhancement of membranous expression of $G\alpha_s$, and, in particular, the shorter but more active 45 kDa $G\alpha_s$. The role of Gβ/γ was not determined but in the kidney we found that the decreased inhibitory effect of $D_1$ receptors on the sodium hydrogen exchanger type 3 is caused by increased expression and linkage of the G protein subunit Gβ/γ *(44)*.

#### Catecholamines and Other Vasoactive Agents

Catecholamines can influence blood pressure not only by direct effects on resistance vessels, but also indirectly by modulating the secretion of other vasoactive agents such as ANG II (via renin), vasopressin, prostaglandins, substance P, and other neuropeptides. In addition to direct chronotropic and inotropic effects on the heart, catecholamines can modulate CO indirectly by affecting blood volume and venous return. Blood volume can be regulated by direct effects on sodium and water transport through renal nerves, by antagonizing effects of other hormones (e.g., vasopressin), and indirectly by modulating vasopressin and aldosterone secretion.

## ADRENERGIC SYSTEM DURING DEVELOPMENT

The low systolic BP at birth, owing to low CO and peripheral resistance, increases rapidly in the first 6 wk of life, remains at a constant level until age 6, and increases gradually until age 18 yr. The pattern is similar for diastolic BP, except that there is a slight decrease in diastolic BP in the first 6 mo of life (relative to the BP in the first week of life). The increase in BP with age in preterm infants occurs as a function of postconceptional age. With advanced age (>60 yr), systolic BP continues to increase. Diastolic BP declines somewhat, leading to an increase in pulse pressure. Increased pulse pressure has been thought to play an independent role in the pathogenesis of the complications of high BP *(45)*. The increase in BP accompanying age is owing to a rise in both CO and total peripheral resistance. The age-related changes in vascular resistance are selective, because in the perinatal period there is a rapid fall in resistance in the lungs, small intestines, brain, and kidney while resistance increases in the femoral vessels *(46)*. The increase in femoral resistance accompanying age is most likely related to an increase in vascular reactivity to vasoconstrictors, with no differential effects of vasodilators (NO and bradykinin). The decrease in regional vascular resistance may be caused by an increase in vessel growth, and changing sensitivities and reactivities to vasoconstrictor and vasodilator agents. The increase in regional blood flow accompanying age cannot be accounted for by an increase in BP. Indeed, in the immediate perinatal period, the increase in regional blood flow with postnatal age is independent of BP *(47)*. In the first 6 mo of life, systolic BP increases, but diastolic BP actually decreases after the first 2 wk of life. This transient decrease in diastolic BP in the first few months of life is associated with a low intestinal vascular resistance *(48)*. This is apparently mediated by NO. Interestingly, increased NO production in the neonatal renal arterial bed *(49,50a)* also dampens the increased vasoconstriction afforded by ANG II early in perinatal life, and catecholamines later in prenatal life *(51)*. NO however, does not play an important role in cerebrovascular responses in the newborn.

The newborn infant increases its CO mainly by increasing its HR. The high HR may be owing to differential sympathetic and parasympathetic effects, hypersensitivity of the cardiac receptors, and peripheral vasodilatation. The low precapillary resistance, and low venous capacitance, are conducive to high systemic blood flow per unit body weight, and provide increased tissue perfusion for growth.

Study of the role of the adrenergic nervous system in the control of cardiovascular dynamics is complicated by species differences. Some studies have suggested that pigs and dogs provide the closest model to the newborn human in terms of cardiovascular development *(52,53)*. On the other hand, the sheep fetus is a very useful model for chronic-conscious studies *(12,54)*.

## DEVELOPMENT OF THE SYMPATHETIC NERVOUS SYSTEM

The development of the sympathetic nervous system can be divided into three stages *(55)*. In the first stage, the neural crest cells migrate to their positions within the body tissues. In the second stage, the cell number and type is refined by cell death (apoptosis). The third stage is concerned with the maturation of synaptic connections and selection of the neurotransmitter. Cholinergic development generally takes place prior to adrenergic differentiation; however, transition from adrenergic to cholinergic function can also occur. In the neonatal rat heart, perinatal β-adrenergics positively regulate the development of sympathetic innervation and suppress the development of $m_2$ muscarinic acetyl choline receptors *(56)*. A critical event in the development of the adrenergic nervous system is the establishment of functional innervation of the different organs. Function requires that central nervous pathways to the preganglionic neurons be established, that information be relayed to postganglionic neurons, and that neurotransmitter synthesis, release, and reuptake, and postreceptor mechanisms be operative. Effector organ innervation involves the outgrowth of new axons, appearance of intense fluorescence, and differentiation of adrenergic nerve varicosities. Maturation of the nerve-terminal-effector complex occurs before ganglionic transmission is fully developed and is largely independent of neural connections. In the heart, the development of β-adrenergic receptors and their responsiveness to catecholamines is not closely linked to innervation. Nonsympathetic hormonal factors appear to control early maturation of receptors and the growth and development of the nervous system.

### Plasma Catecholamines

Plasma norepinephrine and dopamine levels decrease gradually with the advance of gestational weeks *(57)*. Birth is associated with an increase in circulating catecholamines. Umbilical arterial epinephrine and norepinephrine concentrations in infants delivered vaginally are greater than those in infants delivered by cesarean section *(58–60)*. Because there are some studies showing no difference in plasma concentrations between infants delivered vaginally and those by cesarean section *(61,62)*, stress *per se* may not responsible for the high catecholamine levels with vaginal delivery. Studies in the fetal sheep indicate a surge in plasma catecholamines with the onset of parturition that is accentuated by cord-cutting *(63)*. The half-life of circulating catecholamines in the preterm infant may be longer than in older children, owing in part to lower levels of catecholamine-degrading enzymes. However, children may metabolize catecholamines more rapidly than adults. Preterm infants have greater levels of epinephrine in umbilical arterial plasma than full-term human infants. Preterm fetal sheep also have higher circulating catecholamine levels than their full-term counterparts. The circulating levels of catecholamines decrease with maturation, but beyond 20 yr of age plasma norepinephrine increases. Adrenal medullary activity is lower than adrenergic nervous activity at birth and increases with maturation.

### Urinary Catecholamines

Urinary catecholamines are low at birth and increase with gestational and postnatal age *(64–66)*. Small-for-gestational-age babies have greater sympathoadrenal activity than babies of the same gestational age *(64)*. Newborn preterm infants excrete less norepinephrine and more dopamine than term infants, and epinephrine excretion is comparable. At 2 wk of age, urinary dopamine and metabolites are greatly increased in preterm infants. Beyond 1 yr of life, the developmental patterns of adrenergic nervous and adrenal medullary activity are similar, and reach mature values at 5 yr of age. When expressed as a function of surface area or weight, no changes in urinary catecholamines and metabolites occur after 1 yr of age. In the first 5 yr of life, however, sympathoadrenal activity is less in girls than in boys. It should be kept in mind, though, that circulating and urinary levels of catecholamines are only rough indices of adrenergic activity.

### Catecholamines and Adaptation to Extrauterine Life

Catecholamine secretion at birth may be important in the adaptation of the fetus to extrauterine life *(63,67)*. Complete ganglionic blockade before delivery of the lamb does not attenuate the normal postnatal rise in BP, indicating that the autonomic nervous system may not play a significant role in the increase in systemic pressure after birth. However, although clamping of adrenal vessels did not alter mean BP of very young puppies *(68)*, in the newborn dog adrenalectomy leads to hypotension and bradycardia. In addition, adrenergic blockade in the newborn lamb reduces systemic pressure whereas no effect is seen in adult sheep. More evidence of the importance of the adrenergic nervous system during the neonatal period includes impaired myocardial contractile responses to adrenergic agents and hypoxia following adrenalectomy.

The time of development of adrenergic innervation, and responses to adrenergic stimulation, vary not only with species, but also among vessels in the same animal. Some of the reported differences in results may also be due to experimental conditions (anesthetized versus unanesthetized state, in vitro versus in vivo studies). In the heart, responses to β-adrenergic and dopamine stimulation increase with age while the response to α-adrenergic stimulation decreases with age. While the decreasing responsiveness to α-adrenergic stimulation with maturation has been linked to similar directional changes in myocardial $\alpha_1$-adrenergic receptors, the changes in myocardial β-adrenergic receptors are not linked. For example, in the dog heart there is an increased β-adrenergic receptors density in the newborn period. The decline in cardiac β-adrenergic receptors density with age is accompanied by decreased β-adrenergic responsive adenylyl cyclase activity. Other studies (in other species), however, have shown that cardiac β-adrenergic receptors increase with age, but that the proportions of β-adrenergic subtypes do not.

In the mature heart, responsiveness to β-adrenergic agonists can be regulated transsynaptically by neurotransmitter concentrations in the synaptic cleft. High levels of β-adrenergic stimulation result in depressed cardiac responsiveness and reduction in receptor density (down-regulation), while the converse occurs with low levels of stimulation with up-regulation of receptor density. However, this does not occur during the period in which receptor numbers and cardiac sensitivity to agonists are undergoing marked developmental increases. The developmental changes in cardiac responsiveness to dopamine have not been correlated with dopamine receptor density or adenylyl cyclase activation.

### Regional Vascular Flow and Resistance During Development

The development of renal and intestinal circulation is discussed in some detail because splanchnic vascular resistance contributes significantly to peripheral vascular resistance. β-adrenergic relaxation of the aorta of rabbits increases with age, reaching a maximal level at 1 mo; thereafter a decline in responsiveness occurs. In dogs, stimulation of lumbar sympathetics induces femoral vasodilatation early in life; after 2 mo a greater vasoconstriction is noted. This corresponds to a marked increase in adrenergic innervation. In the piglet, the renal vascular response to β-adrenergic stimulation is also less in the immediate newborn period compared to adults but may be markedly increased some time before maturation *(68)*. These changes in renal β-adrenergic responsiveness have been correlated with β-adrenergic receptor density in the dog *(69)*. However, $\beta_2$-adrenergic vasodilatory effects are enhanced in the renal vascular bed of the fetal lamb *(70)*.

The maturation of blood vessel reactivity to α-adrenergic stimulation is regional bed-dependent. In general, the response of the canine aorta and sheep carotid to norepinephrine is less pronounced in the newborn than in the adult. This occurs in spite of comparable responsiveness to KCl *(71)*. The vasoconstrictor effects of α-adrenergic drugs are also less pronounced in immature than in mature animals. In the neonatal rat femoral artery, norepinephrine causes a vasodilation, not vasoconstriction, an effect that is mediated by NO *(72)*. In baboons, the maximum vasoconstrictor response to norepinephrine, thromboxane mimetic, and potassium increased with gestational age but the sensitivity to these vasoconstrictors was similar *(46)*.

### Renal Vascular Bed

Renal blood flow increases progressively with conceptional age, reaching term values by about 35 wk postconception. Forty weeks postconception, renal blood flow, expressed as a function of surface area, increases with postnatal age, reaching middle-age adult values by 1–2 yr of life. The increase in renal blood flow is associated with a fall in renal vascular resistance. Color Doppler ultrasonography has been used to determine renal resistive index, which correlates with renal vascular resistance. In general, the values obtained using clearance methods (e.g., para-aminohippurate) have correlated well by the renal resistive index *(73)*. The increase in renal blood flow associated with age is due to renal growth, an increase in BP, and a decrease in renal vascular resistance. The high renal vascular resistance in the perinatal period has been shown to be caused by alterations in renal vascular smooth muscle reactivity, and sensitivity to vasodilators and vasoconstrictors. After the immediate newborn period, the neonatal renal and cerebral circulation is more sensitive to α-adrenergic stimulation in dogs, pigs, guinea pigs, and baboons *(51,74,75)*. The isolated renal vessels of fetal lamb studied in vitro and in vivo are also more reactive to α-adrenergic stimulation than their newborn or adult counterparts *(76)*. The increased renal $\alpha_1$- and $\alpha_2$-adrenergic effects in fetal sheep are related to increased α-adrenergic receptor density. Competition experiments and rank adrenergic antagonist potency suggested the presence of only the $\alpha_{1B}$-adrenergic receptor in fetal and adult sheep kidneys. However, the $\alpha_{1B}$-adrenergic receptor does not mediate vasoconstriction in adults. The $\alpha_2$-adrenergic receptor that was found only in the fetal sheep studied had a low affinity to rauwolscine, which is unlike that described in most species for $\alpha_2$-adrenergic receptors *(77)*. The molecular biological class of these receptors during development has not been studied.

Inherent renal vascular hypersensitivity or hyperreactivity may be masked by counter-regulatory vasodilator mechanisms. In the fetal sheep studied, renal vascular $\beta_2$-adrenergic receptor-mediated renal vasodilatory capacity is enhanced during fetal life *(78)*. Cerebral arteries from premature and newborn baboons showed a more marked relaxation response to isoproterenol than did arteries from adult animals *(74)*. In the piglet, the renal vasoconstrictor effects of ANG II are counteracted by the vasodilatory action of NO *(49,50,79)*. However, the contribution of specific adrenergic receptors and regulation of NO level or availability to the development of renal circulation remains to be determined.

The neonatal renal circulation is also more responsive to the effects of renal nerve stimulation in some species *(80)*. While renal nerve transection in piglets leads to an increase in renal blood flow *(80)*, this effect is not seen in fetal sheep. Moreover, renal nerve stimulation during α-adrenergic blockade actually increases renal blood flow *(70)*. In the neonatal dog kidney, increased α-adrenergic effects are related to increased α-adrenergic receptor density *(69)*. Dopamine mainly induces a vasoconstrictor response (an α-adrenergic receptor effect) in the early neonatal period *(69)*. Even low dosages, which produce renal vasodilatation in the adult kidney, are associated with renal vasoconstriction in the newborn period. The vasodilator effects of dopamine become evident in the femoral circulation before being noted in the kidney. When α- and β-adrenergic receptors are blocked during dopamine infusion, the renal vasodilator effect of dopamine is still less pronounced in the fetus and the newborn animal than in the adult. In contrast to the correlation between renal vascular responses and α- and β-adrenergic receptor density, no correlation is observed with dopamine receptors and the age-related changes in renal dopamine responsiveness.

The low renal blood flow in the young is due to several factors, including smaller size, decreased number of glomeruli, lower systemic pressure, and higher renal vascular resistance. The increased renal vascular resistance in the newborn is most likely due to increased activity of the RAS, as well as to increased sensitivity to vasoconstrictor catecholamines, itself a product of receptor and postadrenergic receptor mechanisms. Critical vasodilators, such as NO, may act to counterbalance these vasoconstrictor forces. The increase in renal blood flow associated with age presumably occurs, in part, as the vasoconstrictor influences decline.

### Intestinal Vascular Bed

Intestinal blood flow, like renal blood flow, increases with gestational age, postconceptional age, and maturation *(81)*. Fetal intestinal vascular resistance is high during fetal life. In the piglet, there is a decrease in intestinal vascular resistance in the first few days of life, only to progressively increase after the first week of life. This is in contrast with kidneys, which exhibit a progressive decrease in renal vascular resistance in the perinatal period. The neonatal intestinal circulation is controlled by inherent myogenic response and NO similar to that seen in the neonatal renal circulation. Like the neonatal kidney neonatal intestinal circulation may also be regulated by alterations in α-adrenergic receptor *(82)*. However, in contrast to the neonatal kidney, endothelin plays a part in the regulation of neonatal intestinal circulation. In older piglets, regulation of the intestinal circulation does not involve NO or endothelin, the responses being mostly passive in nature *(48,83)*. In contrast to the importance of NO in the renal and intestinal vasodilator response in the newborn, bradykinin and prostanoids perform this role in the neonatal cerebral vascular bed *(84)*. However, with maturation NO assumes a more important role.

## CONCLUSION

Increases in BP with age in the first few months of life are mainly owing to increases in CO. Vascular resistance in many vascular beds may transiently decrease because of increased production of, or the availability of, NO, or prostanoids. Increased sensitivity to β-adrenergic stimulation may also play a role. The involvement of a particular agent is regional bed dependent. While the maturation of receptor classes involved in the regulation of CO and vascular resistance is known, the maturation of specific receptor subtypes in different vascular beds remains to be determined.

## ACKNOWLEDGMENT

Aruna Natarajan is supported by the Mentored Clinical Research Scholar Program Award, grant RR17613 from the National Center for Research Resources, National Institutes of Health, Department of Health and Human Services.

## REFERENCES

1. Tibby SM, Murdoch IA. Monitoring cardiac function in intensive care. Arch Dis Child 2003;88:46–52.
2. Guyton, AC. *Arterial Pressure and Hypertension*. Philadelphia: Saunders, 1980.
3. Veille JC, Hanson R, Steele L, Tatum K. M-mode echocardiographic evaluation of fetal and infant hearts: longitudinal follow-up study from intrauterine life to year one. Am J Obstet Gynecol 1996; 175: 922–928.
4. Phoon CK. Circulatory physiology in the developing embryo. Curr Opin Pediatr 2001; 13: 456–464.
5. Walther T, Schultheiss HP, Tschope C, Stepan H. Natriuretic peptide system in fetal heart and circulation. J Hypertens 2002; 20: 785–791.
6. Aviado DM, Guevara Aviado D. The Bezold-Jarisch reflex. A historical perspective of cardiopulmonary reflexes. Ann NY Acad Sci 2001; 940: 48–58.
7. Mazursky JE, Birkett CL, Bedell KA, Ben-Haim SA, Segar JL. Development of baroreflex influences on heart rate variability in preterm infants. Early Hum Dev 1998; 53: 37–52.
8. Tavernarakis N, Driscoll M. Degenerins. At the core of the metazoan mechanotransducer? Ann NY Acad Sci 2001; 940: 28–41.
9. Drummond HA, Welsh MJ, Abboud FM. ENaC subunits are molecular components of the arterial baroreceptor complex. Ann NY Acad Sci 2001; 940: 42–47.
10. Lanfranchi PA, Somers VK. Arterial baroreflex function and cardiovascular variability: interactions and implications. Am J Physiol Regul Integr Comp Physiol 2002; 283: R815–R826.
11. Chapleau MW, Li Z, Meyrelles SS, Ma X, Abboud FM. Mechanisms determining sensitivity of baroreceptor afferents in health and disease. Ann NY Acad Sci 2001; 940: 1–19.
12. Segar JL. Ontogeny of the arterial and cardiopulmonary baroreflex during fetal and postnatal life. Am J Physiol 1997; 273: R457–R471.
13. Yu ZY, Lumbers ER. Effects of birth on baroreceptor-mediated changes in heart rate variability in lambs and fetal sheep. Clin Exp Pharmacol Physiol 2002; 29: 455–463.
14. Gootman PM, Gootman N. Postnatal changes in cardiovascular regulation during hypoxia. Adv Exp Med Biol 2000; 475: 539–548.
15. Buckley BJ, Gootman N, Nagelberg JS, Griswold PR, Gootman PM. Cardiovascular response to arterial and venous hemorrhage in neonatal swine. Am J Physiol 1984; 247: 8626–8633.
16. Bevan JAA, Su C. Sympathetic mechanisms in blood vessels: nerve and muscle relationships. Annu Rev Pharmacol 1973; 13: 269–285.
17. Piascik MT, Perez DM. $\alpha_1$-Adrenergic receptors: new insights and directions. Pharmacol Exp Ther 2001; 298: 403–410.
18. Guimaraes S, Moura D. Vascular adrenoceptors: an update. Pharmacol Rev 2001; 53: 319–356.
19. Alexander S, Mathie A, Peters J, MacKenzie G, Smith A. TIPs 2001 Nomenclature Supplement. Current Trends, London.
20. Rokosh DG, Simpson PC. Knockout of the $\alpha_{1A/C}$-adrenergic receptor subtype: the $\alpha$-$_{1A/C}$ is expressed in resistance arteries and is required to maintain arterial blood pressure. Proc Natl Acad Sci USA 2002; 99: 9474–9479.
21. Daly CJ, Deighan C, McGee A, Mennie D, Ali Z, McBride M, et al. A knockout approach indicates a minor vasoconstrictor role for vascular $\alpha_{1B}$-adrenoceptors in mouse. Physiol Genomics 2002; 9: 85–91.
22. Tanoue A, Koshimizu TA, Tsujimoto G. Transgenic studies of $\alpha_1$-adrenergic receptor subtype function. Life Sci 2002; 71: 2207–2215.
23. MacDonald E, Kobilka BK, Scheinin M. Gene targeting—homing in on alpha$_2$-adrenoceptor-subtype function. Trends Pharmacol Sci 1997; 18: 211–219.
24. Rohrer DK. Physiological consequences of $\beta$-adrenergic receptor disruption. J Mol Med 1998; 76: 764–772.
25. Chruscinski AJ, Rohrer DK, Schauble E, Desai KH, Bernstein D, Kobilka BK. Targeted disruption of the $\beta$2 adrenergic receptor gene. J Biol Chem 1999; 274: 16694–16700.

26. Rohrer DK, Chruscinski A, Schauble EH, Bernstein D, Kobilka BK. Cardiovascular and metabolic alterations in mice lacking both β1- and β2-adrenergic receptors. J Biol Chem 1999; 274: 16701–16708.
27. Jimenez M, Leger B, Canola K, Lehr L, Arboit P, Seydoux J, et al. $\beta_1/\beta_2/\beta_3$-adrenoceptor knockout mice are obese and cold-sensitive but have normal lipolytic responses to fasting. FEBS Lett 2002; 530: 37–40.
28. Ozono R, O'Connell DP, Wang ZQ, Moore AF, Sanada H, Felder RA, et al. Localization of the dopamine $D_1$ receptor protein in the human heart and kidney. Hypertension 1997; 30: 725–729.
29. Habuchi Y, Tanaka H, Nishio M, Yamamoto T, Komori T, Morikawa J, et al. Dopamine stimulation of cardiac beta-adrenoceptors: the involvement of sympathetic amine transporters and the effect of SKF38393. Br J Pharmacol 1997; 122: 1669–1678.
30. Jose PA, Eisner GM, Felder RA. Role of dopamine receptors in the kidney in the regulation of blood pressure. Curr Opin Nephrol Hypertens 2002; 11: 87–92.
31. Vieira-Coelho MA, Soares-da-Silva P. Ontogenic aspects of $D_1$ receptor coupling to G proteins and regulation of rat jejunal Na+, K+ ATPase activity and electrolyte transport. Br J Pharmacol 2000; 129: 573–581.
32. Schafer JA, Li L, Sun D. The collecting duct, dopamine and vasopressin-dependent hypertension. Acta Physiol Scand 2000; 168: 239–244.
33. Saito O, Ando Y, Kusano E, Asano Y. Functional characterization of basolateral and luminal dopamine receptors in rabbit CCD. Am J Physiol Renal Physiol 2001; 281: F114–F122.
34. Jose PA, Eisner GM, Felder RA. The renal dopamine receptors in health and hypertension. Pharmacol Ther 1998; 80: 149–182.
35. Narkar V, Hussain T, Lokhandwala M. Role of tyrosine kinase and p44/42 MAPK in $D_2$-like receptor-mediated stimulation of Na+, K+-ATPase in kidney. Am J Physiol Renal Physiol 2002; 282: F697–F702.
36. Yasunari K, Kohno M, Kano H, Minami M, Yoshikawa J. Dopamine as a novel antioxidative agent for rat vascular smooth muscle cells through dopamine $D_1$-like receptors. Circulation 2000; 101: 2302–2308.
37. Hogg N. The biochemistry and physiology of S-nitrosothiols. Annu Rev Pharmacol Toxicol 2002; 42: 585–600.
38. Pao CS, Benovic JL. Phosphorylation-independent desensitization of G protein-coupled receptors? Sci STKE 2002; 2002: PE42.
39. Ferguson SS. Evolving concepts in G protein-coupled receptor endocytosis: the role in receptor desensitization and signaling. Pharmacol Rev 2001; 53: 1–24.
40. Kohout TA, Lefkowitz RJ. Regulation of G protein-coupled receptor kinases and arrestins during receptor desensitization. Mol Pharmacol 2003; 63: 9–18.
41. Felder RA, Sanada H, Xu J, Yu P-Y, Wang Z, Watanabe H, et al. G protein-coupled receptor kinase 4 gene variants in human essential hypertension. Proc Natl Acad Sci USA 2002; 99: 3872–3877.
42. Yu P, Asico LD, Eisner GM, Hopfer U, Felder RA, Jose PA. Renal protein phosphatase 2A activity and spontaneous hypertension in rats. Hypertension 2000; 36: 1053–1058.
43. Auman JT, Seidler FJ, Slotkin TA. Beta-adrenoceptor control of G protein function in the neonate: determinant of desensitization or sensitization. Am J Physiol Regul Integr Comp Physiol 2002; 283: R1236–R1244.
44. Li XX, Albrecht FE, Robillard JE, Eisner GM, Jose PA. Gβ regulation of Na/H exchanger-3 activity in rat renal proximal tubules during development. Am J Physiol Regul Integr Comp Physiol 2000; 278: R931–R936.
45. Dart AM, Kingwell BA. Pulse pressure—a review of mechanisms and clinical relevance. J Am Coll Cardiol 2001; 37: 975–984.
46. Anwar MA, Ju K, Docherty CC, Poston L, Nathanielsz PW. Developmental changes in reactivity of small femoral arteries in the fetal and postnatal baboon. Am J Obstet Gynecol 2001; 184: 707–712.
47. Yanowitz TD, Yao AC, Pettigrew KD, Werner JC, Oh W, Stonestreet BS. Postnatal hemodynamic changes in very-low-birthweight infants. J Appl Physiol 1999; 87: 370–380.
48. Reber KM, Nankervis CA, Nowicki PT. Newborn intestinal circulation. Physiology and pathophysiology. Clin Perinatol 2002; 29: 23–39.
49. Simeoni U, Zhu B, Muller C, Judes C, Massfelder T, Geisert J, et al. Postnatal development of vascular resistance of the rabbit isolated perfused kidney: modulation by nitric oxide and angiotensin II. Pediatr Res 1997; 42: 550–555.
50. Solhaug MJ, Wallace MR, Granger JP. Nitric oxide and angiotensin II regulation of renal hemodynamics in the developing piglet. Pediatr Res 1996; 39: 527–533.
50a. Solhaug MJ, Jose PA. Postnatal maturation of renal blood flow. In: Polin R, Fox W, eds. Neonatal and Fetal Medicine. PA: W B Saunders Co, 3rd edition (1242–1249).

51. Jose P, Slotkoff L, Lilienfield L, Calcagno P, Eisner G. Sensitivity of the neonatal renal vasculature to epinephrine. Am J Physiol 1974; 226: 796–799.
52. Duckles SP, Banner W Jr. Changes in vascular smooth muscle reactivity during development. Annu Rev Pharmacol Toxicol 1984; 24: 65–83.
53. Ruggles BT, Murayama N, Werness JL, Gapstur SM, Bentley MD, Dousa TP. The vasopressin-sensitive adenylate cyclase in collecting tubules and thick ascending limb of Henle's loop of human and canine kidney. J Clin Endocrinol Metal 1985; 60: 914–921.
54. Nuyt AM, Segar JL, Holley AT, Robillard JE. Autonomic adjustments to severe hypotension in fetal and neonatal sheep. Pediatr Res 2001; 49: 56–62.
55. Francis NJ, Landis SC. Cellular and molecular determinants of sympathetic neuron development. Annu Rev Neurosci 1999; 22: 541–566.
56. Garofolo MC, Seidler FJ, Auman JT, Slotkin TA. β-adrenergic modulation of muscarinic cholinergic receptor expression and function in developing heart. Am J Physiol Regul Integr Comp Physiol 2002; 282: R1356–R1363.
57. Wang L, Zhang W, Zhao Y. The study of maternal and fetal plasma catecholamines levels during pregnancy and delivery. J Perinat Med 1999; 27: 195–198.
58. Agata Y, Hiraishi S, Misawa H, Han JH, Oguchi K, Horiguchi Y, et al. Hemodynamic adaptations at birth and neonates delivered vaginally and by Cesarean section. Biol Neonate 1995; 68: 404–411.
59. Hirsimaki H, Kero P, Ekblad H, Scheinin M, Saraste M, Erkkola R. Mode of delivery, plasma catecholamines and Doppler-derived cardiac output in healthy term newborn infants. Biol Neonate 1992; 61: 285–293.
60. Irestedt L, Dahlin I, Hertzberg T, Sollevi A, Lagercrantz H. Adenosine concentration in umbilical cord blood of newborn infants after vaginal delivery and cesarean section. Pediatr Res 1989; 26: 106–108.
61. Pohjavuori M, Rovamo L, Laatikainen T, Kariniemi V, Pettersson J. Stress of delivery and plasma endorphins and catecholamines in the newborn infant. Biol Res Pregnancy Perinatol 1986; 7: 1–5.
62. Eliot RJ, Lam R, Leake RD, Hobel CJ, Fisher DA. Plasma catecholamine concentrations in infants at birth and during the first 48 hours of life. J Pediatr 1980; 96: 311–315.
63. Padbury JF, Polk DH, Newham JP, Lam RW. Neonatal adaptation: greater sympathoadrenal response in preterm than full-terns fetal sheep at birth. Am J Physiol 1985; 248: E443–E449.
64. Dahnaz YL, Peyrin L, Dutruge J, Sann L. Neonatal pattern of adrenergic metabolites in urine of small for gestational age and preteen infants. J Neural Trans 1980; 49: 151–165.
65. Nicolopoulos D, Agathopoulos A. Galanakos-Tharouniati M, Stergiopoulos C. Urinary excretion of catecholamines by full term and premature infants. Pediatrics 1969; 44: 262–265.
66. Vanpee M, Herin P, Lagercrantz H, Aperia A. Effect of extreme prematurity on renal dopamine and norepinephrine excretion during the neonatal period. Pediatr Nephrol 1997; 11: 46–48.
67. Heymann MA, Iwamoto HS, Rudolph AM. Factors affecting changes in the neonatal systemic circulation. Annu RevPhysiol 1981; 43: 371–381.
68. Gootman N, Gootman PM. *Perinatal Cardiovascular Punchon*. New York: Marcel Dekker, 1983.
69. Felder RA, Jose PA. Development of adrenergic and dopamine receptors in the kidney. In: Strauss J, ed. *Electrolytes, Nephrotoxins, and the Neonatal Kidney*. The Hague: Martinus-Nihjoff, 1985.
70. Robillard JE, Nakamura KT. Neurohormonal regulation of renal function during development. Am J Physiol 1988; 254: F771–F779.
71. Gray SD. Reactivity of neonatal canine aortic strips. Biol Neonate 1977; 31: 10–14.
72. Nishina H, Ozaki T, Hanson MA, Poston L. Mechanisms of noradrenaline-induced vasorelaxation in isolated femoral arteries of the neonatal rat. Br J Pharmacol 1999; 127: 809–812.
73. Andriani G, Persico A, Tursini S, Ballone E, Cirotti D, Lelli Chiesa P. The renal-resistive index from the last 3 months of pregnancy to 6 months old. BJU Int 2001; 87: 562–564.
74. Hayashi S, Park MK, Kuehl TJ. Higher sensitivity of cerebral arteries isolated from premature and newborn baboons to adrenergic and cholinergic stimulation. Life Sci 1984; 35: 253–260.
75. Fildes RD, Eisner GM, Calcagno PL, Jose PA. Renal alpha-adrenoceptors and sodium excretion in the dog. Am J Physiol 1985; 248: F128–F133.
76. Guillery EN, Segar JL, Merrill DC, Nakamura KT, Jose PA, Robillard JE. Ontogenic changes in renal response to $alpha_1$-adrenoceptor stimulation in sheep. Am J Physiol 1994; 267: R990–R998.
77. Gitler MS, Piccio MM, Robillard JE, Jose PA. Characterization of renal alpha-adrenoceptor subtypes in sheep during development. Am J Physiol 1991; 260: R407–R412.

78. Nakamura KT, Matherne GP, Jose PA, Alden BM, Robillard JE. Ontogeny of renal β-adrenoceptor-mediated vasodilation in sheep: comparison between endogenous catecholamines. Pediatr Res 1987; 22: 465–470.
79. Sener A, Smith FG. Renal hemodynamic effects of L-NAME during postnatal maturation in conscious lambs. Pediatr Nephrol 2001; 16: 868–873.
80. Gootman PM, Buckley NM, Gootman N. Postnatal maturation of neural control of the circulation. In: Scarpelli EM, Cosmi EV eds. *Reviews in Perinatal Medicine vol. 3.* New York: Raven Press, 1979: 1–72.
81. Maruyama K, Koizumi T. Superior mesenteric artery blood flow velocity in small for gestational age infants of very low birth weight during the early neonatal period. J Perinat Med 2001; 29: 64–70.
82. Hoang TV, Choe EU, Lippton HL, Hyman AL, Flint LM, Ferrara JJ. Effect of maturation on alpha-adrenoceptor activity in newborn piglet mesentery. J Surg Res 1996; 61: 330–338.
83. Nankervis CA, Reber KM, Nowicki PT. Age-dependent changes in the postnatal intestinal microcirculation. Microcirculation 2001; 8: 377–387.
84. Willis AP, Leffler CW. Endothelial NO and prostanoid involvement in newborn and juvenile pig pial arteriolar vasomotor responses. Am J Physiol Heart Circ Physiol 2001; 281: H2366–H2377.
85. Jose PA, Martin GR, Felder RA. Cardiovascular and autonomic influences on blood pressure. In: Loggie JMH, ed. Pediatric and Adolescent Hypertension. Oxford, UK: Blackwell Scientific, 1992;p.33.

# 3 Development of Circadian Time Structure and Blood Pressure Rhythms

*Erhard Haus,* MD, PhD
*and Michael H. Smolensky,* PhD

*Contents*



## INTRODUCTION

About 24-h rhythms of systolic and diastolic blood pressure are an expression of numerous neural, endocrine, and vascular circadian rhythms superimposed on which are the differential day–night level of physical and emotional loads *(1,2)*. The human circadian time structure begins to develop in utero. It is completed in infants during the first 2 yr of life coinciding with the maturation of the neural, endocrine, and other systems. The circadian clock, and the rhythms it generates, becomes fully entrained to the 24-h societal routine through daily exposure to cyclic environmental time cues, especially the alternation of light and darkness and the temporal pattern of childcare. This article reviews the development of the human circadian time structure as it pertains to the establishment of 24-h rhythms in BP, the management of childhood hypertension (HTN), and pediatric medicine.

From: *Clinical Hypertension and Vascular Disease: Pediatric Hypertension*
Edited by: R. J. Portman, J. M. Sorof, and J. R. Ingelfinger © Humana Press Inc., Totowa, NJ

## INTRODUCTION TO BIOLOGICAL TIME STRUCTURE

Living matter displays an organization in space, a molecular and anatomic structure, and an organization in time or time structure. The human time structure consists of a spectrum of rhythms of different periods, ranging from milliseconds to years, which are superimposed on one another and on the time-dependent changes that accompany growth, development, and aging. Biological rhythms are genetically fixed with the specific gene and gene products now identified in several mammalian species. Endogenous rhythms under constant ambient conditions are adjusted (entrained or synchronized) in their exact period and staging by environmental time cues, such as the 24-h, lunar, and seasonal light–dark cycles, to optimally meet the demands of the periodic surroundings.

Rhythms with a period of about 24 h are called circadian rhythms. They are ubiquitous in human cells, tissues, and organs. Molecular oscillator mechanisms create the circadian periodicity in these peripheral structures, and are regulated by a master clock located in the paired suprachiasmatic nuclei (SCN) of the anterior hypothalamus. This master clock coordinates the tissue-specific peripheral oscillators by adjusting their period length and time relations in synchrony with the environmental 24-h light–dark cycle *(3)*.

Understanding how the clock genes and their protein products in the central and peripheral oscillators interact to create the human time structure helps to explain 24-h patterns in the pathophysiology and symptoms of disease, both in children and adults. It also lays the foundation for exploring new-generation pharmacologic interventions aimed at manipulating the human timing system to rapidly reset the central clock and peripheral oscillators to different time schedules, e.g., to correct misaligned internal phase relations between central and peripheral oscillators found in certain sleep disorders, endogenous depressions, and cancers. In adult life, they might be used to moderate or avert the side effects of a disturbed time structure following rapid transport across time zones (jet lag) or rapid rotation between day and night work shifts.

## CIRCADIAN OSCILLATOR MECHANISMS

The mammalian central circadian oscillator in the SCN is a multiple-gene mechanism consisting of interacting positive and negative transcription–translation feedback loops *(3–5)*. The clock mechanisms and clock genes in many animal species and human beings are similar *(4,6)*. The central master clock is kept entrained with the solar day–night cycle (or artificial lighting regimen) through non-vision-related ganglion cells in the retina, which serve as slow-acting photoreceptors *(7,8)*. Circadian peripheral oscillators, which possess a molecular composition like that of the master clock, are found in many tissues and typically cycle with a 6–8-h delay with reference to the central pacemaker *(9)*.

Most mammalian peripheral oscillators in the intact organism do not react directly to light, but are instead synchronized by the neuronal and humoral outputs of the SCN *(3,10)*. An exception may be the circadian clock genes of the human skin keratinocytes that can be regulated directly by ultraviolet B-band radiation *(11)*. It is at present unclear if extra-retinal light exposure can exert circadian synchronization *(12,13)*. The central circadian oscillator, when removed from the brain of laboratory animals and placed in organ culture, continues to cycle for more than 31 d *(10)* and presumably as long as the explant can be kept viable. In contrast, peripheral oscillators, when kept in organ culture, typically display a dampening in the circadian amplitude of clock gene expression with subsequent loss of rhythmicity *(10)*.

However, peripheral oscillators can be reactivated by certain manipulations, such as a change in culture media or by biochemical or hormonal stimuli *(10,14)*. In the intact animal, peripheral oscillators possess some autonomy from the central clock and can become uncoupled from central synchronization, e.g., by glucocorticoids *(9)* or atypical restricted time-of-day feeding schedules *(15)*.

The central oscillator adjusts rapidly in response to a sudden advance or delay in the environmental light cycle; however, the peripheral oscillators and the physiologic functions they control adjust slowly, requiring several transient cycles *(10)*. During this time of phase shift, there is transient loss of phase control of the peripheral oscillator by the central oscillator. This results in an internal disruption (desynchronization) of the 24-h time structure, which lasts until the process of phase adaptation and re-entrainment is complete *(10)*. The phase resetting of some peripheral (e.g., heart) tissue oscillators induced in an animal model by light pulses shows a transient phase alteration of the sequence of gene expression within the oscillator. The phase shift in ribonucleic acid (RNA) of one of the oscillator genes (Per 1) precedes that of the other oscillator genes by one day, leading to an internal phase alteration within the oscillator itself *(16)*. Mammals require a certain amount of time to adapt the rhythm of their peripheral oscillators to a new synchronizer schedule. During the time of phase adaptation, which varies among different tissue oscillators, a transient alteration is experienced not only in the relationship between the phasing of the central and peripheral oscillators, but apparently even within the individual oscillators. It is not known if occasional or persistent desynchronization within an oscillator has functional consequences.

Restricting the time of food availability to an atypical 4-h span during the daytime rest span of rats uncouples the normal phase relationships of some peripheral oscillators from the central master clock *(17)*. In a transgenic rat model in which the Per 1 gene promoter is linked to a luciferase reporter *(15)*, the sudden change in feeding from the usual nighttime to atypical daytime hours resets the phase of the rhythmic gene expression in peripheral oscillators only gradually over several consecutive transient cycles. The SCN, in contrast, remains entrained to the ambient light–dark cycle. Food-induced phase resetting of peripheral oscillators proceeds faster in the liver than in the kidney, heart, lung, and pancreas—e.g., the liver oscillator shifts to a new feeding schedule within 2–7 d, while the lung oscillator shifts more slowly and incompletely *(15)*. The phasing of the peripheral oscillators in these organs adapts after one wk of the imposed time-restricted diurnal feeding schedule.

Peripheral oscillators are also found in the heart and blood vessels *(16,18)*. Vascular endothelial cells display circadian oscillations of clock-related genes that regulate the circadian oscillations of plasminogen activator inhibitor-1 (PAI-1) *(19)*. In humans, this circadian variation results in reduced fibrinolysis in the morning *(20)* and is thought to contribute to the elevated risk of thrombotic events at this time of the day. The mouse aorta displays a circadian rhythm in the expression of circadian oscillator genes, and vascular smooth muscle cells in cultures display synchronous cycles of their oscillator genes after brief exposure to angiotensin II *(14)*. In cultured rat fibroblasts, the vasoactive peptide endothelin-1 induces circadian rhythmic gene expression like that in the SCN *(21)*.

The presence and behavior of peripheral oscillators in the cardiovascular system, as components of the organism's circadian time structure, help explain some aspects of cardiovascular physiology and pathology. Such circadian oscillators determine rhythmic changes in the functional state of the heart and blood vessels, which are clinically expressed as rhythms in the responsiveness to various stimuli, including stress and medications, and as 24-h patterns in adult cardiovascular morbidity and mortality *(22,23)*. Desynchronization of the central and peripheral oscillators perhaps constitutes an unappreciated problem in the early developmental stage of the human time organization, especially in preterm infants. Identification of the oscillator genes and their gene products may open the way for environmental (timed light) and pharmacologic (timed medication) manipulations of abnormal rhythmicity *(24)*.

## RHYTHMICITY DURING FETAL LIFE

### *Fetal Clock Functions*

The central circadian clock in the mammalian hypothalamus begins to oscillate in the fetus in utero *(25–27)*. The SCN develops in fetal rodents during the last one-third of intra-uterine life *(26)*. Transplantation of fetal SCN cells into SCN-lesioned animals restores rhythmicity to the recipient *(28–31)*. The human SCN is morphologically recognizable by wk 18 of gestation through labeling the nuclei with $^{125}$I melatonin and SKF38393 *(26,32)*. Functional studies also suggest that primate nuclei oscillate prenatally *(32,33)*. Innervation of the primate SCN by the retina, the anatomic substrate for light activation, is found in baboons at a developmental stage corresponding to approx 25 wk postconception in human infants *(34)*. Moreover, full-term baboon newborns are responsive to light as verified by metabolic changes and gene expression in their SCN *(35)*. The maturation of the SCN continues for some time after birth in human infants, for example, with the vasopressinergic neurons in the SCN reaching adult numbers only about or after 1 yr of age *(36)*.

Various maternal signals time-cue fetal rhythms during prenatal development. Temporal (24-h) patterns in the maternal rest–activity routine, body temperature, nutrient intake *(37)*, and hormones that pass through the placenta (e.g., melatonin *[38]*, cortisol *[39]*, and dopamine *[40]*) act as entraining agents of fetal rhythms. Partial elimination of the maternal light–dark synchronized circadian periodicity in an animal model, achieved by the destruction of the maternal SCN, fails to disrupt the fetal SCN rhythm *(41)*. However, the SCN of the fetus is no longer in phase with the SCN of the mother, as demonstrated by the time patterns of labeled deoxyglucose incorporation into the SCN *(41)*.

### *Activity and Organ Rhythms*

The circadian rhythm in *fetal movement* was reported first by Sterman in 1967 *(42)*. He described a marked increase in fetal activity during maternal sleep, especially during Rapid Eye Movement, or REM, phase. Circadian patterns of fetal movement can easily be recognized from 24 to 30 wk gestation, with an increasingly prominent peak during the night with maturation *(43–46)*. Continuous monitoring of 26 fetuses of gestational age 26–38 wk shows a circadian rhythm in activity in eight (31%), and only a 12-h rhythm in four (15%) *(45)*. High-frequency ultradian (<24-h) rhythms of fetal movement are also described *(47–49)*.

A circadian rhythm in *"breathing" movements* occurs in fetuses by 30–40 wk gestational age. The peak of this circadian rhythm also occurs during maternal sleep, between 2 and 7 AM, and is superimposed on high-frequency ultradian periodicities of between 100 and 500 min. The circadian rhythm in breathing movements is apparently influenced by exogenous factors; maternal meals or glucose intake increases breathing movements 1–2 h later *(47–51)*.

The *fetal heart rate* (HR) displays a circadian rhythm. It is lowest overnight during maternal sleep, between 2 and 6 AM, when the maternal HR is lowest. It shows a prolonged elevation during the daytime with the peak around 2 PM *(46,52,53)*. Ultradian rhythms with periods ranging from less than a minute to as long as 3–4 h also are described in both fetal HR and in HR variability *(54,55)*.

Statistical analysis of continuously monitored fetal HR reveals a circadian rhythm with a superimposed 12-h component in 73% of the fetuses studied. A circadian rhythm with a superimposed prominent 12-h component in the high and low frequency bands of the power spectrum of HR variability is present in 46% and 38%, respectively, of the studied fetuses *(45)*. The amplitude of the fetal HR rhythm is positively correlated with gestational age in fetuses between 26 and 38 wk. The correlation between maternal and fetal HR is also positive, with a time lag between the staging of rhythms ranging from +2 to –4 h. Finally, although there is a positive correlation between the circadian (and 12-h) rhythms of fetal HR and maternal cortisol, it is negative for maternal melatonin *(45)*. The documentation of such correlations in rhythm staging, however, does not imply causality.

Finally, a circadian variation in *fetal bladder volume* is reported with the trough between midnight and 6 AM. This is indicative of circadian rhythmicity in fetal renal, adrenal, and/or cardiovascular function *(56)*.

Circadian and ultradian rhythms in HR, as well as fetal breathing and physical movement, are related to the rhythms of the corresponding period in fetal cortical state or the fetal "sleep–wake" pattern, which, late in pregnancy, is similar to that of newborn infants.

### *Biochemical and Endocrine Rhythms*

In most instances, the study of fetal endocrine rhythms requires invasive techniques. Therefore, most of the available information is derived from investigations of nonhuman primate species. In humans, information about these rhythms is obtained by the study of fetal hormones or their metabolites found in the blood of pregnant women. Estriol is a product of the fetal-placental unit that is produced by the placenta in increasing amounts late during pregnancy, mostly from precursors derived from the fetal adrenal (i.e., dehydroepiandrosterone sulfate). Consequently, the maternal plasma estriol concentration reflects fetal adrenal function. The plasma estriol concentration in the maternal circulation shows a circadian rhythm *(57,58)*, with a peak around midnight *(59–61)*. In women carrying fetuses of 34–35 wk gestation, the prominent circadian rhythms in plasma estriol and plasma cortisol differ in phase by 12 h *(61)*. It appears that the maternal adrenocortical rhythm may have a synchronizing influence on fetal adrenal rhythms through negative feedback on the fetal pituitary–adrenal axis. Interventions that abolish or suppress the maternal adrenocortical rhythms exert a marked effect on fetal adrenal hormones and their metabolic products, such as estriol. Treatment of pregnant women with prednisone or dexamethasone suppresses their circadian rhythm in cortisol, and it abolishes the circadian rhythms of estriol, breathing movement, and HR variability in the fetus *(62–64)*. In a pregnant woman who had an adrenalectomy performed prior to pregnancy and who received adrenal corticosteroid hormone replacement, levels of estriol were low and without recognizable circadian rhythmicity. Similarly, there was an absence of circadian rhythmicity in fetal HR variability *(65)*. It appears, therefore, that the maternal adrenocortical rhythm is a major synchronizer of fetal circadian rhythms.

Certain information about fetal endocrine rhythms can be gained from cord blood sampling. Studies involving maternal and fetal blood sampling done within minutes of delivery reveal in-phase, 24-h rhythms of mothers and fetuses in red blood cell glucose phosphate isomerase and hexosaminidase *(66)*. A circadian rhythm is also seen in cord plasma cortisol *(67)* and dehydroepiandrosterone *(68)*. The cortisol peak occurs between noon and 2 PM, and follows the maternal peak that occurs between 4 AM and noon. A circadian rhythm of prolactin is detected in cord plasma after spontaneous delivery *(69)*, but not in cord blood obtained after elective hysterotomy *(70)*.

The presence or absence of circadian periodicity in the fetus in utero does not seem to be an indicator of fetal health, because the small percentage of fetuses that fail to display detectable circadian rhythms in physiologic variables appear just as healthy at birth as those who do.

### *Rhythm-Dependencies of Fetal Toxicology*

The fetal toxicity of drugs and environmental agents is complex, because it is dependent on gestational age, and maternal and fetal pharamcokinetic and placental transfer phenomena. Susceptibility to teratogenesis varies during gestation, and embryonic tissue is especially sensitive to insult. The most critical period in the development of a particular tissue or organ is the time of its most rapid cell division during organogenesis, which in the human embyro ranges from roughly d 18–60 of gestation. This developmental stage corresponds to gestational d 7–13 in mice. Several studies show that the sensitivity of embryonic tissues to toxicants depends on the circadian time when vulnerable fetal tissue is exposed. Circadian phase-dependent teratogenesis is reported in rodent experiments involving cortisone *(71)*, dexamethasone *(72)*, hydroxyurea *(73)*, 5-fluorouracil *(74)*, cyclophosphamide *(75–77)*, cytosine arabinoside *(78)*, and ethanol *(79–82)*. The number of fetuses per litter developing malformations and/or growth defects and the severity of the fetotoxicity depends both on gestational stage and on the circadian time the agent is injected into the mother.

Glucocorticoids, such as cortisone and dexamethasone, produce cleft palate in rodents at the time of palatal shelf closure—d 11–15 of gestation in mice. In rodents, the number of cleft palates stemming from a steroid injection is significantly greater when timed during the second half of the mother's nocturnal activity span *(71,72)*. In contrast, the incidence of digital and limb defect deformities is greatest when these medications are administered to the mother at the beginning of her daily rest span *(73)*. 5-fluorouracil causes the highest incidence of digital defects and kinky tail when injected into the mother in the second half of the 12-h diurnal rest span on d 11 of gestation *(74,82)*. Also in rodents, cyclophosphamide causes the highest incidence of fetal malformations when given to the mother at the time of the daily transition between nocturnal activity and daytime rest. The severity and number of malformations from cyclophosphamide are lowest when exposure is timed during the middle of the dark span *(82)*. Cyclophosphamide requires extra-embryonic metabolism by the maternal liver to achieve biological activity *(83)*; thus, maternal rhythms likely play a role in the observed circadian variation in its teratogenicity.

The sensitivity of fetal tissue to ethanol also is circadian rhythmic *(79,80,84)*. The incidence of developmental abnormalities and impact on fetal body weight is significantly greater when ethanol is administered maternally during the early to mid-nocturnal activity span. The extent of fetal insult at this circadian time of exposure is positively correlated with the concentration of alcohol achieved in maternal blood. The circadian timing of ethanol results in a differential impact on embryonic fetal tissues *(79–81)* and, although not yet studied, may be a potential determinant of fetal alcohol syndrome development in newborns.

Betamimetic tocolytics apparently exert effects upon the fetal cardiovascular system and its functional status that may persist into childhood and even into adulthood *(85,86)*. The transplacental passage of betamimetics in pregnant women is associated with an increase in the amplitude of the circadian BP rhythm of about 40% compared to nonexposed infants. Forty-eight-hour ambulatory BP monitoring (ABPM) of 11–14-yr-old adolescents previously exposed to betamimetics in utero showed a circadian BP rhythm of higher amplitude than those of similar complicated pregnancies treated with different medications *(86)*. The exposed children also tended to have a larger left ventricular mass index *(86)*. These findings imply that intrauterine exposure to betamimetics can affect the circadian rhythm of BP regulation, not only in newborns at birth but later in adolescence. Elevated circadian BP amplitude (above the 90th percentile of clinically healthy peers) may confer an elevated risk for ischemic stroke later in life *(87)*. Interestingly, elevated circadian BP amplitude has been reported in infants *(88,89)* and children *(90)* with a positive family history of HTN.

## CHRONOBIOLOGY OF THE NEWBORN AND INFANT

The postnatal development of the human 24-h time structure is dependent on the maturation of the inherited central and peripheral clock oscillators, and the exposure of the newborn to periodic and nonperiodic environmental factors that act as entraining agents. In general, the circadian periodicity which develops in concert with the maturation of the newborn's central nervous system and central oscillator is likely to be more poorly expressed and slower to develop in preterm than term infants *(91)*.

The circadian periodicity that is observed in newborns during the first week of life may still represent, at least in part, the influence of the mother's 24-h rhythms *(92–95)*. High-frequency ultradian rhythms predominate at the time of birth and thereafter during the ensuing several weeks of extra-uterine life. Recognizable circadian periodicity in the newborn develops gradually during the first months of life and, in some biological variables and functions, later during the first year of life, presumably with the maturation of the genetically inherited circadian oscillator, and increasing exposure and response capability to 24-h environmental time cues *(96)*. Environmental synchronizers, in addition to the 24-h light–dark cycle, include the temporal pattern of newborn feeding and handling, both in the hospital nursery and in the home. The presence or absence of the mother or other caregivers is also important. In preterm infants and in many full-term babies, endogenously driven circadian rhythms may not be apparent, and if present may be free-running (not exactly 24 h) in period. This becomes obvious only through longitudinal monitoring of single newborns and may not be visible as a group phenomenon. The feeding and handling patterns during the 24 h exert influence on the infant temperature, HR, and activity patterns; it is likely that infant care schedules drive, reinforce, and/or synchronize high-frequency ultradian rhythms in neonates. Individual differences in the maturity of the clock mechanisms between infants and differences in the strength and extent of exposure to environmental time cues and entraining agents, such as the lighting regimen and feeding schedules among others in neonatal and preterm infant care units, account for the great individual variability in their development of time organization in the initial days and weeks of postnatal life.

### *Body Temperature and Heart Rate*

Rhythmicity in body temperature in newborns and infants has been studied since the early 1900s. In 1904, Jundell *(95)* reported temperature variations in children and newborns and described the gradual establishment of its circadian rhythm during the first 9 mo of life. The analysis of Jundell's data by modern statistical techniques used in the field of rhythm study shows that the proportion of the total variance in body temperature ascribable to the circadian rhythm component (the "circadian quotient") in 4–9-d-old newborns is approx 35%. This

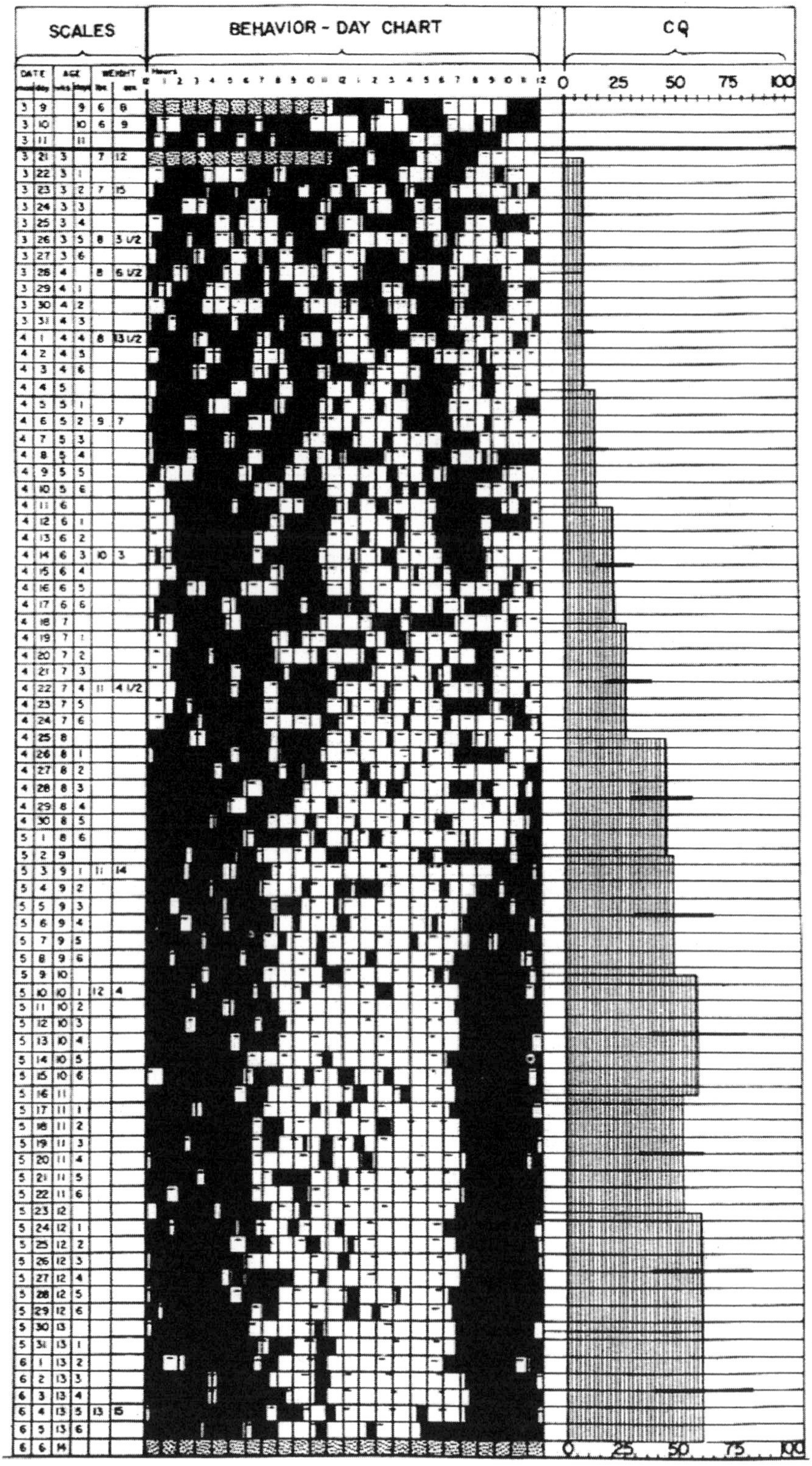


Fig. 1. Development of the sleep (■)–wake (□) and feeding (—) circadian rhythms in a neonate raised on demand from birth to 14 wk of age. The far left two columns of the figure give the calendar mo and d, the middle two columns the age of the newborn in wk and d, and the last two columns body weight in lbs and oz. The column to the far right of the figure is labeled CQ, which depicts the prominence of

variance increases to about 50% by d 10–28 of life, and remains at about this level until age 70 d. At 3–9 mo of age, the circadian rhythm component increases to between 60 and 75%. The circadian rhythm component in children 2.5–4.5 yr of age amounts to between 76 and 90%, which is comparable to that found in older children and adults. The amplitude of the circadian rhythm of body temperature increases up to the age of 3 yr *(97,98)*. The development of the circadian rhythm in HR shows roughly the same pattern as in temperature.

Circadian rhythms in temperature and HR in extremely preterm infants of postconceptional age 24–29 wk are not recognizable and generally are not apparent even at 17 wk after birth *(98)*. The development of the circadian rhythm of sleep and wakefulness in preterm compared to normal-term infants is delayed as well *(92,98–101)*. Infants of postconceptional age 35 wk show high-frequency ultradian temperature and HR rhythms, but not circadian rhythms *(101,102)*.

Although circadian rhythms of HR and temperature are not found in all newborns, they can be detected in more than half of those kept in a normal light–dark environment *(93,102)*. When clinically "healthy" preterm infants are studied under as far as feasible "constant" environmental conditions, statistically significant circadian rhythms with a period in the range of between 22–28 h are detectable in HR and/or body temperature in about 50% of those assessed *(102)*. Neonatal rhythms with periods that are close to, but not precisely, 24 h in length free-run from the calendar day and may go undetected if sampling is inadequate or if data are analyzed on a group rather than individual basis.

### Sleep–Wakefulness

Circadian rhythmicity of sleep and wakefulness and of appetite is absent during the first week of extra-uterine life in full-term babies *(103)*. The circadian sleep–wake cycle establishes itself in infants during the second month of life *(104–106)*, although its development is delayed in preterm babies *(103)*. Higher-frequency ultradian oscillations of 3–4 h duration, which to some extent may be reinforced and/or synchronized by the infant care schedule, are superimposed upon the 24-h sleep–wake rhythm *(107)*. Other studies reveal that the alternation of sleep and wakefulness occurs during the first weeks of life more or less at random *(108,109)*, which in part may be owing to temporal attributes of the infant care regimen.

When the newborn is fed on demand rather than at fixed clock times, the demands often occur at irregular intervals during the day and night *(108)*. However, with the demand feeding schedule, sleep episodes are more common during the night—between 11 PM and 7 AM—than during other times of the day. The elimination of known synchronizers by raising infants under continuous room light and demand feeding shows that bouts of sleep and wakefulness occur at random until age 40 d or so (Fig. 1) *(110)*. After this age, the infant displays one long sleep

the circadian sleep–wake rhythm at the different ages. It is the percent of the total variance explained by 24-h pattern. During the first 5 wk of life episodes of sleeping and waking are at first random and then of high frequency. The low CQ of approx 12% at this age substantiates the low prominence of 24-h periodicity. In the ensuing few wk sleep episodes gradually consolidate to the nighttime with longer spans of waking during the daytime. The CQ reflects this, increasing markedly at approx 8–9 wk of age and more so thereafter until approx 14 wk, the end of record. Early in life, between 3 and 4 wk of age, episodes of feeding occur at short intervals. Feeding episodes are less frequent during the night at approx 8–9 wk of life as the expression of the circadian sleep–wake rhythm strengthens. From Halberg et al. *(110)*.

period every 24 h. After 54 d, this longer sleep period recurs at regular intervals, thereby establishing the circadian rhythm in sleep and wakefulness. The main sleep span under these rearing conditions occurs between 5 and 10 AM, indicating that the infant's behavior is not in phase with environmental or societal cycles. Finally, if after the 80th d of age the infant is exposed to the usual 24-h light–dark cycle, the characteristic environmentally synchronized circadian rhythm in sleep and wakefulness is expressed within a week. These observations on newborns raised in the absence of environmental time cues and synchronizers indicate that this genetically determined circadian rhythm develops progressively with the maturation of the infant and its endogenous time structure.

Longitudinal observation of single newborns was reported by Kleitman and Engelmann *(104)*, Parmelee *(106)*, and Halberg et al. *(110)*, and reviewed by Hellbrügge *(96,99)*. The infant studied longitudinally by Kleitman and Engelmann *(105)* changed its activity rhythm during the first 6 mo of life from a predominantly high-frequency ultradian to a free-running (not exactly 24 h) circadian pattern at about 8 wk of age, and to a day–night synchronized 24-h pattern at about 16 wk of age. Hellbrügge and colleagues *(99)* described the development of circadian rhythms of different physiologic variables as occurring apparently independently from one another, and at progressively different ages after birth. The development of the circadian periodicity of sleep and wakefulness leads to a shift from a higher-frequency ultradian to a circadian time structure. In most infants, it may not be until the second yr of life before they no longer awaken during the nighttime. It appears that only then does the child fully follow environmental synchronizers, the most prominent being the 24-h alternation of light and darkness.

## ENDOCRINE RHYTHMS

Circadian periodicity in adrenal function is absent during the first few months of life as shown by the absence of the expected morning decline in the number of circulating eosinophil leukocytes in peripheral blood. A decrease in eosinophil count between 6:30 and 9:30 AM, similar to that seen in adults, is found in babies older than 15 mo *(111)*. In 3-wk-old infants, the concentration of 17-hydroxycorticosteroids, the principal metabolic product of cortisol in the urine, is higher between 6 AM and 6 PM than between 6 PM and 6 AM. Definite circadian rhythms in plasma *(112,113)* and salivary cortisol *(114)* appear between 3 and 6 mo of age. The circadian rhythm in plasma cortisol, as in that of the adult, is established as a group phenomenon by 3 mo of age *(115,116)*. Zurbrugg *(117)* studied plasma cortisol with 4-h sampling in groups of neonates aged 3–9 d, infants 1–6 mo, children 1.5–11.5 yr, and adults. The mean 24-h cortisol concentration was similar among the groups; however, the circadian amplitude increased with age. The circadian rhythm in plasma cortisol may appear at an earlier postnatal age through the intensive study of individual infants not yet fully synchronized with the surrounding day–night cycle. In this regard, Vermes and colleagues *(115)* identified free-running plasma cortisol circadian rhythms in infants 2–3 wk old.

The circadian rhythm in melatonin is detected at 12 wk of age when day–night differences in activity become more apparent in infants *(118–120)*. Transverse 24-h study of different groups of infants sampled at different hours (e.g., five children sampled at 6 AM, five others at 7 AM, etc.) reveals no recognizable circadian rhythm in growth hormone *(121)*, which may result from the absence of environmental synchronization among the different infants.

### *Cardiovascular Rhythmicity*

Maturation of the neonate results in the transposition of cardiovascular rhythms from a high-frequency ultradian to a circadian time structure *(122–125)*. In newborns, the amplitude of the circadian BP rhythm is small and demonstrable at the 5% probability level only in about 35% of the data series obtained by 48-h ABPM. Nonetheless, circadian rhythmicity can be documented as a group phenomenon, more prominent in full- than preterm infants. On average, the peak in BP occurs early in the morning on the first day of life, with a progressive shift thereafter to an afternoon peak.

Longitudinal and cross-sectional repeat-measures study protocols reveal rhythms in addition to 24 h in BP and HR during the first days of life. High-frequency ultradian rhythms appear to be associated with, or synchronized by, the frequent feeding pattern of the newborn. As a group phenomenon, approx 7-d and approx 1-yr rhythms modulate the circadian system of the infant *(85,126)*. With reference to the date (rather than the day of the week) of birth, a statistically significant approx 7-d pattern in systolic and diastolic BP and in HR emerges as a group phenomenon with an amplitude much greater than that of the circadian or circannual rhythms *(127,128)*. This periodicity is believed to be an expression of the endogenous 7-d clock component of the human time structure. Birth and related processes do not induce the rhythm because the event of birth itself carries no 7-d information, although a 7-d synchronized rhythm in birth is documented *(129)*.

The magnitude of the circadian amplitude of BP in the newborn has been associated with a family history of HTN through a series of small-scale epidemiologic investigations. Moreover, it has been linked to differences in the risk of HTN and cardiovascular disease in adulthood *(88,89,130,131)*. Although the findings of these initial investigations are intriguing, they have not always been consistent. Additional studies of appropriate scale are needed to define the association, if any, between the various characteristics of the BP circadian rhythm of newborns and family history of HTN, as well as the risk of HTN and cardiovascular disease later in life.

Circadian rhythms are discernable in cardiovascular parameters other than HR and BP. Doppler flow-meter studies reveal 24-h rhythms in neonatal aortic blood velocity, aortic blood acceleration, and aortic stroke distance by the first day of life in clinically healthy neonates and in intrauterine growth-retarded mature neonates *(132)*. In contrast, circadian rhythms are not found in preterm newborns. The amplitude of these circadian rhythms increases rapidly between postpartum d 2 and 10. Newborns with positive family histories of HTN and myocardial infarction show a statistically significant, lower 24-h mean level of aortic blood velocity than those with negative family histories, and considerably smaller circadian amplitude of both aortic velocity and stroke distance. The potential pathophysiologic significance of these findings awaits further study.

## CIRCADIAN TIME ORGANIZATION AND INFANT CARE PATTERNS

The development of the circadian time structure in early postnatal life is owing in part to the maturation of the circadian timekeeping system, and in part to entrainment by environmental synchronizers. An increasing body of evidence substantiates the significance of the circadian time organization in normal development. Environmental entrainment is important for normal somatic and behavioral development of the neonate, and warrants appropriate attention in the design of infant care facilities and schedules. The human newborn seems to possess a fully functional mechanism of light perception and photic entrainment, even in environments of relatively low light intensity *(34,133)*. However, in many regular and intensive care neonatal units, newborns are continuously exposed either to continuous light or to very low-intensity 24-h light–dark cycles. Superimposed upon such atypical environmental lighting schedules are the fixed feeding and care routines provided by different personnel during the day and night. Such an arrangement is likely to delay the development of circadian synchronization and/or result in a circadian time organization that is out of phase with the schedule of care. Preterm infants receiving care in a nursery with ambient-like light–dark cycles wean earlier from ventilator support, feed by mouth sooner, gain weight faster, develop more quickly, establish circadian sleep–wake cycling sooner, and are healthier than those cared for in a nursery environment of constant illumination *(134–137)*. Moreover, preterm infants housed in a hospital nursery with a day–night cycle of lighting, in comparison to a matched group housed in an environment of continuous lighting, display better physical and behavioral abilities, including enhanced motor coordination *(136,137)*. Term infants cared for by a single provider and exposed to regular light–dark cycles develop the circadian sleep–wake pattern at an earlier age than those housed in an environment in which there is an irregular and unstructured care pattern *(136,137)*.

The findings of these studies reveal the importance of the environment to the growth and development of newborns. Neonatal care environments that incorporate the 24-h ambient-like light–dark cycle achieve synchronization of the circadian time organization more rapidly, and better promote biological and behavioral development. Such findings call for the reconsideration of the traditional constant-light hospital nursery environment under which premature and term neonates are routinely housed.

## THE BIOLOGIC TIME ORGANIZATION DURING CHILDHOOD

With maturation, the time organization of the newborn gradually shifts from a high-frequency ultradian to a circadian time structure *(91,99)*. However, the development of the circadian time structure seems to proceed at an unequal rate, not only in different tissues and organs, but in individual tissues and organs, as well. For example, Helbrügge *(91,99)* found that renal water excretion, a variable bound to glomerular function, developed circadian periodicity earlier than electrolyte excretion tied to tubular function. A detectable circadian rhythm in electrolyte excretion was found only after weeks of exposure to light–dark and other environmental synchronizers *(91,99)*, substantiating the endogenous nature of this rhythm on which environmental factors provided by the daily care regimen are superimposed. A circadian time organization in clinical, biochemical, and endocrine variables comparable to that of adolescents and adults (with the exception of the gonadal hormones and gonadotrophins, which undergo major change at the time of puberty) is found in children older than 2 yr of age *(138,139)*. During childhood, behavioral rhythms of different (24-h, 7-d, and/or 1-yr) periods also become apparent, e.g., in feeding/eating patterns *(140)*, risk of accident *(141)*, vigilance and sleepiness, and school performance *(142)*.

## TIME-QUALIFIED REFERENCE VALUES IN SCHOOL-AGE CHILDREN

The circadian time structure is expressed as rhythmic variations in reference values of endocrine and other frequently assessed laboratory hematology and blood chemistry parameters. The findings of earlier studies conducted by one of the authors (EH) are of direct rel-

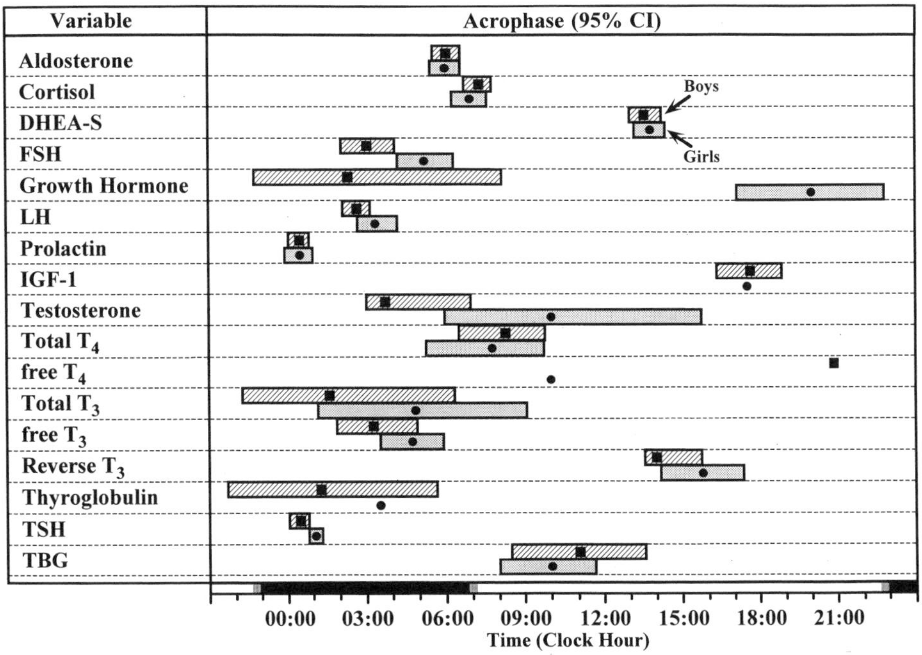


Fig. 2. Acrophase (peak time of the cosine curve best approximating the time series data) and 95% confidence intervals of circadian rhythms of hormones in the blood of children. (When group rhythmicity is not statistically validated, only the acrophase is shown and is indicative of the time of higher values.) 87 boys (■) and 107 girls (•), 11 ± 1.5 yrs of age, were studied in Tirgoviste, Romania with blood sampling every 4 h during a single 24-h study span. Analysis of data by population mean cosinor. Time scale at the bottom is labeled in military units (00:00 = midnight, 12:00 = noon, etc.); shading between approx 23:00 (11 PM, time of retiring to bed) and approx 07:00 (7 AM, time of awakening) and absence of shading between approx 07:00 and approx 23:00 depict the average sleep–wake synchronizer routine of the study sample. After Haus et al., 1992 *(145)*.

evance to pediatrics. A group of clinically healthy Caucasian children living in Tirgoviste, Romania were studied. They were synchronized by their school routine of beginning daytime activity between 6:30 and 7 AM, and retiring to bed at night between 9 and 11 PM. Blood samples were drawn at 4-h intervals during a single 24-h span. All chemical analyses were done in the same laboratory *(143)*.

Circadian rhythms were verified by so-called cosinor analysis, a statistical technique commonly used in the field of chronobiology *(144)*. The circadian acrophase—the peak time of the 24-h cosine curve that best fits the time series data—and its 95% confidence interval are shown for each variable in Figs. 2 and 3. The extent of the circadian variation—the difference between the highest and lowest value (expressed as a percentage of the lowest value)—is shown in Tables 1 and 2. A comparison of the findings concerning these children with findings concerning children of different ages and geographic locations can be found elsewhere *(143,145,146)*.

The manifestation of high-amplitude circadian rhythms in parameters of clinical interest requires the use of time-qualified reference values to best interpret the results of diagnostic tests. Several hormonal variables differ greatly in level according to the time of sampling, e.g., plasma cortisol is much higher in the morning after awakening than late in the afternoon and evening. Other adrenal steroids, such as DHEA, 17-OH-progesterone, and 11-deoxycortisol, show circadian patterns comparable to that of cortisol in clinically healthy children, and in

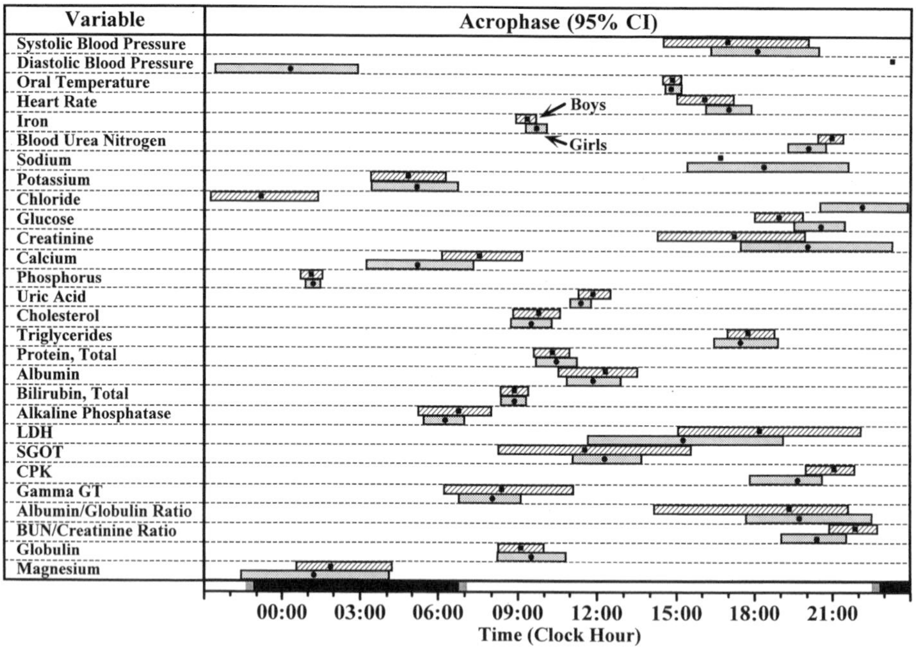


Fig. 3. Acrophase (peak time of the cosine curve best approximating the time series data) and 95% confidence intervals of circadian rhythms of chemical variables in the blood of children. (When group rhythmicity is not statistically validated, only the acrophase is shown and is indicative of the time of day of high values.) Same children, study protocol, and labeling as in Fig. 2. After Haus et al., 1992 *(145)*.

children with congenital adrenal hyperplasia *(147)*. The circadian rhythm of plasma DHEA-S characteristically shows a later acrophase, presumably owing in part to its longer plasma half-life *(143)*.

The high-amplitude circadian rhythms of circulating white blood cells are of clinical importance; however, reference values are presently available only for adults *(143,145, 148,149)*. The acrophases and the extent of the variation of these rhythms are shown in Fig. 4 and Table 3. Circadian rhythm-qualified reference values are useful for certain hematologic variables, e.g., the number of circulating lymphocytes *(145,148)*. The considerable variability in the occurrence of the peak and trough values of other hematologic variables among adults results in these time-qualified references being very broad, which compromises their application in medicine. However, the extent of the circadian variation found in individuals has to be kept in mind, because an unexpectedly large difference in findings between blood samples collected from the same patient at two different times of the day may be caused by circadian periodicity and not by change in clinical condition. Such unexpected and often large changes must be evaluated against the background of the patient's clinical condition. We must emphasize that the peaks and troughs of circadian rhythms are determined by the 24-h synchronizer schedule of the child or adult—principally, the sleep in darkness and activity in light routine. Consequently, the accurate application of laboratory and other reference values qualified according to circadian stage mandates that the time of patient blood sampling be referred to a relevant marker of the sleep–wake synchronizer routine, such as the middle of the sleep span or morning wake-up.

Table 1
Extent of Circadian Variation of Endocrine Parameters

| | *RO* | *RO* | *RO* | *UK* | *US* | *Japan* | *US* | *RO* | *RO* | *RO* | *Site* |
|---|---|---|---|---|---|---|---|---|---|---|---|
| | *11±2* | *11±2* | *11±2* | *22±3* | *24±10* | *35±15* | *36±16* | *77±8* | *77±8* | *77±8* | *Age* |
| *Variables* | *M+F* | *M* | *F* | *M* | *M+F* | *F* | *F* | *M+F* | *M* | *F* | *Sex* |
| ACTH | | | | 356 | 63 | | | 83 | | | |
| Aldosterone | 383 | | | 241 | 195 | 127 | | 109 | | | |
| Cortisol | 165 | | | 634 | 182 | 327 | 261 | 140 | | | |
| DHEA-S | 26 | | | | 21 | 38 | 39 | | 20 | 24 | |
| C-Peptide | | | | | | | | 144 | | | |
| Growth hormone | 107 | | | 152 | 74 | | | | | | |
| Insulin | | | | | 119 | 234 | 366 | 158 | | | |
| Prolactin | 174 | | | | | 350 | 169 | 69 | | | |
| Estrone | | | | | | | 12 | | | | |
| Estradiol | | | | | | | | | | 23 | |
| Estriol | | | | | | | 59 | | | | |
| FSH | 28 | | | | 7 | | | | | | |
| LH | 51 | | | | 38 | | | | 7 | 11 | |
| Progesterone | | | | | | | | | | 76 | |
| 17-OH Prog | | | | | | 66 | 34 | | 77 | 271 | |
| Testosterone | | 128 | 105 | | | | | | 30 | 32 | |

Extent of circadian variation (average of the ratio of the highest to lowest value obtained during the 24 h in each subject expressed in percent of the lowest value) of endocrine variables in clinically healthy, diurnally active subjects grouped by geo-ethnicity (RO = Romania; UK = United Kingdom; US = United States), age, and gender. Blood sampling at 4-h intervals during a single 24-h span. After Haus et al., 1988 *(143)* and Haus and Touitou, 1992 *(145)*.

Pattern analysis of the acrophases of 12 endocrine variables shows the time organization of Romanian children is similar to that of Romanian adults, as well as to American adolescents and adults. However, it differs from Japanese women of varying ages *(150)*. Therefore, the establishment of chronobiologic reference values requires an adjustment for ethnic–geographic differences *(143,150–154)*. Seasonal variations (circannual rhythms) in laboratory variables in adults and young children are also known; these findings are accessible elsewhere *(155,156)*.

## CIRCADIAN RHYTHM-DEPENDENCIES OF MEDICATIONS IN CHILDREN

Chronopharmacology is the study of administration-time differences in the pharamaco-kinetics and dynamics of medications with reference to circadian or other period rhythms *(157)*. Circadian rhythms of the gastrointestinal tract, liver, kidney, and circulation can differentially affect the absorption, distribution, metabolism, and elimination of medications according to the time of dosing *(158)*. Rhythms in the ratio of free drug faction, receptor number/conformation, molecular mediators, and metabolic pathways, among others, can result

Table 2
Circadian Variation of Biochemical Serum Parameters

| | *RO* | *RO* | *UK* | *US* | *US* | *RO* | *Site* |
|---|---|---|---|---|---|---|---|
| | *11±2* | *21±2* | *22±3* | *24±8* | *71±5* | *76±8* | *Age* |
| *Variables* | *M+F* | *M+F* | *M* | *M+F* | *M+F* | *M+F* | *Sex* |
| Alkaline phosphatase | 8 | 10 | | 12 | | 7 | |
| CPK | 28 | 30 | | 40 | 18 | 18 | |
| Gamma GT | 50 | 53 | 37 | | 34 | 15 | |
| LDH | 5 | 17 | 118 | 23 | 22 | | |
| SGOT | 11 | 15 | 28 | | 15 | 9 | |
| Bilirubin, total | 81 | 65 | 67 | 75 | 52 | 42 | |
| Cholesterol | 7 | 6 | 4 | | 4 | 9 | |
| Triglyceride | 82 | 129 | 78 | 73 | 57 | 38 | |
| Uric acid | 14 | 10 | | 6 | | 4 | |
| BUN | 30 | 10 | 11 | 34 | 13 | 9 | |
| Creatinine | 6 | | 29 | 22 | 14 | 7 | |
| BUN/creatinine | 22 | 11 | 32 | 25 | 9 | 9 | |
| Glucose | 21 | 23 | 56 | 14 | | 48 | |
| Calcium | 3 | 4 | | | | 4 | |
| Chloride | 1 | 3 | 2 | 1 | 1 | 2 | |
| Iron | 106 | 54 | 66 | 49 | 60 | 48 | |
| Phosphorus | 24 | 18 | 28 | 33 | | 7 | |
| Potassium | 8 | 8 | | | | 8 | |
| Sodium | 1 | 3 | 1 | | | 2 | |
| Protein, total | 5 | 7 | 5 | 6 | 5 | 8 | |
| Albumin | 5 | 7 | 6 | 6 | 3 | 7 | |
| Globulin | 8 | 6 | | 6 | 9 | 9 | |
| Albumin/globulin | 5 | 6 | 6 | 4 | | 3 | |

Extent of circadian variation (average of the ratio of the highest to lowest value obtained during the 24 h in each subject expressed in percent of the lowest value) of biochemical serum parameters in clinically healthy, diurnally active subjects grouped by geo-ethnicity (RO = Romania; UK = United Kingdom; US = United States), age, and gender. From Haus et al., 1988 *(143)* and Haus and Touitou, 1992 *(145)*.

in administration-time differences in dose–response relationships, as well as the outcome, benefit, and/or tolerance of therapy *(157)*.

Numerous studies, primarily involving young to middle-age adults, reveal that the kinetics and dynamics of various types and classes of medications, including those used to manage HTN, are affected by the circadian time structure *(157,159,160)*. However, there has yet to be a systematic study of administration-time differences in the effects of medications on newborns, young infants, or school-age children. Indeed, only a limited number of studies have explored administration-time differences in the kinetics of medications in children, generally between 6 and 17 yr of age, controlling for meal timings and contents.

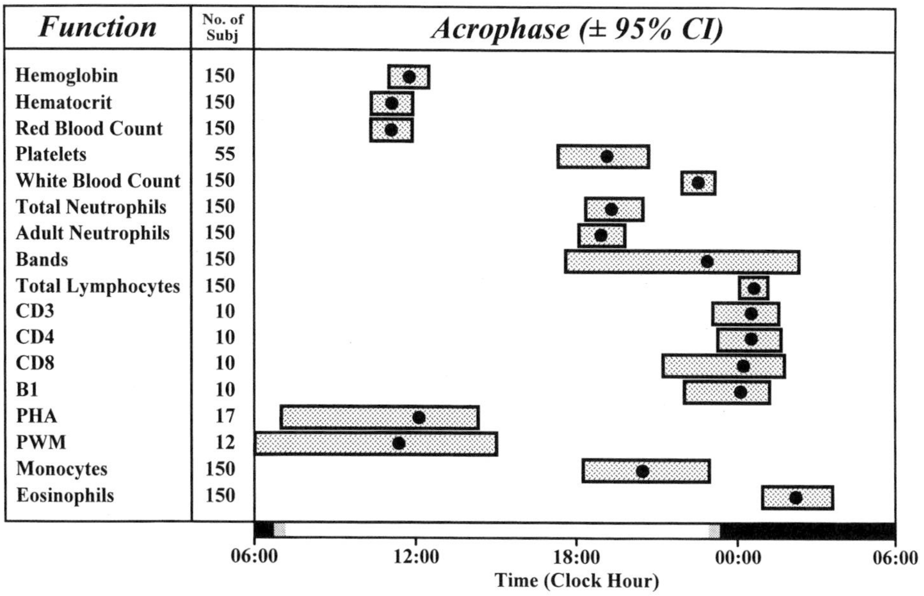


Fig. 4. Acrophase (peak time of the cosine curve best approximating the time series data) and 95% confidence intervals of circadian rhythms of circulating formed elements in the peripheral blood of clinically healthy, diurnally active subjects of both sexes (mean age 24± 10 yr, range 11–57 yr) studied in St. Paul, MN. Blood sampling done at 4-h intervals during a single 24-h span. Analysis by population mean cosinor. Time scale at bottom is labeled in military units (00:00 = midnight, 12:00 = noon, etc.); shading between approx 23:00 (11 PM, time of retiring to bed) and approx 07:00 (7 AM, time of awakening) and absence of shading between approx 07:00 and approx 23:00 depict the average sleep–wake synchronizer routine of the study sample. After Haus et al., 1996 *(148)*.

One of the authors of this chapter (MHS) showed that the kinetics of a once-popular, sustained-release twice-a-day theophylline tablet product in asthmatic children 6–13 yr of age varies markedly after morning vs evening dosing under steady-state (long-term) treatment *(161)*. The rate and extent of drug absorption is significantly greater after the morning than after the evening dose, resulting in the risk of suboptimal protection against nocturnal exacerbations of asthma, which is primarily a nighttime disease in children and adults *(162,163)*. Comparable studies, however, on adult asthmatics with this and other marketed sustained-release twice-a-day theophylline medications, reveal little dosing-time-dependent effect on drug kinetics *(162)*. Another investigation on a once-a-day oral theophylline medication marketed in the US reveals extreme and clinically meaningful administration-time-dependent differences in drug kinetics, both in children and adults *(164)*. The bioavailability (area under the time-drug concentration curve) of this once-a-day formulation in 8–15-yr-old asthmatic children assessed during steady-state treatment conditions is approximately threefold greater with an evening compared to morning once-a-day dosing schedule. Consequently, adverse effects of significant intensity were quite common with evening, but not with morning, dosing of this particular theophylline medication. The dosing-time-dependent differences in the bio-availability of this theophylline medication were identical in children and adults when studied in the same way *(164)*. The extent of the dosing-time effect on theophylline kinetics seems to be determined by the circadian rhythms of the gastrointestinal tract and their impact on the particular drug-delivery

Table 3
Circadian Variation of Hematological Variables

| | *Peak-trough difference* | | *% Range of change* | |
|---|---|---|---|---|
| | *Mean ± SD* | *Range* | *Mean ± SD* | *Range* |
| Total white blood count | 2400 ± 1000 | 400–6100 | 41 ± 18 | 7–133 |
| Total neutrophils | 1840 ± 1025 | 480–7186 | 66 ± 42 | 20–346 |
| Adult neutrophils | 1567 ± 856 | 330–6347 | 72 ± 43 | 18–344 |
| Bands | 563 ± 350 | 56–1790 | 152 ± 114 | 15–780 |
| Lymphocytes | 1616 ± 770 | 331–5556 | 84 ± 41 | 14–234 |
| Monocytes | 366 ± 167 | 80–974 | 277 ± 221 | 30–1560 |
| Eosinophils | 230 ± 110 | 40–816 | 292 ± 190 | 61–1031 |
| Basophils | 105 ± 57 | 0–390 | 315 ± 175 | 27–858 |
| Platelets ($\times 10^3$) | 54 ± 32 | 12–198 | 23 ± 15 | 3–83 |

Extent of circadian variation (average of the ratio of the highest to lowest value obtained during the 24 h in each subject expressed in percent of the lowest value) of hematological variables (cells/cc) in a group of 150 clinically healthy, diurnally active American subjects (mean age 24 ± 10 yr, range 11–57 yr) studied in St. Paul, MN, USA. Note the remarkably large variations encountered within the 24-h span in these clinically healthy subjects, which can give rise to diagnostic errors. SD = standard deviation. After Haus et al., 1996 *(148)*.

system/technology of the individual products. Administration-time-differences in theophylline absorption kinetics seem to be key, because the continuous 24-h infusion of aminophylline reveals no circadian rhythmicity in drug elimination *(165)*. Studies of other medications reveal administration-time differences in the absorption kinetics of trans-cutaneously administered lidocaine in children on average 32 mo of age being prepared for minor surgery *(166)*, and in the elimination kinetics of diphenylhydantin (phenytoin) in overdosed epileptic children 6–11 yr of age *(167)*.

Only a very small number of studies have explored rhythm-dependencies in the effects of medications in children. It is the synthetic corticosteroid medications that were first studied extensively for circadian rhythm-dependencies in their adverse effects *(168)*. Low-to-moderate doses of corticotherapy in the morning at the beginning of the diurnal activity span, which corresponds with the peak of the circadian rhythm in endogenous cortisol, minimizes the risk of adrenal suppression and perhaps other adverse effects *(169,170)*. Corticosteroid dosing in the late afternoon or evening results in moderate to severe dose-dependent, administration-time adrenal suppression in adults of all ages and in children *(168,171)*. Indeed, this circadian rhythm-dependent difference in adrenal suppression is the basis for the nighttime administration schedule of synthetic corticosteroid medication to optimize the treatment of congenital adrenal hyperplasia *(172)*. The beneficial effect of corticotherapy in children also depends on the circadian time of treatment. Reinberg and colleagues *(173)* studied a group of 12 asthmatic boys between 7 and 15 yr of age. They demonstrated that the effect of a single large (40 mg) dose of methylprednisolone on airway patency, as assessed by peak expiratory flow, depends strongly on its injection time. The effect of the corticosteroid, improvement of the 24-h mean peak flow rate, is best when timed in the afternoon at 3 PM, about 8–9 h after the customary time of awakening in the morning from nighttime sleep. Administering the medication at 7 AM is also effective, but less so than at 3 PM. In contrast, the single 40-mg dose has little effect when administered either at 7 PM or 3 AM. Beam and colleagues confirmed these findings by a series of trials on steroid-dependent adult asthmatics *(174)*. The effect of a single oral dose of 50 mg prednisone on nocturnal airways patency and inflammation strongly depends on the circadian time of dosing. Ingestion of the large dose of prednisone at 3 PM (again, about 8–9 h after awakening from nighttime sleep) results in the best response. The effect of the large 50 mg prednisone dose in the morning at 8 AM or in the evening at 8 PM is no better than placebo. It has no effect on nighttime airway patency and inflammation.

Circadian rhythm-dependent differences in the therapeutic effects of a few other often-prescribed medications have been demonstrated in young children, mostly between 6 and 15 yr of age. The increase in airway patency in asthmatic children 15 min after inhaling 2 mg of the β-adrenergic brochodialator aerosol medication orciprenaline is greatest when administered in the morning around 8 AM. The effect of the identical dose is only half as great when dosed at 4 PM *(175)*. Studies on the same group of children show that the effect of inhaling 400 μg of the vagolytic aerosol medication ipratropium bromide is also greatest when dosed around 8 AM, but almost without effect when dosed at 10 PM *(175)*. A plasma theophylline concentration–airway patency response relationship is demonstrable at 4 AM, but not at 4 PM *(162,165)*. Finally, Rivard and colleagues *(176,177)* clearly demonstrated that the response of Canadian children 1–17 yr of age to cancer medications varies significantly according to treatment time. The children were treated for acute lymphoblastic leukemia by a protocol consisting of 6-mercaptopurine daily, methotrexate weekly, and vincristine and prednisone monthly. The disease-free survival is significantly better when mercaptopurine and methotrexate are administered in the evening (after 5 PM) than in the morning (before 10 AM). Indeed, long-term follow-up of the children shows the relative risk of relapsing to be more than 2.5-fold greater with morning than with evening treatment. These findings are substantiated by another, larger study of young German children *(178)*.

A number of studies have explored administration-time differences in the kinetics and effects of various classes of antihypertensive medications in normotensive and hypertensive adults, although not in children *(179,180)*. Briefly, studies show several angiotensin converting enzyme, calcium antagonist, and β-agonist medications exert (sometimes profoundly) stronger BP and/or HR-lowering effects during nighttime sleep and/or in the morning upon awakening when dosed in the evening at bedtime compared to when dosed in the morning upon awakening. We are unaware of any studies on children that have addressed dosing-time-dependent differences of the safety and therapeutic efficiency of antihypertensive medications. The circadian pattern of systolic and diastolic BP in normotensive infants, children, and adults is characterized by an accelerated rise upon awakening in the morning, persisting elevation during diurnal activity, a slight drop in the evening, and maximum decline during nighttime sleep. The 24-h pattern is comparable in uncomplicated essential HTN, but is often quite different in HTN secondary to renal disease, endocrine conditions including diabetes, autonomic nervous system dysfunction, and sleep apnea *(2,181,182)*. In both adults and children with secondary HTN, the 24-h BP pattern displays an attenuated decline during sleep, a more or less constant 24-h level, or even reversed waveform (i.e., with highest values during sleep). In adults, certain characteristics of the BP circadian pattern, in particular the extent of the morning rate of the rise, magnitude of the daytime elevation, and extent of the sleep-time decline are determinants of the risk to target organ injury and morning cardiovascular events *(2,183,184)*.

Conventional treatment of HTN primarily involves the prescription of one or more medications of sufficiently long half-life that are said to exert nearly consistent BP-lowering effect throughout the 24 h. A new generation of antihypertensives called chronotherapies has been introduced during the last decade. These medications rely on sophisticated drug-delivery technologies to synchronize the medication level during the 24 h to the circadian pattern of systolic and diastolic BP. The specific goals of these medications are to attenuate the rate of BP acceleration in the morning and to normalize BP level during daytime activity and nighttime sleep *(184)*. Presently, in the US, the marketed chronotherapies for adult HTN include the β-agonist propranolol and the calcium channel blockers verapamil and diltiazem. Only one outcome trial has been initiated to test the advantage of chronotherapy vs conventional therapy in the treatment of HTN. The CONVINCE trial *(185)* compared the effects of verapamil chronotherapy against standard β-blocker and diuretic therapy in the control of HTN and the prevention of morning cardiovascular accidents in adults. Unfortunately, the CONVINCE trial was never completed; it was terminated prematurely because of lack of interest and financing by the takeover company that acquired the product. Data analysis of the outcome variables does not permit valid conclusions about the value of the verapamil chronotherapy for cardiovascular event risk prevention *(186)*. Present pediatric trials of antihypertensive medications are not designed to explore treatment-time differences in their beneficial and adverse effects; moreover, none of the chronotherapeutic formulations currently marketed for adults have been studied in children. Because medications of various classes are affected by the circadian time structure of children and adults, as discussed above, it is reasonable to expect that administration-time-dependent differences are likely in the effects of some classes of antihypertensive medications in children.

## SUMMARY AND CONCLUSIONS

The human circadian time structure is genetically determined. Its origin is a set of oscillator genes whose activity is rather precisely regulated during the 24 h by a transcriptional–translational feedback system in both the central master oscillator located in the SCN of the hypothalamus and in numerous peripheral oscillators located in most cells and tissues throughout the body. The central oscillator is kept in step with our 24-h periodic surroundings through a non-vision-related mechanism in the retina which coordinates the cycling and staging of peripheral oscillators located in the heart, the vascular endothelia, the vascular smooth muscle, the liver, the lung, and the adrenal cortex, among other tissues.

This clock mechanism develops during fetal life, and it, together with transplacentally transmitted time-of-day signals from the mother, determines fetal rhythmicity. The endogenous and maternally induced rhythms of the fetus give rise to circadian differences in the susceptibility to toxic agents and, most likely, therapeutic interventions. These circadian susceptibilities are superimposed on the better-known fetal-stage-dependent differences in vulnerability. The type and severity of embryopathies owing to fetal toxicity is, in experimental models, determined by the interaction of both the circadian time and the developmental stage of exposure *(81,82)*.

At the time of birth, the newborn is suddenly separated from its inter-uterine environment in which synchronizing signals are provided from the mother via the placenta. The ambient environment presents a foreign set of time cues, resulting in an initial disruption or even loss of circadian synchronization. The circadian oscillator system is not yet mature in normal-term newborns, and it is even less mature in preterm newborns. At birth, high-frequency ultradian rhythms predominate over circadian rhythms. After birth, two processes together determine the establishment of the circadian time organization. One is the ongoing maturation process of the oscillator system, and the other is time structure synchronization provided by the 24-h cycle of light and dark, feeding, and handling, among other periodic aspects of the infant's environment and care regimen. The development of the circadian time organization seems to be dependent on the strength of the 24-h periodic inputs by the nurturing environment; the stronger the inputs, the faster the development of the circadian time structure. Accordingly, many recommend that hospital nurseries be outfitted with a day–night alternating light–dark schedule like that of the natural environment, and that care patterns be redesigned to mimic the diurnal activity–nocturnal sleep routine characteristic of the human species.

Most clinicians, including pediatricians, know little about the circadian time structure or of its relevance to clinical medicine. The field of chronobiology (biological rhythm study) has much to contribute. Several medical conditions display day–night patterns in pathophysiology and symptom intensity in infants and adolescents *(184,187)*. Sudden infant death syndrome (SIDS), which shows the highest incidence at a time when circadian rhythmicity in the infants is evolving, is most frequent in the early morning hours *(188)*. The symptoms of allergic rhinitis are most problematic overnight and in the morning, and exacerbations of asthma are much more frequent and severe during the night than daytime *(163,189)*. Inherited circadian sleep disorders—e.g., delayed sleep phase insomnia and non-24-h sleep–wake cycling—are discernable early in childhood, although they may not be fully appreciated by parents and pediatricians until the age of formal schooling *(190,191)*. Reference values that are time-qualified for circadian rhythm facilitate the accurate interpretation of laboratory studies involving variables that display large circadian change by helping to distinguish between values that are indicative of normal variation and abnormal values indicative of illness. Time-qualified reference values for the 24-h patterns of diastolic and systolic BP have been developed and used by some to better differentiate normotension from HTN in adults *(192)*. They have yet to be accepted and applied in clinical medicine, however. Time-qualified reference values are now being developed for application to infants and children. A substantial number of studies, primarily involving young adults, and fewer studies involving children between 6 and 17 yr of age, clearly demonstrate that the therapeutic efficiency and, in some instances, safety of commonly prescribed medications may be compromised if administered at the wrong biological time. Moreover, in children and adults, the side effects of a medication may be the disruption and desynchronization of the circadian time structure *(193,194)*, evidenced by abnormality of sleep–wake cycle and/or other complaints as reviewed elsewhere *(194)*. The incidence of this newly recognized adverse effect is unknown, because it is not taken into account in clinical trials of medications on adults and children.

The pharmaceutical industry has only recently shown an interest in conducting clinical trials that assess the effects of prescription medications on children. At this time, we know nothing about administration-time differences in the behavior and effects of antihypertensive and most other medications commonly prescribed for children. Nonetheless, it is entirely possible that the results of clinical trials on medications involving dosing at a specified time of day (e.g., morning) will not be indicative of the effectiveness and safety of the same medications when administered at a different time of day (e.g., evening). Adherence entails taking the right medication in the correct dose at the designated time of day as specified by the information contained in package inserts. In everyday life, especially in school-age children, medications may be dosed at times other than those specified. We recommend that potential drug-administration differences in the safety and/or efficiency of medications be assessed, at least in representative subgroups, in future trials.

## REFERENCES


1. Pickering G, Schwartz JE, Stone A. Behavioral influences on diurnal blood pressure rhythms. In: Portaluppi F, Smolensky MH, eds. Time-Dependent Structure and Control of Arterial Blood Pressure. NY Acad of Sci 1996;783:132–140.
2. Portaluppi F, Smolensky MH. Circadian rhythm and environmental determinants of blood pressure regulation in normal and hypertension conditions. In: White B, ed. Blood Pressure Monitoring in Cardiovascular Medicine and Therapeutics. Totowa, NJ: Humana Press, 2001;79–138.
3. Reppert SM, Weaver DR. Molecular analysis of mammalian circadian rhythms. Ann Rev. Physiol 2001;63: 647–676.
4. Dunlap JC. Molecular bases for cellular clocks. Cell 1999;96:271–290.
5. Shearman LP, Sriram S, Weaver DR, et al. Interacting molecular loops in the mammalian circadian clock. Science 2000;288:1013–1019.
6. Bjarnason GA, Jordan RCK, Wood PA, et al. Circadian expression of clock genes in human oral mucosa and skin. Am J Path 2001;158:1793–1800.
7. Benson DM, Dunn FA, Takao M. Phototransduction by retinal ganglion cells that set the circadian clock. Science 2002;295:1070–1073.
8. Ruby NF, Brennan TJ, Sie M, et al. Role of melanopsin in circadian responses to light. Science 2002;298: 2211–2216.
9. Basalobre A, Brown SA, Marcacci L, et al. Resetting of circadian time in peripheral tissues by glucocorticoid signaling. Science 2000;289:2344–2347.
10. Yamazaki S, Numano R, Abe M, et al. Resetting central and peripheral circadian oscillators in transgenic rats. Science 2000;288:682–685.
11. Kawara S, Mydlarski R, Mamelak AJ, et al. Low-dose ultraviolet B rays alter the mRNA expression of the circadian clock genes in cultured human keratinocytes. J Invest Dermatol 2002;119:1220–1223.
12. Lindblom N, Hatonen T, Laakso M, Alila-Johansson A, Laipio M, Turpemen U. Bright light exposure of a large skin area does not affect melatonin or bilirubin levels in humans. Biol Psychiatry 2000;48:1098–1104.
13. Wright KP Jr, Czeisler CA. Absence of circadian phase resetting in response to bright light behind the knees. Science 2002;297:571.
14. Nonaka H, Emoto N, Ikeda K, et al. Angiotensin II induces circadian gene expression of clock genes in cultured vascular smooth muscle cells. Circulation 2001;104(15):1746–1748.
15. Stokkan K-A, Yamazaki S, Tei H, Sakaki Y, Menaker M. Entrainment of the circadian clock in the liver by feeding. Science 2001;291:490–493.
16. Sakamoto K, Ishida N. Light-induced phase-shift in the circadian expression rhythm of mammalian period genes in the mouse heart. Europ J Neursci 2000;12:4003–4006.
17. Damiola F, Minh NL, Preitner N, Kornmann B, Fleury-Oleba F, Schibler U. Restricted feeding uncouples circadian oscillators in peripheral tissues from the central pacemaker in the suprachiasmatic nucleus. Genes and Development 2000;14:2950–2961.
18. Portmann MA. Molecular clock mechanisms and circadian rhythms intrinsic to the heart. Circulation Research 2001;89(12):1184–1186.
19. Maemura K, Layne MD, Watanabe M, Perrell MA, Nagai R, Lee M. Molecular mechanisms of morning onset of myocardial infarction. Ann NY Acad Sci 2001;947:398–402.
20. Andreotti F, Kluft C. Circadian variation of fibrinolytic activity in blood. Chronobiol Int 1991;8:336–351.
21. Yagita K, Tamanini F, van der Horst GTJ, Okamura H. Molecular mechanisms of the biological clock in cultured fibroblasts. Science 2001;292:278–281.
22. Cohen MC, Rohtla KM, Lavery CE, Muller JE, Mittleman MA. Meta-analysis of the morning excess of acute myocardial infarction and sudden cardiac death. Amer J Cardiol 1997;79:1512–1516.
23. Elliott WJ. Circadian timing in the timing of stroke onset. A meta-analysis. Stroke 29:992–996.
24. Richardson G, Tate B. Hormonal and pharmacological manipulation of the circadian clock: recent developments and future strategies. Sleep 2000;23(Suppl 3):S77–S85.
25. Reppert SM, Weaver DR, Rivkees SA. Maternal communication of circadian phase to the developing mammal. Psychoneuroendocrinology 1988;13:63–78.
26. Reppert SM, Weaver DR, Rivkees SA, Stopa EG. Putative melatonin receptors in a human biological clock. Science 1988;242(4875):78–81.

27. Serón-Ferré M, Ducsay CA, Valenzuela GJ. Circadian rhythms during pregnancy. Endocrine Rev 1993;14(5): 594–609.
28. Silver R, Lehman MN, Gibson M, Gladstone WR, Bittman EL. Dispersed cell suspensions of fetal SCN restore circadian rhythmicity in SCN lesioned adult hamsters. Brain Res 1990;525:45–58.
29. Earnest DJ, Sladek CD, Gash DM, Weigand SJ. Specificity of circadian function in transplants of the fetal suprachiasmatic nucleus. J Neurosci 1989;9:2671–2677.
30. Weaver DR. The suprachiasmatic nucleus: a 25-yr retrospective. J Biol Rhythms 1998;13:100–112.
31. Gillette MU, Tischkau SA. Suprachiasmatic nucleus: the brain's circadian clock. Recent Prog Horm Res 1999; 54:33–58.
32. Rivkees SA, Hao H. Developing circadian rhythmicity. Seminar in Perinatology 2000;24(4):232–242.
33. Reppert SM, Schwartz WJ. Functional activity of the suprachiasmatic nuclei in the fetal primate. Neurosci Lett 1984;46:145–149.
34. Hao H, Rivkees SA. The biological clock of very premature primate infants is responsive to light. Proc Natl Acad Sci USA 1999;96:2426–2429.
35. Rivkees SA, Hofman PL, Fortman J. Newborn primate infants are entrained by low intensity lighting. Proc Natl Acad Sci USA 1997;94:292–297.
36. Swaab DF. Development of the human hypothalamus. Neurochem Res 1995;20:509–519.
37. Weaver DR, Reppert SM. Periodic feeding of SCN-lesioned pregnant rats entrains the fetal biological clock. Brain Res Dev Brain Res 1989;46:291–296.
38. Grosse J, Velickovic A, Davis FC. Entrainment of Syrian hamster circadian activity rhythms by neonatal melatonin injections. Am J Physiol 1996;270:R533–R540.
39. Walsh SW, Ducsay CA, Novy MJ. Circadian hormonal interactions among the mother, fetus and amniotic fluid. Am J Obstet Gynecol 1984;150:745–753.
40. Weaver DR, Rivkees SA, Reppert SM. D1 dopamine receptors activate c-fos expression in the fetal suprachiasmatic nuclei. Proc Natl Acad Sci 1992;89:9201–9204.
41. Shibata S, Moore RY. Development of a fetal circadian rhythm after disruption of the maternal circadian system. Dev Brain Res 1988;41:313–317.
42. Sterman MB. Relationship of intrauterine fetal activity to maternal sleep stage. Exp Neurol 1967;19(Suppl): 98–106.
43. DeVries JIP, Visser GHA, Prechtl HFR. The emergence of fetal behavior. II. Quantitative aspects. Early Hum Dev 1983;12:99–120.
44. Nasello-Paterson C, Natale R, Connors G. Ultrasonic evaluation of fetal body movements over twenty-four hours in the human fetus at twenty-four to twenty-eight weeks' gestation. Am J Obstet Gynecol 1988;158:312–316.
45. Lunshof S, Boer K, Wolf H, van Hoffen G, Bayram N, Mirmiran M. Fetal and maternal diurnal rhythm during the third trimester of normal pregnancy. Am J Obstet Gynecol 1998;178:247–254.
46. Patrick J, Fetherston W, Vick H, Voegelin R. Human fetal breathing movements and gross fetal body movements at weeks 34 to 35 at gestation. Am J Obstet Gynecol 1978;130:693–699.
47. Richardson B, Natale R, Patrick J. Human fetal breathing activity during effectively induced labor at term. Am J Obstet Gynecol 1979;133:247–255.
48. Campbell K. Ultradian rhythms in the human fetus during the last ten weeks of gestation: a review. Semin Perinatol 1980;4:301–309.
49. Boddy K, Dawes GS. Fetal breathing. J Physiol 1974;243:559–603.
50. Patrick J, Challis J. Measurement of human fetal breathing movements in healthy pregnancies using a real-time scanner. Semin Perinatol 1980;4(4):275–286.
51. Patrick J, Campbell K, Carmichael L, Probert C. Influence of maternal HR and gross fetal body movements on the daily pattern of fetal HR near term. Am J Obstet Gynecol 1982;144:533–538
52. Visser GHA, Goodman JDS, Levine DH, Dawes GS. Diurnal and other cyclic variations in human fetal heart rate near term. Am J Obstet Gynecol 1982;142:535–544.
53. Visser GHA, Carse EA, Goodman JDS, Johnson P. A comparison of episodic heart-rate patterns in the fetus and newborn. Br J Obstet Gynecol 1982;89;50–55.
54. Happenbrowers T, Ugartechca JC, Combs D, Hodgman JE, Harpe RM, Sterman MB. Studies of maternal-fetal interaction during the last trimester of pregnancy: ontogenesis of the basic rest-activity cycle. Exp Neurol 1978;61:136–153.

55. Dalton KJ, Denman DW, Dawson AJ, Hoffman HJ. Ultradian rhythms in human fetal HR: a computerized time series analysis. Int J Biomed Comput 1986;18:45–60.
56. Chamberlain PF, Manning FA, Morrison I, Lange IR. Circadian rhythm in bladder volumes in the term human fetus. Obstetrics and Gynecology 1984;64:657–660.
57. Townsley JD, Dubin IVH, Grannis GF, Gortman J, Crystle CD. Circadian rhythms of serum and urinary estrogens in pregnancy. J Clin Endocrinol 1973;36:289–295.
58. Honnebier MBOM, Swaab DF, Mirmiran M. Diurnal rhythmicity during early human development. In: Reppert SM, ed. Development of Circadian Rhythmicity and Photoperiodism in Mammals. Ithaca: Perinatology, 1989;221–244.
59. Meis PJ, Buster JE, Kundu N, Magyar D, Marshall JR, Halberg F. Individualized cosinor assessment of circadian hormonal variation in third trimester human pregnancy. Chronobiologia 1983;10:1–11.
60. Meis PJ. Chronobiology of pregnancy and the perinatal time span. In: Touitou Y, Haus E, eds. Biologic Rhythms in Clinical and Laboratory Medicine. New York: Springer-Verlag, 1992;158–166.
61. Patrick J, Challis J, Natale R, Richardson B. Circadian rhythms in maternal plasma cortisol, estrone, estradiol and estriol at 34 to 35 weeks' gestation. Am J Obstet Gynecol 1979;135:791–798.
62. Patrick J, Challis J, Campbell K, Carmichael L, Richardson B, Tevaarwerk G. Effects of synthetic glucocorticoid administration on human fetal breathing movements at 34 to 35 weeks' gestational age. Am J Obstet Gynecol 1981;139:324–328.
63. Challis JRG, Patrick J, Richardson B, Tevaarwerk G. Loss of diurnal rhythm in plasma estrone, estradiol, and estriol in women treated with synthetic glucocorticoids at 34 to 35 weeks' gestation. Am J Obstet Gynecol 1981;139:338–343.
64. Arduini D, Rizzo G, Parlati E, et al. Modification of ultradian and circadian rhythms of fetal heart rate after fetal-maternal adrenal gland suppression: a double blind study. Prenat Diagn 1986;6:409–417.
65. Arduini D, Rizzo G, Parlati E, dell' Acqua S, Romanini C, Mancuso S. Loss of circadian rhythms of fetal behavior in a totally adrenalectomized pregnant women. Gynecol Obstet Invest 1987;23:226–229.
66. Wilf-Miron R, Peleg L, Goldman B, Ashkenazi IE. Rhythms of enzymatic activity in maternal and umbilical cord blood. Experientia 1992;48:520–523.
67. Riffo R, Germain AM, Wild R, Badia J, Vergara M, Serón-Ferré M. The human term fetus produces cortisol in a circadian fashion. Program of the 71st Annual Meeting of The Endocrine Society, Seattle, WA: 1989;157 (Abstract).
68. Germain AM, Correa R, Wild R, Bustos L, Vergara M, Serón-Ferré M. Adrenal function during a 24 hour period in human term fetuses. Program of the 36th Annual Meeting of the Society for Gynecologic Investigation, San Diego, CA: 1989;116 (Abstract).
69. Yaginuma T. Possible circadian periodicity of foetal prolactin secretion in late gestation. Acta Endocrinol (Copenh) 1981;98:106–111.
70. Correa R, Germain AM, Wild R, Vergara M, González A, Serón-Ferré M. Plasma concentration of cortisol and prolactin during a 24 hour period in human term fetuses. Program of the Liggins Symposium of Fetal Physiology and Medicine. Rotorua, New Zealand: 1988;38 (Abstract).
71. Isaacson RJ. Investigation of some of the factors involved in the closure of the secondary palate. Thesis, University of Minnesota, Minneapolis, 1959.
72. Sauerbier I. Circadian variation in teratogenic response to dexamethasone in mice. Drug Chem Toxicol 1986;9:25–31.
73. Clayton DL, Mullen AW, Barnett CC. Circadian modification of drug-induced teratogenesis in rat fetuses. Chronobiologia 1975;2:210–217.
74. Sauerbier I. Circadian modification of 5-fluorouracil-induced teratogenesis in mice. Chronobiol Int 1986;3: 161–164.
75. Schmidt R. Zur zirkadianen Modifikation der pränataltoxischen Wirkung von Cyclophosphamid. Biol Rundsch 1978;16:243–248.
76. Sauerbier I. Circadian system and teratogenicity of cytostatic drugs. Prog Clin Res 1981;59C:143–149.
77. Sauerbier I. Embryotoxishe Wirkung von Zytostatika in Abhängigkeit von der Tageszeit der Applikation bei Mäusen. Verh Anat Ges 1983;77:147–149.
78. Endo A, Sakai N, Ohwada K. Analysis of diurnal differences in teratogen (Ara-C) susceptibility in mouse embryos by a progressive phase-shift method. Teratogensis Carcinog Mutagen 1987;7:475–482.
79. Sauerbier I. Circadian modification of ethanol damage in utero in mice. Am J Anat 1987;178:170–174.

80. Sauerbier I. Circadian influence on ethanol-induced intrauterine growth retardation in mice. Chronobiol Int 1988;5:211–216.
81. Sauerbier I. Rhythms in drug-induced teratogenesis. In: Touitou Y, Haus E, eds. Biologic Rhythms in Clinical and Laboratory Medicine. New York: Springer-Verlag, 1992;151–157.
82. Sauerbier I. Embryotoxicity of drugs: possible mechanisms of action. In: Lemmer B, ed. Chronopharmacology. Cellular and Biochemical Interactions. New York: Dekker, 1989;683–697.
83. Hales BF, Slott VL. The role of reactive metabolites in drug-induced teratogenesis. Prog Clin Biol Res 1987;253:181–191.
84. Sturtevant RP, Garber SL. Circadian exposure to ethanol affects the severity of cerebellar cell dysgenesis. Anat Rec 1985;211:187.
85. Halberg F, Wang Z, Cornélissen G, et al. SIDS about-weekly patterns in vital signs of premature babies. In: Yoshikawa M, Uono M, Tanabe H, Ishikawa S, eds. New Trends in Autonomic Nervous System Research: Basic and Clinical Interpretations. Selected Proc 20th Int Cong Neurovegetative Research, Tokyo, Sept 10–14, 1990. Amsterdam: Excerpta Medica, 1990;581–585.
86. Syutkina EV, Cornélissen G, Halberg F, et al. Effects lasting into adolescence of exposure to Betamimetics In Utero. Clin Drug Invest 1995;354–362.
87. Otsuka K, Cornélissen G, Halberg F. Elevado riesgo de nefropatias en normotensos con excesive amplitud circadiena de la tension arterial (TA). IV Reunion Nacional de Grupos de Chronobiologia, La Coruna, Spain. 1994;67–68 (Abstract).
88. Halberg F, Cornélissen G, Wilson D, Ferencz C. Circadian systolic amplitude separates boys of parents with or without a high blood pressure. Int Symp Chronobiology and VI Conf Indian Soc Chronobiology, Osmania University, Hyderabad, India, Nov 19–21, 1986;23–24.
89. Halberg F, Cornélissen G, Bingham C, et al. Neonatal monitoring to assess risk for hypertension. Postgrad Med 1986;79:44–46.
90. Scarpelli PT, Marz W, Cornélissen G, et al. Blood pressure self-measurement in schools for rhythmometric assessment of hyperbaric impact to gauge pressure "excess." Proceedings of the International Symposium Ambulatory Monitoring: March 29–30, 1985, Padua, CLEUP Editore. 1986;229–237.
91. Hellbrügge T. The development of circadian rhythms in infants. Cold Spring Harbor Symp on Quant Bio 1960;25:311–323.
92. Updike PA, Accurso FJ, Jones RH. Physiologic circadian rhythmicity in preterm infants. Nursing Res 1985; 34:160–163.
93. Mirmiran M, Kok JH. Circadian rhythms in early human development. Early Human Dev 1991;26:121–128.
94. Rivkees SA, Reppert RM. Perinatal development of day-night rhythms in humans. Horm Res 1992;37(Suppl 3):99–104.
95. Jundell J. Über die nykthemeralen Temperaturschwankungen im I Lebensjahr des Menschen. J Kinderhk 1904;59:521–619.
96. Hellbrügge T. The development of circadian and ultradian rhythms of premature and full term infants. In: Scheving LE, Halberg F, Pauly JE, eds. Chronobiology. Tokyo: Igaku Shoin, 1974;339–341.
97. Abe K, Fukui S. The individual development of circadian temperature rhythm in infants. J Interdisc Cycle Res 1979;10:227–232.
98. D'Souza SW, Tenreiro S, Minors D, Chiswick ML, Sims DG, Waterhouse J. Skin temperature and HR rhythms in infants of extreme prematurity. Arch Dis Child 1992;67(7 Spec No.):784–788.
99. Hellbrügge T, Ehrengut Lange J, Rutenfranz J, Stehr K. Circadian periodicity of physiological functions in different stages of infancy and childhood. Ann NY Acad Sci 1964;117:361–373.
100. Glotzbach SF, Edgar DM, Boeddiker M, Ariagno RL. Biological rhythmicity in normal infants during the first 3 months of life. Pediatrics 1994;94(4 Pt 1):482–488.
101. Glotzbach SF, Edgar DM, Ariagno RL. Biological rhythmicity in preterm infants prior to discharge from neonatal intensive care. Pediatrics 1995;95:231–237.
102. Mirmiran M, Lunshof S. Perinatal development of human circadian rhythms. Progr in Brain Res 1996;111: 217–226.
103. Anders TF, Keener M. Developmental course of night-time sleep-wake patterns in full-term and premature infants during the first year of life. I. Sleep 1985;8:173–192.
104. Kleitman N, Engelmann TG. Sleep characteristics of infants. J Appl Physiol 1953;6:269–282.
105. Kleitman N. Sleep and wakefulness. Chicago: University of Chicago, 1963.

106. Parmelee AH Jr. Sleep cycles in infants. Dev Med Child Neurol 1969;11:794–795.
107. Menna-Barreto L, Benedito-Silva AA, Marques N, Morato de Andrade MM, Louzada F. Ultradian components of the sleep-wake cycle in babies. Chronobiol Int 1993;10:103–108.
108. Sander LW, Stechler G, Burns P, Julia H. Early mother-infant interaction and 24-hour patterns of activity and sleep. J Am Acad Child Psychiatry 1970;9:103–123.
109. Martin du Pan R. Some clinical applications of our knowledge of the evolution of the circadian rhythm in infants. In: Scheving LE, Halberg F, Pauly JE, eds. Chronobiology. Tokyo: Igaku Shoin, 1974;138–144.
110. Halberg F, Diffley M, Stein M, Panofsky H, Adkins G. Computer techniques in the study of biologic rhythms. NY Acad of Sciences 1964;115(2):695–720.
111. Halberg F, Ulstrom RA. Morning changes in number of circulating eosinophils in infants. Acta Paediatr 1952;50:160–170.
112. Beitins IZ, Kowarski A, Migeon CJ, Graham GG. Adrenal function in normal infants and in marasmus and kwashiorkor. Cortisol secretion, diurnal variation of plasma cortisol, and urinary excretion of 17-hydroxycorticoids, free corticoids, and cortisol. J Pediatr 1975;86(2):302–308.
113. Onishi S, Miyazawa G, Nishimura Y, et al. Postnatal development of circadian rhythm in serum cortisol levels in children. Pediatrics 1983;72:399–404.
114. Price DA, Close GC, Fielding BA. Age of appearance of circadian rhythm in salivary cortisol values in infancy. Arch Dis Child 1983;58:454–456.
115. Vermes I, Dohanics J, Toth G, Pongracz J. Maturation of the circadian rhythm of the adrenocortical functions in human neonates and infants. Horm Res 1980;12:237–244.
116. Spangler G. The emergence of adrenocortical circadian function in newborns and infants and its relationship to sleep, feeding and maternal adrenocortical activity. Early Hum Dev 1991;25:197–208.
117. Zurbrügg RP. Hypothalamic-pituitary-adrenocortical regulation: a contribution to its assessment, development and disorders in infancy and childhood with special reference to plasma circadian rhythm. Monographs in paediatrics, Vol 7. Basel: Karger, 1976.
118. Kennaway DJ, Stamp GE, Goble FC. Development of melatonin production in infants and the impact of prematurity. J Clin Endocrinol Metab 1992;75:361–369.
119. Kennaway DJ, Goble FC, Stamp GE. Factors influencing the development of melatonin rhythmicity in humans. J Clin Endocrinol Metab 1996;81:1525–1532.
120. Attanasio A, Borrelli P, Gupta D. Circadian rhythms in serum melatonin from infancy to adolescence. J Clin Endocrinol Metab 1995;61:388–390.
121. Sisson TRC, Root AW, Kendall N. Biologic rhythm of plasma human growth hormone in newborns of low birth weight. In: Scheving LE, Halberg F, Pauly JE, eds. Chronobiology. Igaku Shoin. Tokyo: 1974; 348–352.
122. Anderson S, Cornélissen G, Halberg F, et al. Age effects upon the harmonic structure of human blood pressure in clinical health. Proc 2nd Ann IEEE Symp on Computer-Based Medical Systems. Minneapolis, June 26–27, 1989. Washington DC: Computer Society Press, 1989;238–243.
123. Halberg F, Halberg E, Halberg J, et al. Womb to tomb blood pressure monitoring: are single or even 24 hour measurements enough? Proc Assn Adv Med Instr, Washington DC, May 11–15, 1991;38.
124. Cornélissen G, Haus E, Halberg F. Chronobiologic blood pressure assessment from womb to tomb. In: Touitou Y, Haus E, eds. Biologic Rhythms in Clinical and Laboratory Medicine. New York: Springer-Verlag, 1992;428–452.
125. Cornélissen G, Sitka U, Tarquini B, et al. Chronobiologic approach to blood pressure during pregnancy and extra-uterine life. Prog Clin Bio Res 1990;341A:585–594.
126. Hillman DC, Wang ZR, Rigatuso J, et al. Circadian-circaseptan ratios for vital signs and ventilation in human prematurity. Biochim Clin 1991;15:151–154.
127. Wu J, Cornélissen G, Tarquini B, et al. Circaseptan and circannual modulation of circadian rhythms in neonatal blood pressure and heart rate. In: Hayes DK, Pauly JE, Reiter RJ, eds. Chronobiology: Its Role in Clinical Medicine, General Biology, and Agriculture, Part A. New York: Wiley-Liss, 1990;643–652.
128. Wrbsky P, Mills M, Cornélissen G, Johnson D, Halberg F. Circadian and circaseptan variations of systolic blood pressure (SBP) and heart rate (HR) in preterm babies. Chronobiologia 1993;20:135–136.
129. Marazzi A, Wang Z, Paccaud F, Hillman DC, Cornélissen G, Halberg F. Circadian, circaseptan and secular variation in human birth and stillbirth. Abstract, 2nd World Conf on Clinical Chronobiology, Monte Carlo, April 10–13, 1990. Chronobiologia 1990;17:1777.

130. Halberg F, Cornélissen G, Kopher R, et al. Chronobiologic blood pressure and ECG assessment by computer in obstetrics, neonatology, cardiology and family practice. In: Computers and Perinatal Medicine. Proc 2nd World Symp Computers in the Care of the Mother, Fetus, and Newborn, Kyoto, Japan, Dec 23–26, 1989. Amsterdam: Excerpta Medica, 1990;3–18.
131. Cornélissen G, Wilson D, Halberg F, Ferencz F. Age and sex effects upon circadian characteristics in children of parents with and without high blood pressure. Int Symp Chronobiology and VI Conf Indian Soc Chronobiology, Osmania University, Hyderabad, India, Nov 19–21, 1986;25–27.
132. Wang Z, Sun X, Cornélissen G, et al. Doppler flowmeter-assessed circadian rhythms in neonatal cardiac function, family history and intrauterine growth retardation. Am J Perinatology 1993;10:119–125.
133. Rivkees SA. Developing circadian rhythmicity. Pediatrics Clinics North Am 1997;44:467–487.
134. Mann NP, Haddow R, Stokes L, Goodley S, Rutter N. Effect of night and day on preterm infants in a newborn nursery: randomized trial. Br Med J (Clin Res Ed) 1986;293(6557):1265–1267.
135. Miller CL, White R, Whitman TL, O'Callaghan MF, Maxwell SE. The effects of cycled versus non-cycled lighting on growth and development in preterm infants. Infant Behavior and Development 1995;18:87–95.
136. Miller CL, White R, Whitman TL. The effect of cycled versus non-cycled lighting on the growth and development or preterm infants. Infant Behav Devel 1995;18:95–102.
137. Sander LW, Julia HL, Stechler G, et al. Continuous 24-hour interactional monitoring in infants reared in two caretaking environments. Psychosom Med 1972;34:270–282.
138. Miller WL, Styne DM. Female puberty and its disorders. In: Yen SSC, Jaffe RB, Barbieri RL, eds. Reproductive Endocrinology. Philadelphia: WB Sanders, 1999;388–412.
139. Veldhuis JD. Male hypothalamic pituitary-gonadal axis. In: Yen SSC, Jaffe RB, Barbieri RL, eds. Reproductive Endocrinology. Philadelphia: WB Sanders, 1999;622–631.
140. Debry G, Bleyer R, Reinberg A. Circadian, circannual and other rhythms in spontaneous nutrient and caloric intake in healthy 4-yr olds. Diabete Metabolisme (Paris) 1975;1:91–99.
141. Reinberg O, Reinberg A, Téhard B, Mechkouri M. Accidents in children do not happen at random: predictable time-of-day incidence of childhood trauma. Chronobiol Int 2002;19(3):615–631.
142. Montagner H, de Roquefeuil G, Djakovic M. Biological, behavioral and intellectual activity rhythms of the child during its development in different educational environments. In: Touitou Y, Haus E, eds. Biologic Rhythms in Clinical and Laboratory Medicine. New York: Springer-Verlag, 1992;214–229.
143. Haus E, Nicolau GY, Lakatua D, Sackett-Lundeen L. Reference values for chronopharmacology. Ann Rev Chronopharmacol 1988;4:333–424.
144. Nelson WL, Tong YL, Lee JK, Halberg F. Methods for cosinor rhythmometry. Chronobiologia 1979;6:305–325.
145. Haus E, Touitou Y. Chronobiology in laboratory medicine. In: Touitou Y, Haus E, eds. Biologic Rhythms in Clinical and Laboratory Medicine. New York: Springer-Verlag, 1992;673–708.
146. Haus E, Reinberg A. Chronobiologie clinique: rythmes des valeurs de référence. In: Reinberg A, ed. Chronobiologie Médicale. Paris: Flammarion, 2003;41–64.
147. Nicolau GY, Haus E, Marinesscu I, Lakatua DJ, Sackett-Lundeen L, Petrescu E. Circadian timing of ACTH, beta endorphin, adrenal steroids and testosterone in patients with Adrenogenital Syndrome (21-hydroxylase deficiency). Prog Clin Biol Res 1990;341A:483–491.
148. Haus E. Biologic rhythms in hematology. Path Biol 1996;44 (7):618–630.
149. Haus E, Lakatua D, Swoyer J, Sackett-Lundeen L. Chronobiology in hematology and immunology. Am J Anat 1983;168:467–517.
150. Ticher A, Sackett-Lundeen L, Ashkenazi IE, Haus E. Human circadian time structure in subjects of different gender and age. Chronobiol Int 1994;11(6):349–355.
151. Haus E, Lakatua DJ, Halberg F, et al. Chronobiological studies of plasma prolactin in women in Kyushu, Japan and Minnesota. J Clin Endocr Metab 1980;51:632–640.
152. Haus E, Halberg F, Kawasaki T, et al. Ethnic-geographic differences in the pulsatile secretion of cortisol and prolactin in Japanese and American Women. Presented at the 1st World Congress of Chronobiology, Sept 9–12, 2003, Sapporo, Japan.
153. Kawasaki T, Uezono K, Ueno M, et al. Comparison of circadian rhythms of the renin-angiotensin-aldosterone system and electrolytes in clinically healthy young women in Fukuoka (Japan) and Minnesota (USA). Acta Endocrinol (Copenl.) 1983;102:246–251.
154. Wetterberg L, Halberg F, Halberg E, et al. Circadian characteristics of urinary melatonin from clinically healthy young women at different civilizations disease risks. Acta Med Scandinav 1986;220:71–81.

155. Haus E, Nicolau GY, Lakatua D, et al. Circannual variations in blood pressure, urinary catecholamine excretion, plasma aldosterone and serum sodium, potassium and magnesium in children 11 ± 1.5 yrs of age. In: Advances in Chronobiology: Part B. New York: Liss, 1987;3–19.
156. Haus E, Lakatua DJ, Sackett-Lundeen L, et al. Interaction of circadian, ultradian, and infradian rhythms. In: Touitou Y, ed. Biological Clocks. Amsterdam: Elsevier Science, 1988;141–150.
157. Reinberg A. Clinical chronopharmacology. An experimental basis for chronotherapy. In: Reinberg A, Smolensky MH, eds. Biological rhythms and medicine. Cellular, Metabolic, Physiopathologic, and Pharmacologic Aspects. New York: Springer-Verlag, 1983;211–263.
158. Bélanger PM, Bruguerolle B, Labrecque G. Rhythms in pharmacokinetics; absorption distribution, metabolism and excretion. In: Redfern PH, Lemmer B, eds. Physiology and Pharmacology of Biological Rhythms. Berlin: Springer, 1997;177–204.
159. Lemmer B, ed. Chronopharamcology. Cellular and biochemical interactions. New York: Dekker, 1989.
160. Redfern PH, Lemmer B, eds. Physiology and Pharmacology of Biological Rhythms. Berlin: Springer, 1997.
161. Smolensky MH, Scott PH, Kramer WG. Clinicial significance of day-night differences in serum theophylline concentration with special reference to TheoDur. J Asthma Clin Immunol 1986;78:716–722.
162. Smolensky MH, D'Alonzo GE. Progress in the chronotherapy of nocturnal asthma. In: Redfern PH and Lemmer B, eds. Physiology and Pharmacology of Biological Rhythms. Berlin: Springer, 1997;205–249.
163. Martin RJ, ed. Nocturnal asthma. Mechanisms and treatment. Mt. Kisco, NY: Futura, 1993.
164. Smolensky MH, Scott PH, Harrist RB, et al. Administration-time-dependency of the pharmacokinetic behavior and therapeutic effect of a once-a-day theophylline in asthmatic children. Chronobiol Int 1987;4:435–448.
165. Smolensky MH, Scott PH, Albright D, McGovern JP. Circadian differences in theophylline effect during constant-rate infusion with aminophylline. Ann Rev Chronopharmacol 1986;3:139–142.
166. Bruguerolle B, Giaufre, Prat M. Temporal variations in transcutaneous passage of drugs: the example of lidocaine in children and rats. Chronobiol Int 1991;8:277–282.
167. Garretson LK, Jusko WJ. Diphyenylhydantoin elmination kinetics in overdosed children. Clin Pharmacol Ther 1975;17:481–491.
168. Reinberg A. Chronopharmacology of corticosteroids and ACTH. In: Lemmer B, ed. Chronopharamcology. Cellular and Biochemical Interactions. New York: Dekker, 1989;137.
169. Angeli A. Circadian ACTH-adrenal rhythm in man. In: Aschoff J, Ceresa F, Halberg F, eds. Chronobiological Aspects of Endocrinology. Chronobiologia 1974;1(Suppl 1):253–268.
170. Ceresa F, Angeli A, Boccuzzi G, Molino G. Once-a-day neurally stimulated and basal ACTH secretion phases in man and their responses to corticoid inhibition. J Clin Endocinol Metab 1969;29:1074–1082.
171. Grant SD, Forsham PH, DiRaimondo VC. Suppression of 17-hydroxycorticosteroids in plasma and urine after single and divided doses of triamcinolone. N Engl J Med 1985;273:1115–1118.
172. Moeller H. Chronopharmacology of hydrocortisone and 9-fluorohydrocortisone in the treatment of congential adrenal hyperplasia. Eur J Pediatr 1985;144:370–373.
173. Reinberg A, Halberg F, Faillers C. Circadian timing of methylprednisolone effects in asthmatic boys. Chronobiologia 1974;1:333–347.
174. Beam WR, Weiner DE, Martin RJ. Timing of prednisone and alteration of airways inflammation in nocturnal asthma. Am Rev Respir Dis 1992;146:1524–1530.
175. Gaultier C, Reinberg A, Girard F. Circadian rhythms in lungs resistance and dynamic lung compliance of healthy children. Effects of two bronchodilators. Respir Phsiol 1977;31:169–182.
176. Rivard GE, Infante-Rivard C, Hoyoux C, Champagne J. Maintenance chemotherapy for childhood acute lymphoblastic leukemia better in the evening. Lancet 1985;ii:1264–1266.
177. Rivard GE, Infante-Rivard C, Dresse M-F, Champage J. Circadian time-dependent response of childhood lymphoblastic leukemia to chemotherapy: a long-term follow study of survival. Chronobiol Int 1993;10: 201–204.
178. Schmiegelow K. Impact of morning versus evening schedule for oral methotrexate and 6-mercaptopurine on relapse risk for children with acute lymphoblastic leukemia. Nordic Society for Pediatric Hematology and Oncology (NSPHO). J Pediatr Hematol Oncol 1997;19:102–109.
179. Lemmer B, Poraluppi F. Chronopharmacology of cardiovascular disease. In: Redfern PH, Lemmer B, eds. Physiology and Pharmacology of Biological Rhythms. Berlin: Springer, 1997;251–297.
180. Lemmer B. Cardiovascular chronobiology and chronopharmacology. Importance of timing of dosing. In: White B, ed. Blood pressure monitoring in cardiovascular medicine and therapeutics. Totowa, NJ: Humana, 2001;255–271.

181. Cortelli P, Pierangeli G, Provini F, Plazzi G, Lugaresi E. Blood pressure rhythms in sleep disorders and dysautonomia. In: Portaluppi F, Smolensky MH, eds. Time-dependent structure and control of arterial blood pressure. Ann NY Acad Sci 1996;783:204–221.
182. Anwar YA, White WB. Ambulatory monitoring of blood pressure. Devices, analysis and clinical utility. In: White B, ed. Blood Pressure Monitoring in Cardiovascular Medicine and Therapeutics. Totowa, NJ: Humana, 2001;57–75.
183. Kario K, Pickering TG, Umeda Y, et al. Morning surge in blood pressure as a predictor of silent and cerebrovascular disease in elderly hypertensives. A prospective study. Circulation 2003;107:1401–1406.
184. Smolensky MH, Haus E. Circadian rhythm in clinical medicine with applications to hypertension. Am J Hyperten 2001;14(9, pt 2):S280–S290.
185. Black HR, Elliot WJ, Neaton JD, et al. Rationale and design for the controlled onset verapamil investigation of cardiovascular endpoints (CONVINCE) trial. Control Clin Trials 1998;19:370–390.
186. Black HR, Elliott WJ, Grandits G, et al., CONVINCE Research Group. Principal results of the Controlled Onset Verapamil Investigation of Cardiovascular Endpoints (CONVINCE) trial. JAMA 2003;289:2073–2082.
187. Smolensky MH, Lamberg L. Body Clock Guide to Better Health. NY: Henry Holt, 2000.
188. Kelmanson IA. Circadian variation in the frequency of sudden death syndrome and of sudden death from life-threatening conditions in infants. Chronobiologia 1991;18:181–186.
189. Smolensky MH, Reinberg A, Labrecque G. Twenty-four hour pattern in symptom intensity of viral and allergic rhinitis: treatment implications. J Allergy Clin Immunol 1995;95:1084–1096.
190. Wagner D. Disorders of the circadian sleep/wake cycle. Neurologic Clinics 1996;14:651–670.
191. International classification of sleep disorders: diagnostic and coding manual. American Sleep Disorders Association. Rochester, MN: Davis Publishing, 1997:118–140.
192. Hermida RC, Mojón A, Fernández JR, Ayala DE. Computer-based medical system for the computation of blood pressure excess in the diagnosis of hypertension. Biomed Instrument Technol 1996;30:267–283.
193. Reindl K, Falliers C, Halberg F, Chai H, Hillman D, Nelson W. Circadian acrophase in peak expiratory flow and urinary electrolyte excretion of asthmatic children: phase shifting of rhythms by prednisone given at different circadian system phases. Rass Neurol Veg 1969;23:5–26.
194. Hermesh H, Lemberg H, Abadi J, Dagan Y. Circadian rhythm sleep disorders as a possible side effect of fluvoxamine. CNS Spectrums 2001;6:511–513.

# II

# Assessment of Blood Pressure in Children: Measurement, Normative Data, Epidemiology

# 4 Casual Blood Pressure Measurement Methodology

*Bruce Z. Morgenstern,* MD
*and Lavjay Butani,* MD

***Contents***



## HISTORICAL BACKGROUND

The concept of measuring blood pressure (BP) has significantly evolved over the past two centuries, overcoming the challenge posed by the well-established, but clearly subjective, art of palpation of the pulse for "measures" other than simply determining heart rate (HR). In the US, the BP cuff was introduced by Cushing in Baltimore in 1901, and in Boston in 1903 *(1,2)*, when he returned from a trip to Italy with a version of a Riva-Rocci mercury sphygmomanometer. Recognizing the obstacles to be overcome, Cushing noted, "The belief is more or less prevalent that the powers of observation so markedly developed in our predecessors have, to a large extent, become blunted in us, owing to the employment of instrumental aids to exactness, and the art of medicine consequently has always adopted them with considerable reluctance. *(2)*"

Cook and Briggs, two resident house officers, quickly introduced the new cuff into clinical practice at the Johns Hopkins Hospital *(3)*. They apparently had a single-sized rubber bladder covered by a canvas case that was fitted with hook and eye attachments so that it could be "fitted to any arm from that of an infant to that of a large adult." Interestingly, despite the one-size fits-all bladder, they felt that arm size was a "very small factor" in obtaining pressure using their device. They reported the first "normal" values in children, systolic BPs between 75 and 90 mmHg during the first 2 yr of life and 90–110 mmHg during early childhood. This compared with their reported normal systolic BP of 130 mmHg in young adult males, and 115–120 mmHg

From: *Clinical Hypertension and Vascular Disease: Pediatric Hypertension*
Edited by: R. J. Portman, J. M. Sorof, and J. R. Ingelfinger © Humana Press Inc., Totowa, NJ

in young women. In their extensive report, they demonstrated BP responses during surgery, shock, hemorrhage, postoperative recovery, obstetrics, hypertension, and sepsis. They also documented the response of BP to pressor agents and volume *(3)*. It should be noted that this early technique was based on palpation of the brachial pulse.

At roughly the same time, Korotkoff was describing sounds that could be heard by placing a stethoscope over the brachial artery at the elbow below a BP cuff as the cuff pressure was slowly released (Korotkoff NC, as translated in ref. *4*). The original report by Korotkoff was in fact only one paragraph long, followed by a discussion. This auscultatory method was rapidly adopted with data in adults from the US reported in 1910 *(5)*.

The value of BP determination was quickly recognized; by 1925 the first reports of the association between BP and mortality among US life insurance policyholders appeared *(6)*. Despite this, coordinated studies of BP in children were slow to be developed. The Specialized Centers of Research-Atherosclerosis (SCOR-A) studies in Bogalusa, LA, Miami, FL, and Muscatine, IA were among the earliest, starting in the late 1960s and early 1970s *(6)*. These studies were all based on the auscultatory method.

## IMPORTANCE OF BLOOD PRESSURE MEASUREMENT

The critical need for a standard methodology for BP measurement in children stems from the recognition that both high BP and frank hypertension are pervasive problems in the present era *(7)*. The Third National Health and Nutrition Examination Survey (NHANES) showed the prevalence of frank hypertension (BP > 140/90 mmHg) in adults in the US to be as high as 25%, with an even higher prevalence of suboptimal BP *(7)*. While the epidemiology of childhood hypertension is less well-defined, the reported prevalence of pediatric hypertension varies from a low of 0.8% *(8)* to a high of 5% *(9)*. Notwithstanding the lower prevalence of hypertension in children, the clinical impact of BP monitoring in children should by no means be considered negligible. This is based on the premise that BP tracks from childhood into adulthood and that, with intervention, the long-term adverse consequences of hypertension are almost entirely preventable. Tracking, which will be addressed in a subsequent chapter in greater detail, is defined as the tendency of an individual to maintain his or her percentile rank for a given parameter with age. While there is ongoing controversy as to how predictive childhood BP, as measured by casual methods, is for adult hypertension, it certainly appears that children who might be expected to be at greatest risk of cardiovascular complications—i.e., those with persistently elevated BP readings, high body mass index, excessive weight gain, and a family history of hypertension, especially in the older age groups—have higher coefficients of tracking of BP into adulthood, and are, therefore, more likely to remain hypertensive as adults *(10–12)*. Moreover, childhood BP remains, to date, the strongest identified predictor of adult hypertension *(13)*.

Extrapolating from the adult medical literature, it has long been believed that children with hypertension are at high risk of long-term morbidity and mortality. Clearly high BP, and even less than "optimal" BP *(14)* in adults has been shown to be a risk factor for cardiovascular morbidity (heart failure and myocardial infarction) *(15,16)*, cerebrovascular events (stroke) *(17)*, and end-stage renal disease *(18)*. Not only that, studies in both adults *(19)* and children *(20)* have demonstrated that hypertension is an important marker. Its presence is strongly associated with the co-existence of other metabolic abnormalities such as dyslipidemia, obesity, and insulin resistance, all of which compound the risk of cardiovascular and cerebrovascular morbidity. Even if one considers the link between childhood BP and adult hypertension suspect, the more short-term adverse effects of severe hypertension (which is often clinically silent) on organ function can lead to life-threatening complications, such as aortic dissection *(21)*, intra-cranial hemorrhage, heart failure *(22)*, and encephalopathy *(23)*. Left ventricular hypertrophy is a less devastating, but possibly equally worrisome, effect of hypertension, and a major risk factor for morbid cardiac events in adults *(24)*.

When one considers that hypertension is prevalent in epidemic proportions in adults, that its origins can be traced back, at least to some extent, to childhood, and that it is associated with adverse short- and long-term consequences (most of which, hypothetically, can be prevented with early detection and treatment), it should come as no surprise that periodic and accurate measurement of BP is of critical importance. Recognizing the importance of BP monitoring, the National Heart, Lung, and Blood Institute (NHLBI) and the American Academy of Pediatrics (AAP) have long advocated routine monitoring of BP in all children above the age of 3 yr on an annual basis *(25)*, or at least at the time of routine examinations. Consequently, BP measurements in children have become commonplace. However, at the same time, so has the number of different devices being employed for its measurement, causing confusion and lack of uniformity in the method of BP determination. This raises important questions regarding the validity and accuracy of these devices, and also highlights the need for a standardized means of testing and monitoring their performance to avoid errors in measurement that could have egregious consequences.

The use of the term "casual" in this chapter refers to the more conventional practice of obtaining BP readings on an episodic or intermittent basis, such as readings during an office visit, as opposed to the more "continuous" technique of ambulatory BP monitoring, which is addressed in a more comprehensive manner in a later chapter.

## GENERAL ISSUES IN THE MEASUREMENT OF BLOOD PRESSURE

There are certain general issues in the measurement of BP that apply to both children and adults. These are discussed quite thoroughly in the American Heart Association (AHA) Guidelines for the Measurement of BP *(26)* and a review by Gillman *(27)*. Basically, these issues can be categorized into those that relate to the equipment, the patient, and the observer.

### *Equipment*

Obviously, the equipment must be maintained, calibrated, and functional. All devices for measuring BP require ongoing maintenance. Even mercury columns can be inaccurate *(28)*.

Perhaps the most important source of error related to the equipment in the measuring process pertains to selection of the proper size cuff. This remains an area of controversy, since most suggestions as to what constitutes an appropriate cuff size are based on a great deal of opinion and very limited evidence. The present viewpoint is that the "proper" cuff is one in which the inflatable bladder either has a width which is at least 38% of the arm circumference and/or a length that encircles at least 90% of the upper arm, if not the entire upper arm *(27)*. The British have suggested that three cuffs with bladders measuring 4 × 13 cm, 10 × 18 cm, and the adult dimensions 12 × 26 cm are sufficient for the range of arm sizes likely to be encountered in children from 0–14 yr of age *(29)*. This degree of standardization of commercially available cuffs is not the case in the US. It is interesting to note that the British cuffs have width:length ratios that (1) are variable and (2) would not allow the combination of a width:arm circumference ratio of 0.4 at the same time that they allow a length:arm circumference ratio of 0.9–1.0.

It is well established that undercuffing, i.e., the use of too small a cuff, leads to erroneously high BP measurements. Less well established is the converse, overcuffing. A few papers suggest that a cuff that is too large for the arm will underestimate true BP. Too large in this context generally implies widths that exceed the recommended 0.38–0.4 ratio to arm circumference. Overly long cuffs, which of necessity will overlap, do not seem to generate significant errors *(27,30)*.

The problem of cuff size selection is aggravated by the lack of standards in the US. Although the Association for the Advancement of Medical Instrumentation (AAMI) and AHA standards call for cuffs that allow a cuff width to arm circumference ratio of 0.4, and also call for a bladder length to arm circumference ratio of 0.8, they do not take the logical step of establishing a minimal bladder width to length ratio of 0.5. As a result of the lack of standards, there is a wide variability in commercially available cuffs that are designed for children. In a 1996 survey of BP cuff manufacturers by one of the authors (BZM), cuff sizes, given names suggesting the population for which they were intended, were tabulated (Table 1).

### *Patient Factors*

Several issues relating to the patient are seemingly self-evident and therefore often overlooked. For a proper BP measurement, the subject should have sat calmly for 5 min, and not have used caffeine or tobacco products for at least 30 min (alcohol and food are also often included on this list). In addition, the use of vasoactive medications should be noted. In children, this includes decongestants, while for adolescents nutritional supplements, some of which contain ephedrine or related compounds, should be kept in mind.

It has been established in adults, and extrapolated to children, that the proper position for the patient during BP measurements is sitting, with the back supported and the feet flat on the floor. Of course, for infants and toddlers, the supine posture, by necessity, is also appropriate *(27)*. The arm to be used should be elevated to heart level *(26)*. Blood pressures also vary with time of day and ambient room temperature *(27)*.

**Table 1**
**Commercially Available BP Cuffs for Infants and Children in 1996**

| | *Newborn/Premature* | |
|---|---|---|
| *Company* | *Cuff (W × L)* | *Bladder (W × L)* |
| W.A./TYCOS | 5.3 × 18.8 | |
| BAUM | 4.5 × 23 | 2.5 × 5 |
| SICOA | 5.2 × 18 | 4 × 8 |
| GRAHAM FIELD | 5.2 × 18.5 | 4 × 8 |
| KOSAN/BRESCO | 5.5 × 20 (prem) | 4 × 9 |
| | 4 × 15 (sm prem) | 2.5 × 7 |
| K-T-K | 5 × 23 | |
| | 5 × 16 | |
| RIESTER | 5 × 15.5 (NB) | 3 × 5 |
| ERKA | 4.5 × 25 | 2.5 × 15 |
| CREST-PYMA | | 2.8 × 8.4 |
| ACCOSON | | 2.5 × 10.2 |

(continued)

## *Observer*

There are many device/method-specific issues that relate to the observer. Suffice it to state that the observer needs to be trained in the proper use of the device and understand the method sufficiently to differentiate between valid and invalid readings. It is the observer's responsibility to determine if the patient issues listed above are in fact accounted for. The observer also needs to properly select the cuff and apply it to the upper arm. This includes making sure that the cuff is placed on the bare arm, and that no restricting clothes are placed above the cuff (e.g., a tightly rolled sleeve).

**Table 1 (continued)**

| *Company* | *Infant cuff (w × l)* | *Bladder (w × l)* |
|---|---|---|
| W.A./TYCOS | 7.4 × 26.1 | 5.6 × 11.9 |
| BAUM | 8 × 29 | 6 × 12 |
| SICOA | 7.5 × 26 | 5.5 × 11.5 |
| GRAHAM FIELD | 7.5 × 26.1 | 5.5 × 11.5 |
| PROPPER | 7.6 × 25.4 | 5.7 × 11.4 |
| WINMED | 7.5 × 25.4 | 5.7 × 11.4 |
| K-T-K | 7 × 29 | |
| RIESTER | 7.2 × 23 | 5 × 8 |
| ERKA | 7 × 28 | 5.5 × 15 |
| CREST-MABIS | | 6.4 × 12.1 |
| CREST-PYMA | | 5.3 × 11.4 |
| ACCOSON | | 5.1 × 10.2 |
| | *Child* | |
| W.A./TYCOS | 10.4 × 35.3 | 8.6 × 17.8 |
| BAUM | 11 × 41 | 9 × 18 |
| SICOA | 10.5 × 34.2 | 8.5 × 17 |
| SAMMONS-PRESTON | | 10.2 × 17.9 |
| GRAHAM FIELD | 10.5 × 34.2 | 8.5 × 17 |
| PROPPER | 10.8 × 34.3 | 8.9 × 17.5 |
| KOSAN/BRESCO | 11 × 35 (Child) | 9 × 18 |
| | 8 × 26 (Peds) | 6 × 12 |
| | 9.5 × 30 (Sm Child) | 7.5 × 15 |
| WINMED | 11 × 33.5 | 7.6 × 17.7 |
| K-T-K | 11 × 40 | |
| | 9.5 × 33 | |
| RIESTER | 10 × 35.5 | 8 × 13 |
| ERKA | 9 × 39 | 8 × 20 |
| CREST-MABIS | | 8.3 × 17.8 |
| CREST-PYMA | | 7.9 × 15.2 |
| ACCOSON | | 10.2 × 19.1 |
| | | 7.6 × 15.2 (young) |
| | | 8.0 × 18.0 (new) |
| | | 4 × 13 (new sm) |

There is a wide range of bladder sizes for each category. Bladders which do not have a length = twice the width are unlikely to meet AAMI and AHA criteria for a width to arm circumference ratio of 0.4, while encircling 80% of the upper arm. (Data reported to Bruce Morgenstern by the manufacturers, 1996.) Dimensions are in centimeters.

## METHODS OF BLOOD PRESSURE MEASUREMENT

### *Auscultatory Methods of Blood Pressure Measurement*

Both mercury and aneroid devices are subject to significant observer issues. Of course, the observer must be able to hear and interpret the Korotkoff sounds accurately. This requires training, which is often accomplished with taped recordings of Korotkoff sounds or stethoscopes with two sets of earpieces. The correct performance of the auscultatory method requires that the systolic pressure first be approximated by palpation. The suggested proper bleed rate is 2 mmHg/s. This technique is even more critical when the patient's pulse rate is slow *(26)*.

Although extensive data are lacking, extant data suggest that in children, as in adults, the auscultatory method be performed with the bell of a stethoscope. The proponents of the use of the bell feel that this helps to augment the Korotkoff sounds. This brings us to yet another area of controversy, with auscultation-determining which Korotkoff sound, K4 or K5, represents the diastolic BP more accurately.

In the original report of the Task Force on Blood Pressure control in children *(26,31)*, K4 was accepted as the measure of diastolic BP for children less than 13 yr of age. In the 1987 update *(25)*, this was changed to K5, because data were available to report normal K5 values in younger children, and because this obviated the step in BP values that otherwise occurred at age 13. However, this recommendation has not been universally accepted *(32–34)*. One study, in fact, has suggested that K4 diastolic BP measured in childhood is a better predictor of adult hypertension *(35)*.

A final and critical observer issue is observer bias. At its simplest, this occurs when the observer has a terminal digit preference, and tends to report many BP values ending in that number (e.g., if it's zero, the majority of reported systolic BP and diastolic BP will end in zero). Also, there is the matter of whether K5, disappearance, is the last sound heard, or two mmHg below that value. More complex observer biases can occur when the observer has been informed of his or her digit preference and then overcompensates, avoiding reporting values with that digit. Finally, there is the bias introduced by the knowledge of a patient's previous values, described more fully in the section on random zero sphygmomanometers below.

### *Conventional Mercury Sphygmomanometry*

Mercury sphygmomanometry has been considered the "gold standard" against which other noninvasive measures are compared. The process is straightforward, but not necessarily easy. The components of the system include the bladder and cuff, tubing, a bulb with a screw-controlled bleed valve, a mercury reservoir, and the manometer, which has a filter at the top. Regular maintenance of the tubing, the bulb, the mercury in the reservoir, and the manometer is necessary to maintain accuracy. If the filter atop the manometer becomes clogged, the mercury will not move well in the column *(28)*.

Despite its status as the gold standard, mercury manometers, when systematically evaluated, have a significant number of problems that may preclude accurate use, even if the observer and patient issues are overcome. In a study at St George's Hospital Medical School in London, UK, of 444 devices studied, 167 (38%) had dirty columns. Ninety-five (21%) of these were owing to oxidization of the mercury so that the calibration markings were obscured, making it difficult to read the level of the mercury column. In 81 (18%), the column containing the mercury had either been rotated or the markings on the columns were badly faded, again making it difficult to read the level of the mercury meniscus. In three, mercury had leaked into the metal box. One machine had so little mercury in the column that when it was inflated, air bubbled through the mercury in the column, yet it was still in use *(28)*.

In a number of other studies, between 12 and 21% of evaluated mercury sphygmomanometers were not accurate when tested, but they were still being used clinically *(36,37)*. In a systematic evaluation of sphygmomanometers in a health district in the UK, *none* of the 356 instruments tested met all of the standards compiled for the project (project standards) or all of the relevant British regulatory standards; 14 (39.3%) met less than half of the British standards. Only 220 (61.8%) instruments tested were accurate at all six pressure levels in a calibration check; 12 sphygmomanometers met the accuracy standard at only three pressure levels, while 13 were inaccurate at all pressure levels tested. The authors also developed health and safety standards for the use and handling of mercury manometers. Eighty-six percent of the devices studied did not meet any of the five health and safety related standards *(38)*.

It appears that mercury manometers are likely to be phased out over the next few years, not for reasons of inaccuracy or device failure, although these are not uncommon *(28)*, but for environmental reasons. This process is already taking place to a greater or lesser degree in Europe, and several states in the US have passed regulations concerning the handling of mercury that make it far too expensive to use mercury manometers *(39)*. Although the AHA has taken a position against the elimination of the mercury manometer, it remains to be seen if they can slow this movement *(40)*.

### *Aneroid Manometry*

The aneroid manometer functions in the process of auscultatory BP measurement in essentially the same way as the mercury column. The system is comprised of a metal bellows, a mechanical amplifier, springs, and a gauge that displays the pressure in the cuff and tubing of the sphygmomanometer. Aneroid devices are often felt to be less accurate than mercury columns *(26,41)*.

Aneroid manometers were evaluated in many of the same studies cited for the assessment of mercury manometers. Mion demonstrated that 44% of devices in the hospital and 61% of devices in outpatient settings differed by more than 3 mmHg from the standard *(37)*. In the Canadian study of Vanasse, 17.7% of aneroid manometers were off by ≥ 5 mmHg, and 15% had at least one malfunctioning component (but 52.3% of the mercury devices did) *(36)*. Knight et al., as part of the same systematic study in the UK described for mercury manometers, found that none of the aneroid instruments tested met all of the project standards or all of the British regulatory standards. Seven (6.1%) of 114 devices met fewer than half of the British regulatory standards. The authors combined 14 standards against which aneroid manometers were compared for accuracy. Twenty-nine (25%) of the instruments met all 14 standards and two (1.7%) met seven or less *(38)*.

Additional data also demonstrate that aneroid devices can be inaccurate. In one study, using the very rigid standard of ± 3 mmHg concordance with the mercury standard, 35% of devices were considered "intolerant" at 2 of 5 pressures measured *(42)*. In another assessment of accuracy, Jones found that 34% of devices were not accurate to within 4 mmHg, but only 10% were not accurate to within 8 mmHg *(43)*. In a recent study, using 10 mmHg as the criteria for accuracy, 1% of mercury manometers and 10% of aneroid devices were deemed inaccurate *(44)*.

The underlying reason for this apparent inaccuracy of aneroid devices is likely the lack of a regular program of calibration and maintenance. When practitioners in Humberside and Yorkshire were surveyed in 1988, 23.5% of the 1223 respondents admitted to never servicing the sphygmomanometers in their practices over a mean of 5.75 yr (45). However, it has been established that, with proper calibration, aneroid devices are quite accurate manometers, and therefore subject only to the errors inherent to the auscultatory method *(42,46)*. Accuracy rates with mean differences from a mercury standard of ± 0.2 mmHg have been reported *(47)*. In the Mayo Clinic experience, with a program of regular maintenance and calibration, more than 99% of actively used aneroid devices remain within 3 mmHg of a digital pressure gage standard over 6 mo periods *(46)*.

### *Random-Zero Sphygmomanometry*

The random-zero sphygmomanometer (RZS) was devised in 1970 as a modification of Garrow's "zero-muddler sphygmomanometer," in an attempt to eliminate observer biases related to terminal-digit preference and to previous knowledge of recorded BPs, both of which are common during conventional sphygmomanometry *(48)*. Therefore it has been considered by many to be the "gold standard" for epidemiological studies, and has been employed in studies such as the Multiple Risk Factor Intervention Trial (MRFIT) *(49)*, and the Hypertension Prevention Trial *(50)* in adults.

The machine works on the basic principle that each time a BP reading is obtained, the observer is "blinded" to the reading until after the measurement has been completed. This comes about as a result of the incorporation of a mercury reservoir that fills randomly and to a variable degree during each inflation of the cuff, and adds a random amount of mercury to the manometer column. The amount of mercury added to the reservoir and to the column is unknown to the person using the machine until after the BP cuff has been deflated, at which point this "random-zero" number can be read and subtracted from the uncorrected systolic and diastolic readings. While experience with the RZS is more limited in children, at least one group of investigators has used it for the so-called "Study of Cardiovascular Risk in Young Finns" *(51)*.

The RZS does indeed reduce observer bias, but it does not completely eliminate it. Both the Hypertension Prevention Trial and the MRFIT demonstrated a marked reduction in terminal digit preference of the corrected BP readings (compared to the uncorrected measurements), and also a roughly bell-shaped distribution of the random-zero values *(49,50)*. Compared to conventional sphygmomanometry, use of the RZS in adults has also been shown to result in a greater intra-observer variability in BP readings *(52)*. While this may seem counter-productive to some, in fact it more likely indicates the elimination of the bias caused by observer prejudice with the conventional sphygmomanometer, which artificially causes multiple BP readings by a single observer to be very close to each other owing to knowledge of the previous reading. Identical findings have been reported in children, albeit in a smaller study, when the RZS was compared head-to-head with the conventional sphygmomanometer *(27)*. While the "Study of Cardiovascular Risk in Young Finns" did not simultaneously compare the RZS to any other casual method of BP measurement, the design of this longitudinal study was such that on the first two occasions BPs were measured, in a cohort of randomly selected children between 6 and 18 yr, using a conventional sphygmomanometer. For the third survey, which was conducted on a subset of the original cohort, the RZS was used *(53)*. Therefore, while the study does not allow one to comment directly on the comparability of the two methods, the results are quite interesting and are in line with the previously-mentioned adult data. First of all, this study also demonstrated that, in spite of adequate training, terminal-digit preference was almost universally observed in all personnel obtaining BPs (using the conventional sphygmomanometer) during the initial two surveys, while this was almost completely eliminated using the RZS in the third trial. Secondly, the investigators made an interesting observation that the age-related curves obtained by the two methods differed significantly, with an apparently nonlinear rise in BP (as measured by the conventional method) with age, probably related to observer bias. A more continuous rise in BP with age, as might be expected on a biological basis, was seen when the RZS data were plotted; this was especially noticeable at low BP values. Based on these findings, the study investigators concluded that BPs in children, especially in the lower ranges, are measured more accurately with the RZS compared to the conventional sphygmomanometer, and that the RZS should be the preferred instrument used for epidemiological surveys of BP in this age group.

Notwithstanding all the advantages of the RZS, especially in clinical epidemiology, several concerns have been raised about the accuracy of this instrument, including its impracticality owing to the bulky design, expense, extent of training needed for personnel to use it accurately, and high maintenance costs. From a practical standpoint, it also shares with the conventional sphygmomanometer the disadvantage of having mercury as an intrinsic component of its design. Many studies have also shown that the RZS, when compared to the conventional sphygmomanometer, systematically underestimates diastolic and systolic BP in both adults and in children *(49,53)*. The degree of underestimation varies quite considerably from one study to another. Several studies demonstrated a small and consistent difference of 1–3 mmHg between the two methods *(54,55)*. Others found a much larger and significant difference *(56)*. This has resulted in contentious debate among investigators; some find the instrument acceptable for use according to the guidelines of the British Hypertension Society (BHS) *(54)*, while others strongly advise against its use without further study *(56)*. Whether the "underestimation" of BP by the RZS is real, or owing more to an "overestimation" of BP by the conventional sphygmomanometer, is unclear. Numerous reports have emphasized that these differences can be minimized, or even eliminated, by rigorous attention to the details of the measurement technique, intensive training of personnel *(57)*, and meticulous maintenance of the equipment, which is apparently prone to subtle malfunction *(54,58)*.

In conclusion, although the blinded nature of BP readings using the RZS makes it an ideal candidate instrument for epidemiological studies, the limited data in children and the aforementioned contradictory findings of its accuracy among different investigators, along with the practical issues related to expense, maintenance costs, and need for intensive personnel training, make the use of the RZS very impractical, certainly for routine clinical care, and perhaps also for epidemiological studies pending further research. Ultimately, however, the demise of this instrument will most likely be owing more to environmental concerns than to any issues related to its accuracy.

### *Oscillometric Blood Pressure Measurement*

Oscillometric devices have all but replaced the mercury manometer in a large number of medical centers, especially in European countries where concern about environmental contamination with mercury has been greater *(39)*. Development of the first commercial oscillometric device for BP measurement started in the early 1970s and resulted in the Dinamap, an acronym for "device for indirect noninvasive mean arterial pressure" *(59)*. Since that time, a plethora of oscillometric devices for automated BP measurement have flooded the market, including several new modifications of the original Dinamap Model 825 (Critikon division of Johnson & Johnson, Tampa, FL). The basic principle underlying these devices is the same as that of other cuff-based BP measuring devices, in that compression of the arm by an inflatable cuff allows indirect determination of the intra-arterial vascular pressure. The difference between conventional sphygmomanometry and the oscillometric devices is that, in the latter, cuff inflation and deflation are automated, and that BP determination is made by a microprocessor using information sent to it from a pressure transducer; this has the potential of being tremendously advantageous by eliminating all observer biases. Only a short summary of the process of BP measurement is described herein. More details are available in the article by Ramsey *(59)*. In brief, the BP cuff is automatically inflated to between 160 and 180 mmHg (or 70 and 125 mmHg in the neonatal mode), depending on the specific device, for the first BP determination, and subsequently to 35 mmHg above the previously recorded systolic value. After a brief holding period, the cuff pressure is reduced in a step-wise manner in 5–10 mmHg decrements. As the cuff pressure decreases, oscillations of the arterial wall increase in amplitude and reach a maximum when the cuff pressure approaches the mean arterial pressure. With further deflation of the BP cuff, oscillations of the arterial wall diminish and eventually stop altogether. The monitor uses this information to compute and display values for the mean, and for the systolic and diastolic BP. The precise method of BP determination is far more complicated and is determined by a complex algorithm that varies from one device to another; the pressures displayed on the monitor, therefore, may be calculated rather than actually measured values, at least for some of the oscillometric devices in the market. These algorithms have been considered proprietary information and are therefore kept in confidence, making it impossible for investigators to verify the accuracy of their underlying physiological principals. In addition, since the algorithms are proprietary, the devices may not be interchangeable. In fact, in one study, two different devices used simultaneously yielded different results *(60)*.

Many studies have evaluated the comparability of oscillometric readings with BP readings obtained by invasive means. Park et al. *(61)* compared the Dinamap model 1846 and a conventional mercury sphygmomanometer with radial artery pressures in a group of infants and children admitted to the intensive care unit. While both the Dinamap 1846 and the conventional mercury sphygmomanometer readings correlated well with intra-arterial BP measurements (*see* Figs. 1 and 2), the correlation coefficient was better for BP readings obtained using the Dinamap 1846. The difference between the Dinamap 1846 and intra-arterial BP readings was small and ranged from –7 to +7 mmHg, –9 to +10 mmHg, and –10 to + 8 mmHg for systolic, diastolic and mean BP, respectively. Similarly, BP readings obtained in infants using the Dinamap 847 neonatal and Dinamap 845 vital signs monitor were found to correlate well with BP values obtained using a central aortic catheter, with even smaller mean absolute pressure differences than seen in the previous study *(62)*.

However, comparisons between BP readings using a mercury sphygmomanometer and some oscillometric devices, especially the newer models, demonstrate that the two methods are not comparable. A large single-center study evaluating the newer Dinamap model 8100 against the conventional mercury sphygmomanometer in over 7000 children found that the mean Dinamap 8100 readings were higher for both systolic (by 10 mmHg) and diastolic (by 5 mmHg) values. However, the 95th percentile confidence intervals for differences in systolic and diastolic BPs between the two methods were quite large and ranged from – 4 to +24 mmHg and – 4 to + 23 mmHg respectively, making the "error" nonsystematic and unpredictable *(63)*. Similarly, in the Bogalusa Heart Study, significant differences were noted in BPs obtained using the Dinamap 8100 and a conventional sphygmomanometer. While the mean systolic pressure with the Dinamap 8100 was higher than that obtained using a conventional sphygmo-

Table 2
**Protocols for Assessment of the Accuracy of BP Measuring Devices**

| *BHS grading criteria* | | | |
|---|---|---|---|
| | *Percent that do not differ between test and "standard" device readings (%)* | | |
| *Grade* | *≤5 mmHg* | *≤10 mmHg* | *≤15 mmHg* |
| A | 60 | 85 | 95 |
| B | 50 | 75 | 90 |
| C | 40 | 65 | 85 |
| D | Worse | Worse | Worse |

| *AAMI criteria* | | |
|---|---|---|
| *Grade* | *Mean difference between devices* | *Standard deviation* |
| Pass | ≤ 5 mmHg | ≤ 8 mmHg |
| Fail | > 5 mmHg | > 8 mmHg |

manometer, similar to the study by Park et al., the mean diastolic pressure was, in fact, lower with the Dinamap 8100 *(64)*. Moreover, an age-related difference was noted in the discrepancies between the two devices for diastolic BP. In children under 8 yr of age, the Dinamap 8100 diastolic BPs were higher compared to the conventional sphygmomanometer readings, while in children over 8 yr, the Dinamap 8100 underestimated diastolic BP.

Two different validation standards are currently in use to ensure accuracy of oscillometric BP measuring devices. These are the BHS protocol *(65)* and the guidelines put forth by AAMI *(66)* (Table 2). Since these two protocols can be reconciled, fulfillment of both sets of criteria should be used in validating any oscillometric device. Briefly, the BHS protocol looks at the absolute difference between BPs obtained simultaneously by the oscillometric device and a standard sphygmomanometer in different phases of use (before-use calibration, in-use phase, after-use calibration and static validation). The grade assigned to the device (Grades A and B are acceptable while Grades C and D are unacceptable) improves as the percentage of paired readings that are close to each other increases. The AAMI criteria, on the other hand, require that the device being tested be compared either to a standard sphygmomanometer or to direct intra-arterial readings (especially in neonates, in whom it is often very difficult to hear the Korotkoff sounds). In order to get a passing grade from the AAMI, the test device measurements should not differ from the reference standard by a mean of >5 mmHg and a standard deviation of >8 mmHg. These standards are based upon the assumption, albeit unproven, that the physiologic principles which underlie the oscillation of the arterial wall and its relation to BP are somehow identical to the Korotkoff sounds and their relation to BP. While many concerns have been raised about the reproducibility, complexity, and cumbersome nature of these two guidelines, they remain, to date the "gold-standard" for testing new devices in the market *(67)*. As environmental and other pressures increase the prominence of oscillometric devices, it is quite likely that a new set of distinct criteria will be established, much like the standards applied to direct intra-arterial measurements of BP versus auscultatory methods.

Based on the aforementioned guidelines, O'Brien et al. recently reviewed several oscillometric devices available in the market and found that only a few fulfilled accuracy criteria for both protocols *(68)*. Some of the devices that are recommended in this report for use in children are the CAS Model 9010 (CAS Medical Systems, Branford, CT) for in-hospital use, the Omron

Table 3
Comparison of the Various Methodologies for Casual BP Measurement

| | *Advantages* | *Problems* |
|---|---|---|
| **Conventional sphygmomanometry (CS)** | Easy to use<br>Inexpensive<br>Commonly available<br>Pediatric BP normative data based on it | Operation: Observer biases.<br>Output: Affected by technique, environmental and mechanical factors (e.g., cuff size).<br>Debate over use of K4 vs K5 as being representative of diastolic BP.<br>Environmental issues re handling, spills, disposal. |
| **Mercury** | Perhaps the "gold" standard<br>Minimal maintenance required to maintain calibration | Often not maintained.<br>Easily loses calibration. |
| **Aneroid** | Portable; inexpensive<br>Accurate<br>Measures same parameters as mercury | Gage more subject to bias/misread than Hg column?<br>Often not calibrated. |
| **RZS** | Reduces observer biases | Design: Bulky and difficult to use. Expensive. Uses mercury.<br>Operation: Extensive training required for correct use.<br>Output: BP readings lower than with CS. |
| **Oscillometry** | Easy to use<br>No mercury in the instrument<br>Frees user to allow more than 1 thing to be done at the same time<br>Eliminates observer biases<br>Easier to use in infants and young children compared to CS | Design: Expensive and requires periodic maintenance.<br>Many devices in the market, few of which have been validated for use in children.<br>Output: Affected by technique, environmental and mechanical factors (e.g., cuff size).<br>1st reading effect.<br>High initial inflation pressure may cause anxiety and motion artifacts.<br>Limited normative data available for children.<br>BP reading not equivalent to CS readings. |

RZS, random zero sphygmomanometer.

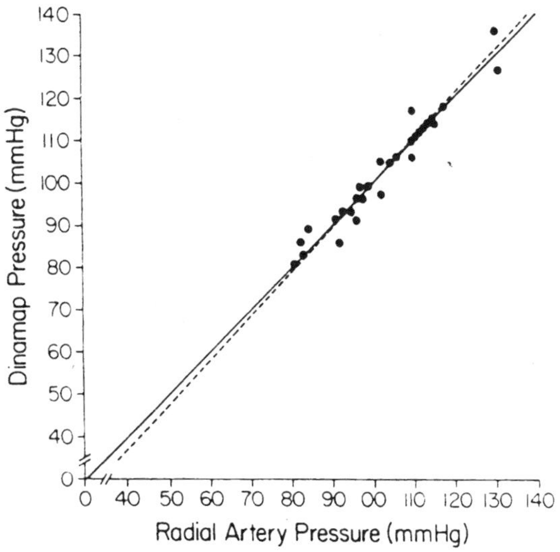


Fig. 1. Relationship between systolic pressure measured by Dinamap and by radial artery catheter. Linear regression equation is $y = 1.05x - 5.36$, and $r = 0.970$, where $y$ = the Dinamap and $x$ = radial artery pressures. Broken line is calculated regression line; solid line is line of identity *(25)*. Reproduced with permission from ref. *61*.

HEM-750CP (Omron Health Care, Inc., Vernon Hills, IL) for self-measurement, and the Daypress 500 (Neural Instruments, Florence, Italy) for ambulatory BP monitoring, although only at rest. One of the more commonly used oscillometric devices in the US, the Dinamap model 8100, has yielded varying results when tested for accuracy. Few pediatric studies have followed the strict guidelines of the AAMI and BHS protocols to evaluate the Dinamap 8100. In a small study in a cohort of prepubertal children (8–13 yr old), compared to the conventional sphygmomanometer, the Dinamap 8100 was found to overestimate systolic BP and underestimate diastolic BP. These differences, however, were within the range acceptable by both the aforementioned validation standards *(70)*. The mean difference (standard deviation) between the BP readings obtained by the Dinamap 8100 and the conventional sphygmomanometer was 4.8 (7.5) mmHg for systolic and –1.9 (7.5) mmHg for diastolic BP, making the device acceptable to the AAMI. Similarly, using the BHS criteria, the Dinamap 8100 achieved a grade of B since more than 50% of its readings were within 5 mmHg, and more than 90% were within 15 mmHg of the conventionally obtained measurements. Other studies, however, have not been as flattering. In a study by O'Brien et al. in 1993, the Dinamap 8100 was evaluated for accuracy in an adult population according to the strict guidelines of the BHS protocol, and found to achieve a grading of D (unacceptable) for diastolic BP and B (acceptable) for systolic BP *(69)*. Therefore, in the absence of further study in a larger group of children, the use of the Dinamap 8100 cannot be recommended without reservation.

Certainly, athough there are discrepancies between auscultatory and oscillometric measurements they are not necessarily errors. Whether the source of the discrepancy is mechanical and in the oscillometric device, or owing to observer error with the conventional sphygmomanometer is, at best, speculative. It is also certainly possible that the "error" arises from a more accurate determination of BP (especially the diastolic BP) by the oscillometric device which detects a "true" intra-arterial BP, thereby eliminating the error inherent in the conventional sphygmomanometer, which must necessarily rely on the Kortokoff sounds as an indirect and

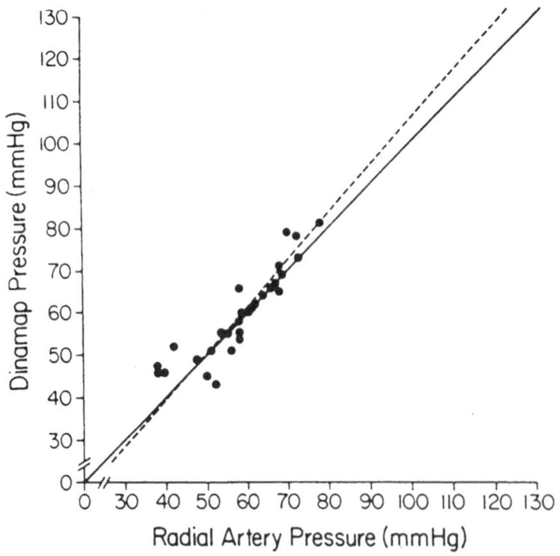


Fig. 2. Relationship between diastolic pressure obtained by Dinamap and by radial artery catheter. Linear regression equation is $y = 1.10x - 4.65$, and $r = 0.903$. Broken line is calculated regression line; solid line is line of identity *(25)*. Reproduced with permission from ref. *61*.

approximate surrogate indicator of true vascular pressure *(71)*. What is clear from studies comparing oscillometric devices with conventional sphygmomanometers is that these two methods of BP measurement should not be used interchangeably, and that they may be measuring different biological parameters.

There are many potential advantages of using oscillometric devices over conventional sphygmomanometry. First and foremost, they are felt to be convenient, easy to use, and to eliminate the need for highly trained personnel, although this may not really be the case *(72)*. Moreover, by avoiding terminal digit preference and bias related to prior knowledge of recorded BPs, the use of these devices, if accurate, can improve measurement precision and substantially lower the sample size required in clinical trials on hypertension. Oscillometric devices are also easier to use in younger children, neonates and infants, in whom movements of the arm may make it difficult to use auscultation to accurately hear the Korotkoff sounds; the success of oscillometric devices in obtaining BPs has been demonstrated in this age group by Park et al. *(73)*. The use of such devices also eliminates the K4-K5 controversy mentioned previously *(35)*, since the oscillometric devices correlate very well with direct intra-arterial pressures *(61)* (Figs. 1 and 2). However, the greatest advantage of these devices may turn out to be an ecological one. Since oscillometric devices do not use mercury, they may eventually supplant all mercury manometers as a result of the previously mentioned concern about the environmental hazard posed by this element *(39)*.

While oscillometric devices, when correctly chosen, can greatly add to the management of patients with hypertension and improve clinical trials, their use is not without problems. As mentioned before, caution must be advised before a particular device is chosen for use, since the accuracy of many newer devices has not been tested in an unbiased manner. In addition, these are expensive pieces of equipment and require continued upkeep and servicing to ensure optimal functioning, which add to their cost. Certain drawbacks also exist in the design of these machines. While perhaps not applicable to any great extent in pediatrics, it is noteworthy that the upper limit of systolic pressure that these devices can measure is limited and varies from 240–280 mmHg (or about 160 mmHg in the neonatal mode) *(61,74)*.

Difficulties may also arise in BP measurements in children with cardiac arrhythmias and in children who are uncooperative and cannot sit still, leading to motion artifacts *(59)*. Moreover, the rapid rate of inflation of the cuff by the machine to a pressure of 160 mmHg may be uncomfortable and disconcerting to children, and may cause them to resist the BP measurement, leading to erroneously high readings. In fact, a "first-reading" effect, in which the first of several BP readings is 3–5 mmHg higher than subsequent readings a few minutes later, has been noted by several investigators using oscillometric devices in children *(64,73)*. Therefore, repeat measurements of BP are important in children to avoid over-diagnosis of hypertension. The optimal number of measurements, per patient and per visit, for oscillometric devices, may vary from machine to machine. For one particular device, the Dinamap 845 XT, the reliability was noted to increase quite significantly when the number of BP measurements went from 3 to 4 per visit, and the number of visits went from 1 to 2 *(27)*. Lastly, an issue that has irked clinical investigators for long is the knowledge that the algorithms used for determination of BP by oscillometric devices vary from one manufacturing company to another, and between different models of the same device. These algorithms have been considered to be proprietary information, and being confidential, have never been subjected to scientific scrutiny. As a consequence, health-care professionals tend to be somewhat skeptical of their validity *(75)*.

Users of oscillometric devices need to be aware of a few other issues. As mentioned earlier, BPs obtained by conventional sphygmomanometry and using oscillometric devices should not be used interchangeably for study purposes because, even with the most accurate of devices, differences exist between the two. Also, since normative data in use at present in children are based on BP measurements obtained by conventional sphygmomanometry *(25)*, using these norms to determine if the BP, measured in a particular child using an oscillometric device, is normal, may not be appropriate. Nevertheless, it must be noted that some normative reference data on BPs using an oscillometric device are available for children younger than 5 yr of age *(73)*. It is also interesting to note that, in spite of the aforementioned concerns with the use of oscillometric devices, some epidemiological studies of BP in adults, and even one in children (the CATCH trial), are using such devices for BP determination *(76,77)*. Furthermore, it has recently been documented that the Dinamap has been programmed in such a way that it specifically cannot report certain values of BP *(78)*. Finally we must all remember that, although oscillometric devices eliminate observer bias, they share with the mercury sphygmomanometer the likelihood that BP readings may be affected by environmental (e.g., ambient temperature) and patient factors (e.g., stress and arm size–cuff size discrepancy).

## PROBLEMS WITH CASUAL BLOOD PRESSURE MEASUREMENTS

Having reviewed the various individual methods of casual BP determination in children, we should recognize that these methods are not infallible, and that there are many concerns related to the use of BPs obtained by such methods (*see* Table 3). Possible problems for each method have already been discussed in earlier sections of this chapter, and the reader can refer to these sections for more specific details. Suffice it so say that with meticulous attention to detail, and by choosing the instrument appropriate to one's purpose, many of these problems and errors can be avoided.

The second concern with casual BP readings is perhaps a more important and fundamental one. Although cross-sectional normative data on BP in children are routinely used in clinical management, there are no direct studies evaluating the validity of these norms in predicting the risk of adverse events in adulthood. Longitudinal epidemiological studies of BP starting in children have not had sufficient time to extend into late adulthood to establish if, as in adults, childhood hypertension or even high BP is predictive of cardiovascular and cerebrovascular morbidity and mortality. More importantly, it has not been shown for certain that early intervention is of any measurable benefit in reducing morbidity and mortality later in life. Indirectly, however, it seems biologically plausible and likely that hypertension begins in childhood and, if persistent, may be a predictor of adult onset morbidity. It would seem equally plausible that BP control in hypertensive children would reduce morbidity later in life. Resolution of left ventricular hypertrophy in children is seen when hypertension is treated.

There is direct evidence of a possible impact of high BP (either alone or by virtue of its being a surrogate marker for children with dyslipidemia, overweight or insulin resistance). This evidence is found in the autopsy studies of the Bogalusa trial and the Pathobiological Determinants of Atherosclerosis in Youth (PDAY) trial, and in the cardiac imaging in participants in the Muscatine study. A subset of children who had participated in the Muscatine trial underwent electron beam computed tomography *(79)* to look for coronary artery calcification, which has previously been established to correlate well with the presence of atherosclerotic plaques in postmortem specimens *(80)*. An odds ratio (OR) of 3.0 (95% confidence interval [CI] 1.3–6.7) for coronary artery calcification at the age of 33 yr was noted for adults who were at the highest decile of body mass index in childhood. Although having high BP as a child (8–18 yr) was not significantly associated with coronary calcification, the diastolic BP as a young adult (20–34 yr) certainly was, with an OR of 4.2 (95% CI 1.9–9.6). The Collaborative Pathology Study, a program of the Bogalusa Heart Study, reported autopsy data in 93 children and young adults (2–39 yr of age) who had died of traumatic causes *(81)*. These investigators found that the extent of raised fibrous plaques in the coronary arteries, which are known to be precursors of progressive atherosclerosis, correlated positively with ante-mortem diastolic and systolic BP. Moreover, the findings indicated a positive correlation between the number of cardiovascular risk factors present at the time of autopsy (body mass index, BP, dyslipidemia), and the extent of early atherosclerosis. Lastly, the PDAY study showed that hypertension augments atherosclerosis in young men and women (15–34 yr of age) by accelerating the conversion of fatty streaks in the coronary arteries to raised plaques beginning in the third decade of life, and that this effect of hypertension increases with age *(82)*.

So, while logic and a significant body of literature support the contention that hypertension in children, as determined by casual methods, is a bad thing and worthy of intervention to prevent adverse events in the future, as of this writing the medical literature offers no direct evidence to support this contention. A second consideration, while interpreting casual BP readings obtained by any method, is the appropriateness of using such isolated and intermittent observations to make therapeutic decisions, especially those that could have a significant impact on the perceived quality of life of an individual. This brings us back to the question of validity. How valid are casual, as compared to ambulatory, BP readings, in predicting adverse long-term outcomes? While this issue is discussed in greater depth in a subsequent chapter (see Chapter 6), it is important to point out here that discrepancies clearly exist in BP determinations made in an office setting compared to those obtained at home. A significant body of literature in adults *(83)*, and some in children *(84)*, indicates that a great majority of children with elevated casual BP readings, who would otherwise be classified as hypertensive by current norms, may actually have "white-coat" hypertension when ambulatory BP readings are used.

This subgroup of children could possibly be at lower or zero risk of adverse outcomes, and therefore not merit extensive, expensive, and invasive work-ups, or require long-term therapy. Preliminary studies have also shown that, as in adults, hypertension in children, when determined by ambulatory methods, has a more significant correlation with risk factors for cardiovascular adverse outcomes, such as left ventricular hypertrophy *(85)*.

## CONCLUSIONS

The concept that there is a "true" BP is probably more obfuscating than illuminating. At any given moment, each of us has a BP, but the force of that pressure will register differently as different systems are used to measure it. Moments later, the pressure is different. Korotkoff himself reported that the first sound heard (K1) appeared before the radial pulse could be palpated as the occluding cuff is deflated *(86)*. K1, on the other hand, is heard after systolic pressure is detected by an indwelling line *(87)*. Mercury and aneroid devices, as discussed earlier, when calibrated properly, agree quite closely on the pressure that they detect. Conversely, oscillometry seems to differ by device and certainly differs from the auscultatory methods, but perhaps comes closest to intra-arterial determinations. All of these methods, if consistently applied, will correlate with the other, but they are rarely likely to be identical.

The use of casual BP measurements, when performed carefully by trained personnel using calibrated and well-maintained devices, remains the primary screening tool to assess populations for hypertension. The largest pool of normative data in children exists for values obtained by auscultatory methods (albeit the data pooled first BP readings). Auscultatory methods are accurate, but subject to many confounding issues. Oscillometric measures will likely replace auscultatory measures as the primary method of BP determination, but they do not measure the same variables as auscultatory measures, and they pose their own unique set of confounding variables. Additional normal values based upon oscillometry are needed.

## REFERENCES


1. Crenner CW. Introduction of the blood pressure cuff into U.S. medical practice: technology and skilled practice. Ann Intern Med 1998;128(6):488–493.
2. Cushing H. On routine determinations of arterial tension in operating room and clinic. Boston Med Surg J 1903;148:250–252.
3. Cook H, Briggs J. Clinical observations of blood pressure. Johns Hopkins Hospital reports 1903;11:451–534.
4. Lewis W. The evolution of clinical sphygmomanometry. Bull NY Acad Med 1941;17:87–881.
5. Gittings J. Auscultatory blood-pressure determinations. Arch Intern Med 1910;6:196–204.
6. Labarthe DR. Overview of the history of pediatric blood pressure assessment and hypertension: an epidemiologic perspective. Blood Press Monit 1999;4:197–203.
7. Burt VL, Whelton P. Prevalence of hypertension in the US adult population. Results from the Third National Health and Nutrition Examination Survey, 1988–1991. Hypertension 1995;25:305–313.
8. Sinaiko AR, Gomez-Marin O. Diastolic fourth and fifth phase blood pressure in 10–15-year-old children. The Children and Adolescent Blood Pressure Program. Am J Epidemiol 1990;132(4):647–655.
9. Mehta SK. Pediatric hypertension. A challenge for pediatricians. Am J Dis Child 1987;141:893–894.
10. Mahoney LT, Clarke WR, Burns TL, Lauer RM. Childhood predictors of high blood pressure. Am J Hypertens 1991;4:608S–610S.
11. Lauer RM, Clarke WR, Mahoney LT, Witt J. Childhood predictors for high adult blood pressure. The Muscatine Study. Pediatr Clin North Am 1993;40(1):23–40.
12. Burke V, Beilin LJ, Dunbar D. Tracking of blood pressure in Australian children. J Hypertens 2001;19(7):1185–1192.
13. Lauer RM, Clarke WR. Childhood risk factors for high adult blood pressure: the Muscatine Study. Pediatrics 1989;84(4):633–641.

14. Vasan RS, Larson MG, Leip EP, et al. Impact of high-normal blood pressure on the risk of cardiovascular disease. N Engl J Med 2001;345(18):1291–1297.
15. Stamler J, Stamler R, Neaton JD. Blood pressure, systolic and diastolic, and cardiovascular risks. US population data. Arch Intern Med 1993;153(5):598–615.
16. Fiebach NH, Hebert PR, Stampfer MJ, et al. A prospective study of high blood pressure and cardiovascular disease in women. Am J Epidemiol 1989;130(4):646–654.
17. Kannel WB, Wolf PA, Verter J, McNamara PM. Epidemiologic assessment of the role of blood pressure in stroke. The Framingham study. JAMA 1970;214(2):301–310.
18. Klag MJ, Whelton PK, Randall BL, et al. Blood pressure and end-stage renal disease in men. N Engl J Med 1996;334(1):13–18.
19. Kannel WB. Blood pressure as a cardiovascular risk factor: prevention and treatment. JAMA 1996;275(20): 1571–1576.
20. Srinivasan SR, Myers L, Berenson GS. Predictability of childhood adiposity and insulin for developing insulin resistance syndrome (syndrome X) in young adulthood: the Bogalusa Heart Study. Diabetes 2002;51(1):204–209.
21. Vogt BA, Birk PE, Panzarino V, Hite SH, Kashtan CE. Aortic dissection in young patients with chronic hypertension. Am J Kidney Dis 1999;33(2):374–378.
22. Hari P, Bagga A, Srivastava RN. Sustained hypertension in children. Indian Pediatr 2000;37(3):268–274.
23. Cooney MJ, Bradley WG, Symko SC, Patel ST, Groncy PK. Hypertensive encephalopathy: complication in children treated for myeloproliferative disorders—report of three cases. Radiology 2000;214(3):711–716.
24. Sorof JM, Cardwell G, Franco K, Portman RJ. Ambulatory blood pressure and left ventricular mass index in hypertensive children. Hypertension 2002;39(4):903–908.
25. Report of the Second Task Force on Blood Pressure Control in Children—1987. Task Force on Blood Pressure Control in Children. National Heart, Lung, and Blood Institute, Bethesda, Maryland. Pediatrics 1987;79(1): 1–25.
26. Perloff D, Grim C, Flak J, et al. Human blood pressure determination by sphygmomanometry. Circulation 1993;88(5 Pt 1):2460–2470.
27. Gillman MW, Cook NR. Blood pressure measurement in childhood epidemiological studies. Circulation 1995; 92(4):1049–1057.
28. Markandu ND, Whitcher F, Arnold A, Carney C. The mercury sphygmomanometer should be abandoned before it is proscribed. J Hum Hypertens 2000;14(1):31–36.
29. Beevers G, Lip GY, O'Brien E. ABC of hypertension. Blood pressure measurement. Part I-sphygmomanometry: factors common to all techniques. BMJ 2001;322(7292):981–985.
30. Vyse TJ. Sphygmomanometer bladder length and measurement of blood pressure in children. Lancet 1987; 1(8532):561–562.
31. Blumenthal S, Epps RP, Heavenrich R. Report of the task force on blood pressure control in children. Pediatrics 1977;59(5 2 suppl):I–II, 797–820.
32. Sinaiko AR, Gomez-Marin O, Prineas RJ. Prevalence of "significant" hypertension in junior high school-aged children: the Children and Adolescent Blood Pressure Program. J Pediatr 1989;114(4 Pt 1):664–669.
33. Uhari M, Nuutinen M, Turtinen J, Pokka T. Pulse sounds and measurement of diastolic blood pressure in children. Lancet 1991;338(8760):159–161.
34. Alpert BS, Marks L, Cohen M. K5 = diastolic pressure. Pediatrics 1996;98(5):1002.
35. Elkasabany AM, Urbina EM, Daniels SR, Berenson GS. Prediction of adult hypertension by K4 and K5 diastolic blood pressure in children: the Bogalusa Heart Study. J Pediatr 1998;132(4):687–692.
36. Vanasse A, Courteau J. Evaluation of sphygmomanometers used by family physicians practicing outside the hospital environment in Bas-Saint-Laurent. Can Fam Physician 2001;47:281–286.
37. Mion D, Pierin AM. How accurate are sphygmomanometers? J Hum Hypertens 1998;12(4):245–248.
38. Knight T, Leech F, Jones A, et al. Sphygmomanometers in use in general practice: an overlooked aspect of quality in patient care. J Hum Hypertens 2001;15(10):681–684.
39. O'Brien E. Has conventional sphygmomanometry ended with the banning of mercury? Blood Press Monit 2002;7(1):37–40.
40. Jones DW, Frohlich ED, Grim CM, Grim CE, Taubert KA.. Mercury sphygmomanometers should not be abandoned: an advisory statement from the Council for High Blood Pressure Research, American Heart Association. Hypertension 2001;37(2):185–186.

41. Sloan PJ, Zezulka A, Davies P, Sangal A, Beevers M, Beevers DG. Standardized methods for comparison of sphygmomanometers. J Hypertens 1984;2(5):547–551.
42. Bailey RH, Knaus VL, Bauer JH. Aneroid sphygmomanometers. An assessment of accuracy at a university hospital and clinics. Arch Intern Med 1991;151(7):1409–1412.
43. Jones JS, Ramsey W, Hetrick T. Accuracy of prehospital sphygmomanometers. J Emerg Med 1987;5(1): 23–27.
44. Ali S, Rouse A. Practice audits: reliability of sphygmomanometers and blood pressure recording bias. J Hum Hypertens 2002;16(5):359–361.
45. Hussain A, Cox JG. An audit of the use of sphygmomanometers. Br J Clin Pract 1996;50(3):136–137.
46. Canzanello VJ, Jensen PL, Schwartz GL. Are aneroid sphygmomanometers accurate in hospital and clinic settings? Arch Intern Med 2001;161(5):729–731.
47. Yarows SA, Qian K. Accuracy of aneroid sphygmomanometers in clinical usage: University of Michigan experience. Blood Press Monit 2001;6(2):101–106.
48. Wright BM, Dore CF. A random-zero sphygmomanometer. Lancet 1970;1(7642):337–338.
49. Dischinger P, DuChene AG. Quality control aspects of blood pressure measurements in the Multiple Risk Factor Intervention Trial. Control Clin Trials 1986;7(Suppl 3):137S–157S.
50. Canner PL, Borhani NO, Oberman A, et al. The Hypertension Prevention Trial: assessment of the quality of blood pressure measurements. Am J Epidemiol 1991;134(4):379–392.
51. Uhari ME, Nuutinen M, Turtinen J, et al. Blood pressure in children, adolescents and young adults. Ann Med 1991;23(1):47–51.
52. Variability of blood pressure and the results of screening in the hypertension detection and follow-up program. J Chronic Dis 1978;31(11):651–667.
53. Nuutinen M, Turtinen J, Uhari M. Random-zero sphygmomanometer, Rose's tape, and the accuracy of the blood pressure measurements in children. Pedirtr Res 1992;32(2):243–247.
54. Mackie A, Whincup P, McKinnon M. Does the Hawksley random zero sphygmomanometer underestimate blood pressure, and by how much? J Hum Hypertens 1995;9(5):337–343.
55. Brown WC, Kennedy S, Inglis GC, Murray LS, Lever AF. Mechanisms by which the Hawksley random zero sphygmomanometer underestimates blood pressure and produces a non-random distribution of RZ values. J Hum Hypertens 1997;11(2):75–93.
56. O'Brien E, Mee F, Atkins N, O'Malley K. Inaccuracy of the Hawksley random zero sphygmomanometer. Lancet 1990;336(8729):1465–1468.
57. Conroy RM, Shelley E, O'Brien E, Atkins N. Ergonomic problems with the Hawksley Random Zero Sphygmomanometer and their effect on recorded blood pressure levels. Blood Press 1996;5(4):227–233.
58. McGurk C, Nugent A, McAuley D, Silke B. Sources of inaccuracy in the use of the Hawksley random-zero sphygmomanometer. J Hypertens 1997;15(12 Pt 1):1379–1384.
59. Ramsey M, 3rd. Blood pressure monitoring: automated oscillometric devices. J Clin Monit 1991;7(1):56–67.
60. Kaufmann MA, Pargger H, Drop LJ, et al. Oscillometric blood pressure measurements by different devices are not interchangeable. Anesth Analg 1996;82(2):377–381.
61. Park MK, Menard SM. Accuracy of blood pressure measurement by the Dinamap monitor in infants and children. Pediatrics 1987;79(6):907–914.
62. Colan SD, Fujii A, Borow KM, MacPherson D, Sanders SP. Noninvasive determination of systolic, diastolic and end-systolic blood pressure in neonates, infants and young children: comparison with central aortic pressure measurements. Am J Cardiol 1983;52(7):867–870.
63. Park MK, Menard SW, Yuan C. Comparison of auscultatory and oscillometric blood pressures. Arch Pediatr Adolesc Med 2001;155(1):50–53.
64. Wattigney WA, Webber LS, Lawrence MD, Berenson GS. Utility of an automatic instrument for blood pressure measurement in children. The Bogalusa Heart Study. Am J Hypertens 1996;9(3):256–262.
65. O'Brien E, Petrie J, Littler W, et al. The British Hypertension Society protocol for the evaluation of automated and semi-automated blood pressure measuring devices with special reference to ambulatory systems. J Hypertens 1990;8(7):607–619.
66. American National Standard for manual, electronic or automated sphygmomanometers. Arlington, Virginia, Association for the Advancement of Medical Instrumentation 2002: 1–78.
67. O'Brien E. Proposals for simplifying the validation protocols of the British Hypertension Society and the Association for the Advancement of Medical Instrumentation. Blood Press Monit 2000;5(1):43–45.

68. O'Brien E, Waeber B, Parati G, Staessen J, Myers MG. Blood pressure measuring devices: recommendations of the Eurpoean Society of Hypertension. BMJ 2001;322(7285):531–536.
69. O'Brien E, Mee F, Atkins N, O'Malley K.. Short report: accuracy of the Dinamap portable monitor, model 8100 determined by the British Hypertension Society protocol. J Hypertens 1993;11(7):761–763.
70. Jin RZ, Donaghue KC, Fairchild J, Chan A, Silink M. Comparison of Dinamap 8100 with sphygmomanometer blood pressure measurement in a prepubertal diabetes cohort. J Paediatr Child Health 2001;37(6):545–549.
71. Moss AJ, Adams FH. Index of indirect estimation of diastolic blood pressure. Am J Dis Child 1963;106:364–367.
72. Smith GR. Devices for blood pressure measurement. Prof Nurse 2000;15(5):337–340.
73. Park MK, Menard SM. Normative oscillometric blood pressure values in the first 5 years in an office setting. Am J Dis Child 1989;143(7):860–864.
74. O'Brien E, Mee F, Atkins N, Thomas M. Evaluation of three devices for self-measurement of blood pressure according to the revised British Hypertension Society Protocol: the Omron HEM-705CP, Philips HP5332, and Nissei DS-175. Blood Press Monit 1996;1(1):55–61.
75. O'Brien E. Replacing the mercury sphygmomanometer. Requires clinicians to demand better automated devices. Brit Med Jrnl 2000;320(7238):815–816.
76. Kelder SH, Osganian SK, Feldman HA, et al. Tracking of physical and physiological risk variables among ethnic subgroups from third to eighth grade: the Child and Adolescent Trial for Cardiovascular Health cohort study. Prev Med 2002;34(3):324–333.
77. Staessen JA, Celis H, Hond ED, et al. Comparison of conventional and automated blood pressure measurements: interim analysis of the THOP trial. Blood Press Monit 2002;7(1):61–62.
78. Rose KM, Arnett DK, et al. Skip patterns in DINAMAP-measured blood pressure in 3 epidemiological studies. Hypertension 2000;35(5):1032–1036.
79. Mahoney LT, Burns TL, Stanford W, et al. Coronary risk factors measured in childhood and young adult life are associated with coronary artery calcification in young adults: the Muscatine Study. J Am Coll Cardiol 1996;27(2):277–284.
80. Simons DB, Schwartz RS, Edwards WD, Sheedy PF, Breen JF, Rumberger JA. Noninvasive definition of anatomic coronary artery disease by ultrafast computed tomographic scanning: a quantitative pathologic comparison study. J Am Coll Cardiol 1992;20(5):1118–1126.
81. Berenson GS, Srinivasan SR, Bao W, Newman WP 3rd, Tracy RE, Wattigney WA. Association between multiple cardiovascular risk factors and atherosclerosis in children and young adults. The Bogalusa Heart Study. N Engl J Med 1998;338(23):1650–1656.
82. McGill HC Jr, McMahan CA, Tracy RE, et al. Relation of a postmortem renal index of hypertension to atherosclerosis and coronary artery size in young men and women. Pathobiological Determinants of Atherosclerosis in Youth (PDAY) Research Group. Arterioscler Thromb Vasc Biol 1998;18(7):1108–1118.
83. Pickering TG, Coats A, Mallion JM, Mancia G, Verdecchia P. Blood pressure monitoring. Task force V: White-coat hypertension. Blood Press Monit 1999;4(6):333–341.
84. Sorof JM, Portman RJ. White coat hypertension in children with elevated casual blood pressure. J Pediatr 2000;137(4):493–497.
85. Chamontin B, Amar J, Barthe P, Salvador M. Blood pressure measurements and left ventricular mass in young adults with arterial hypertension screened at high school check-up. J Hum Hypertens 1994;8(5):357–361.
86. Shevchenko YL, Tsitlik JE. 90th Anniversary of the development by Nikolai S. Korotkoff of the auscultatory method of measuring blood pressure. Circulation 1996;94:116–118.
87. McAlister FA, Straus SE. Measurement of blood pressure: an evidence-based review. BMJ 2001;322:908–911.

# 5 Development of Blood Pressure Norms in Children

*Bonita Falkner,* MD

*Contents*



## INTRODUCTION

It is only in the past decade that blood pressure (BP) assessment in children and adolescents has become a routine clinical practice. BP was rarely measured in very young children prior to the 1970s, because it was too difficult to obtain reliable measurements. Additionally, it was generally believed that hypertension (HTN) was a rare problem in children *(1)*. Since BP measurement had not yet become routine, high BP was detected only when significant clinical signs or symptoms were present. Because there were no age-appropriate data available, clinicians used available adult criteria for reference information. We now know that early descriptions of hypertension in the young represented only the most severe cases of childhood HTN.

Looking back on this practice, and considering what we now know about BP in the young, one can understand how some beliefs in medicine develop. With regard to childhood hypertension, the belief had been that hypertension in children was secondary to an underlying cause, and that primary, or essential, hypertension did not exist in children. This belief has changed with the development and understanding of reference data on BP in children, relative to physical development. We now have BP data and a body of clinical experience that enable clinicians to evaluate BP levels in children relative to age, sex, body size, and other clinical parameters. Moreover, the clinician can use available reference BP data and the child's clinical characteristics to determine the child's overall health in terms of future risk or a BP level that warrants further evaluation. We now know that hypertension in some children is secondary to an underlying disorder, such as renal disease. We also know that essential HTN can be detected

From: *Clinical Hypertension and Vascular Disease: Pediatric Hypertension*
Edited by: R. J. Portman, J. M. Sorof, and J. R. Ingelfinger © Humana Press Inc., Totowa, NJ

in the young, and that recognizing the early phase of HTN increases our ability to modify the cardiovascular outcome.

Clinical trials, research, and analysis have furthered our knowledge of childhood hypertension over the past thirty years. One outcome is the BP normative distribution data on which we base our current definitions of normotension and hypertension in children and adolescents. This chapter will review that process, and, consequently provide an historical reflection. The questions and concerns expressed by the authors of the early reports are important to note as a catalyst that propelled the process, and provided a model for future progress.

## OUTCOME OF CHILDHOOD HYPERTENSION

HTN is a significant health problem in that adverse clinical outcomes can be attributed to, or associated with, BP levels that exceed an acceptable level. Little had been known about the health consequences of HTN in childhood. Still and Cottom *(2)* provided one of the first descriptions on the outcome of severe HTN in children by reviewing cases treated at the Hospital for Sick Children, Great Ormond Street, from 1954 to 1964. All reviewed had sustained diastolic BP greater than 120 mmHg. Of the 55 cases reviewed, 31 died, 18 survived with treatment that achieved a reduction in BP, and 6 were cured of HTN following corrective surgery for an identifiable lesion (coarctation repair, unilateral nephrectomy, pheochromocytoma removal). Of the 56% of children who died, the average duration of survival following diagnosis of HTN was 14 mo. The analysis of this sample of severe childhood HTN indicated a 90% mortality rate within one year, a rate that is the *same* as that of malignant HTN in adults. While these numbers are shocking by today's standards, the clear message at the time was that severe HTN in children could be as deadly as in adults.

The Still and Cottom report, and others of that era was limited to children with quite severe HTN. In the absence of BP data on normal children at that time, the standard adult cut point of 140/90 mmHg was generally used to define HTN in children. This then limited the diagnosis of HTN in children to those with the most extreme elevations of BP, and severe HTN is frequently associated with renal disease or some other disorder that causes the HTN. As a result, for some time the issue of childhood HTN focused on the evaluation for underlying disease, and search for secondary cause. Subsequent efforts to develop normative data on BP in childhood were a necessary prelude for a shift from the narrow focus of secondary HTN to a broader perspective that high levels of BP could indicate an early phase of a chronic process. It was established that severe HTN had an adverse outcome if left untreated. What was yet to be determined was how frequent did HTN occur, and what level of BP elevation in a given child conferred risk for target organ or vessel injury.

## PREVALENCE OF HYPERTENSION IN CHILDHOOD

In the last half of the 20th century, HTN was established as a significant health problem in adults, and efforts were underway, from both a public health and clinical care perspective, to improve its detection and management. To a large extent, HTN was regarded as a component of aging and a reflection of chronic atherosclerosis. Consequently, HTN appeared to have little relevance in the young. Jennifer Loggie was one of the first to consider the possibility that "essential" HTN could be detected in adolescents *(3)*. In a review article in 1974, Loggie discussed the reports available at that time on the prevalence of HTN in persons 25 yr of age or younger. Of the five published reports *(4–8)* that attempted to determine the incidence of

**Table 1**
**Reported Prevalence of HTN in Persons 25 Yr of Age or Less Prior to Normative Data**

| *Authors* | *Subjects age (yr)* | *Number screened* | *Position in which pressure was taken* | *Definition of HTN (mmHg)* | *Prevalence (%)* |
|---|---|---|---|---|---|
| Masland et al., 1956 *(4)* | "Adolescents" | 1795 | Not Stated | 140/90 | 1.4 |
| Boe et al., 1957 *(5)* | 15–19 | 3833 | Sitting | 150/90 | 3.01 Males<br>1.04 Females |
| Heyden et al., 1969 *(6)* | 15–25 | 435 | Sitting | 140/90 | 11.0 |
| Londe, 1966 *(7)* | 4–15 | 1473 | Supine | Systolic or Diastolic >90th% | 12.4 Males<br>11.6 Females |
| | | | | Systolic or Diastolic >95th% (Repeated Measures) | 1.9 |
| Wilber et al., 1972 *(8)* | 15–25 | 799 | Sitting | Systolic>160<br>Diastolic>90 | 1.0<br>1.5 |

Adapted from Loggie, 1974 *(3)*

HTN in the young by conducting BP screening on large samples of healthy individuals, the prevalence of HTN in the young ranged from 1% *(8)* to 12.4% *(7)*. Table 1 summarizes these reports and denotes the differences in the criteria used to define HTN, methods of measurement (sitting vs supine), and the age of the sample examined. Those reports that examined adolescents and young adults defined HTN by a set level of BP, similar to values used for adults *(4–6,8)*, and reported rates of HTN between 1 and 3%. The report by Londe *(6)* was based on an examination of younger children, aged 4–15 yr, and used a different definition of HTN. Londe measured BP in his own practice and observed that BP rises with age, concurrent with growth and development *(6,7)*. He then analyzed the BP data to determine the range of systolic and diastolic BP stratified by age, and selected the 90th percentile for each age that defined HTN. His reported rates of HTN were slightly above 10% and consistent with his definition. He also noted that on repeated measurement, there is regression toward the mean, and that the prevalence of persistent systolic or diastolic BP greater than the 95th percentile was 1.9%. Little attention was given to Londe's work for some time. His findings, however, are remarkably similar to contemporary data that measured a much larger sample.

## DEFINITION OF HYPERTENSION IN CHILDHOOD

The fundamental problems facing researchers was to discover what constituted normal BP, and what level of BP defined HTN in the young person. The approach to defining abnormal BP in adulthood uses, as the definition of HTN, the approximate level of BP that marks an increase in mortality above the average level. The cut-point numbers for BP were largely derived from actuarial data from life insurance mortality investigations. These data indicated an increase in death rates when the systolic BP exceeded 140 mmHg, or the diastolic BP exceeded 90 mmHg.

This method was challenged by Master et al. *(9)* in a report published in 1950. These authors argued that defining HTN by a single number was arbitrary, because HTN occurred far more frequently in the elderly and was commonly associated with atherosclerosis. They contended that an increase in BP was a reflection of aging, and that the use of one number to define a disorder for all ages resulted in an over-diagnosis of HTN in the elderly. They proposed a statistical definition based on the distribution of BP readings around the mean, according to sex and age. BP, like most human characteristics, demonstrates a frequency distribution that yields a fairly normal curve. In a normal distribution, roughly two-thirds of the observations will occur within the range of the statistical mean plus or minus one standard deviation from the mean, and 95 percent of the observations will be within the range of the mean plus or minus two standard deviations. Master et al. proposed that BP that reached a level two standard deviations beyond the statistical mean, or greater than the 95th percentile, should be considered abnormal. They supported their position by examining data obtained from industrial plants in various sections of the country on approx 7400 persons who were stated to be in "average good health and able to work." Using a statistical method to define the normal range of BP, they described the normal range of systolic BP in males to be 105–135 mmHg at age 16, and rising progressively with age to reach 115–170 mmHg at age 60–64 yr. They also noted a gender difference in the normal range, with females having a normal range of systolic BP of 100–130 mmHg at 16 yr of age, and rising to a normal range of 115–175 mmHg at age 60–64 yr. The conclusion of the authors was that HTN was over diagnosed in adults, particularly in the elderly. Their conclusion was supported, they believed, by their ability to demonstrate that large numbers of persons were living with BP above 140/90 mmHg and were "in average good health and able to work."

A large body of subsequent epidemiological and clinical investigations on HTN in adults has clearly dismissed the conclusion by Master et al. *(9)* that HTN is over-diagnosed because the normal range of BP increases with age. Based on extensive data, the clinical consensus in adults is that the risk for cardiovascular events that are associated with BP is continuous, and that the risk rises concurrently with BP levels *(10)*. However, the report by Master et al. is the earliest to show that the normal range of BP is lower in persons aged 16–19 yr than in persons 20 yr and older *(9)*. The authors also demonstrated gender differences in the normal range of BP. Most significantly, they provided a statistical method to define the normal range. Abnormal BP could then be defined in the absence of mortality or morbidity end points.

The question that remained unanswered until the early 1970s was that of the prevalence of HTN in children and adolescence. This question could not be answered without a clear and consistent definition of HTN in the young. Moreover, the definition of HTN could not be developed in the absence of knowledge about what constituted normal BP in children and adolescents. There were some quite limited data on BP levels in normal children *(6,11–14)*. The available data indicated that the BP level was considerably lower in young children than in adults, and that there appeared to be a normal rise in BP with age that was concurrent with growth *(15)*. It was also recognized that owing to difficulty in measurement techniques, there was likely to be considerable variability in what data were available.

Efforts to gain a better understanding of the occurrence of hypertension in the young initially tended to focus on adolescents. Based on a careful examination of her own clinical data on cases she had evaluated for BP elevation, Loggie *(3)* suggested that essential HTN was more common in adolescents than had been previously believed. Kilcoyne et al. *(16)* made an effort to determine if asymptomatic HTN could be detected in healthy adolescents. These investigators conducted BP screening on urban high school students. They observed that female students of all races had lower systolic pressures than males. Using 140/90 mmHg as a definition of HTN, they detected an overall prevalence of 5.4% systolic and 7.8% diastolic HTN at the initial screening; followup screening of those with elevated measurements demonstrated a decline in prevalence to 1.2% systolic and 2.4% diastolic HTN. They also noted higher rates of sustained HTN among the black males. These investigators examined their data further by creating frequency distributions of systolic BP in the males at successive age levels of 14 yr, 16 yr, and 18 yr. These distribution curves demonstrated a progressive rightward displacement with increasing age, that, the authors suggested, indicated a transition to adult characteristics. However, they also noted that this shift in distribution did not occur in females between 14 and 19 yr of age. Based on their data, these investigators suggested that the criteria used to define BP elevations in adolescents would be more meaningful if they were based on the frequency distributions of BP in an adolescent sample, and proposed that values exceeding one standard deviation above the mean would more appropriately define HTN. From their data, one standard deviation above the mean would be 132/85 mmHg for males and 123/82 mmHg for females. It is of note that, although one standard deviation above the mean, as oppposed to two, was proposed, these values are reasonably close to the numbers that Master et al. *(9)* reported to be at the top of the normal range for persons 16–19 yr of age (males 135 mmHg; females 130 mmHg).

Similar efforts to investigate BP in healthy adolescents were conducted by other investigators, largely in the context of high school screening projects *(17–20)*. These studies detected initial rates of HTN at approx 5%; the rate declined on repeat examination when adult measurement criteria were used. These reports also noted lower BP levels in adolescent females compared to males. Some differences in BP by race were reported, with higher levels and more HTN reported among African-Americans *(16,17)*. An effect of weight on BP was also described *(17,20)*. Seen together, these reports emphasized a need to develop a better definition of HTN in the young, based on more representative data that were derived from a large sample of healthy children.

This need was recognized by the National Heart, Lung, and Blood Institute (NHLBI), which directed the National High Blood Pressure Education Program to appoint a Task Force on Blood Pressure Control in Children. The Task Force published its first report in 1977 *(21)*, and in that report described the results of its proceedings. The goal of the report was to (1) describe a standard methodology for measurement of BP in the young; (2) provide BP distribution curves by age and sex; (3) recommend a BP level that is the upper limit of normal; and (4) provide guidelines for detection, evaluation, and treatment of children with elevated or at risk BP measurements. The BP distribution curves were based on data gathered from three studies conducted in Muscatine, Iowa; Rochester, Minnesota; and Miami, Florida. The total size of the sample was 9283 children from age 5 through 18 yr, with an additional 306 children aged 2–5 yr (Miami). The BP data were presented as distribution curves, by age, for systolic and diastolic BP in males and females, similar to the standard pediatric growth curves for weight and height.

These BP distribution curves were clearly an advancement, particularly for clinicians who cared for children. Although based on cross-sectional data, the curves indicated a normal increase in BP level with age, which was concurrent with an increase in height and weight. The BP curves also established a normative range for BP in early childhood that was different from that of adults. Using a statistical definition, the 95th percentile for each age and sex was the recommended BP level for ascertainment of hypertension, if verified on repeated measurement. These distribution curves, for the first time, provided a clear view on the levels of BP that were outside the normal range in young children. However, by age 13 yr in boys the 95th percentile had reached 140 mmHg systolic and 90 mmHg diastolic pressure, with a progressive rise to 18 yr, at which age the 95th percentile was over 150 mmHg systolic and at 95 mmHg diastolic. These numbers seemed to indicate that by early adolescence the adult criteria to define hypertension would be appropriate. However, the 95th percentile delineated BP levels that seemed to be high, particularly in view of the data that had been collected in the preceding high school screening studies. This discrepancy raised concern as to how well these distribution curves truly reflected the normative BP distribution in children and adolescents.

## NORMATIVE BLOOD PRESSURE DISTRIBUTION IN CHILDREN AND ADOLESCENTS

The first Task Force on Blood Pressure Control in Children and Adolescents established the importance of BP in childhood as an indicator of health status. It provided a clear methodology for measurement of BP in children and encouraged clinicians to measure BP in the young. It also provided a definition of HTN that could be applied to children. What was not clear was whether or not the BP distribution curves were an accurate reflection of the normative distribution. The NHLBI recognized the need to obtain a larger body of data on BP in the young within the context of childhood growth, and subsequently supported several epidemiological studies that prospectively investigated BP and growth in children and adolescents. These projects were conducted at several sites, applied rigorous detail to the methodology of BP measurement, and examined the anthropometric determinants of BP level relative to physiological development.

As these data emerged, a second Task Force on Blood Pressure Control in Children and Adolescents was convened to re-examine the data on BP distribution throughout childhood, and prepare distribution curves of BP by age accompanied by height and weight information *(22)*. With this new information, the second Task Force also updated the guidelines for detection, evaluation, and management of HTN in the young in its 1987 report. Table 2 provides the sites that contributed data that were used to develop the new BP distribution curves. BP data were available for more than 65,000 children. This sample included an age range from infancy to 20 yr of age, and a substantial representation of different racial and ethnic groups. The BP distribution curves *(23–36)* published in the Second Task Force Report again demonstrated a progressive rise in BP that was concurrent with age. Gender differences in BP during adolescence were verified. The BP in males continued to increase from age 13 through 18 yr, whereas the BP in females tended to plateau after age 13 yr; the normal distribution was somewhat higher in adolescent males compared to females. Moreover, the entire distribution was lower and, consequently, the 95th (and 90th) percentile delineated a level of BP that was substantially lower than that described in the previous report. The second Task Force Report applied the same definition of HTN that was used in the first Task Force Report, which was systolic or diastolic BP that was repeatedly equal to or greater than the 95th percentile. However, in consideration of how much lower the 95th percentile appeared to be at that time, along with the concern about possibly over-diagnosing HTN in the young, this report included a classification table for *significant* and *severe* HTN. According to age strata, the BP values that approximated the 95th to 99th percentiles were designated significant HTN, and the BP values

Table 2
Data Sources for the Second Task Force Report

| *Source* | *Age (yr)* | *N* |
|---|---|---|
| Muscatine, IA *(23–25)* | 5–19 | 4208 |
| University of South Carolina *(26)* | 4–20 | 6657 |
| University of Texas, Houston *(27)* | 3–17 | 2922 |
| Bogalusa, LA *(28,29)* | 1–20 | 16,442 |
| Second National Health and Nutrition Examination Survey *(30)* | 6–20 | 4563 |
| University of Texas, Dallas *(31,32)* | 13–19 | 24,792 |
| University of Pittsburgh *(33)* | Newborn–5 | 1554 |
| Providence, RI *(34)* | Newborn–3 | 3487 |
| Brompton, England *(35,36)* | Newborn–3 | 7804 |

that exceeded the 99th percentile were designated as severe HTN. At the time the report was developed, it could seem that the authors were hedging on the definition of HTN in the young. However by intention or not, the concept of staging HTN, on the basis of degree of BP elevation, was novel and had not yet been considered in the field of adult HTN. It was not until publication of The Sixth Report of the Joint National Committee in 1998 *(10)* that the HTN stage was introduced as a method to guide patient care and clinical management decisions in adults.

Subsequent to the 1987 Task Force Report, additional childhood BP data were developed from the National Health and Nutrition Examination Survey III *(37)*. There was also evidence that children with elevated BP in childhood often developed HTN in early adulthood *(38)*. As the contention that the origins of HTN exhibited themselves early in life gained increasing support, the prevailing opinion was that there should be an emphasis on BP surveillance in children, along with early preventive efforts. It required a re-examination of the national data on childhood BP to provide substance to these recommendations. Therefore, a third Task Force was convened to update the normative data as well as the guidelines for management, including preventive guidelines.

The addition of the new BP data, and re-analysis of the entire childhood database resulted in BP distribution curves that were slightly lower than, but generally consistent with, the findings of the second Task Force *(39)*. The third report, which was termed "Update on the 1987 Task Force Report," provided further details on the relationship of body size to BP. The contribution of body size was considered in the analysis that was conducted by the second Task Force, as well as the analysis of the data from individual sites by the investigators who had developed the data. Analysis of those data indicated that height and body weight, as well as age, were major determinants of BP. Height was considered to be the best determinant of BP within the normal range. Therefore, it was recommended that height adjustment be applied in the evaluation of BP level. To support this practice, the second Task Force Report contained information on the 90th percentile for height at the 90th for BP. It was assumed that pediatricians, who were accustomed to making weight-for-height adjustments, could figure out how to make the height adjustment for BP. The third or Update Report expanded the presentation of the data by providing tables with the systolic and diastolic BP level at the 90th and 95th percentile for each height percentile, and each age from 1 through 17 yr. These tables provide a better view on the variation of BP according to height, as well as to age. The revised tables also render more precisely the ability to determine if the BP level in a given child is normal, high normal, or abnormally elevated for sex, age, and height.

The current BP norms are based on data developed from over 70,000 children and adolescents and collected according to a rigorous and uniform methodology. The sample represented diverse racial and ethnic groups from several areas of the US, and an additional sample from England. The analysis of these data, and the production of BP norms, provide a framework upon which to identify children and adolescents with HTN and ascertain risk for future hypertension. The development of childhood normative BP data has been underway for many years. The process has benefited from additional information from other areas in the field of hypertension. The process itself has been informative. The current state of knowledge on BP level and BP criteria for HTN in the young is the result of persistent inquiry by many thoughtful clinicians, the demands of clinical investigators for accurate data on which to base definitions, and the skills of epidemiologists and biostatisticians who developed and analyzed the data. This process must continue. Consideration of the substantial progress that has occurred should provide encouragement to continue.

## REFERENCES


1. McCrory W, Nash FW. Hypertension in Children: A Review. Am J Med Sci 1952;223:671.
2. Still JL, Cottom D. Severe Hypertension in Childhood. Arch Dis Child 1967:42:34–39.
3. Loggie J. Essential hypertension in adolescents. Postgraduate Medicine 1974;56:133–141.
4. Masland RP Jr., Heald FP Jr., Goodale WT, Gallagher JR. Hypertensive vascular disease in adolescence. N Engl J Med 1956;255:894.
5. Boe J, Humerfeit S, Wedervang F. The blood pressure in a population. Acta Med Scand Suppl 1957;321:1.
6. Heyden S, Bartel AG, Hames CG, McDonough JR. Elevated blood pressure levels in adolescents, Evans County, Georgia: seven year follow-up of 30 patients and 30 controls. JAMA 1969;209:1683.
7. Londe S. Blood pressure in children as determined under office conditions. Clin Pediatr 1966;5:71.
8. Wilber JA, Millward D, Baldwin A, et al. Atlanta community high blood pressure program: methods of community hypertension screening. Circ Res 1972;3(Suppl 2):101.
9. Master AM, Dublin LI, Marks HH. The normal blood pressure range and its clinical implications. JAMA 1950;143:1464.
10. The sixth report of the joint national committee on prevention, detection, evaluation and treatment of high blood pressure. Arch Intern Med 1977;157:2413–2446.
11. Graham AW, Hines EA, Gage RP. Blood pressures in children between the ages of five and sixteen years. Am J Dis Child 1945;69:203.
12. Londe S. Blood pressure standards for normal children as determined under office conditions. Clin Pediatr 1968;7:400.
13. Vital Health Stat. Blood pressure levels of children 6–11 years: relationship to age, sex, race and socioeconomic status. 1973;11:135.
14. Allen-Williams GM. Pulse-rate and blood pressure in infancy and early childhood. Arch Dis Child 1945; 20:125.
15. McLain LG. Hypertension in childhood: a review. American Heart Journal 1976;92:634–647.
16. Kilcoyne MM, Richter RW, Alsup PA. Adolescent hypertension. I. detection and prevalence. Circulation 1974;50:758–764.
17. Kotchen JM, Kotchen TA, Schwertman NC, Kuller LH. Blood pressure distributions of urban adolescents. Amer J Epidem 1974;99:315–324.
18. Reichman LB, Cooper BM, Blumenthal S, et al. Bureau of chronic disease control and maternal and child health services of the New York City Department of health and the New York City Medical Advisory Committee on Hypertension, New York. Hypertension testing among high school students—surveillance procedures and results. J Chron Dis 1975;28:161–171.

19. Miller RA, Shekelle RB. Blood pressure in tenth grade students: results from the Chicago Heart Association pediatric heart screening project. Circulation 1976;54:993–1000.
20. Garbus SB, Garbus SB, Young CJ, Hassinger G, Johnson W. Screening for hypertension in adolescents. Southern Medical Journal 1980;73:174–182.
21. NHLBI Report of the task force on blood pressure control in children. Pediatrics 1977;59 (Suppl): 797–820.
22. NHLBI Report of the second task force on blood pressure control in children, task force on blood pressure control in Children. Pediatrics 1987;79:1–25.
23. Clarke WR, Schrott HG, Leaverton PE, Connor WE, Lauer RM. Tracking of blood lipids and blood pressure in school age children: the muscatine study. Circulation 1978;58:626–636.
24. Lauer RM, Clarke WR, Beaglehole R. Level, Trend and variability of blood pressure during childhood: the muscatine study. Circulation 1984;69:242–249.
25. Lauer RM, Burns TL, Clarke WR. Assessing children's blood pressure—considerations of age and body size: the muscatine study. Pediatrics 1985;75:1081–1090.
26. Lackland DT, Riopel DA, Shepard DM,Wheeler FC. Blood pressure and anthropometric measurement results of the South Carolina dental health and pediatric blood pressure study. South Carolina Dental Health and Blood Pressure Study, January 1985.
27. Gutgesell M, Terrell G, LaBarthe DR. Pediatrics blood pressure: ethnic comparison in a primary care center. Hypertension 1980;3:39–47.
28. Berenson GS, McMahan CA, Voors AW, et al. Cardiovascular risk factors in children—the early natural history of atherosclerosis and essential hypertension. New York: Oxford University Press, 1980.
29. Voors AW, Foster TA, Frerichs RR, Webber LS, Berenson GS. Studies of blood pressure in children ages 5–14 years in a total biracial community—the bogalusa heart study. Circulation 1976;54:319–327.
30. McDowell A, Engel A, Massey J, Maurer KR. The plan and operation of the second national health and nutrition examination survey, 1976–1980. Department of Health and Human Services Publication No. (PHS) 81-1317, series 1, No. 15. Government Printing Office, July 1981.
31. Fixler DE, Laird WP. Validity of mass blood pressure screening in children. Pediatrics 1983;72:459–463.
32. Baron, AE, Freyer, B, Fixler, DE. Longitudinal blood pressures in blacks, whites and mexican americans during adolescence and early adulthood. Am J Epidem 1986;123:809–817.
33. Schachter J, Kuller LH, Perfetti C. Blood pressure during the first five years of life: relation to ethnic group (black or white) and to parental hypertension. Am J Epidem 1984;119:541–553.
34. Zinner SH, Rosner B, Oh WO, Kass EH. Significance of blood pressure in infancy. Hypertension 1985;7:411–416.
35. de Swiet M, Fayers P, Shinebourne EA. Blood pressure survey in a population of newborn infants. Br Med J 1976;2:9–11.
36. de Swiet M, Fayers P, Shinebourne EA. Systolic blood pressure in a population of infants in the first year of life: the brompton study. Pediatrics 1980;65:1028–1035.
37. Centers for Disease Control and Prevention, National Center for Health Statistics. National Health and Nutrition Survey (NHANES III), 1988–1991, Data computed for the NHLBI. Atlanta, GA: Centers for Disease Control and Prevention.
38. Lauer RM, Clarke WR. Childhood risk factors for high adult blood pressure: the muscatine study. Pediatrics 1984;84:633–641.
39. Update on the 1987 Task force report on high blood pressure in children and adolescents: a working group report from the National High Blood Pressure Education Program. Pediatrics 1996;98:649–658.

# 6 Ambulatory Blood Pressure Methodology and Norms in Children

*Empar Lurbe,* MD *and Josep Redon,* MD, FAHA

*CONTENTS*



## INTRODUCTION

Casual blood pressure (BP) measurement is the basis of present knowledge about the risks associated with hypertension *(1)* and has guided patient management for many years *(2)*. Nevertheless, casual BP is characterized by high variability, and the small number of measurements obtained in medical settings may not necessarily reflect the usual BP of an individual *(3)*. The possibility of carrying out repeated measurements with ambulatory BP monitoring (ABPM) using invasive *(4)* or noninvasive devices *(5)* provides more representative values of BP, and permits the observation of the behavior of BP during activity and sleep.

Over the last few years, ABPM has been introduced into pediatric populations. In spite of a number of publications *(6–11)* that have raised numerous important methodological questions, the interpretation of the results and the definition of normal ambulatory BP remain to be clarified. These questions are important when monitoring subjects in a range of ages and body sizes and whose levels of physical activity and fitness differ. It is possible that ambulatory BP in children could provide the basis for an easier and earlier recognition of abnormal BP values and/or behavior than is presently possible *(7,8)*, mainly in older children with persistent casual mild hypertension.

The proper clinical use of ABPM requires understanding of the monitors and methods available, the best protocol for the monitoring procedure, and the potential of the information obtained.

From: *Clinical Hypertension and Vascular Disease: Pediatric Hypertension*
Edited by: R. J. Portman, J. M. Sorof, and J. R. Ingelfinger © Humana Press Inc., Totowa, NJ

Table 1
Characteristics of the Methods

| | *Oscillometric* | *Auscultatory* |
|---|---|---|
| Placement | Easy and stable | Difficult |
| Percentage of errors | Low | High |
| Compliance | High | Low |
| Accuracy | SBP medium<br>DBP low | SBP high<br>DBP medium-low |
| Inacuracy in low pulse oscillation | High | Low |

## MONITORS AND METHODS FOR MEASURING AMBULATORY BLOOD PRESSURE

### *Monitors*

Each type of monitor used to measure ambulatory BP uses either the auscultatory or the oscillometric method of BP assessment. Each monitor's features are shown in Table 1. Auscultatory methods are based on the detection of Korotkoff sounds by microphonic sensors, while oscillometric methods determine mean BP directly from the point of maximum oscillation. Neither systolic nor diastolic BP is measured directly by monitoring devices, but is calculated using an algorithm based on a putative relationship between oscillations. Although both methods have problems, the oscillometric device is the one most often used in a pediatric population, primarily because the percentage of erroneous readings for oscillometric devices is low compared to the auscultatory devices. Although the oscillometric method should simulate a clinical reading with a sphygmomanometer, it is prone to microphone errors when used in an ambulatory setting. In one study comparing the two methods, 30% of all ambulatory readings using the Korotkoff system received an error code, compared to 4% using the oscillometric system *(12)*. The most common errors of the Korotkoff method were owing to noise detected by the microphone or the inability to detect Korotkoff sounds clearly. The difficulties inherent in microphone placement and maintaining the microphone position are at least partly responsible for these errors *(13)*.

The monitors available on the market differ in their key components and, as a consequence, in BP assessment. For auscultatory devices, differences in microphone sensibility exist among the different manufacturers. Among oscillometric devices, different algorithms to calculate systolic and diastolic BP from the point of maximal oscillation are used by different devices.

Many of the devices used with children had previously been validated with adults, but the pediatric population differs from the adult population in a number of important ways which affect both methods. In the technique that utilizes Korotkoff sound, the inability to clearly distinguish Korotkoff sounds, and the absence of the fifth sound in some children, gives a very poor estimate of BP. With oscillometry, the narrow pulse pressure present in some children does not fit the predictable relationship between vessel and cuff pressure oscillations and subsequent systolic and diastolic pressure, the basis for the algorithms for each manufacturer's oscillometric devices. Even though these differences do not permit extrapolating the data obtained from adults and applying it to children, few studies have attempted to validate moni-

Table 2
Monitors Validated Following AAMI or BHS Protocol

| *Monitor* | *Mode* | *AAMI* | *BHS* | *Grade* |
|---|---|---|---|---|
| Quiet Track *(17)* | Auscultatory | SBP passed | SBP | A |
| | | DBP passed | DBP | A |
| Spacelabs 90207 *(15)* | Oscillometric | SBP passed | SBP | C |
| | | DBP passed | DBP | D |
| Takeda 2421 *(13)* | Oscillometric | Not performed | SBP | C/D |
| | | | DBP | C/D |
| Takeda 2421 *(13)* | Auscultatory | Not performed | SBP | A |
| | | | DBP (IV) | |
| | | | DBP (V) | B/C |
| Dynapulse 5000A *(16)* | Oscillometric | Failed | Not performed | |

AAMI, Association for the Advancement of Medical Instrumentation; BHS, British Hypertension Society Validation Protocol

tors in the children. Although the British Hypertension Society (BHS) Protocol *(14)* used in the validation of BP measurement devices describes what is essential to the validation protocol, and specifically addresses the characteristics of the children to include as subjects, some difficulties remain. Problems measuring diastolic BP in some children make evident the difficulty in validating the diastolic readings provided by these devices.

The published validation studies in pediatric populations are shown in Table 2. In general, the oscillometric monitors tested passed with grades of B and C for systolic BP. The diastolic BP grades are lower, achieving grades of C and D *(13,15,16)*. The auscultatory method achieves a grade of A for systolic BP and B for diastolic BP *(13,17)*, similar to the grades for adults, according to one validation study concerning the QuietTrak monitor *(17)*. The QuietTrak monitor, however, does not include the percentage of erroneous measurements. This last aspect is important because, although the auscultatory method achieved better grades, another study *(12)* shows this method to have a high percentage of erroneous measurements, diminishing its potential for use in monitoring children. The development of oscillometric devices with tailored algorithms for this specific age group is necessary for improving device accuracy.

Recently, the European Working Group in Ambulatory Blood Pressure *(18)* released a new validation protocol that reduced the number of subjects necessary for the validation procedure without losing the capacity to detect potential inaccuracies in the tested devices. Simplifying the validation procedure without reducing accuracy may permit a larger number of validations than presently feasible. The present protocol, however, does not introduce specific procedures to validate devices in such special populations as pediatrics.

### *Monitoring Procedure*

The characteristics of the pediatric population dictate the careful application of standardized recording techniques in order to achieve successful measurements with ambulatory devices. Successful techniques include providing adequate cuff size, simple tailored instructions, and a short period of adaptation. As in clinical measurements, the length of the bladder should be at least 90% of the arm circumference, and the width should be about 40% of the arm circumference. Ambulatory BP monitoring has been performed while permitting normal recreational activities, although the children were advised against participating in excessively vigorous physical activities or contact sports. In addition, age-tailored instructions concerning the meaning and importance of the monitoring were also addressed.

Frequency of BP readings is the major determinant in achieving the best information from the procedure. If the objective is to assess only a reproducible 24 h BP average, the number of readings to program may be as low as 20; if, however, the circadian variability needs to be assessed, a larger number of readings should be preset. This should include enough readings to cover each hourly period throughout the day and night. In the protocol used for our group, the mean of valid readings over a 24-h period is 62 ± 7, obtained by programming a reading frequency of every 20 min from 6 AM to midnight, and every 30 min from midnight to 6 AM. When interference or error in a reading occurs, the process automatically repeats after 2 min, while retaining the pre-established sequence. During the awake period (8 AM to 10 PM) an acoustic signal prior to the measurement is automatically programmed to remind the child to relax the arm.

One of the clinically useful aspects of ambulatory BP has been the monitoring quality and those factors that are related to the achievement of good monitoring quality in children. This might be important in a population with substantial physical activity. In an unselected pediatric population aged 3–18 yr, 84% of the BP monitorings obtained with an oscillometric method attained a high standard, defined as those with successful measurements greater than or equal to 80% of the total *(19)*.

Age and BP values were the main factors independently related to optimal monitoring. The highest percentage of successful measurements was obtained in the oldest children and in those with the highest BP. Success was attributed to a better understanding of, and adherence to, the instructions given, and the higher BP values in older children, which, owing to their relatively large oscillations, decreased the potential for erroneous measurements *(19)*. Nevertheless, age and 24 h systolic BP combined account for only a small variance, an indication that other nonmeasurable factors also influence the monitoring. Accepting the device and complying with the monitoring process may be the variables most important to achieving the best recordings.

### *Data Analysis*

After the monitoring procedure, data analysis can be performed in a number of ways. We have discussed the convenience of editing recordings before analyzing data. Generally, it is convenient to automatically reject BP measurements by establishing BP value limits. The limits most used are systolic BP >220 mmHg or <70 mmHg, diastolic BP >140 mmHg or <40 mmHg, pulse pressure (systolic BP minus diastolic BP) <20 mmHg or >120 mmHg *(19,20)*. Manual editing, the removing of measurements after visual inspection, is not recommended, since it does not offer a significant improvement to the information obtained. A typical BP recording plot is shown in Fig. 1A.

In general, the information is gathered in periods which correspond to different activities throughout the day. The most common is to divide the monitoring into three different time periods: the 24-h period, the daytime, or awake, period and the nighttime, or sleep, period. The daytime, or awake, period includes all readings obtained from 8 AM to 10 PM, while the nighttime, or sleep, period includes all those taken from midnight to 6 AM, because these periods more closely correspond to stretches of activity and sleep in the majority of the subjects. Data from 10 PM to midnight and from 6 AM to 8 AM are not included as part of the sleep or awake periods to minimize overlaps, but are included as part of the 24-h ambulatory BP data. The 24-h period includes all valid readings performed during monitoring, although a more precise assessment of awake and sleep periods may be obtained by using a mini-diary. No differences, however, were present when fixed time periods similar to those described above were analyzed against the mini-diary in a mixed population of 402 normo- and hypertensive subjects ranging from 3 to 84 yr of age *(21)*.

There are several parameters that can be calculated when analyzing ambulatory BP from the measurements obtained during the monitoring: the total number of readings and the percentage of those that are erroneous, the average of systolic BP, mean BP, diastolic BP, and heart rate (HR) over the 24 h, awake, sleep, and hourly periods. Systolic BP and diastolic BP load, defined as the percentage of BP readings exceeding the upper limit of normalcy during a 24-h period, can be calculated, although their significance and clinical utility have been debated. Recently, the average of 24 h pulse pressure, calculated as the average of the differences between systolic and diastolic BP, has received attention as an indirect estimate of elasticity of the great vessels.

Besides the averages of BP values, variability can be assessed by using ambulatory BP monitoring. Blood pressure fluctuates continuously over time, either spontaneously or in response to a variety of external stimuli, of which activity is a major determinant *(22)*. Blood pressure changes following the activity–sleep cycle (circadian variability) and variation between BP values measured by each reading (intrinsic variability) has received attention. The occurrence of continuous, and often pronounced BP fluctuation, is not only of pathophysiological interest, but it may also have clinical relevance *(23)*. Recent interest in the study of circadian variability was raised by the fact that deviations from the usual diurnal rhythm may have pathological relevance *(24)*. Likewise, it has been shown that high BP variability has been linked to the development of high BP values and/or to the presence of hypertension-related organ damage *(25)*.

The diurnal part of the circadian BP profile, which many experts would agree is largely dependent on physical and mental activity, may be described by various mathematical approaches ranging from simple statistics such as the difference between the awake and the sleep BP to more complex derivations such as Fourier analysis. In one study *(26)*, the diurnal BP curve and the nocturnal blood pressure fall in normotensive children and adolescents was analyzed. More than 80% of the children showed a diurnal BP rhythm that differed significantly from random variation. The observation that the nocturnal BP fall followed a unimodal distribution suggests that the distinction between subjects with and without reduction in the sleep BP above or below a given level (so-called dippers and nondippers) is quite arbitrary. The threshold most often used to define nondippers is a BP fall from awake to sleep lower than 10%. An example of the nondipper pattern is shown in Fig. 1B.

Although limited, intrinsic variability, estimated as the standard deviation from discontinuous noninvasive BP monitoring techniques, may represent important information about cardiovascular regulation. Measuring BP at intervals greater than 10 min cannot provide information on rapid BP fluctuations and may provide a distorted assessment of slow BP changes *(27,28)*. Although there may be some degree of inaccuracy in the absolute values of variability, previous studies using the same methodology have demonstrated the relationship between BP variability and the presence of early organ damage owing to hypertension *(25,29)*, the progression of early carotid atherosclerosis *(30)*, and the risk for developing cardiac dysfunction *(31)*. The highest variability seems to reflect a higher vascular reactivity, which could

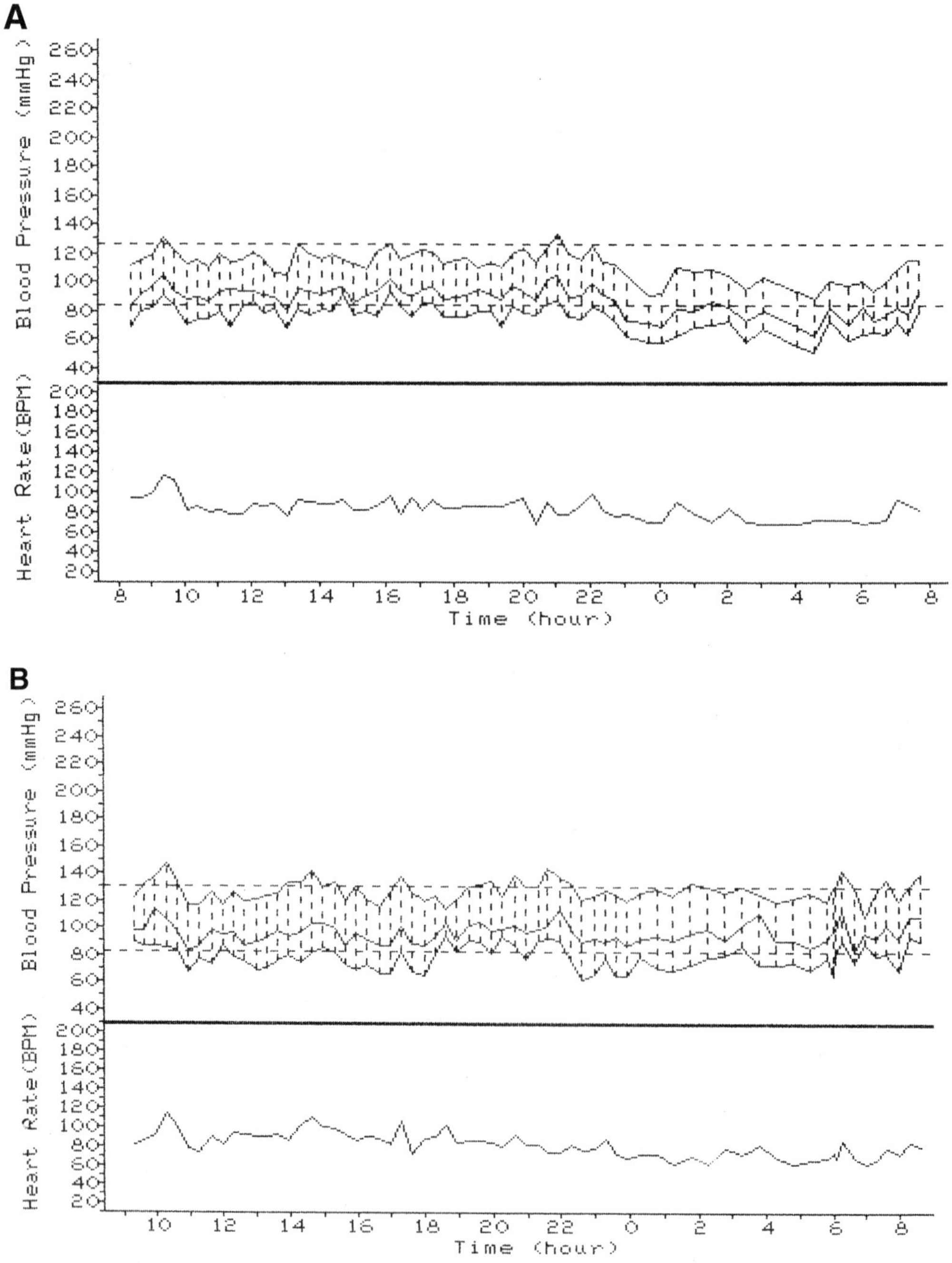


Fig. 1. (A) Circadian pattern of ambulatory blood pressure through the 24-h period. A circadian variation is present with lower values during the night period. (B) Circadian pattern of a patient with blunted decline of the physiological nocturnal fall, nondipper pattern. (C) Circadian pattern of a patient with high intrinsic variability.

Fig. 1. *(continued)*

C

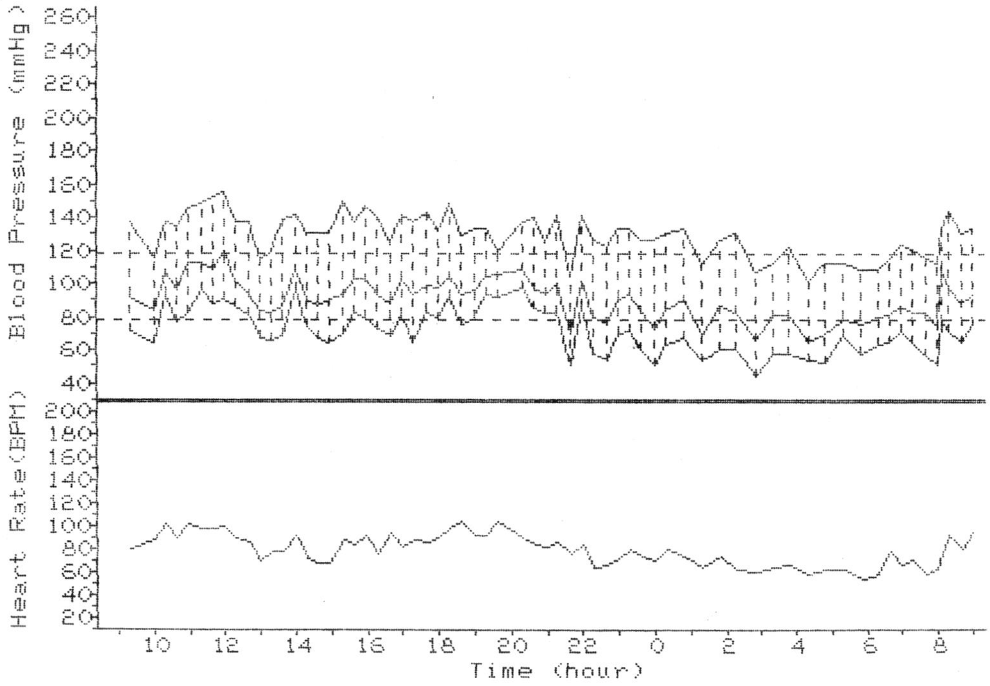


result from sympathetic overdrive, enhancement of smooth muscle cell contractility, or abnormal baroreflex sensitivity. An example of high variability is shown in Fig. 1C.

### *Reproducibility of Ambulatory Blood Pressure*

One advantage inherent in ambulatory BP recording is better reproducibility. In both normotensive and hypertensive subjects, ambulatory monitoring is more reliable and reproduceable than estimates of casual BPs, independent of age *(32)*. The reproducibility between BP measurements performed two days apart depends mainly on the number of measurements performed during the monitorings. Intra-individual variability, estimated as the standard deviation of the difference between the two measurements, decreased progressively as an increasing number of ambulatory readings were averaged, reaching the lowest value with 20 measurements *(33)*; no further improvement was observed by increasing the number of measurements. When the reproducibility of BP was studied in children and adolescents *(34,35)*, casual BP measurements were poorly reproducible. In contrast, the averages of ambulatory BP during 24 h awake and sleep time were more reproducible, especially for systolic BP.

## AMBULATORY BLOOD PRESSURE MONITORING AND REFERENCE VALUES

The clinical use of ambulatory BP depends on the normal BP ranges available as reference values, the compilation of which is a difficult and laborious task. In adults, the most meaningful reference values for both casual and ambulatory BP have been produced by long-term prospective studies; they are based on cardiovascular morbidity and mortality rates and not the BP distribution in the general population *(36)*. In children it is very difficult, if not impossible, to validate diagnostic reference values based on morbidity and mortality, because in childhood, incidence rates are too low to be used in a meaningful way *(37)*. Since it is not possible to assess cardiovascular outcomes in children and adolescents, reference casual BP data have been developed from the BP distribution of thousands of children, grouped by age and sex *(38)* or age, sex, and height *(39)*. Presently available ambulatory BP data are insufficient to create similar reference tables. However, functional, rather than distribution-based, definitions of ambulatory hypertension, must be further developed. Functional definitions may be validated by correlating intermediary signs of target organ involvement, such as left ventricular mass *(40)*, with the BP levels obtained by conventional and automated measurements, or by studying the relationship of these BP levels with pediatric risk factors that predict the development of hypertension in adulthood *(41)*.

In the meantime, more information regarding ambulatory BP values and early target organ damage is being compiled. Some preliminary data may be useful as a departure point. These data have been obtained from the simultaneous monitoring of casual and ambulatory BP, and from the distribution of ambulatory BP values in healthy pediatric populations.

### *Casual vs Ambulatory Blood Pressure*

The first tentative approach to obtaining reference values has been to relate the values of ambulatory BP with those of casual BP. This is done in an attempt to identify the average ambulatory BP that corresponds to a given value of casual BP, and the upper limit of normalcy for age and sex. When both casual and ambulatory values are plotted, there is a wide dispersion of points around the regression lines, unfortunately suggesting difficulty in inferring ambulatory BP from casual BP. This first attempt to obtain reference values from the relationship between office and ambulatory BP proved to be misleading *(20)*.

The distribution of points on both sides of the regression lines indicates that there are subjects for whom ambulatory BP is significantly lower than for their office counterparts, and there are others in which the opposite situation is observed. How common and important the intra-individual differences are is a keystone to the use of ABPM as a diagnostic tool.

The ambulatory BP values obtained have generally been higher than those of their casual BP counterparts. The differences observed in children could be attributable, at least in part, to several factors. First, this population actively carries out its everyday activities during the ambulatory BP monitoring, whereas the subjects are quiet and relaxed for the casual BP monitoring. Furthermore, casual BP is obtained using an auscultatory method, while ambulatory BP is measured by an oscillometric device for which the overestimation of BP values in the range of low BP values has been described *(20)*. Whether these reasons fully explain the differences observed between casual BP and ambulatory BP needs to be clarified.

### *Distribution of Ambulatory Blood Pressure Values*

One method used to obtain an approach to reference values is that of evaluating the distribution of the averages of 24 h ambulatory BP values with age and/or height in children. Unfortunately, there are few studies which report the distribution of ambulatory BP values in healthy children *(12,20,42)*, and some methodological aspects differ among the studies, making it difficult to pool data. Furthermore, while one of the studies included only healthy and normotensive children *(20,43)*, another multicenter study that did not have uniformity of monitoring devices included an unselected population of children from different schools *(42)*. Finally, one of the studies used the auscultatory technique *(12)*. With such differences in the

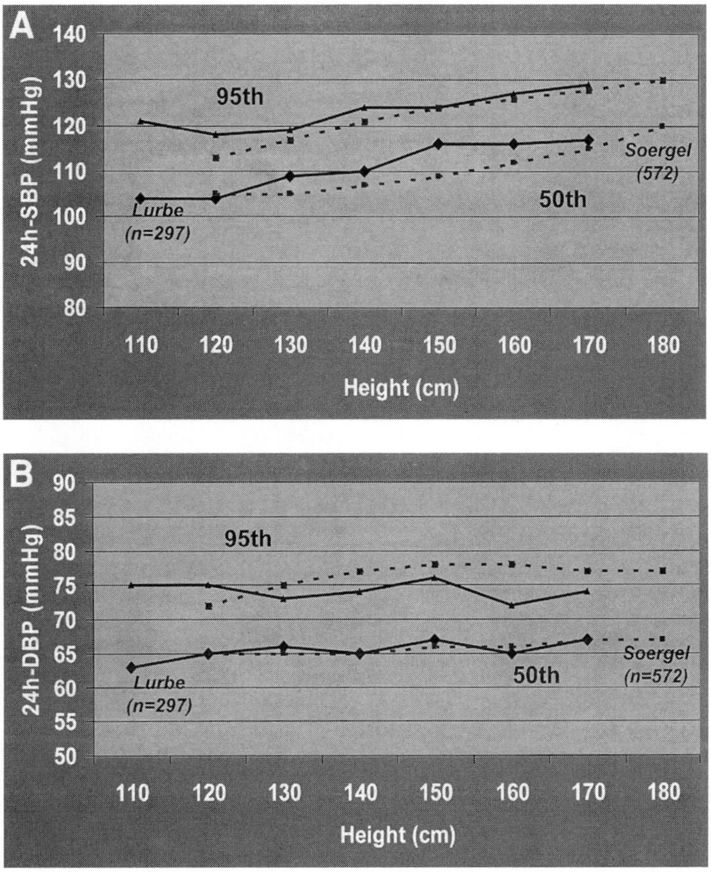


Fig. 2. Distribution of ambulatory blood pressure over a 24-h period in a pediatric population in relation to height in two studies *[42]*, dotted lines and *[43]*, continuous lines), (A) systolic BP in males; (B) diastolic BP in males; (C) systolic BP in females; (D) diastolic BP in females.

methodological approach as the use of different monitors, which employ neither the same algorithm nor the same frequency of measurements, data are not comparable. In two of the studies using the oscillometric technique *(42,43)*, the 95th percentile for systolic and diastolic BP is used as the upper limit of normality, and since a circadian variability is present, the BP percentiles for awake and sleep are also reported. Despite some methodological differences between the two studies, the 95th percentiles are close to each other. A progressive increase in the values of the 50th percentile and the 95th percentile with height is observed in the averages of systolic BP during the 24 h, awake, and sleep periods in both boys and girls. In contrast, there is no increase of diastolic BP with height. The average of 24 h systolic and diastolic BP corresponding to the two studies is plotted in Fig. 2.

In addition to the importance of height in determining BP levels, the influence of gender on BP throughout adolescence also merits attention. The mean for awake systolic BP grouped by age and sex progressively increased in boys from 10 to 16 yr of age. In contrast, awake systolic BP remains stable or even decreases in girls older than 13 yr (*see* Fig. 3). Changes in awake systolic BP during adolescence may reflect the effect of growth and hormonal maturation *(44)*.

Another study *(12)* collected ambulatory BP data from 1121 schoolchildren using a dual monitor which permits measuring BP both by oscillometric and by auscultatory methods. From

Fig. 2. *(continued)*

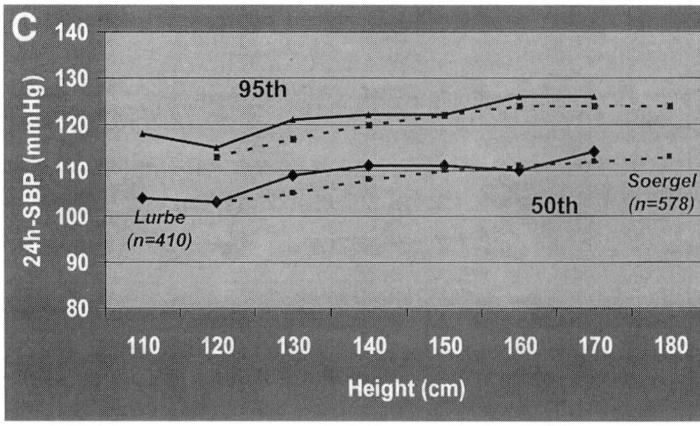


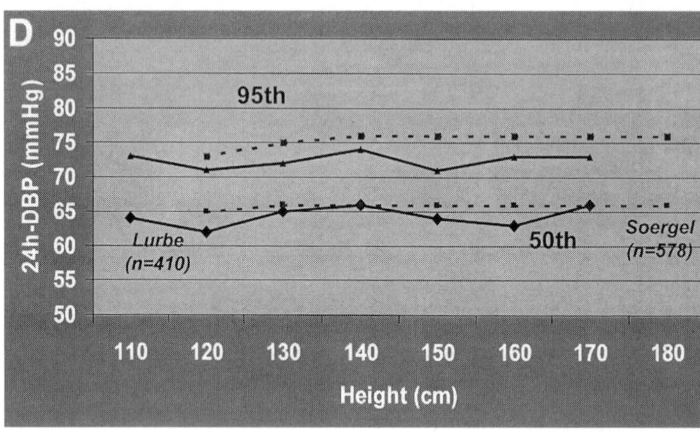


the values obtained with the auscultatory method, the authors plotted the mean and the mean plus two standard deviations for six groups based on height from 120 to 170 cm. The values were plotted separately for resting conditions, school, home, and sleep periods. Although it is difficult to evaluate the BP values from the reported plot, a similar trend to the other studies for systolic BP can be observed. In contrast to the data from oscillometric studies, however, the increase in diastolic BP values by height is more evident during resting conditions and school hours.

Finally, racial differences in ambulatory BP patterns may be important, as reported by Harshfield, who consistently found that African-American youths have higher sleep BP values than Caucasians, despite similar awake BP *(45)*. This ethnic difference in ambulatory BP patterns appears stable over a 2-yr period *(46)*.

### *White Coat Effect and the Inverse Phenomenon*

Differences between the BP values measured in clinical and ambulatory settings may have relevance in terms of whether or not a subject is diagnosed with hypertension. How common and important the intra-individual differences are within clinical and ambulatory BP is the keystone to the use of ABPM as a diagnostic tool. Casual BP measurements can lead to an overestimation of BP owing to the so-called white coat phenomenon. This can lead to an erroneous diagnosis of hypertension when office BP is high but ambulatory BP is below

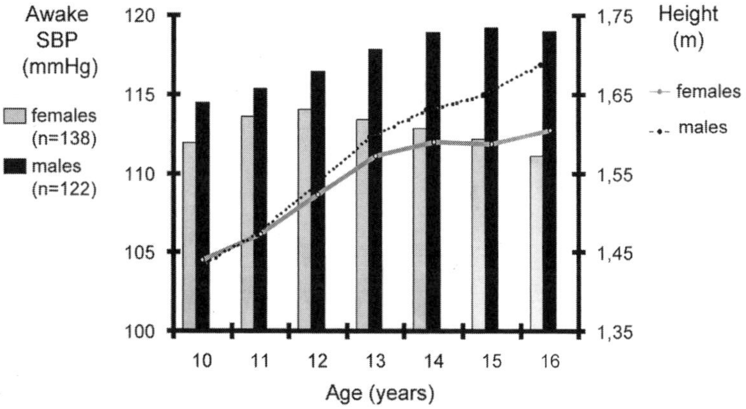


Fig. 3. Awake systolic blood pressure and height in male and female adolescents grouped by age *(44)*.

conventional thresholds, termed white coat hypertension (WCH), or the more appropriately termed isolated clinical hypertension *(47)*. The few studies of WCH in children report a high prevalence, ranging from 44–88% *(48–52)*. The elevated figures for the white coat phenomenon are dependent on the threshold defined as the upper limit of normality for ambulatory BP. The higher the ambulatory BP threshold, the greater the prevalence of the white coat phenomenon. Sometimes the thresholds used in the cited papers are the same for both ambulatory and office BP. If not, they are arbitrarily selected by comparing age- and height-based reference values for office BP with height-based values for ambulatory BP. Questions concerning whether the white coat phenomenon in adolescents is innocuous or a prelude to future permanent adult hypertension needs to be clarified.

The opposite phenomenon, normal conventional BP and high ambulatory BP, has also been observed. Although a juxtaposition of BP values has been described in adolescents in the highest rank of normal casual BP, it is less frequent and has received less attention. Once again, problems with choosing the thresholds underlie the phenomenon. The significance of having ambulatory BP values in the hypertension range with conventional BP values below the upper limit of normalcy, however, remains elusive. Whether or not treatment should be initiated in such cases must await supporting evidence.

## CLINICAL SIGNIFICANCE OF AMBULATORY BLOOD PRESSURE

The measurement of BP must be considered as nothing more than a screening test that alerts the physician to initiate investigation, but it is not necessarily a diagnostic test leading to treatment. The best estimation of BP values benefits clinical decisions. Labeling a child as hypertensive when casual BP consistently exceeds the 95th percentile ignores the changes that occur in BP over the 24-h period. Experience in adults has shown that ambulatory BP is a better predictor of prognosis than casual BP readings. It is possible that ambulatory BP in children could provide the basis for an easier and earlier recognition of abnormal BP values and/or behavior than is presently possible. The fact that ambulatory BP values in children are characterized by a reasonable reproducibility, one better than that observed for casual BP, argues in favor of this hypothesis.

The use of ambulatory BP monitoring in the pediatric population is increasing, and some aspects regarding its use need to be improved over the next few years. Such improvements may facilitate the early identification of hypertension, 24 h control of hypertension, and the detection of subtle BP abnormalities *(53)*. Bringing these abnormalities, potential predictors of future hypertension, to light is important in the prevention of hypertension and the subsequent cardiovascular and renal risk in a population where intervention leads to greater benefits for the individual subject and for the community at large. Likewise, a blunted physiological nocturnal fall has been described frequently in hypertension with renal disease, or in Type 1 diabetes, even in the absence of hypertension *(24)*. This blunted circadian variability not only contributes to increasing the 24 h BP average, but is also itself a marker of high risk of BP-induced organ damage. The refinement of ambulatory BP monitoring for the management of hypertension and for clinical research should be mandatory for the pediatric age. Only multicenter, cooperative studies using uniform methodology may provide enough data to obtain valuable norms.

## REFERENCES

1. MacMahon S, Peto R, Cutler J, et al. Blood pressure, stroke and coronary heart disease (Part I). Lancet 1990;335:765–774.
2. The 1988 Report of the Joint National Committee on Detection, Evaluation, and Treatment of High Blood Pressure. Arch Intern Med 1988;148:1023–1038.
3. Weber MA. Whole-day blood pressure. Hypertension 1988;11:288–298.
4. Littler WA, Honour AH, Pusgley DJ, Sleight P. Continuous recording of direct arterial pressure in unrestricted patients: its role in the diagnosis and management of high blood pressure. Circulation 1975;51:1101–1106.
5. Mancia G, Parati G, Pomidossi G, Di Rienzo M. Validity and usefulness of non-invasive ambulatory blood pressure monitoring. J Hypertens 1985;3(Suppl 2):S5–S11.
6. Daniels SR, Loggie JMH, Burton T, Kaplan S. Difficulties with ambulatory blood pressure monitoring in children and adolescents. J Pediatr 1987;111:397–400.
7. Portman RJ, Yetman RJ, West SM. Efficacy of 24 hour ambulatory blood pressure monitoring in children. J Pediatr 1991;118:842–849.
8. Schwartz GL, Turner ST, Sing ChF. Twenty-four hour blood pressure profiles in normotensive sons of hypertensive parents. Hypertension 1992;20:834–840.
9. Lurbe E, Alvarez V, Liao Y, et al. The impact of obesity and body fat distribution on ambulatory blood pressure in children and adolescents. Am J Hypertens 1998;11:418–424.
10. Lurbe E, Redón J, Tacons J, Torró I, Alvarez V. Current and birth weights exert independent influences on nocturnal pressure-natriuresis relationship in normotensive children. Hypertension. 1998;31(part 2):546–551.
11. Calzolari A, Giordano U, Matteucci MC, et al. Hypertension in young patients after renal transplantation. Ambulatory blood pressure monitoring versus casual blood pressure. Am J Hypertens 1998;11:497–501.
12. O'Sullivan JJ, Derrick G, Griggs P, Foxall R, Aitkin M, Wren C. Ambulatory blood pressure in schoolchildren. Arch Dis Child 1999;80:529–532.
13. O'Sullivan JJ, Derrick G, Griggs PE, Wren C. Validation of the Takeda 2421 ambulatory blood pressure monitor in children. J Med Eng Technol 1998;22:101–105.
14. O'Brien E, Petrie J, Litter WA, et al. British Hypertension Protocol: evaluation of automated and semi-automated blood pressure measuring devices. J Hypertens 1993;11(Suppl 2):S43–S63.
15. Belsha CW, Wells TG, Bowe Rice H, Neaville WA, Berry PL. Accuracy of the SpaceLabs 90207 ambulatory blood pressure monitor in children and adolescents. Blood Press Monit 1996;1:127–133.
16. Goonasekera CD, Wade AM, Slattery M, Brennan E, Dillon MJ. Performance of a new blood pressure monitor in children and young adults: the difficulties in clinical validation. Blood Press 1998;7:231–237.
17. Modesti PA, Costoli A, Cecioni I, Toccafondi S, Carnemolla A, Serneri GG. Clinical evaluation of the QuietTrak blood pressure recorder according to the protocol of the British Hypertension Society. Blood Press Monit 1996;1:63–68.
18. O'Brien E, Pickering T, Asmar R, et al. on behalf of the Working Group on Blood Pressure monitoring of the European Society of Hypertension. Blood Press Monit 2002;7:3–17.
19. Lurbe E, Cremades B, Rodriguez C, Torro MI, Alvarez V, Redon J. Factors related to quality of ambulatory blood pressure monitoring in a pediatric population. Am J Hypertens 1999;12:929–933.

20. Lurbe E, Redon J, Liao Y, Tacons J, Cooper R, Alvarez V. Ambulatory blood pressure monitoring in normotensive children. J Hypertens 1994;12:1417–1423.
21. Redon J, Vicente A, Alvarez V, et al. [Circadian variability of blood pressure: Methodological aspects]. Med Clin 1998;112:285–289 (in Spanish).
22. Pickering TG, Harshfield GA, Kleinert HD, Blank S, Laragh JH. Blood pressure during normal daily activities, sleep and exercise. JAMA 1982;247:992–996.
23. Parati GF, Di Rienzo M, Ulian L, Santucciu C, Girard A, Elghozi JL, et al. Clinical relevance of blood pressure variability. J Hypertens 1998;16(suppl 3):S25–S33.
24. Lurbe E, Redon J, Pascual JM, Tacons J, Alvarez V, Batlle DC. Altered blood pressure during sleep in normotensive subjects with type 1 diabetes. Hypertension 1993;21:227–235.
25. Mancia G, Giannasttasio C, Failla M, Sega R, Parati G. Systolic blood pressure and pulse pressure: role of 24-h mean value and variability in the determination of organ damage. J Hypertens 1999;17(suppl 5):S55–S61.
26. Lurbe E, Thijs L, Redon J, Alvarez V, Tacons J, Staessen J. Diurnal blood pressure curve in children and adolescents. J Hypertens 1996;14:41–46.
27. Di Rienzo M, Grassi G, Pedotti A, Mancia G. Continuous intermittent blood pressure measurements in estimating 24-hour average blood pressure. Hypertension 1983;5:264–269.
28. Frattola A, Parati G, Cuspidi C, Albini F, Mancia G. Prognostic value of 24 hour blood pressure variability. J Hypertens 1993;11:1133–1138.
29. Palatini P, Penzo M, Racioppa A, et al. Clinical relevance of nighttime blood pressure and of daytime blood pressure variability. Arch Intern Med 1992;152:1855–1860.
30. Sander D, Kukla C, Klingelhofer J, Winbeck K, Conrad B. Relationship between circadian blood pressure patterns and progression of early carotid atherosclerosis: a 3-year follow-up study. Circulation 2000;102: 1536–1541.
31. White WB, Dey HM, Schulman P. Assessment of the daily blood pressure load as a determinant of cardiac function in patients with mild to moderate hypertension. Am Heart J 1989;118:782–795.
32. Staessen J, Bulpitt ChJ, O'Brien E, et al. The diurnal blood pressure profile. A population study. Am J Hypertens 1992;5:386–392.
33. Coats A. Reproducibility or variability of casual and ambulatory blood pressure data: implications for clinical trials. J Hypertens 1990;8(suppl 6):S17–S20.
34. Lurbe E, Aguilar F, Gomez A, Tacons J, Alvarez V, Redon J. Reproducibility of ambulatory blood pressure monitoring in children. J Hypertens 1993;11(suppl 5):S288–S289.
35. Lurbe E, Redon J. Reproducibility and validity of ambulatory blood pressure in children. Am J Hypertens 2002;15:69S–73S.
36. The sixth report of the Joint National Committee on prevention, detection, evaluation and treatment of high blood pressure. Arch Intern Med 1997;157:2413–2447.
37. Sinaiko A. Measurement of blood pressure in children. Am J Hypertens 2001;14:976–977.
38. Second task force on blood pressure control in children. Report of the second task force on blood pressure control in children 1987. Pediatrics 1987;79:1–25.
39. Update on the 1987 task force report on high blood pressure in children and adolescents: a working group report from the national high blood pressure education program. Pediatrics 1996;98:649–658.
40. Belsha CW, Wells TG, McNiece KL, Seib PM, Plummer JK, Berry PL. Influence of diurnal blood pressure variations on target organ abnormalities in adolescents with mild essential hypertension. Am J Hypertens 1998;11:410–417.
41. Sorof JM, Portman RJ. Ambulatory blood pressure monitoring in the pediatric patient. J Pediatr 2000;136:578–586.
42. Soergel M, Kirschstein M, Busch C, et al. Oscillometric twenty-four-hour ambulatory blood pressure values in healthy children and adolescents: a multicenter trial including 1141 subjects. J Pediatr 1997;130:178–184.
43. Lurbe E, Cremades B, Torro I, Rodríguez C, Alvarez V, Redon J. Reference values of ambulatory blood pressure in children and adolescents. Am J Hypertens 2000;13:265A.
44. Lurbe E, Cremades B, Torró I, Alvarez V, Tacons J, Redón J. Gender modifies the relationship between awake systolic blood pressure and growth in adolescents. Am J Hypertens 1998;11(part 2):20A.
45. Harshfield GA, Barbeau P, Richey PA, Alpert B. Racial differences in the influence of body size on ambulatory blood pressure in youths. Blood Press Monit 2000;5:59–63.
46. Harshfield GA, Treiber FA, Wilson M, Kapuku GK, Davis HC. A longitudinal study of ethnic differences in ambulatory blood pressure in youth. Am J Hypertens 2002;15:525–530.

47. Parati G, Ulian L, Santuccio C, Omboni S, Mancia G. Difference between clinic and daytime blood pressure is not a measure of the white coat effect. Hypertension 1998;31:1185–1189.
48. Hornsby JL, Mongan PF, Taylor AT, Treiber FA. "White-coat" hypertension in children. J Fam Pract 1991;33:617–623.
49. Kouidi E, Fahadidou-Tsiligiroglou A, Tassoulas E, Deligiannis A, Coats A. White coat hypertension detected during screening of male adolescent athletes. Am J Hypertens 1999;12:223–226.
50. Koch VH, Furusawa EA, Saito MI, et al. White coat hypertension in adolescents. Clin Nephrol 1999;52:297–303.
51. Sorof JM, Portman RJ. White coat hypertension in children with elevated casual blood pressure. J Pediatr 2000;137:493–497.
52. Sorof JM, Poffenbarger T, Franco K, Portman RJ. Evaluation of white-coat hypertension in children: importance of the definitions of normal ambulatory blood pressure and the severity of casual hypertension. Am J Hypertens 2001;14:855–860.
53. Lurbe E, Redon J. Ambulatory blood pressure monitoring in children and adolescents: The future. J Hypertens 2000;18:1351–1354.

# 7 Epidemiology of Essential Hypertension in Children

## *The Bogalusa Heart Study*

*Elaine M. Urbina,* MD, *Sathanur R. Srinivasan,* PhD, *and Gerald S. Berenson,* MD

*Contents*



## INTRODUCTION

Cardiovascular diseases, including heart attack and stroke, remain the leading causes of death and disability in the US *(1)*. However, the adult heart diseases begin decades earlier *(2)*. Observations from many well established epidemiologic studies in adults have implicated risk factors such as high blood pressure (BP), hypercholesterolemia, and obesity, along with lifestyles of poor diet, smoking, and sedentary behavior, as related to the development of clinical heart disease *(3–5)*. Unfortunately, hypertension (HTN) is a major public health problem involving as much as 40% of the black adult population *(3)*. Furthermore, a strong relationship has been proven to exist between cardiovascular risk factors and underlying atherosclerotic, hypertensive, vascular abnormalities at autopsy, in adults, children and adolescents *(6)*. The occurrence of anatomic changes at a young age is the most compelling evidence that the adverse effects of risk factors such as HTN are not limited to adult heart disease, but that hypertensive cardiovascular–renal diseases begin in childhood *(3,4,7)*. Epidemiologic studies at a young age now provide considerable understanding of the early natural history of high BP and the hypertensive disease leading to clinical events.

From: *Clinical Hypertension and Vascular Disease: Pediatric Hypertension*
Edited by: R. J. Portman, J. M. Sorof, and J. R. Ingelfinger © Humana Press Inc., Totowa, NJ

Table 1
Median and 90th Percentile for BP Levels in Children
(The Bogalusa Heart Study)

| | *Systolic (mmHg)* | | *Diastolic (4th phase, mmHg)* | | *Diastolic (5th phase, mmHg)* | |
|---|---|---|---|---|---|---|
| *Age* | *Median* | *90% percentile* | *Median* | *90% percentile* | *Median* | *90% percentile* |
| 5–6 | 93 | 103 | 52 | 62 | 42 | 54 |
| 7–8 | 97 | 108 | 58 | 67 | 48 | 58 |
| 9–10 | 100 | 112 | 61 | 69 | 51 | 61 |
| 11–12 | 103 | 113 | 63 | 71 | 53 | 63 |
| 13–14 | 107 | 118 | 66 | 75 | 57 | 68 |
| 15–16 | 109 | 121 | 68 | 77 | 61 | 71 |
| 17–18 | 111 | 124 | 71 | 81 | 64 | 75 |

## PREVALENCE OF HYPERTENSION

The prevalence of HTN in children is influenced by the definition of what may be considered normal in growing children and methods used to obtain BP levels. Indirect measurement is the accepted form and proper cuff size that is essential for valid measurements *(8,9)*. Because of considerable variations and limitations of observations in children, replicating the measures of BP in the resting state have been found to best reflect an individual's BP level *(10)*. However, the precise level defining HTN in childhood is controversial. Early recommendations listed normal and elevated percentiles of BP by gender and age (Table 1) *(11)*. An update of the Second Task Force on Blood Pressure in Children improved the definition of HTN in growing children by evaluating BP levels as a function of height *(12)*. The importance of height as a determinant of BP was shown in the Bogalusa Heart Study, where 39% of the variability in systolic BP was related to body size and not age *(13)*. Because children mature at different rates, taller children of the same age equate with a distribution at higher levels (Fig. 1). Based on this finding, it is recommended that BP levels be related to height for defining abnormality.

Additional controversy exists surrounding which gender- and height-derived percentiles are abnormally high. Anatomic changes in target organs suggest that levels above the 90th percentile could be considered abnormal *(12)*. Epidemiologic evidence demonstrates that the ability to predict future HTN (by adult definitions) is 33.3% if the 90th percentile of BP is defined as childhood HTN *(14)*.

The definition of diastolic HTN has also varied over time. Some have advocated abandoning diastolic BP measurements in children altogether *(15)*. Others suggest reporting both K4 and K5 *(16)*, using K4 up to a certain age and then shifting to K5 *(11)*, or using only K4 or K5 diastolic BP measurements *(17,18)*. Although the use of K5 diastolic BP would provide continuity between reporting of childhood and adult values, studies in children have demonstrated a large difference between K4 and K5 levels, particularly in young children. One study found that 27% of all children 5–8 yr of age had at least one of six measurements of K5 near zero, a value with limited physiological significance *(17)*. A measure of K4 diastolic BP is more reproducible in childhood and is a better predictor of adult HTN (Fig. 2) *(19)*.

Other considerations for choice of childhood BP norms exist. The most recent published guidelines for BPs in children base normal values on data averaged from multiple epidemiologic studies *(12)*. However, only a single measurement, often the first and only measurement,

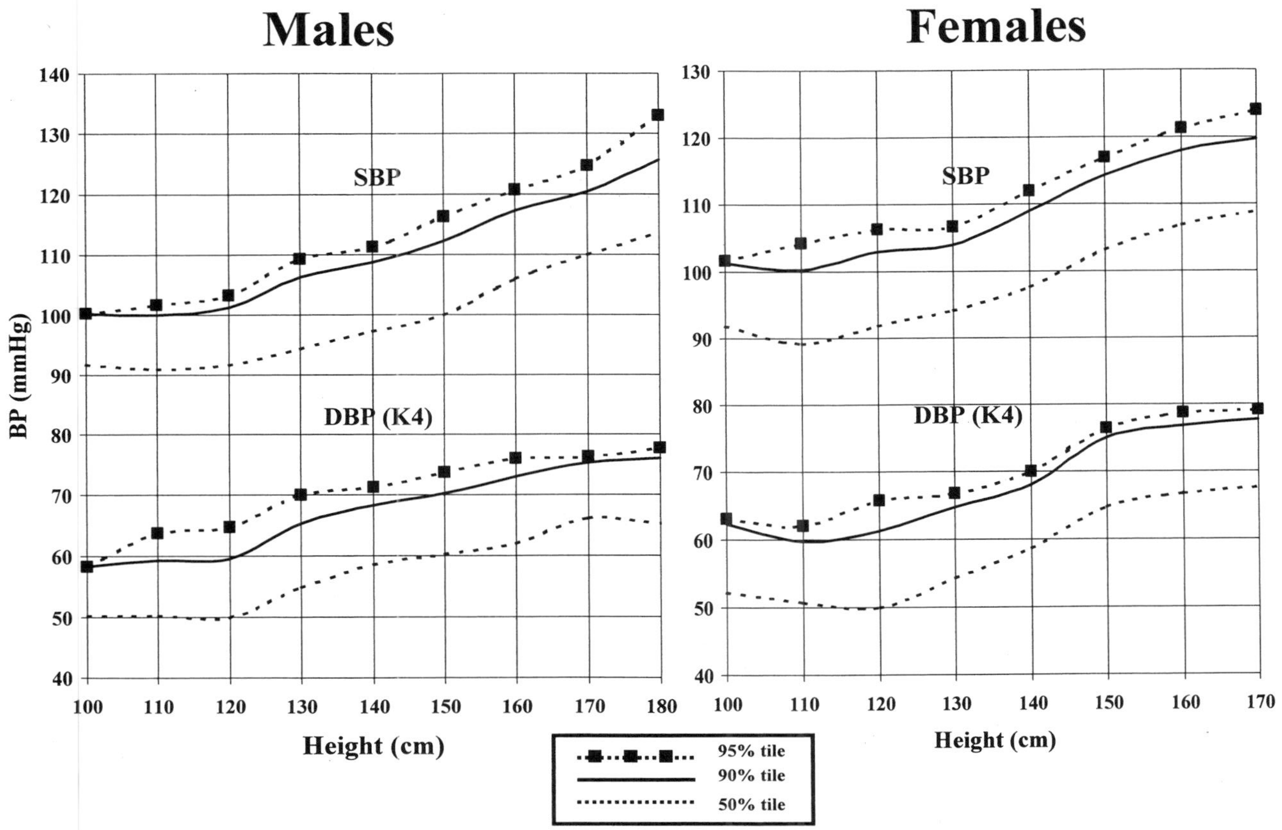


Fig. 1. Percentile levels for blood pressure (BP) by height for males and females (The Bogalusa Heart Study) ($N = 3352$). Abbreviations: SBP = systolic BP; DBP = diastolic BP *(106)*.

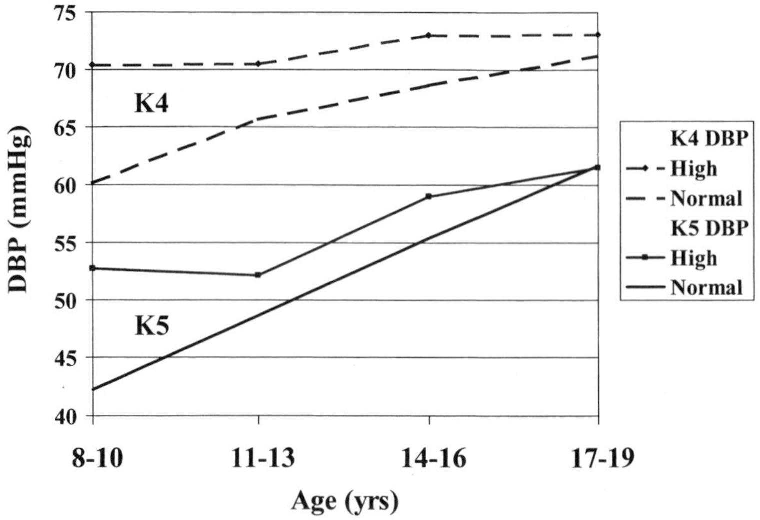


Fig. 2. Childhood K4 and K5 related to normo and hypertensive adults (The Bogalusa Heart Study) (*N* = 1017). P values for difference between levels of DBP measured in childhood for normo- and hypertensive adults are ≤0.05 for ages 8–16.

is used. The use of a single measurement to define normal BP levels is markedly limited by the observed and significant within subject variation in BP levels. Four to six replicate and serial measurements are needed to obtain levels characteristic of a given individual. Otherwise, subjects may be misclassified *(10,20)*. Furthermore, a single BP recording may be subject to the "first reading effect." With both automatic Dinamap-type devices *(10,21)* and the mercury sphygmomanometer, the first reading may be higher than an individual's intrinsic BP *(20)*. "White coat" HTN is another phenomenon that may be observed with the use of a single BP recording *(22)*. For these reasons, studies, including the Bogalusa Heart Study, have published BP norms that are lower by 5–10 mmHg for systolic BP (slightly less for diastolic BP) *(23)*. Nighttime levels have been found to be even lower *(24)*. Further studies revealed that at least two repeat 24-h ambulatory recordings are needed to account for 90% of the variability in BP recordings *(24)*. Since African-American children in Bogalusa have been shown to have higher BP levels than white children *(8)*, insufficient numbers of non-white participants in nationally published averages may make these data less readily applicable to minority populations.

## CHARACTERISTICS OF THE HYPERTENSIVE CHILD

The characteristics of the hypertensive child represent the underlying determinants of HTN.

### *Anthropometrics*

Although height relates strongly to BP levels in growing children, body fatness influences childhood BP levels, even after adjustment for height *(25)*. This relationship between obesity and BP is stronger in white children than black, especially in black males *(13)*. Central body fat distribution may be important and significantly related to systolic BP in children 5–17 yr of age, even after adjustment for peripheral body fat *(26)*. The reverse was not true. Furthermore, male children and adolescents with total body fat levels greater than 25% were found to be 2.8 times more likely to have higher BP levels than lean children. This remained significant even after adjusting for potential confounding factors such as age, race, and truncal fat pattern

Table 2
Plasma Renin Activity, Urine Potassium Excretion, and Serum Dopamine-β-Hydroxylase Levels by BP Stratum in Children
(The Bogalusa Heart Study) *(32)*
($N$ = 272)

| | *Race* | *Gender* | *1 (Low BP)* | *2* | *3* | *4* | *5 (High BP)* |
|---|---|---|---|---|---|---|---|
| *Plasma* | White | Male | 5.7 (±1.7) | 7.1 (±1.7) | 6.6 (±1.9) | 7.6 (±2.1) | 8.6 (±2.4) |
| *renin* | | Female | 7.4 (±1.1) | 6.5 (±1.3) | 5.9 (±1.6) | 7.7 (±2.3) | 8.0 (±2.4) |
| *activity* | Black | Male | 6.1 (±3.1) | 6.9 (±2.2) | 4.2 (±1.1) | 4.1 (±1.3) | 3.7 (±2.5) |
| *(ng/mL/min)* | | Female | 3.5 (±2.0) | 6.2 (±1.9) | 5.0 (±1.2) | 7.0 (±2.1) | 4.5 (±1.1) |
| *24-h Urine* | White | No | 33.2 (±4.9) | 42.0 (±5.6) | 34.2 (±7.2) | 44.7 (±10.2) | 38.8 (±6.8) |
| *potassium* | Black | gender | 24.8 (±5.7) | 26.5 (±4.2) | 27.4 (±4.4) | 29.4 (±5.0) | 29.8 (±11.6) |
| *excretion* | | differences | | | | | |
| *(meq/24 h)* | | found | | | | | |
| *Serum* | White | Male | 37 (±6) | 29 (±7) | 32 (±8) | 28 (±7) | 33 (±8) |
| *dopamine-β-* | | Female | 30 (±12) | 25 (±8) | 27 (±8) | 29 (±7) | 35 (±6) |
| *hydroxylase* | Black | Male | 26 (±13) | 23 (±5) | 17 (±5) | 24 (±6) | 23 (±13) |
| *(Mmol/min/L)* | | Female | 17 (±7) | 20 (±7) | 22 (±5) | 22 (±6) | 19 (±18) |

*(27)*. Data in females were similar. With the trend towards increasing prevalence of overweight children well documented *(28,29)*, obesity may be the most important, preventable cause of elevated BP in young people, especially in whites.

### *Renal Function and Electrolytes*

Perturbations in renal hemodynamics have long been postulated to be an etiology for adult HTN *(30)*. Only recently have these hypotheses been tested in children. Researchers have shown a positive relationship between 24-h sodium excretion, 24-h urine sodium to potassium ratio, and BP for black adolescents with higher resting BP levels *(31)*. Interestingly, these relationships were not seen in whites. Additional racial contrasts are seen in factors related to BP. Black children, especially those with higher BPs for age, size, and gender, have lower plasma renin activity than white children (Table 2). Blacks were also found to have less urine potassium excretion and slightly lower creatinine clearance *(32)*. Young black adults also demonstrate greater natriuresis with a negative stool and urine sodium balance, as well as a cumulative potassium balance in response to an oral potassium challenge. These results were not found for whites *(33)*. It should be noted that additional studies proved no significant difference among the two races in overall sodium to potassium dietary intake *(34)*. Unfortunately, two-thirds of these school age children had sodium intakes above the recommended 2 g/d, and 50–70% had potassium intakes below the recommended daily allowance (2 meq/kg/d) *(35)*. It is clear that dietary modification may be an important step in preventing HTN in genetically salt sensitive individuals, especially in blacks.

### *Neural Mechanisms*

While the HTN in black adolescents from the above observations seems to be driven by renal mechanisms, elevated BP in whites may have neural—specifically, sympathomimetic—

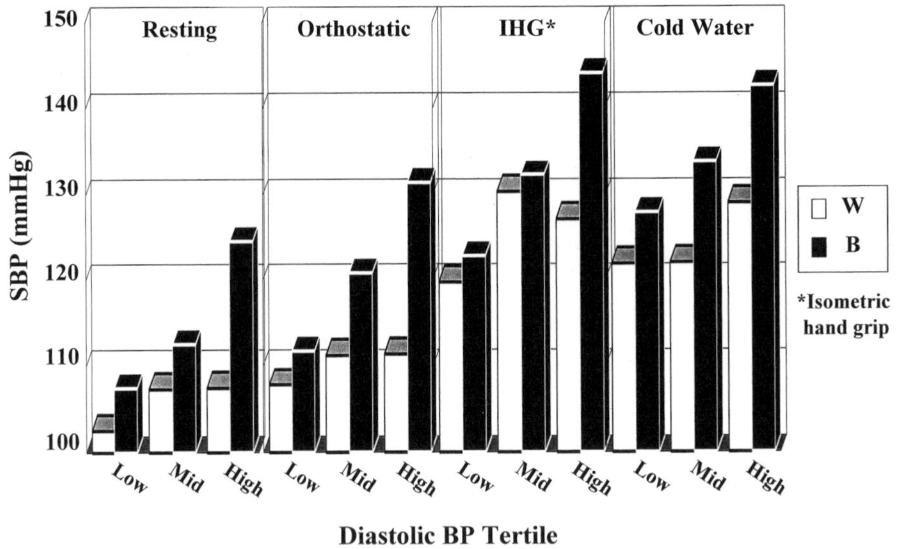


Fig. 3. Resting and maximal stress systolic blood pressure (SBP) levels in boys aged 7–15 yr by race and resting diastolic blood pressure tertile. The Bogalusa Heart Study ($N$ = 136). All $p$ values for race difference in maximal stressed SBP are ≤0.01 *(42)*.

origins. White children demonstrate higher dopamine-β-hydroxylase levels regardless of resting BP levels (Table 2) *(31)*. This suggests sympathetic predominance in white children *(32)*. The faster heart rates seen at higher levels of BP in white children, especially in boys, support this theory *(31)*. Other supportive data are found in studies of heart rate variability in adults where sympathetic predominance at rest is found as compared to age-matched controls, with the degree of abnormality correlating with severity of HTN *(36)*. Adult patients with HTN also demonstrate loss of the circadian rhythm of the low frequency component measured by heart rate variability *(37)*. In one of the few studies using heart rate variability in children, healthy white male adolescents, regardless of BP levels, demonstrated higher sympathetic tones and lower parasympathetic tones than blacks. A trend toward sympathetic predominance in the higher BP group was noted for both races *(38)*. Again, it was hypothesized that variations in sympathetic nervous system function that occur among the races are related to the initiation of essential HTN.

### *Stress Responses*

Not only do racial differences exist in resting autonomic tone, but there are also demonstrated differences in response to stress for both children *(39)* and adults *(40)*. Black children performing cardiovascular response tests have higher maximal stressed systolic BP than whites, regardless of resting BP levels (Fig. 3) *(32,39,41)*. For black adolescents with elevation of resting BP, systolic levels of BP, especially during orthostatic and cold pressor testing, exceeded those of other race–sex groups *(32,42)*. Peripheral vasoconstriction is also much more pronounced in black children in response to α-adrenergic stimulation, such as that produced by cold stress *(43,44)*, a finding that has been noted in normotensive black adults *(45)*. In addition, mental stress in hypertensive blacks results in diminished cardiac sympathomimetic tone with higher peripheral vascular response *(46)*. In contrast, white males with borderline high BPs have a greater increase in cardiac index in response to stress *(44)*, while black subjects exhibit

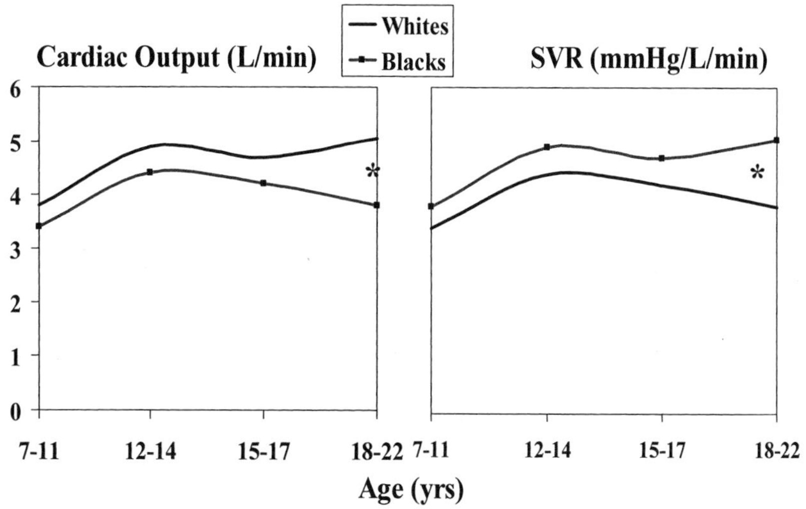


Fig. 4. Cardiac output and systemic vascular resistance (SVR) measured by echocardiography in males by race and age (The Bogalusa Heart Study). **p* for race difference ≤0.01 *(49)*.

increases in vascular tone *(47–49)*. Sympathetic predominance in white children has also been shown by heart rate variability data collected during reactivity testing, with a trend towards sympathetic predominance in hypertensives of both races *(50)*. These data show racial differences occur in response to stress even in early borderline HTN. There may be underlying black–white differences in autonomic tone or response of the nervous system to stress with different types of adrenergic receptors stimulated to different degrees. BP responses to stress may also be a marker for the individual genetically predisposed to adult HTN. Parker et al. found that peak BP in children during orthostatic stress, isometric handgrip, and cold pressor testing helped predict future BP even after adjusting for baseline BP levels *(48)*. Furthermore, BP reactivity has been found to be predictive of future left ventricular mass corrected for body size, especially in blacks *(51)*. Interestingly, both BP response to exercise and left ventricular mass have also been found to predict future BP *(52)*. Left ventricular mass likely represents the sum of long term effects of BP, both at rest and during stress *(52)*. A combination of resting and peak exercise BP levels, along with measurement of left ventricular mass, may prove to be an excellent predictor of adult HTN.

### *Hyperdynamic Circulation*

Black–white contrasts have been demonstrated in resting measures of cardiovascular function. White children have been found to have higher resting heart rates *(42)* and higher cardiac output as measured by echocardiography (Fig. 4) *(49)*. Black children were found to have higher peripheral vascular resistance, and BP levels were positively correlated with resting cardiac output and stroke volume *(49)*. These findings in children are notable, since studies in adults have suggested that a hyperdynamic state with increased cardiac output, owing to enhanced contractility, occurs early in persons genetically susceptible to HTN *(53)*. Later, cardiac output may become normalized, because of a sustained increase in peripheral vascular resistance occurring with a progressive down regulation of beta-receptors. This may eventually result in clinical HTN *(44)*.

Obesity, well known to increase the risk of HTN, may also increase risk for development of a hyperdynamic circulatory pattern. The "double product," or heart rate times BP, has been

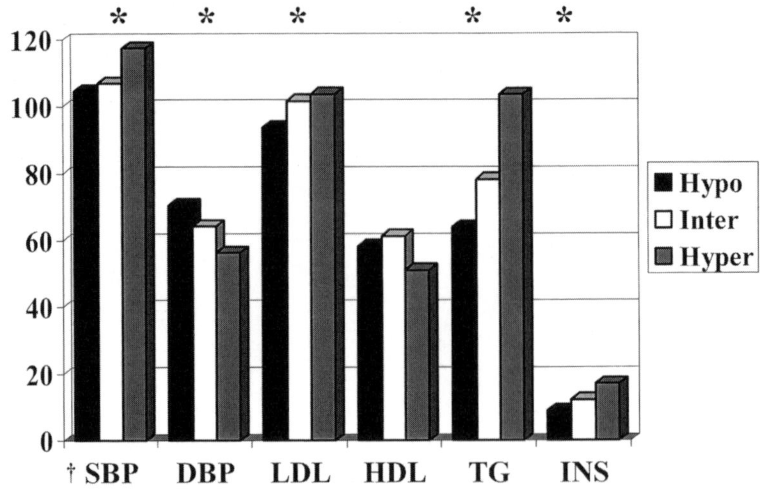


Fig. 5. Hyperdynamic circulation in obese boys (body fat > 75%) aged 8–17 yr: effect on blood pressure (BP), lipids, and insulin. The Bogalusa Heart Study ($N = 96$). †Units are as follows: systolic and diastolic BP = mmHg; LDL-C, HDL-C and TG mg/dl; insulin μU/mL. *$p$ values for slope of linear regression of variables on hemodynamic status after adjusting for age and race are ≤ 0.003.

described as a measure of hyperdynamic circulation *(54)*. Boys with obesity were found to have a higher double product, suggesting a link between weight and chronic cardiac stress through an effect on myocardial oxygen consumption *(54)*. Investigators have also found that obese boys (percent body fat >75th percentile) with hyperdynamic circulation (high pulse pressure and heart rate) have higher systolic BP, triglyceride, VLDL-cholesterol, and fasting insulin levels, regardless of age and race (Fig. 5) *(55)*. These features of adult type Syndrome X persisted when the subjects were followed over three years ("tracking") *(55)*. These data suggest that an obesity-insulin induced hyperdynamic circulation may be an early feature of Type II diabetes of adult onset, and that it occurs even at young ages.

## *Effect of Insulin on Hemodynamics*

Glucose loading experiments in children have been performed to further investigate the relationships between carbohydrate metabolism and cardiovascular function. White children had higher 1-h plasma glucose levels than blacks, and fasting glucose levels in whites were seen to increase with each successively higher quintile of resting BP (Fig. 6) *(32)*. A trend for increasing fasting insulin levels with higher levels of BP was also seen in white boys, even after adjusting for body weight *(32)*. When the "peripheral insulin resistance" product was calculated for white boys (1 h glucose in mg/dL multiplied by the 1-h insulin level in μUnits/mL), there was a significant increase at higher levels of BP *(56)*. Additionally, white males with a higher insulin resistance product demonstrated a positive relationship between fasting glucose and resting BP adjusted for body size *(56)*. Further study has confirmed racial differences in carbohydrate metabolism, with black children demonstrating significantly higher insulin and lower glucose levels than whites *(57)*. This study also found a positive relationship between metabolic measures, such as insulin and glucose, and BP levels *(57)*. The independent nature of these relationships was confirmed with multivariate models showing a significant relationship between fasting insulin and both systolic and diastolic BP in children (5–12 yr) and young adults (18–26 yr), even after controlling for glucose level and body fatness (Table 3) *(58)*.

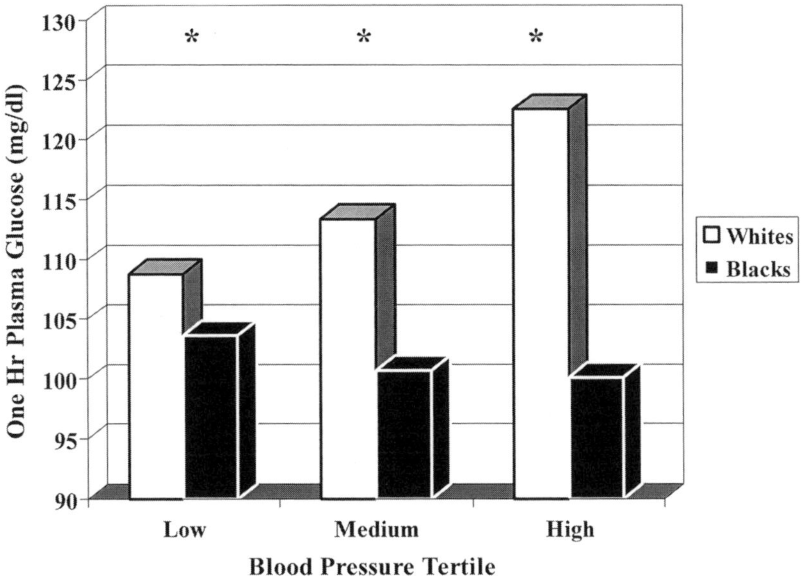


Fig. 6. One hour plasma glucose levels by race and blood pressure (BP) level in children 7–15 yr (the Bogalusa Heart Study) ($N = 270$). For white children the slope of the linear regression of 1-h glucose on BP stratum was significantly positive ($p \leq 0.05$) *(32)*.

Weaker relationships were found during puberty (13–17 yr), which may have been caused by the complex and variable rates of change of sex hormones and growth velocity during these ages *(58)*. The stronger relationship between insulin and systolic, rather than diastolic, BP has been postulated to be a result of the effect of insulin on pulse pressure *(59)*. The importance of these findings was confirmed with longitudinal analyses demonstrating a positive relationship between baseline fasting insulin and glucose and follow-up systolic BP adjusted for body size *(60)*. Racial contrast was again noted, as these relationships were significant only for white children *(60)*. The relationship between insulin and BP may differ between individuals of different genetic/racial makeup, resulting in variable alterations in sympathetic tone, sodium reabsorption by the distal renal tubules, or an amount of vascular hypertrophy leading to distinct etiologies for the same manifestation (HTN) *(58,61)*. Regardless of ethnicity, levels of fasting insulin demonstrate tracking (persistence of relative rank over time with $r = 0.23$–$0.36$) *(62)*. This is significant because subjects in the highest quartile of insulin demonstrated higher levels of systolic BP (+7 mmHg), diastolic BP (+3 mmHg), body mass index (+9 kg/m$^2$), triglycerides (+58 mg/dL), LDL cholesterol (+11 mg/dL), VLDL cholesterol (+8 mg/dL), and glucose (+9 mg/dL). Lower levels of HDL cholesterol (–4 mg/dL) were noted. They were 3.3 times more likely to report a parental history of diabetes and 1.2 times more likely to report a family history of HTN *(62)*. The prevalence of adult HTN was increased 2.5-fold in subjects with persistently high insulin levels, with increased rates for obesity (3.6-fold) and dyslipidemia (threefold) also reported *(62)*. These data introduce the concept of "clustering" of cardiovascular risk factors, where elevated levels of multiple risk factors are found to exist together in many adults, and leading to a multiplicative risk of cardiovascular diseases. Clustering has also been demonstrated in children with persistently higher levels of BP, contributing most strongly to the prediction of multiple risk factor clustering as an adult *(63)*.

Table 3
Independent Variables Associated With BP by Age[a]
(The Bogalusa Heart Study)

| *5–8 yr (N = 717)* | *9–12 yr (N = 939)* | *13–17 yr (N = 1048)* | *18–26 yr (N = 814)* |
|---|---|---|---|
| *Systolic BP* | | | |
| BMI | BMI | Age | Gender |
| Subscapular skinfold | Insulin | Gender | BMI |
| Insulin | Glucose | BMI | Insulin |
| Glucose | | Race | Race |
| | | Glucose | |
| $R^2 = 0.27$ | $R^2 = 0.25$ | $R^2 = 0.13$ | $R^2 = 0.16$ |
| *Diastolic BP* | | | |
| BMI | Subscapular skinfold | Gender | BMI |
| Age | Insulin | Age | Gender |
| Subscapular skinfold | Glucose | Glucose | Age |
| Race | Gender | | Insulin |
| | BMI | | |
| $R^2 = 0.13$ | $R^2 = 0.16$ | $R^2 = 0.10$ | $R^2 = 0.06$ |

[a]Listed in order of acceptance by the stepwise regression model. BMI indicates body mass index. All $p \leq 0.05$.

## *Family History*

Predicting and preventing adult heart and kidney diseases are the major motivations for examining children with potential HTN. Family history is an important component of these evaluations, as parental history provides a surrogate measure of future cardiovascular disease. In a study of 3312 children aged 5–17 yr, significant correlations were found between levels of risk factors in children and family history, even after adjusting for age, race, and gender *(64)*. However, independent associations between childhood risk factor levels and family history were only found for combinations of parental diseases, such as heart attack and high BP or diabetes in the fathers *(64)*. In contrast, when childhood BP rank was analyzed longitudinally over 9 yr, family history of HTN alone was found to be an independent predictor of future systolic BP in these children *(65)*. Similar relationships between childhood BP levels and parental history of HTN were found in the Muscatine Study *(66)*. When younger children were studied (birth to 7 yr of age), the strongest relationships were found between parental and child height and weight *(67)*. However, significant relationships were found when the parents' systolic BP levels were related to their childrens' levels with regression coefficients. These relationships tended to increase with the child's age *(67)*. It seems logical that as parents age, they begin to develop morbidity from elevated levels of risk factors that were not apparent earlier. In fact, in a study of 8276 subjects, the prevalence of parental cardiovascular disease was greater in subjects aged 25–31 compared to the 5–10-yr-old group *(68)*. This included an increase in reporting of a positive family history of HTN by up to 32%, depending on race *(68)*. Furthermore, children of hypertensive parents had higher BP after 10 yr of age, regardless of weight, and also demonstrated increased prevalence of dyslipidemias *(68)*. Racial differences were also seen with white children, especially boys, demonstrating higher LDL-cholesterol levels and reporting a parental history of heart attack. Blacks had higher insulin levels and were

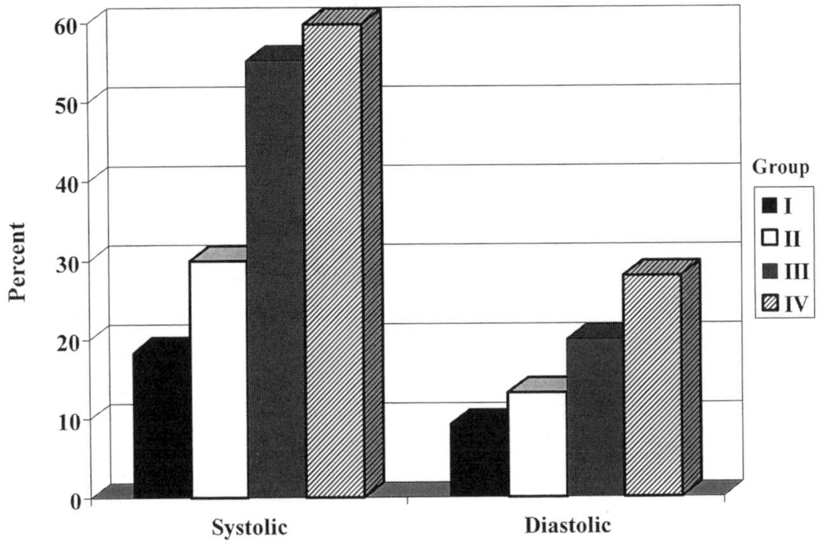


Fig. 7. Frequency of ambulatory blood pressure (BP) readings greater than the 90th percentile by BP and parental history group in children 12–21 yr (The Bogalusa Heart Study [$N = 57$; 42% male, 60% white]). I = Low BP Group, No Parental Hypertension; II = Low BP Group, +Parental Hypertension; III = High BP Group, No Parental Hypertension; IV = High BP Group, +Parental Hypertension *(24)*.

more likely to report parental HTN *(68)*. Ambulatory BP studies have also demonstrated the importance of a family history of HTN *(24)*. When ambulatory BP load was calculated, the percentage of readings above the race-, gender-, and height-specific 90th percentile for systolic and diastolic BP was found to be greatest in children with high resting BP and a family history of HTN. However, children with low resting BP and a positive family history of HTN also had a higher ambulatory BP load than normotensive children without a family history (Fig. 7) *(24)*.

### *Birthweight*

Retrospective studies of adults have found an association between adult HTN and low birthweight *(69,70)*. The "fetal origins" hypothesis suggests that fetal programming by under nutrition in utero may initiate processes such as reduced numbers of nephrons in the kidney or changes in other organs, resulting in chronic diseases like HTN later in life *(71)*. Postnatal influences, such as the increased metabolic demands imposed by the development of obesity, may amplify the effects of fetal programming *(72)*. However, data from epidemiologic studies show inconsistent relationships between birth weight and adult BP levels *(73,74)*. Additional prospective studies are planned (The National Children's Study cosponsored by the National Institute of Child Health and Human Development, the National Institute of Environmental Health Sciences, the Centers for Disease Control and Prevention, and the US Environmental Protection Agency). These studies may shed more light on this issue by factoring in influences such as gestational age *(75)*, disproportionate, head-sparing low birth weight *(69)*, and maternal factors *(76)*.

## SUBCLINICAL TARGET ORGAN DAMAGE

Subclinical target organ damage occurs in the hypertensive child and can be measured by invasive and non-invasive techniques.

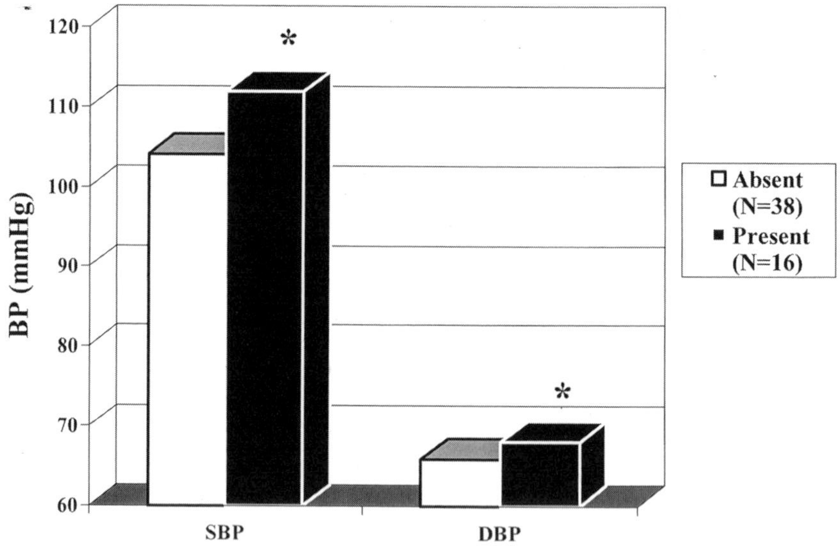


Fig. 8. Levels of blood pressure (BP) adjusted for age with and without coronary artery fibrous plaques (The Bogalusa Heart Study). *$p$ level for BP difference is ≤0.04 *(106)*.

## *Autopsy Studies*

Since 1978, autopsies have been performed on participants in the Bogalusa Heart Study in Louisiana who died between the ages of 3 and 31 yr *(2,4,77)*. Most deaths resulted from vehicular accidents, homicides, or suicides, with only 10% related to natural causes. Tissue samples collected from 85 autopsies included coronary arteries, aorta, kidney, adrenals and blood. Aortas and coronary arteries were stained with Sudan IV. Gross evaluation of fatty streaks and fibrous lesions were performed according to protocols developed in the International Atherosclerosis Project. Histological evaluations were also performed, with anatomic results compared to antemortem cardiovascular risk factor data.

A consistent pattern of associations between lesions and risk factors emerged. Antemortem levels of total and LDL cholesterol were strongly related to the extent of fatty streak lesions in the aorta *(2,77)*. Fatty streaks in the aorta and coronary arteries were also related to systolic BP. However, after adjustment for age, the relationship was found to be significant only for the coronaries *(2,78)*. Importantly, fibrous plaques in coronary arteries, the type of lesions felt to be prone to progression, were also correlated with age-adjusted antemortem systolic and diastolic BP levels (Fig. 8) *(77,78)*. Observations of increased prevalence of fibrous plaques in the coronary arteries of hypertensive men and its relationship to risk factors has been extended in the Pathologic Determinants of Atherosclerosis in Youth study *(79)*.

Once again, race and gender differences were found. Black subjects demonstrated larger areas of the aorta staining for fatty streaks *(7)*. Males had more fatty streaks in the aorta, and more progression-prone fibrous lesions in both the aorta and coronary arteries. These relationships were strongest for white males *(2,4)*. Furthermore, males demonstrated the strongest relationship between antemortem cholesterol levels and aorta fat streaks, with white males showing the greatest correlation between systolic and diastolic BP and coronary artery lesions *(4)*. In all subjects, age-adjusted BP levels correlated strongly with aortic foam cell infiltration on histologic evaluations, and the extent and intensity of lipid staining in that great vessel *(78)*. However, only males, especially black males, showed significant correlations between BP levels and foam cell infiltration and lipid staining in the coronary arteries *(78)*. When intimal thickening of the coronary arteries was studied, a weak relationship was found with antemortem BP levels. The coronary artery thickening was found to be strongly related to hyalinization of renal arterioles *(78)*.

Additional studies have been conducted exploring the relationship between BP and renal microvascular abnormalities. A mathematical model was developed to relate quantity of lesions found in renal arteries measuring 50–400 μm to mean BP *(80)*. A linear relationship, mean BP = 1.60 × microvascular lesions +79.7, with correlation coefficient 0.698, was found for all ages *(80)*. The study sample came from a population with a mean age of less than 20 yr. These data strongly confirm that the atherosclerotic-hypertensive process begins in youth, and the degree of vascular involvement correlates with antemortem levels of cardiovascular risk factors, including BP levels.

### *Cardiac Structure and Function*

Even before echocardiography was in wide usage, investigators demonstrated that subtle ECG changes, possibly representing early left ventricular hypertrophy, were apparent in children with higher BP levels *(81)*. Later, epidemiology studies measuring left ventricular thickness by M-mode analyses confirmed this hypothesis by showing a positive correlation between the wall thickness and systolic BP, even after adjusting BP for body size *(82)*. Other epidemiologic studies in children relating BP levels to left ventricular mass, particularly in males, have confirmed these relationships *(83–85)*. Possibly the best way to identify hypertensive children at high risk of target organ damage may be a calculation of ambulatory BP load *(24)*. The percentage of BP recordings higher than the 95th percentile correlates significantly to left ventricular mass index *(86)*. When left ventricular size is studied longitudinally, linear growth (i.e. height) emerges as the major determinant of heart growth in children *(87)*. However, development of obesity was shown to lead to increased left ventricular mass in children and in females; this increased mass may actually precede the development of high BP *(87)*. Additionally, left ventricular mass was shown to demonstrate tracking through late childhood and adolescence, confirming the importance of measuring heart size in hypertensive children *(87)*. Exploration was also made of the relationships between obesity, metabolic syndrome, and left ventricular mass. Although no direct, independent effect of insulin on left ventricular mass was found in healthy adolescents and young adults of normal weight, in obese persons, measured by increasing subscapular skinfold thickness, increasing fasting insulin level was associated with greater heart mass (Fig. 9) *(88)*. These data suggest that syndrome X phenotype may relate to target organ damage, even in adolescents prior to the development of clinical type II diabetes.

The effect of BP level on cardiac function has also been examined. In a sample of children taken from across the entire BP distribution, left ventricular stroke volume and cardiac output were found to be positively correlated with systolic and diastolic BP, while ejection fraction and peripheral vascular resistance related significantly to diastolic BP levels *(49)*. With increasing systolic BP and age, an increase in left ventricular output and stroke volume were seen regardless of race or gender. However, further analyses did demonstrate race-gender differences. White males, compared to black males, demonstrated greater cardiac output and stroke volume after adjustment for systolic BP and measures of body size (1.25 L/min for ages 18–22 yr, and 10 mL greater, respectively) *(49)*. Conversely, black males had higher peripheral resistance (4.5 mmHg/L/min) than white males. These findings were confirmed in a recent study of over 200 children in Cincinnati, Ohio *(89)*. It is clear then, that racial differences in

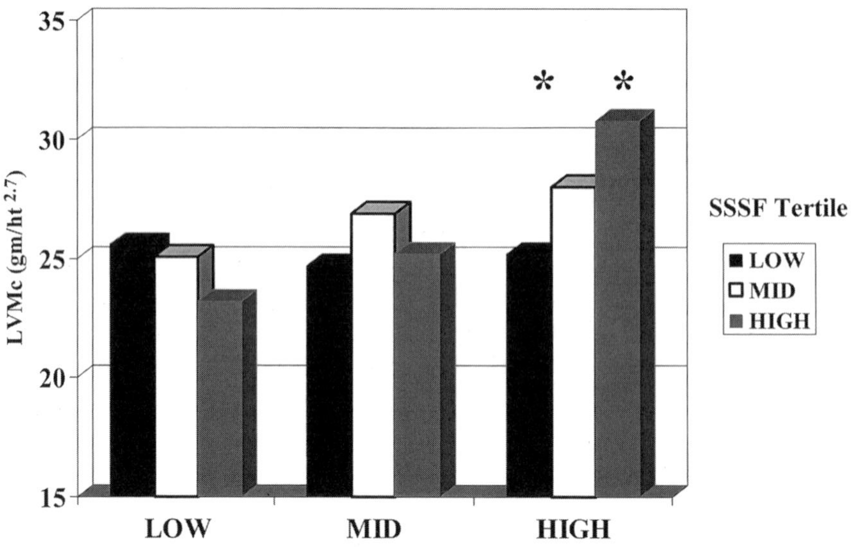


Fig. 9. Left ventricular mass by insulin and subscapular skinfold thickness in children aged 13 to 17 yr (The Bogalusa Heart Study) ($N = 216$). SSSF indicates subscapular skinfold thickness. *$p \leq 0.05$ Low SSSF vs High SSSF and Mid SSSF vs High SSSF *(88)*.

the hemodynamic mechanisms operate in the early phase of HTN *(49)*. Muscle sympathetic nerve activity (MSNA) measured by microneurography also demonstrated racial differences. An enhanced BP was seen in blacks associated with augmented MSNA, suggesting enhanced alpha-adrenergic sensitivity *(45)*. In contrast, the natural history of HTN in whites may involve an initial increase in cardiac output, followed by down regulation of β-adrenergic receptors, and leading to the transition to a progressive increase in systemic vascular resistance *(90)*.

### *Vascular Abnormalities*

One of the earliest studies of the effect of cardiovascular risk factors on the cardiovascular tree was conducted in the early 1980s *(91)*. In this study, ultrasounds of the carotid artery were performed to measure maximal and minimal diameters during the cardiac cycle. From these data the pressure-strain elastic modulus ($E_p$), a measure of stiffness that is the inverse of distensibility, was calculated. The study subjects were divided into a low and high risk group based on race, gender, and age-specific tertiles for total serum cholesterol and systolic BP. The high risk group of children had stiffer carotid arteries, with a mean $E_p$ 5.1 kPa higher than in the low risk group, even after controlling for race, sex, and age *(91)*. Subjects with a positive family history for HTN or diabetes tended to have higher $E_p$ values, and those with a history of parental myocardial infarction had a statistically significant increase in carotid artery stiffness *(91)*. Therefore, functional changes in great vessels can be detected in asymptomatic children and adolescents at risk for the development of adult heart disease. Structural changes may be more difficult to detect owing to the limited resolution of ultrasonograph machines, making it difficult to precisely measure small differences in a given individual. However, when a subset of this population was studied as young adults, increases in intima-media thickness of the carotid artery were seen with increasing numbers of risk factors (higher systolic BP,

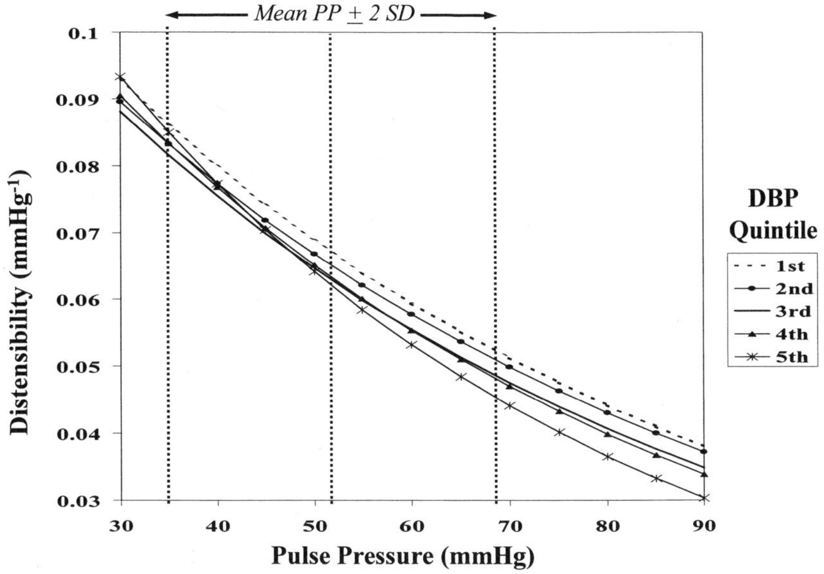


Fig. 10. Brachial artery distensibility as a function of pulse pressure by quintiles of DBP (The Bogalusa Heart Study). ($N$ = 920). *Distensibility decreased for the fifth as compared to the first and second quintiles ($p \leq 0.03$) *(93)*.

cigarette smoking, higher total cholesterol to HDL-cholesterol ratio, greater level of obesity, and higher insulin levels) *(92)*.

Studies of the vascular function of other portions of the vascular tree have also been conducted. Distensibility of the brachial artery was measured on 920 healthy young adults who had been followed from childhood as part of the Bogalusa Heart Study. As expected, distensibility tended to decrease with age, reaching significance in females *(93)*. However, race and gender differences existed (whites > blacks; females > males) even after adjustment for age. When distensibility was plotted as a function of pulse pressure to control for distending pressure, subjects with higher systolic, diastolic and mean arterial pressure had lower distensibility of the brachial artery (Fig. 10) *(93)*. The independent effects of measures of BP on distensibility were confirmed in multivariate analyses *(93)*. Longitudinal analyses are needed to explore the effects of childhood levels of risk factors on adult measures of non-invasive, subclinical vascular changes related to arteriosclerosis.

### *Renal Function*

Microalbuminuria may result from increased intraglomerular pressure as a result of HTN. In diabetic subjects, urine protein may correlate with BP levels *(94)*. Importantly, studies in healthy young individuals have confirmed the significant and positive relationship between urine albumin excretion and systolic and diastolic BP, especially in blacks (Fig. 11) *(94)*. Furthermore, in blacks with diagnosed HTN, elevated urine albumin excretion occurred with greater frequency than those considered normotensive *(94)*. These associations were not significant in whites and it has been postulated that black individuals may be more susceptible to renal damage from relatively low levels of BP increases *(94)*. Another method that was used to explore the subtle renovascular disease that occurs with HTN measures levels of urinary activity of *N*-acetyl-β-D-glucosaminidase (NAG) *(95)*. In a study of asymptomatic young

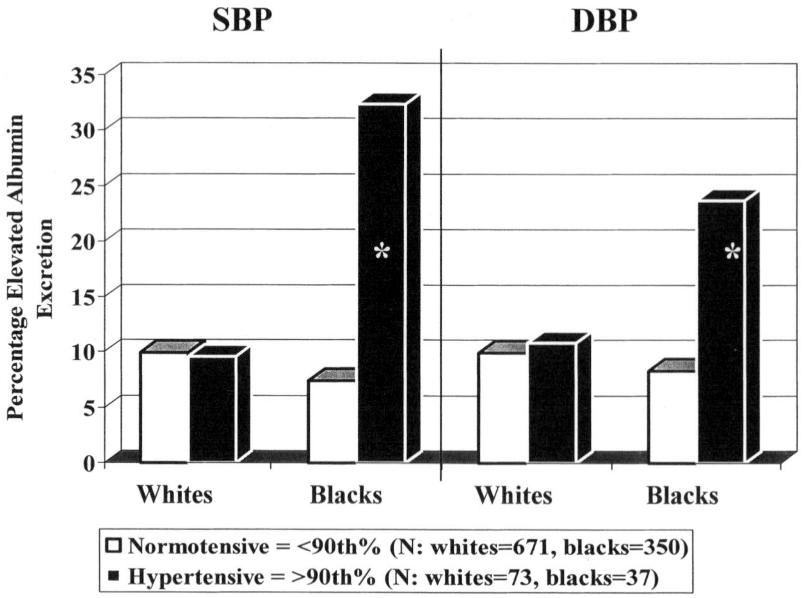


Fig. 11. Percentage of elevated albumin excretion in young adults by race and blood pressure classification (The Bogalusa Heart Study). **p* for difference between normo- and hypertensive subjects is $\leq 0.01$ *(94)*.

people, elevated urinary NAG/creatinine ratios were found as systolic BP levels increased (4 mmHg from lowest to highest quintile). This effect was strongest in black women *(95)*. Again, these observations point to the fact that subclinical kidney damage occurs with HTN, and that the effects are more extensive in the black race.

## RESULTS OF INTERVENTION

No longer are HTN and coronary heart disease thought of as adult diseases. The studies of cardiovascular risk factors in children described in this chapter have clearly proven that hypertensive disease and atherosclerosis begin in youth. It is paramount to begin prevention efforts early to obtain maximum benefit and attempt to break the vicious cycle of developing hypertensive disease. Physicians should encourage screening of high-risk groups, in addition to promoting a population-based approach to achieving healthy life styles.

Guidelines for identifying and screening high-risk families should be followed by measuring risk factor levels of all family measures and implementing both primary and secondary prevention *(12,96,97)*. If lifestyle modification as the initial therapy for HTN in a child fails, behavior change, combined with low-dose medication, will likely prove to be both safe and effective *(12,98–101)*.

Many population-based models of prevention have proven effective. The DASH diet in adults shows how lifestyle changes can help broadly modulate BP levels in a population *(102)*. The Health Ahead/Heart Smart Program was developed as an outgrowth of data collected from the Bogalusa Heart Study as a public health approach to prevention of heart disease *(103)*. This is a coordinated and comprehensive health education program for kindergarten through sixth grade that addresses the entire school, community and home environment. Traditional classroom training in health-promoting behaviors is combined with education in nutrition and physical activity in a noncompetitive setting. School workers are taught healthier cooking methods while parents and teachers acting as role models are encouraged to engage in healthy lifestyles. Family and community support are encouraged through free screenings at "health fairs" where nutrition and exercise are promoted as a family lifestyle. Studies have proven the effectiveness of these programs in changing adverse health habits in both children and adults, leading to measurable decreases in BP levels in parents *(104)*. This program of educating children to become more aware of the need to take care of their own health has implications for physicians to provide leadership to bring this message to their own communities *(105)*.

## SUMMARY

It is clear that HTN with target organ damage begins in youth. HTN is a complex syndrome mediated by multiple mechanisms and lifestyles *(106)*. Proven methods for primary prevention should be a major goal for all health professionals, along with more aggressive management of elevated BP in early life.

## ACKNOWLEDGMENT

This research was supported by the National Heart, Lung, and Blood Institute (NHLBI) Grant HL-38844,and National Institutes of Health (NIH) grant AG-16592. The authors wish to acknowledge the children and families in Bogalusa who made this research possible. The joint effort of the many individuals who have contributed to this study is gratefully acknowledged.

## REFERENCES

1. Smaha LA. Is cardiovascular disease going away? CVR & R 2000;21:67–68.
2. Berenson GS, Wattigney WA, Tracy RE, et al. Atherosclerosis of the aorta and coronary arteries and cardiovascular risk factors in persons aged 6 to 30 years and studied at necropsy (The Bogalusa Heart Study). Am J Cardiol 1992;70:851–858.
3. St. Clair, RW. Biology of atherosclerosis. In: Pearson TA, ed. Primer in Preventive Cardiology. American Heart Association: 1994;11–24.
4. Newman WP 3rd, Freedman DS, Voors AW, et al. Relation of serum lipoprotein levels and systolic blood pressure to early atherosclerosis the Bogalusa Heart Study. N Engl J Med 1986;314:138–144.
5. Wilson PWF. Established risk factors and coronary artery disease: the Framingham Study. Am J Hypertens 1994;7:7S–12S.
6. Solberg LA, Strong JP. Risk factors and atherosclerosis lesions: a review of autopsy studies. Arteriosclerosis 1983;3:187–198.
7. Freedman DS, Newman WP 3rd, Tracy RE, et al. Black/white difference in aortic fatty streaks in adolescence and early adulthood: The Bogalusa Heart Study. Circulation 1988;77:856–964.
8. Voors AW, Foster TA, Frerichs RR, Webber LS, Berenson GS. Studies of blood pressures in children, ages 5–14 years, in a total biracial community, The Bogalusa Heart Study. Circulation 1976;54:319–327.
9. Perloff D, Grim C, Flack J, Frohlich ED, Hill M, McDonald M, Morgenstern BZ. Human blood pressure determination by sphygmomanometry. Circulation 1993;88:2460–2470.
10. Gillman MW, Cook NR. Blood pressure measurement in childhood epidemiological studies. Circulation 1995; 92:1049–1057.
11. Report of the Second Task Force on Blood Pressure Control in Children. Pediatrics 1987;79:1–25.
12. Update on the 1987 Task Force Report on high blood pressure in children and adolescents: a working group report from the National High Blood Pressure Education Program, National Heart, Lung, and Blood Institute. Pediatrics 1996;98:649–658.
13. Voors AW, Webber LS, Berenson GS. Relationship of blood pressure levels to height and weight in children. J Cardiovasc Med 1978;3:911–918.
14. Shear CL, Burke GL, Freedman DS, Webber LS, Berenson GS. Designation of children with high blood pressure—considerations on percentile cut points and subsequent high blood pressure: the Bogalusa Heart Study. Am J Epidem 1987;125:73–84.

15. Weisman DN. Systolic or diastolic blood pressure significance. Pediatrics 1988;82:112–114.
16. Kirkendall WM, Burton AC, Epstein FH, Freis ED. Recommendation for human blood pressure determinations by sphygmomanometer. Circulation 1967;36:980–988.
17. Hammond IW, Urbina EM, Wattigney WA, Bao W, Steinmann WC, Berenson GS. Comparison of fourth and fifth Korotkoff diastolic blood pressures in 5 to 30 year old individuals. The Bogalusa Heart study. Am J Hypertens 1995;8:1083–1089.
18. Uhari M, Nuutinen M, Turtinen J, Pokka T. Pulse sounds and measurement of diastolic blood pressure in children. Lancet 1991;338:159–161.
19. Elkasabany AM, Urbina EM, Berenson GS. The validity and reliability of k4 versus k5 as a measure of diastolic blood pressure in children: the Bogalusa Heart Study. J Invest Med 1997;45:71A.
20. Burke GL, Webber LS, Shear CL, Zinkgraf SA, Smoak CG, Berenson GS. Sources of error in measurement of children's blood pressure in a large epidemiologic study: Bogalusa Heart Study. J Chron Dis 1987;40:83–89.
21. Wattigney WA, Webber LS, Lawrence MD, Berenson GS. Utility of an automatic instrument for blood pressure measurements in children. The Bogalusa Heart Study. Am J Hypertens 1996;9:256–262.
22. Hornsby JL, Mongan PF, Taylor T, Treiber FA. 'White coat' hypertension in children. J Fam Pract 1991;33: 617–623.
23. Bronfin DR, Urbina EM. The role of the pediatrician in the promotion of cardiovascular health. Am J Med Sci 1995;310(Suppl 1):S42–S47.
24. Berenson GS, Dalferes ER Jr, Savage D, Webber LS, Bao W. Ambulatory blood pressure measurements in children and young adults selected by high and low casual blood pressure levels and parental history of hypertension: the Bogalusa Heart Study. Am J Med Sci 1993;305(6):374–382.
25. Lauer RM, Clarke WR. Childhood risk factors for high adult blood pressure: the Muscatine Study. Pediatrics 1984;84:633–641.
26. Shear CL, Freedman DS, Burke GL, Harsha DW, Berenson GS. Body fat patterning and blood pressure in children and young adults. The Bogalusa Heart Study. Hypertension 1987;9:236–244.
27. Williams DP, Going SB, Lohman TG, et al. Body fatness and risk for elevated blood pressure, total cholesterol, and serum lipoprotein ratios in children and adolescents. Am J Pub Health 1992;82:358–363.
28. Gidding SS, Bao W, Srinivasan SR, Berenson GS. Effects of secular trends in obesity on coronary risk factors in children: the Bogalusa Heart Study. J Pediatr 1995;127:868–874.
29. Freedman DS, Srinivasan SR, Valdez RA, Williamson DF, Berenson GS. Secular increases in relative weight and adiposity among children over two decades: the Bogalusa Heart Study. Pediatrics 1997;99:420–426.
30. Ruilope LM, Lahera V, Rodicio JL, Romero JC. Are renal hemodynamics a key factor in the development and maintenance of arterial hypertension in humans? Hypertension 1994;23:3–9.
31. Voors AW, Berenson GS, Dalferes ER, Webber LS, Shuler SE. Racial differences in blood pressure control. Science 1979;204:1091–1094.
32. Berenson GS, Voors AW, Webber LS, Dalferes, ER Jr., Harsha DW. Racial differences of parameters associated with blood pressure levels in children—The Bogalusa Heart Study. Metabolism 1979;28:1218–1228.
33. Voors AW, Dalferes ER, Frank GC, Aristimuno GG, Berenson GS. Relation between ingested potassium and sodium balance in young blacks and whites. Am J Clin Nutr 1983;37:583–594.
34. Frank GC, Voors AQ, Berenson GS, Webber LS. A simplified inventory method for quantitating dietary sodium, potassium and energy. Am J Clin Nutr 1983;38:474–480.
35. Nicklas TA, Farris RP, Webber LS, Berenson GS. Dietary studies in children and hypertension. Cardiovascular Research Update 1989;3:13–19.
36. Guzzetti S, Piccaluga E, Casati R, et al. Sympathetic predominance in essential hypertension: a study employing spectral analysis of heart rate variability. J Hypertension 1988;6:711–717.
37. Guzzetti S, Dassi S, Pecis M, et al. Altered pattern of circadian neural control of heart period in mild hypertension. J Hypertension 1991;9:831–838.
38. Urbina EM, Bao W, Pickoff AS, Berenson GS. Ethnic (black–white) contrasts in twenty-four hour heart rate variability in male adolescents with high and low blood pressure: the Bogalusa Heart Study. A.N.E. 2000;5(3): 207–213.
39. Murphy JK, Alpert BS, Walker SS. Consistency of ethnic differences in children's pressor reactivity, 1987–1992. Hypertension 1994;23 (Suppl I):I-152–I-155.
40. Anderson NB, McNeilly M, Myers H. Autonomic reactivity and hypertension in blacks: a review and proposed model. Ethnicity & Disease 1991;1:154–170.

41. Treiber FA, Strong WB, Arensman FW, Forrest T, Davis H, Musante L. Family history of myocardial infarction and hemodynamic responses to exercise in young black boys. AJDC 1991;145:1029–1033.
42. Voors AW, Webber LS, Berenson GS. Racial contrasts in cardiovascular response tests for children from a total community. Hypertension 1980;2:686–694.
43. Treiber FA, Musante L, Braden D, et al. Racial differences in hemodynamic responses to the cold face stimulus in children and adults. Psychosom Med 1990;52:286–296.
44. Sherwood A, Hinderliter AL, Light KC. Physiological determinants of hyperreactivity to stress in borderline hypertension. Hypertension 1995;25:384–390.
45. Calhoun DA, Mutinga ML, Collins AS, Wyss JM, Oparil S. Normotensive blacks have heightened sympathetic response to cold pressor test. Hypertension 1993;22:801–805.
46. Fredrickson M. Racial differences in cardiovascular reactivity to mental stress in essential hypertension. J Hypertens 1986;4:325–331.
47. Sherwood A, May CW, Siegel WC, Blumenthal JA. Ethnic differences in hemodynamic responses to stress in hypertensive men and women. Am J Hypertens 1995;8:552–557.
48. Parker FC, Croft JB, Cresanta JL, et al. The association between cardiovascular response tasks and future blood pressure levels in children: Bogalusa Heart Study. Am Heart J 1987;113:1174–1179.
49. Soto LF, Kikuchi DA, Arcilla RA, Berenson GS. Echocardiographic functions and blood pressure levels in children and young adults from a biracial population: the Bogalusa Heart Study. Am J Med Sci 1989;296:271–279.
50. Urbina EM, Bao W, Pickoff AS, Berenson GS. Ethnic (black–white) differences in heart rate variability measured during cardiovascular reactivity testing in healthy male adolescents: the Bogalusa Heart Study. Am J Htn, 1998;11:196–202.
51. Murdison KA, Treiber FA, Mensah G, Davis H, Thompson W, Strong WB. Prediction of left ventricular mass in youth with family histories of essential hypertension. Am J Med Sci 1998;315:118–123.
52. Mahoney LT, Schieken RM, Clarke WR, Lauer RM. Left ventricular mass and exercise responses predict future blood pressure. The Muscatine Study. Hypertension 1988;12:206–213.
53. Hinderliter AL, Light KC, Willis PW IV. Patients with borderline elevated blood pressure have enhanced left ventricular contractility. Am J Hypertens 1995;8:1040–1045.
54. Voors AW, Webber LS, Berenson GS. Resting heart rate and pressure-rate product of children in a total biracial community—The Bogalusa Heart Study. Am J Epidem 1982;116:276–286.
55. Jiang X, Srinivasan SR, Urbina EM, Berenson GS. Hyperdynamic circulation and cardiovascular risk in children and adolescents—The Bogalusa Heart Study. Circulation 1995;91:1101–1106.
56. Voors AW, Radhakrishnamurthy B, Srinivasan SR, Webber LS, Berenson GS. Plasma glucose level related to blood pressure in 272 children, ages 7–15 years, sampled from a total biracial population. Am J Epidem 1981;113:347–356.
57. Burke GL, Webber LS, Srinivasan SR, Radhakrishnamurthy B, Freedman DS, Berenson GS. Fasting plasma glucose and insulin levels and their relationship to cardiovascular risk factors in children: Bogalusa Heart Study. Metabolism 1986;35:441–446.
58. Jiang X, Srinivasan SR, Bao W, Berenson GS. Association of fasting insulin with BP in young individuals—The Bogalusa Heart Study. Arch Intern Med 1993;153:323–328.
59. Rowe JW, Young JB, Minaker KL, Stevens AL, Pallotta J, Landsberg L. Effect of insulin and glucose infusions on sympathetic nervous system activity in normal men. Diabetes 1981;30:219–225.
60. Jiang X, Srinivasan SR, Bao W, Berenson GS. Association of fasting insulin with longitudinal changes in blood pressure in children and adolescents—The Bogalusa Heart Study. Am J Hypertens 1993;6:564–569.
61. Berenson GS, Bao W, Wattigney WA, Webber LS. Primary hypertension beginning in childhood. Cardiol Rev 1993;1:239–249.
62. Bao W, Srinivasan SR, Berenson GS. Persistent elevation of plasma insulin levels is associated with increased cardiovascular risk in children and young adults—The Bogalusa Heart Study. Circulation 1996;93:54–59.
63. Myers L, Coughlin SS, Webber LS, Srinivasan SR, Berenson GS. Prediction of adult cardiovascular multifactorial risk status from childhood risk factor levels, The Bogalusa Heart Study. Am J Epidemiol 1995;142:918–924.
64. Shear CL, Webber LS, Freedman DS, Srinivasan SR, Berenson GS. The relationship between parental history of vascular disease and cardiovascular disease risk factors in children: The Bogalusa Heart Study. Am J Epidemiol 1985;122:762–771.

65. Shear CL, Burke GL, Freedman DS, Berenson GS. Value of childhood blood pressure measurements and family history in predicting future blood pressure status: results from 8 years of follow-up in the Bogalusa Heart Study. Pediatrics 1986;77:862–869.
66. Clarke WR, Schrott HG, Burns TL, Sing CF, Lauer RM. Aggregation of blood pressure in the families of children with labile high systolic blood pressure. The Muscatine Study. Am J Epidemiol 1980;123:67–80.
67. Rosenbaum PA, Elston RC, Srinivasan SR, Webber LS, Berenson GS. Predictive value of parental measures in determining cardiovascular risk factor variables in early life. Pediatrics 1987;80(Suppl):807–816.
68. Bao W, Srinivasan SR, Wattigney WA, Berenson GS. The relation of parental cardiovascular disease to risk factors in children and young adults—The Bogalusa Heart Study. Circulation 1995;91:365–371.
69. Barker DJP, Bull AR, Simmonds SJ. Fetal and placental size and risk of hypertension in adult life. BMJ 1990; 301:259–262.
70. Law CM, Shiell AW. Is blood pressure inversely related to birth weight? The strength of evidence from a systematic review of the literature. J Hypertens 1996;14:935–941.
71. Barker DJP. Fetal origins of coronary heart disease. BMJ 1995;311:171–174.
72. Barker DJP. Early growth and cardiovascular disease. Archives of Diseases in Children 1999;80:305–306.
73. Falkner B. Birth weight as a predictor of future hypertension. AJH 2002;15:43S–45S.
74. Donker GA, Labarthe DR, Harrist RB, Selwyn BJ, Wattigney W, Berenson GS. Low birth weight and blood pressure at age 7–11 years in a biracial sample. Am J Epidemiol 1997;145:387–397.
75. Siewert-Delle A, Ljungman S. The impact of birth weight and gestational age on blood pressure in adult life: a population-based study of 49-year-old men. A J Hypertens 1998;II:946–953.
76. Shu XO, Hatch MC, Mills J, Clemens J, Susser M. Maternal smoking, alcohol, drinking, caffeine consumption and fetal growth: results from a prospective study. Epidemiol 1990;60:115–120.
77. Tracy RE, Newman III, WP, Wattigney WA, Berenson GS. Risk factors and atherosclerosis in youth—autopsy findings of the Bogalusa Heart Study. Am J Med Sci 1995;310(Suppl 1):S37–S41.
78. Newman WP 3rd, Wattigney W, Berenson GS. Autopsy studies in United States children and adolescents—relationship of risk factors to atherosclerotic lesions. Ann NY Acad Sci 1991;623:16–25.
79. McGill, Jr. HC, Strong JP, Tracy RE, McMahan A, Oalmann MC. Relation of a postmortem renal index of hypertension to atherosclerosis in youth. Arterioscler Thromb Vasc Biol 1995;15:2222–2228.
80. Tracy RE, Mercante DE, Moncada A, Berenson GS. Quantitation of hypertensive nephrosclerosis on an objective rational scale of measure in adults and children. Am J Clin Pathol 1986;85:312–318.
81. Aristimuno GG, Foster TA, Berenson GS, Akman D. Subtle electrocardiographic changes in children with high levels of blood pressure. Am J Cardiol 1984;54:1272–1276.
82. Burke GL, Arcilla RA, Culpepper WS, Webber LS, Chiang RA, Berenson GS. Blood pressure and echocardiographic measures in children: the Bogalusa Heart Study. Circulation 1986;75:106–114.
83. Goble MM, Mosteller M, Moskowitz B, Schieken RM. Sex differences in the determinants of left ventricular mass in childhood. The Medical College of Virginia Twin Study. Circulation 1992;85:1661–1665.
84. Daniels SR, Kimball TR, Morrison JA, Khoury P, Witt S, Meyer RA. Effect of lean body mass, fat mass, blood pressure and sexual maturation on left ventricular mass in children and adolescents. Statistical, biological and clinical significance. Circulation 1995;92:3249–3254.
85. Malcolm DD, Burns TL, Mahoney LT, Lauer RM. Factors affecting left ventricular mass in childhood: The Muscatine Study. Pediatrics 1993;92:703–709.
86. Sorof JM, Cardwell G, Franco K, Portman RJ. Ambulatory blood pressure and left ventricular mass index in hypertensive children. Hypertension 2002;39:903–908.
87. Urbina EM, Gidding SS, Bao W, Pickoff AS, Berdusis K, Berenson GS. Effect of body size ponderosity and blood pressure on left ventricular growth in children and young adults, The Bogalusa Heart Study. Circulation 1995;91:2400–2406.
88. Urbina EM, Gidding GS, Bao W, Elkasabany A, Berenson GS. Correlation of fasting blood sugar & insulin with left ventricular mass in healthy children & adolescents: The Bogalusa Heart Study. Am Heart J 1999;138(1 pt 1):122–127.
89. Daniels SR, Kimball TR, Khoury P, Witt S, Morrison JA. Correlates of the hemodynamic determinants of blood pressure. Hypertension 1996;28:37–41.
90. Sherwood A, Hinderliter AL. Responsiveness to α- and β-adrenergic receptor agonists: effects of race in borderline hypertensive compared to normotensive men. Am J Hypertens 1993;6:630–635.
91. Riley WA, Freedman DS, Higgs NA, Barnes RW, Zinkgraf SA, Berenson GS. Decreased arterial elasticity associated with cardiovascular disease risk factors in the young: Bogalusa Heart Study. Arteriosclerosis 1986;6: 378–386.

92. Urbina EM, Srinivasan SR, Tang R, Bond MG, Kieltyka L, Berenson GS. Impact of multiple coronary risk factors on the intima-media thickness of different segments of carotid artery in healthy young adults (The Bogalusa Heart Study). Am J Cardiology 2002;90(9):953–958.
93. Urbina EM, Brinton TJ, Elkasabany A, Berenson GS. Brachial artery distensibility and relation to cardiovascular risk factors in healthy young adults (The Bogalusa Heart Study). Am J Cardiology 2002;89:946–951.
94. Jiang X, Srinivasan SR, Radhakrishnamurthy B, Dalferes, Jr, ER, Bao W, Berenson GS. Microalbuminuria in young adults related to blood pressure in a biracial (black–white) population, The Bogalusa Heart Study. Am J Hypertens 1995;7:794–800.
95. Agirbasli M, Radhakrishnamurthy B, Jiang X, Bao W, Berenson GS. Urinary N-acetyl-β-D-glucosaminidase changes in relation to age, sex, race, and diastolic and systolic blood pressure in a young adult biracial population, The Bogalusa Heart Study. Am J Hypertens 1996;9:157–161.
96. National Cholesterol Education Program. Report of the Expert Panel on Blood Cholesterol Levels in Children and Adolescents. Pediatrics 1992;89:525–584.
97. Cardiovascular health in childhood. Position Statement of the Committee on Atherosclerosis, Hypertension and Obesity in the Young of the Council on Cardiovascular Disease in Youth. Circulation 2002;106:143–160.
98. Berenson GS, Shear SL, Chiang YK, Webber LS, Voors AW. Combined low-dose medication and primary intervention over a 30-month period for sustained high blood pressure in childhood. Am J Med Sci 1990;299: 79–86.
99. Farris RP, Frank GC, Webber LS, Berenson GS. A nutrition curriculum for families with high blood pressure. J Sch Health 1985;55:110–113.
100. Cunningham RJ, Urbina EM, Hogg RJ, Sorof JM, Moxey-Mimms M, Eissa MA, Representing the Ziac Pediatric Hypertension Study Group. A double-blind, placebo-controlled, dose escalation safety, and efficacy study of ziac in patients, ages 6–17 years, with hypertension. Am J Hypertens 2000;13(Suppl 1): S38–S39.
101. Falkner B, Sadowski RH. Hypertension in children and adolescents. Am J Hypertens 1995;8:106S–110S.
102. Sacks FM, Svetkey LP, Vollmer VM, et al. Effects on BP of reduced dietary sodium and the Dietary Approaches to Stop Hypertension (DASH) diet. DASH-Sodium Collaborative Research Group. N Engl J Med 2001;344:3–10.
103. Downey AM, Frank GC, Webber LS, et al. Implementation of "Heart Smart:" a cardiovascular school health promotion program. J Sch Health 1987;57:98–104.
104. Johnson CC, Nicklas TA, Arbeit ML, et al. Cardiovascular intervention for high-risk families: the Heart Smart Program. So Med J 1991;84:1305–1312.
105. Downey AM, Greenberg JS, Virgilio SJ, Berenson GS. Health promotion model for "Heart Smart": the medical school, university, and community. Am J Hlth Promotion 1989;13:31–46.
106. Urbina EM, Berenson GS. Hypertension studies in the Bogalusa Heart Study. In: *Development of the Hypertensive Phenotype: Basic and Clinical Studies* (McCarty R, Blizard D, Chevalier B, eds.). Amsterdam: Elsevier, 1999; pp 607–637.

# III

# Hypertension in Children: Definitions, Predictors, Risk Factors, and Special Populations

# 8 Definitions of Hypertension in Children

*Jonathan M. Sorof, MD*

*CONTENTS*



## INTRODUCTION

The manner in which hypertension (HTN) is defined in children has undergone substantial changes over the last several decades. Prior to the availability of statistical data on the normal distribution of blood pressure (BP) during childhood, adult thresholds of BP normality were generally applied to children. Although the specific values recommended to define HTN in adults have migrated downwards in recent years, in general a single set of values is applied to adults regardless of age. In fact, the most recent clinical advisory statement from the Coordinating Committee of the National High Blood Pressure Education Program categorically states that the use of age-adjusted BP targets in adults is "discouraged." This recommendation has no validity for the evaluation of hypertensive children. Children predictably undergo an age- and height-related rise in BP as they mature, thus requiring the threshold of normality to be continually redefined throughout childhood. This fundamental issue has created confusion among primary care providers who care for hypertensive children, and confounded the clinical investigation of pediatric HTN by researchers.

There are important conceptual differences between the adult and pediatric definitions of HTN. In adults, the BP values to define HTN in adults advocated by the Joint National Committees have been validated by association with outcome. Specifically, the recommendations regarding the threshold values for defining HTN in adults are based on the associations between BP values that exceed these thresholds and subsequent morbidity or mortality. These associations are difficult to establish in children, since overt morbid events such as stroke, myocardial infarction, and congestive heart failure are rare except in cases of severe HTN. In lieu of an

From: *Clinical Hypertension and Vascular Disease: Pediatric Hypertension*
Edited by: R. J. Portman, J. M. Sorof, and J. R. Ingelfinger © Humana Press Inc., Totowa, NJ

outcome-based approach, the current standard for defining HTN in children is based on BP values that exceed the 95th percentile, derived from population percentiles of the normal distribution of BP within a specific age, gender, and height-percentile combination. This approach has provided the foundation for virtually all current research and clinical practice in the evaluation of pediatric HTN.

Although these normative data have proved critical to furthering our ability to evaluate BP in children, the current definitions of pediatric HTN suffer from several important weaknesses. The upper BP limit of normotension has been chosen somewhat arbitrarily as the 95th percentile of the population. This limit is statistical rather than functional and categorizes the upper 5th percentile of all children as hypertensive on initial screening. HTN defined in this manner does not correlate well with sequelae in the form of end-organ injury. No longitudinal studies in children have investigated whether normalization of BP to less than the 95th percentile prevents or reverses end-organ injury. Furthermore, recent data suggest that many children with elevated clinic BP may have white coat hypertension (WCH) by ambulatory BP criteria. Thus, there are few data to support early pharmacological treatment in children with borderline or moderate HTN by current criteria. This chapter will review the strengths and weaknesses of these criteria, as well as potential future strategies for defining HTN in children.

## TASK FORCE DEFINITION

Prior to the report of the National Heart, Lung, and Blood Institute (NHLBI) of the Task Force on Blood Pressure Control in Children published in 1977 *(1)*, there were no normative data for interpretation of BP values in children. In the absence of normative data, adult definitions of HTN (usually greater than 140/90 mmHg) were applied to children. After publication of the 1977 Task Force Report, new and more extensive epidemiological data on normal BP distributions and the natural history BP throughout the pediatric age range became available. The report of the Second Task Force for Blood Pressure Control in Children and Adolescents provided additional data that described the distribution of BP values in over 70,000 normal children *(2)*. The incorporation of BP measurement into the routine pediatric examination, as well as the publication of the Task Force national norms for BP in children *(1,2)*, enabled not only detection of significant asymptomatic secondary HTN, but also confirmed that mild elevations in BP during childhood were more common than previously recognized, particularly in adolescents. These reports have provided the foundation for virtually all current research and clinical practice in the evaluation of pediatric HTN.

The Working Group Update in 1996 incorporated the NHANES III data and, for the first time, incorporated height percentile as well as gender and age in the calculation of normative percentile values for BP in children *(3)*. Height percentiles were added with the recognition that the physical stature of a child within a chronological year increment has substantial effects on BP. In fact, the difference in BP between children at the 5th percentile of height and the 95th percentile is consistently 8–9 mmHg. This wide difference based on height has obvious practical clinical implications for the diagnosis of HTN in children. It is important to note that there are no normative BP standards that account for weight or body mass index (BMI) in children. There is compelling evidence that overweight status and elevated BP are closely related and synergistically increase cardiovascular risk. Adjustment of BP norms based on increased weight would therefore inappropriately control for the pathologic influence of overweight on BP.

It is important to note, however, that the reliability of the measurement of diastolic BP has been identified as an important issue in the study of BP in children. In particular, the use of the

Korotkoff (K)4 or the K5 sound to define the auscultatory diastolic BP is controversial and has been found to affect the prevalence of diastolic HTN. Sinaiko et al. compared K4 with K5 in 19,274 children aged 10–15 yr and found that the K4–K5 difference was 5–10 mmHg in 20 percent, 11–20 mmHg in 11 percent, and greater than 21 mmHg in 3 percent of the children *(4)*. In this study, the choice of K4 or K5 to define diastolic BP changed the prevalence for significant diastolic HTN by 2–3%. Uhari et al. studied 3012 randomly selected children and found that K4 was absent in a higher percentage of individuals than K5, leading to the conclusion that reliable and repeatable BP measurements in children are best achieved with K5 as the indicator of diastolic blood pressure *(5)*. Investigators from the Bogalusa Heart Study evaluated differences between K4 and K5 from 4633 subjects 5–30 yr of age and found an overall mean difference between K4 and K5 of 9.9 ± 5.6 mmHg (mean ± standard deviation [SD]) *(6)*. Based on the finding that K5 was zero in a relatively high percentage of individuals, they concluded that K4 was the more reproducible measure of diastolic BP. Biro et al. performed a cross-sectional analysis of BP from 2379 9-yr-old children in the NHLBI Growth and Health Study (NGHS) *(7)*. Of the 159 subjects potentially classified with elevated diastolic BP, 60% would be classified differently in terms of diastolic HTN, depending on whether K4 or K5 was used to define elevated diastolic BP. Therefore, the choice of the onset of K4 or K5 for determining diastolic BP in children may have important implications for defining diastolic HTN.

The most recent Task Force report defines HTN not only on the distribution of BP in healthy children, but on "clinical experience and consensus." Normal BP is defined as systolic and diastolic BP less than the 90th percentile for age, gender, and height percentile. High-normal BP (prehypertension) is defined as systolic or diastolic BP greater than or equal to the 90th percentile, but less than the 95th percentile. HTN is defined as systolic or diastolic BP greater than or equal to the 95th percentile. By this definition, one in twenty children would be considered hypertensive. However, the Task Force norms are based on a single set of BP measurements. It is critical for elevated BP to be confirmed on repeated visits before characterizing an individual as having HTN. This is because BP at high levels tends to fall on subsequent measurement as the result of accommodation to the act of having BP measured and regression to the mean. Ideally, BP should be measured over a period of weeks to months in order to more precisely characterize an individual's BP status. According to the Task Report, with repeated measurement of BP only about 1% of children and adolescents will be found to have HTN.

The importance of repeated measures has been illustrated in multiple epidemiological and interventional studies in children. Several screening programs have collected repetitive BP data to determine the prevalence of HTN in an unselected population of school-aged children. One of the earliest and largest studies was by Fixler et al., who screened over 10,000 school-aged children for HTN defined as BP greater than 140/90 mmHg *(8)*. After three sets of measurements, the overall prevalence of HTN decreased from approx 9% initially to less than 2% by the third set of measurements. However, the reliance on adult definitions rather than on currently accepted pediatric definitions from the Task Force data makes the validity of this early study less clear. A more current study by Sinaiko et al. in 1989 reported the prevalence of HTN in approx 15,000 school children using the age- and gender-specific percentile values from the Task Force *(9)*. After only two sets of measurements, the prevalence of HTN decreased from approx 4% to 1%. Sorof et al. recently performed HTN screening in approx 2500 predominantly ethnic minority adolescents *(10)*. Students with initial BP greater than the 90th percentile underwent additional BP measurements. After three sets of school-based BP mea-

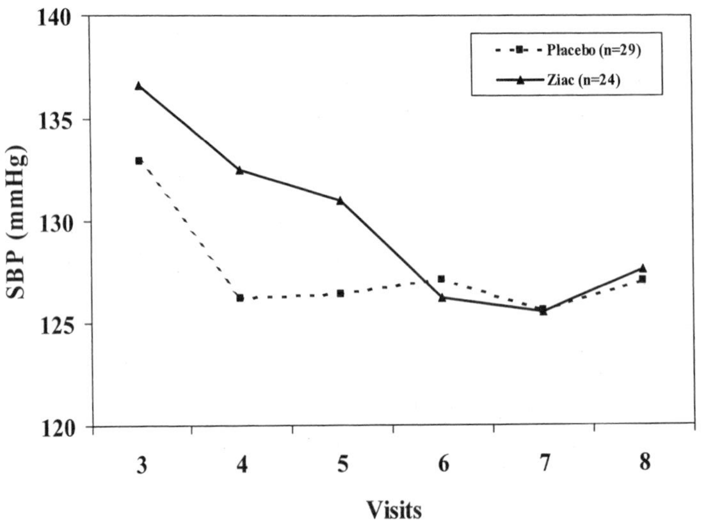


Fig. 1. Systolic blood pressure at study visits 3–8 in subjects treated with all dose levels of study drug and in subjects treated with placebo. From ref. *59*, with permission.

surements, the estimated prevalence of HTN decreased from 24% to 9%. Among the 30 adolescents with persistent HTN who were subsequently evaluated in a HTN clinic, 11 were no longer hypertensive on follow-up.

The phenomenon of normalization of elevated BP with repeated measurements has been documented in the context of pediatric antihypertensive medication trials. Berenson et al. randomly assigned 95 children whose BP was persistently above the 90th percentile over a 4-mo period to either pharmacological treatment or usual care *(11)*. Although the treated group showed a significantly greater reduction in BP relative to the comparison group, patients in the untreated comparison group showed progressive reductions in BP during follow-up despite the prolonged confirmatory period of observation prior to study entry. Comparable results were obtained from the Ziac pediatric HTN trial, a double-blind, multicenter, parallel, dose-escalation study comparing bisoprolol fumarate/hydrochlorothiazide to a placebo *(12)*. The study consisted of three phases: a 2-wk single-blind, placebo-screening phase, a 10-wk double-blind, randomized-treatment phase, and a 2-wk dose-tapering phase. Despite confirmation of HTN on multiple occasions prior to study entry, the most common reason for early study termination was normalization of BP during the placebo-screening phase (17% of all study subjects). Among the subjects qualified for randomized treatment, placebo-treated patients continued to have progressive reductions in BP (Fig. 1). Ultimately, 34% of those treated with placebo had BP less than the 90th percentile at the end of the trial. These studies suggest that children with mild to moderate HTN often have normalization of BP without pharmacological therapy, and, therefore, observation for several months without antihypertensive medications may be indicated before labeling them "hypertensive."

## AMBULATORY BLOOD PRESSURE DEFINITION

Although the Task Force data have added immeasurably to our understanding of the normal distribution of BP throughout the pediatric age range, it may be argued that any definition of HTN based on casual BP measurements is fundamentally flawed. The most important limitation of casual BP measurements in general is that they provide only a glimpse of the entire 24-h circadian BP pattern. BP is a constantly changing hemodynamic variable whose pattern may be altered in a number of ways that cannot be detected by intermittent daytime casual BP measurements, even when repeated on several occasions over an extended period of time. In addition, some patients may repeatedly manifest a transient stress response when BP is measured in the presence of a medical professional (i.e., WCH). This phenomenon may cause overdiagnosis of persistent HTN leading to potentially unnecessary diagnostic studies and treatment.

Ambulatory BP monitoring (ABPM) addresses several of the limitations associated with casual BP measurements. ABPM measures BP multiple times during a predefined time period, which more accurately captures the continuous nature of BP. ABPM provides a measurement of BP in the patient's normal environment during both awake and sleep periods. This reduces the potential for transient stress-induced elevations in BP. In addition, ABPM measures both awake and sleeping BP, and thus evaluates not only diurnal but also nocturnal BP patterns. Among patients receiving antihypertensive therapy, ABPM also allows determination of the efficacy and dosing of antihypertensive medications over the entire 24-h period.

The utility and tolerability of ABPM has been documented in multiple pediatric studies. A study by Portman et al.—one of the first to report on the use of ABPM in children—demonstrated excellent tolerability among 99 fifth-grade children *(13)*. Similarly, Reusz et al. also reported excellent tolerability in 123 healthy and hypertensive children ranging from 9.5 to 14.5 yr of age *(14)*. Gellerman et al. recently reported successful performance of ABPM in 77% of 101 children less than 6 yr of age *(15)*. Sorof et al. reported on the successful use of ABPM in 115 children ranging from age 2 to 20 yr *(16)*. These studies provide evidence that ABPM can be performed successfully in children throughout the pediatric age range.

Critical to the interpretation of ABPM data is the availability of normative data against which ABPM results may be compared. Staessen at al. reported the results of an international database of 4577 normotensive adults from which normative ABPM data was derived *(17)*. Based on these data, the recommended thresholds for defining ambulatory HTN were (systolic and diastolic, respectively) 135 and 85 mmHg for 24-h ambulatory BP, 140 and 90 mmHg for daytime ambulatory BP, and 125 and 75 mmHg for nighttime ambulatory BP, respectively. They also studied the distribution of ambulatory BP in normotensive and untreated hypertensive subjects initially classified by casual BP. From these data, thresholds of normality were defined and validated by correlating ambulatory BP to end-organ damage and cardiovascular morbidity and mortality.

Few similar studies exist in pediatric subjects. The largest study to date on normative pediatric ambulatory BP comes from a European multicenter collaborative study group. Soergel et al. studied 1141 healthy children stratified by height to establish the 50th, 90th, and 95th percentile for 24-h day and night mean BP by ABPM *(18)*. Another large study by O'Sullivan et al. collected data on 1121 English school-aged children to determine the range and variability of ambulatory BP *(19)*. While very useful for the interpretation of pediatric ABPM data, these studies are limited to some extent by the presence of only mid-European Caucasian children. Whether these normative data are applicable to children from other ethnic and/or racial backgrounds is uncertain. Harshfield et al. studied a biracial group of 300 normal children using both ausculatory and oscillometric ABPM equipment to establish reference values for ABPM data by gender, age, and race *(20)*. However, the relatively small sample size, as low as 5–10 subjects per age group, limits the utility of these data for use as normal reference values.

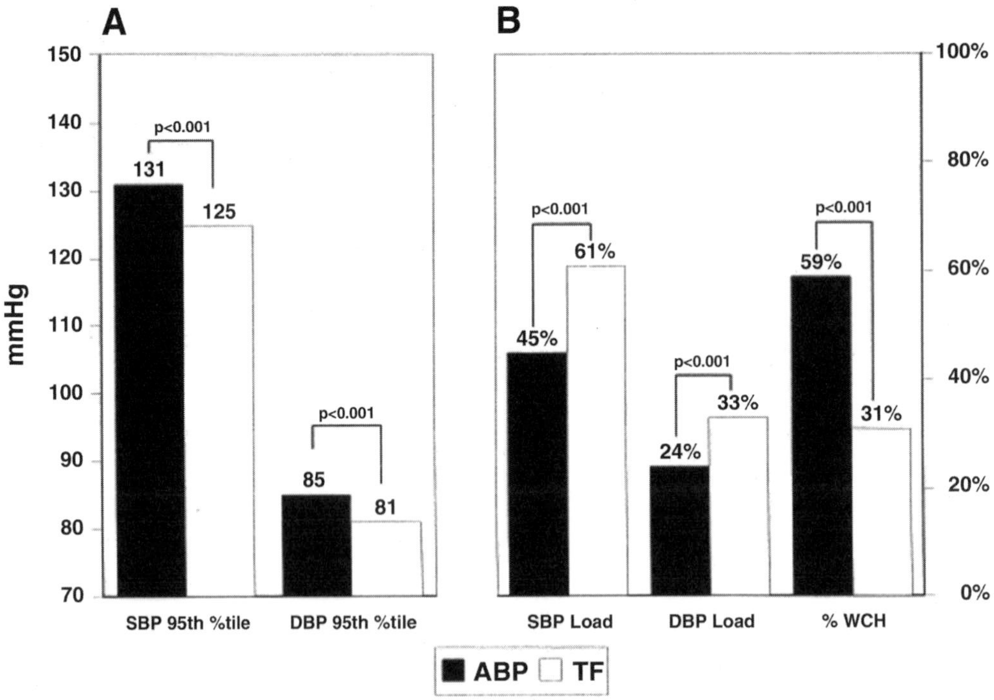


Fig. 2. (A) Comparison of patient-specific 95th percentile threshold limits derived from the normative data from the ambulatory blood pressure *(18)* and Task Force (TF) *(3)* datasets. (B) Comparison of calculated blood pressure load and prevalence of white coat hypertension based on the different threshold limits. From ref. *60*, with permission.

Furthermore, none of these studies include definitions of "normal" pediatric values for BP load or nocturnal BP decline defined by the population 95th percentile.

Many early studies of ABPM in children relied on Task Force values to define HTN, while recent studies have increasingly used the data from the German collaborative group. Sorof et al. investigated the specific clinical implications of using Task Force data compared to the German data for 71 children undergoing evaluation for HTN *(21)*. Because the Task Force data include no measurements of nighttime BP, the analyses of ambulatory BP for the current study were restricted to daytime BP measurements only. Pairwise comparisons of the same patients showed that the 95th percentile for ambulatory daytime BP compared to the Task Force BP was on average 6 mmHg higher for systolic BP and 3.5 mmHg higher for diastolic BP (Fig. 2). Interpretations of ABPM data from the same 24-h period were then compared using the two normative datasets. Corresponding to the higher ambulatory BP limits, daytime BP load was lower by ambulatory criteria than by Task Force criteria for systolic BP (45% vs 61%) and for diastolic BP (24% vs 33%) ($p < 0.001$). Based on Task Force criteria, ambulatory HTN was defined as mean daytime systolic BP and/or diastolic BP greater than the 95th percentile by gender, age, and height percentile. Based on ambulatory BP criteria, ambulatory HTN was defined as mean daytime systolic BP and/or diastolic BP greater than the ambulatory daytime 95th percentile by gender and height. Using these two sets of criteria, ABPM confirmed persistent HTN in 41% of patients by ambulatory criteria and 69% by Task Force criteria ($p < 0.001$).

These results confirm the importance of the choice of threshold BP values used to define ambulatory HTN in children. Direct comparison of the patient-specific BP limits showed that the ambulatory BP limits were significantly higher than the corresponding Task Force limits. Although this systematic difference might be attributed to differences in measurement methodology used to generate the BP datasets (oscillometric for ambulatory BP vs auscultatory for Task Force), excellent reliability of the oscillometric monitoring used to generate the ambulatory BP limits has been reported *(22)*. In addition, these monitors have been validated in children by simultaneous auscultatory measurements from trained observers using K5 criteria for diastolic BP *(23)*. Alternatively, the systematic difference in the limit values may be explained by the fact that the Task Force measurements were made in seated subjects after 5 min of rest, while the ambulatory BP measurements were made in the midst of a normal and active day. It is therefore expected that the 95th percentile limits from the normative ambulatory BP dataset are higher than those from the Task Force. Accordingly, the lower Task Force limits resulted in a higher calculated BP load and a higher prevalence of ambulatory HTN. These data suggest the possibility that using Task Force limits to interpret ambulatory BP may lead to overdiagnosis of ambulatory HTN in children.

## SYSTOLIC VS DIASTOLIC BLOOD PRESSURE

The issue of the appropriate definition of HTN in children may also be addressed from the standpoint of whether systolic or diastolic HTN should be prioritized. In adults, the paradigm has clearly shifted to an emphasis on systolic BP. Systolic HTN in older patients is more common. It is also a marker for vascular disease and a predictor for cardiovascular morbidity and mortality. When treated, systolic HTN results in decreased morbidity and mortality. However, in regard to the evaluation and management of pediatric HTN, the reasons cited in adults for emphasizing systolic BP are unclear. The increased stiffness of large arteries from atherosclerotic disease, identified as one of the major etiological factors for isolated systolic HTN in adults, is less common in children. Furthermore, the low rate of overt morbidity or mortality in the majority of hypertensive children has effectively prevented the linkage of treated or untreated to mildly to moderately elevated BP with poor outcome. Nonetheless, data that support a similar pattern of disease in children and adolescents are emerging *(24)*.

Systolic HTN is more common in children, whether examining an unselected sampling of patients by routine screening, or a selected sampling of referred hypertensive patients. The largest study to date by Rosner et al. combined the data from eight large studies, dating from 1978 to 1991, and taken from different geographic regions in the US *(25)*. Overall, systolic BP data were available for 47,196 children (68,556 visits). Diastolic BP (K5) data were available for 38,184 children (52,053 visits). Using Task Force definitions, there was a 4.4% rate of systolic HTN, and a 3.2% rate of diastolic HTN after pooling the data from all visits. Further analysis showed a higher rate of systolic HTN for virtually every subgrouping of race, gender, and age. These findings were corroborated by data from the Ziac Pediatric Hypertension Study, a multicenter study conducted through subject recruitment from 22 centers that care for children with HTN in the US and Brazil *(12)*. To qualify for randomization, subjects were required to have an average sitting systolic and/or diastolic BP above the Task Force's 95th percentile at the last visit of the screening placebo phase. Of 140 children initially screened for the study, 110 qualified for randomization. At the screening visit, 71% of subjects had systolic HTN (isolated or in combination with diastolic HTN) and 51% had diastolic HTN (isolated or in combination with systolic HTN). At randomization, 83% had systolic HTN and 53% had diastolic HTN. Among the randomized patients, the rate of isolated systolic HTN was 47%, compared to a 17% rate of isolated diastolic HTN. Thus, systolic HTN was found to be more common than diastolic HTN in children specifically referred for evaluation and treatment of elevated BP.

Studies of children also suggest that end-organ changes are more closely related to systolic than to diastolic BP. Several studies of echocardiography in normotensive children have revealed that systolic BP is more highly correlated with left ventricular mass index than diastolic BP *(26–29)*. Similar findings are reported in hypertensive children *(30,31)*. These data indicate that systolic BP may be more important than diastolic BP in defining HTN in children. This assertion has practical implications. Specifically, treatment of HTN should be directed at normalization of systolic BP, even when diastolic BP is within the normal range.

## PROBLEMS WITH CURRENT HYPERTENSION DEFINITIONS

The availability of large datasets of BP values in healthy children has substantially improved the ability to define HTN in children. However, the principle of using population percentiles to define BP normality is inherently problematic for several reasons. One of the most important problems relates to the predictable evolution in the epidemiology of the reference pediatric population. Percentile-based definitions are derived from data collected over a finite time span in a population with a particular ethnic distribution. As the demographics and clinical characteristics of the reference population evolve, it is unclear whether the percentile values used to define normality should also evolve. As an example, updates of weight, height, and BMI percentiles of children in the US have recently been published to account for new trends in the population *(32)*. These updated growth curves raise some important and provocative questions regarding the current definition of pediatric HTN. Since the most recent Task Force update incorporates height percentile into the determination of the BP 95th percentile, it will need to be resolved whether the Task Force tables should be completely regenerated to accommodate the transition to the new height percentile data.

Anthropometric trends in the US pediatric population raise concerns beyond simply the inconvenience of regenerating BP tables. In the US, the prevalence and severity of overweight status is clearly increasing among children. National surveys from the 1960s to the 1990s show that the rate of overweight children grew from 5% to 11% *(33)*. Furthermore, Morrison et al. showed that most of the increase in BMI in grade school-aged children between the 1970s and 1990 occurred in children between the 50th and 100th percentiles *(34)*. In concert with the increasing prevalence of obesity in children, BP values have shifted upwards. Leupker et al. found a concordant increase in BMI and systolic BP in middle school students, aged 10–14 yr, from 1986 to 1996 *(35)*. This association between adiposity and HTN in children has been reported in numerous studies among a variety of ethnic and racial groups, with virtually all studies finding higher blood pressures and/or higher rates of HTN in obese compared to lean children *(10,36–44)*. These trends and associations strongly suggest that BP values are creeping upwards in the pediatric population. If so, as new epidemiological data on BP in children are collected and analyzed, the 95th percentile values used to define HTN for a given gender, age, and height percentile combination will also increase. This will effectively allow higher BPs to be considered "normal" based on a pathological increase in overweight status among US children.

Similar questions may be raised regarding the issue of ethnicity. Hispanics are the fastest-growing ethnic group in the US and are expected to surpass African-Americans as the second largest ethnic group after whites. Recent data suggest that Hispanic children are more prone to obesity and the resultant complication of HTN than are white children *(10)*. Furthermore, African-Americans are at greater risk of HTN and its sequelae than other ethnic groups, a trend that has its roots in late childhood and adolescence. Based on these ethnic differences, it might be argued that separate criteria for normality should be applied to each ethnic group. However, careful consideration suggests that this approach would be flawed. HTN should be defined by comparison with the group at the lowest risk of cardiovascular morbidity and mortality, not by comparison with societal and ethnic peers. To do otherwise would, in effect, "control" for the cardiovascular risk associated with obesity and/or ethnic predispositions to HTN and its sequelae.

The Task Force definition also does not account for the possibility of transient, stress-induced elevations in BP (i.e., WCH). In the largest pediatric study to date, Sorof et al. reported in children referred for evaluation of HTN that the frequency of WCH by ABPM was 35% (40/115) for all patients and 22% (11/51) for those with HTN confirmed in the clinic *(16)*. While these results suggest that the phenomenon of WCH occurs commonly in children, it should be emphasized that WCH may not be an entirely benign condition and, in fact, may represent a prehypertensive state. In adults, 37% of patients with WCH evolved to persistent HTN over a period of follow-up as brief as 0.5–6.5 yr *(45)*. There are currently no data on the long-term follow-up of children found to have WCH on initial assessment. Thus, there is insufficient evidence to assert that elevated casual BP with normal ambulatory BP in children is reassuring.

ABPM address some of the limitations associated with casual BP for diagnosing HTN. However, HTN definitions based on normative ambulatory BP data in children still rely on population percentiles. The collaborative German data published by Soergel et al. provide 50th and 95th percentile values of ambulatory BP based on gender and height range (not height percentile as for the Task Force Update) *(18)*. Age is not factored into the derived percentile values. Although this is the largest dataset of ambulatory BP in healthy children (approx 1100), subdividing subjects by gender and height range results in a relatively small number of subjects per category for establishing population-based percentiles. Since other large datasets of ambulatory BP in healthy children exist, a merger of the available data might improve the reliability of the derived percentile values. The advantage of this approach must be balanced against the fact that different datasets were collected using different methodologies, using auscultatory techniques instead of oscillometric techniques, for example. The issue of methodology could make the merger of independently-created datasets suspect. The conceptual problems associated with defining HTN by population percentiles remain, regardless of the size of the dataset. This may be particularly true for the German data, which consist entirely of Caucasian children of European descent.

The validity of this normative ambulatory BP dataset has also been questioned. To a large extent, the data were generated using oscillometric monitors. Oscillometric monitors rely on an algorithm to calculate systolic and diastolic BP, based on the measured mean arterial pressure. A detailed examination of the BP tables contained in the report reveals a lack of variability in the diastolic BP values. In direct contrast to the Task Force data derived from auscultatory methodology, diastolic BP is reported to be virtually fixed and, therefore, independent of height across a range of 60 cm (Fig. 3). This lack of variability is counterintuitive and raises the question of the reliability of the proprietary algorithm used to calculate diastolic BP in children. Consequently, defining ambulatory diastolic HTN based solely on percentile values from this report is problematic.

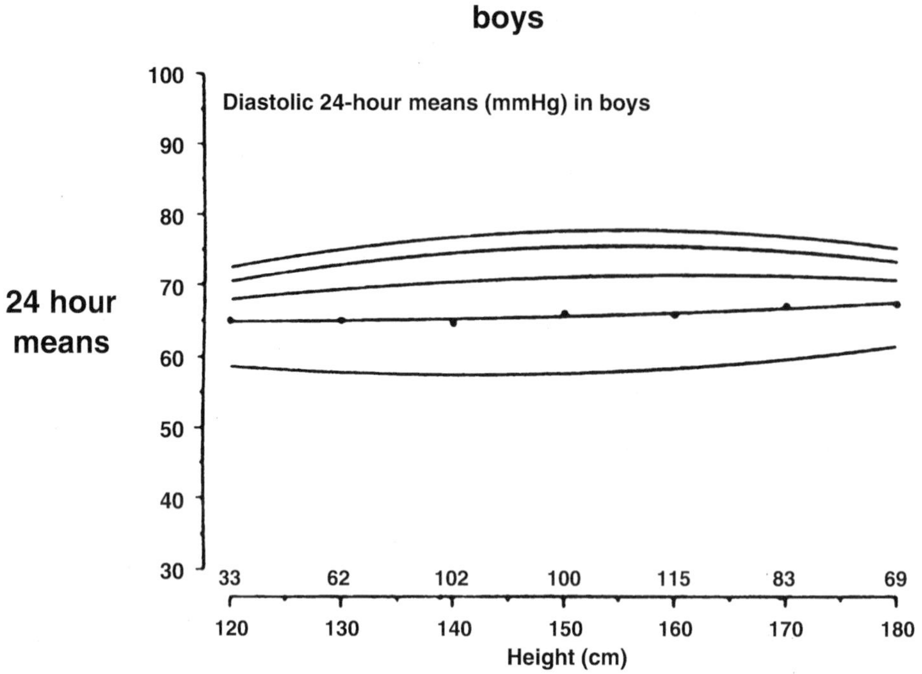


Fig. 3. Diastolic ambulatory blood pressure in boys related to height: 24-h (top), daytime (middle), and nighttime (bottom) means. The points show the raw median values for each height group. The lines represent the fitting polynomials for the 10th, 50th, 75th, 90th, and 95th percentiles. The smaller numbers on the *x*-axis indicate the number of subjects for each height group. From ref. *61*, with permission.

## FUNCTIONAL HYPERTENSION DEFINITIONS

To some extent, indirect BP measurements at the brachial artery are arbitrary numeric representations of a hemodynamic state. In the absence of a linkage of these numeric values to the risk of specific disease outcomes, physicians are treating the numbers but not the disease. The paucity of data linking statistically based definitions of HTN in children with evidence of hypertensive end-organ injury results in uncertainty regarding the indications for initiating antihypertensive medication in children whose BP exceeds these threshold values. Since overt morbid cardiovascular events are rare in the majority of hypertensive children, more attention has been paid to other markers of hypertensive injury, such as increased left ventricular mass index, and the presence of left ventricular hypertrophy (LVH).

Studies of normal and hypertensive children have found that BP and left ventricular mass index are positively correlated across a wide range of BP values *(27–30,46–48)*. Furthermore, elevated left ventricular mass may also be present in patients whose BP values fall within the so-called "normotensive" range. It has been suggested that, although a child's current BP may fall within the population-based range of normality, a previously undetected pattern of relative increases in BP across percentile lines over time may still effectively render that patient "hypertensive" *(49)*. Among patients with HTN by conventional definitions, the reported prevalence of LVH defined by pediatric standards ranges widely, from 30 to 70% *(30,47,48,50–55)*. A recent multicenter study of LVH of 115 hypertensive children with a mean age of approx 14 yr found that the prevalence of LVH was 38% by pediatric criteria and 16% by adult criteria (consistent with severe LVH) *(56)*. Although these data suggest that children with elevated BP do suffer end-organ injury during childhood, its prediction using current HTN definitions is unreliable.

Casual BP values are reliable in their detection of children with elevated BP. However, they do not allow differentiation among patients who have WCH, persistent HTN, or persistent HTN with target organ injury. In hypertensive adults, ambulatory BP parameters are reported to be better correlated with left ventricular mass index, and more predictive of LVH than casual BP values *(57)*. Recent studies in children have found similar relationships between ambulatory BP and left ventricular mass *(31,54)*. To determine whether ambulatory BP is a better predictor of LVH in hypertensive children than casual BP, Sorof et al. performed echocardiography and ambulatory BP in 37 untreated hypertensive children *(31)*. Left ventricular mass index correlated with several ambulatory systolic BP parameters, but did not correlate with clinic BP values. The overall prevalence of LVH was 27%. The prevalence of LVH was 47% (8/17) in patients with both systolic BP load greater than 50% and 24-h systolic BP above the 95th percentile, compared to 10% (2/20) in patients without those criteria ($p = 0.015$). By demonstrating a stronger association with hypertensive sequelae, these data provide preliminary evidence that HTN definitions in children should incorporate ambulatory BP, as well as clinic BP, to identify patients at risk for the development of end organ injury.

## CONCLUSIONS

When very young children have extreme BP elevation, secondary HTN is strongly suspected and an aggressive approach to BP management is required. However, the changing epidemiology of pediatric HTN has made these types of patients increasingly less common in the face of a growing epidemic of childhood obesity. In a large pediatric HTN practice, the typical patient demographic is that of an otherwise healthy adolescent with mild to moderate HTN and some combination of other cardiovascular disease risk factors. In this context, the indications for pharmacological treatment and the target BP values to aim for in response to treatment are unclear based on the current definitions of HTN in children. Incorporating ambulatory BP data into the definition of HTN may increase the definition's reliability for clinical decision-making. However, more robust normative ambulatory BP data are needed for such reliability. In addition, earlier and more sensitive markers of HTN sequelae, such as carotid intimal-medial thickness, or measures of vascular compliance, may allow for the development of functional definitions of HTN that link specific BP values with outcomes. Only then can these definitions be considered evidence-based. Although the medical community has made significant progress in recent years in defining HTN in children, in recognizing that the sequelae of HTN begin in childhood, and in developing evidence-based guidelines for the pharmacological treatment of HTN in childhood, much work remains to be done.

The Working Group on The National High Blood Pressure Education Program Working Group on Children and Adolescents is releasing a fourth report this month *(58)*. The new report discusses the striking increase in obesity and the metabolic syndrome in children and adolescents, and notes the importance of intervention. Tables from that new report are found in the Appendix.

## REFERENCES

1. Blumenthal S, Epps RP, Heavenrich R, et al. Report of the task force on blood pressure control in children. Pediatrics 1977;59:797–820.

2. Task force on blood pressure control in children: report of the second task force on blood pressure control in children—1987. Pediatrics 1987;79:1–25.
3. Update on the 1987 Task Force Report on High Blood Pressure in Children and Adolescents: a working group report from the National High Blood Pressure Education Program. National High Blood Pressure Education Program Working Group on Hypertension Control in Children and Adolescents. Pediatrics 1996;98:649–658.
4. Sinaiko AR, Gomez-Marin O, Prineas RJ. Diastolic fourth and fifth phase blood pressure in 10–15-year-old children. The Children and Adolescent Blood Pressure Program. Am J Epidemiol 1990;132:647–655.
5. Uhari M, Nuutinen M, Turtinen J, et al. Pulse sounds and measurement of diastolic blood pressure in children. Lancet 1991;338:159–161.
6. Hammond IW, Urbina EM, Wattigney WA, et al. Comparison of fourth and fifth Korotkoff diastolic blood pressures in 5 to 30 year old individuals. The Bogalusa Heart Study. Am J Hypertens 1995;8:1083–1089.
7. Biro FM, Daniels SR, Similo SL, et al. Differential classification of blood pressure by fourth and fifth Korotkoff phases in school-aged girls. The National Heart, Lung, and Blood Institute Growth and Health Study. Am J Hypertens 1996;9:242–247.
8. Fixler DE, Laird WP, Fitzgerald V, et al. Hypertension screening in schools: results of the Dallas study. Pediatrics 1979;63:32–36.
9. Sinaiko AR, Gomez-Marin O, Prineas RJ. Prevalence of "significant" hypertension in junior high school-aged children: the Children and Adolescent Blood Pressure Program. J Pediatr 1989;114:664–669.
10. Sorof JM, Poffenbarger T, Franco K, et al. Isolated systolic hypertension, obesity, and hyperkinetic hemodynamic states in children. J Pediatr 2002;140:660–666.
11. Berenson GS, Shear CL, Chiang YK, et al. Combined low-dose medication and primary intervention over a 30-month period for sustained high blood pressure in childhood. Am J Med Sci 1990;299:79–86.
12. Sorof JM, Urbina EM, Cunningham RJ, et al. Screening for eligibility in the study of antihypertensive medication in children: experience from the Ziac Pediatric Hypertension Study. Am J Hypertens 2001;14:783–787.
13. Portman RJ, Yetman RJ, West MS. Efficacy of 24-hour ambulatory blood pressure monitoring in children. J Pediatr 1991;118:842–849.
14. Reusz GS, Hobor M, Tulassay T, et al. 24 hour blood pressure monitoring in healthy and hypertensive children. Arch Dis Child 1994;70:90–94.
15. Gellermann J, Kraft S, Ehrich JH. Twenty-four-hour ambulatory blood pressure monitoring in young children. Pediatr Nephrol 1997;11:707–710.
16. Sorof JM, Portman RJ. White coat hypertension in children with elevated casual blood pressure. J Pediatr 2000;137:493–497.
17. Staessen JA, O'Brien ET, Amery AK, et al. Ambulatory blood pressure in normotensive and hypertensive subjects: results from an international database. J Hypertens Suppl 1994;12:S1–S12.
18. Soergel M, Kirschstein M, Busch C, et al. Oscillometric twenty-four-hour ambulatory blood pressure values in healthy children and adolescents: a multicenter trial including 1141 subjects. J Pediatr 1997;130:178–184.
19. O'Sullivan JJ, Derrick G, Griggs P, et al. Ambulatory blood pressure in schoolchildren. Arch Dis Child 1999;80:529–532.
20. Harshfield GA, Alpert BS, Pulliam DA, et al. Ambulatory blood pressure recordings in children and adolescents. Pediatrics 1994;94:180–184.
21. Sorof JM, Poffenbarger T, Franco K, et al. Evaluation of white coat hypertension in children: importance of the definitions of normal ambulatory blood pressure and the severity of casual hypertension. Am J Hypertens 2001;14:855–860.
22. Baumgart P, Kamp J. Accuracy of the SpaceLabs Medical 90217 ambulatory blood pressure monitor. Blood Press Monit 1998;3:303–307.
23. Portman RJ, Yetman RJ, West MS. Efficacy of 24-hour ambulatory blood pressure monitoring in children. J Pediatr 1991;118:842–849.
24. Sorof JM. Systolic hypertension in children: benign or beware? Pediatr Nephrol 2001;16:517–525.
25. Rosner B, Prineas R, Daniels SR, et al. Blood pressure differences between blacks and whites in relation to body size among US children and adolescents. Am J Epidemiol 2000;151:1007–1019.
26. Burke GL, Arcilla RA, Culpepper WS, et al. Blood pressure and echocardiographic measures in children: the Bogalusa Heart Study. Circulation 1987;75:106–114.
27. Malcolm DD, Burns TL, Mahoney LT, et al. Factors affecting left ventricular mass in childhood: the Muscatine Study. Pediatrics 1993;92:703–709.

28. Daniels SR, Kimball TR, Morrison JA, et al. Effect of lean body mass, fat mass, blood pressure, and sexual maturation on left ventricular mass in children and adolescents. Statistical, biological, and clinical significance. Circulation 1995;92:3249–3254.
29. Treiber FA, McCaffrey F, Pflieger K, et al. Determinants of left ventricular mass in normotensive children. Am J Hypertens 1993;6:505–513.
30. Daniels SR, Meyer RA, Loggie JM. Determinants of cardiac involvement in children and adolescents with essential hypertension. Circulation 1990;82:1243–1248.
31. Sorof JM, Cardwell G, Franco K, et al. Ambulatory blood pressure and left ventricular mass index in hypertensive children. Hypertension 2002;39:903–908.
32. Ogden CL, Kuczmarski RJ, Flegal KM, et al. Centers for Disease Control and Prevention 2000 growth charts for the United States: improvements to the 1977 National Center for Health Statistics version. Pediatrics 2002;109:45–60.
33. Ogden CL, Troiano RP, Briefel RR, et al. Prevalence of overweight among preschool children in the United States, 1971 through 1994. Pediatrics 1997;99:E1.
34. Morrison JA, James FW, Sprecher DL, et al. Sex and race differences in cardiovascular disease risk factor changes in schoolchildren, 1975–1990: the Princeton School Study. Am J Public Health 1999;89:1708–1714.
35. Luepker RV, Jacobs DR, Prineas RJ, et al. Secular trends of blood pressure and body size in a multi-ethnic adolescent population: 1986 to 1996. J Pediatr 1999;134:668–674.
36. Elcarte LR, Villa EI, Sada GJ, et al. [The Navarra study. Prevalence of arterial hypertension, hyperlipidemia and obesity in the infant-child population of Navarra. Association of risk factors.] An Esp Pediatr 1993;38:428–436.
37. Verma M, Chhatwal J, George SM. Obesity and hypertension in children. Indian Pediatr 1994;31:1065–1069.
38. Guillaume M, Lapidus L, Beckers F, et al. Cardiovascular risk factors in children from the Belgian province of Luxembourg. The Belgian Luxembourg Child Study. Am J Epidemiol 1996;144:867–880.
39. Macedo ME, Trigueiros D, de Freitas F. Prevalence of high blood pressure in children and adolescents. Influence of obesity. Rev Port Cardiol 1997;16:27–28.
40. Freedman DS, Dietz WH, Srinivasan SR, et al. The relation of overweight to cardiovascular risk factors among children and adolescents: the Bogalusa Heart Study. Pediatrics 1999;103:1175–1182.
41. Morrison JA, Barton BA, Biro FM, et al. Overweight, fat patterning, and cardiovascular disease risk factors in black and white boys. J Pediatr 1999;135:451–457.
42. Zweiker R, Eber B, Schumacher M, et al. "Non-dipping" related to cardiovascular events in essential hypertensive patients. Acta Med Austriaca 1994;21:86–89.
43. Shigematsu Y, Hamada M, Ohtsuka T, et al. Left ventricular geometry as an independent predictor for extracardiac target organ damage in essential hypertension. Am J Hypertens 1998;11:1171–1177.
44. Ziegler MG, Mills P, Dimsdale JE. Hypertensives' pressor response to norepinephrine. Analysis by infusion rate and plasma levels. Am J Hypertens 1991;4:586–591.
45. Verdecchia P, Schillaci G, Borgioni C, et al. Identification of subjects with white-coat hypertension and persistently normal ambulatory blood pressure. Blood Press Monit 1996;1:217–222.
46. Harshfield GA, Koelsch DW, Pulliam DA, et al. Racial differences in the age-related increase in left ventricular mass in youths. Hypertension 1994;24:747–751.
47. Laird WP, Fixler DE. Left ventricular hypertrophy in adolescents with elevated blood pressure: assessment by chest roentgenography, electrocardiography, and echocardiography. Pediatrics 1981;67:255–259.
48. Culpepper WS, Sodt PC, Messerli FH, et al. Cardiac status in juvenile borderline hypertension. Ann Intern Med 1983;98:1–7.
49. Goonasekera CD, Dillon MJ. Measurement and interpretation of blood pressure. Arch Dis Child 2000;82:261–265.
50. Goldring D, Hernandez A, Choi S, et al. Blood pressure in a high school population. II. Clinical profile of the juvenile hypertensive. J Pediatr 1979;95:298–304.
51. Schieken RM, Clarke WR, Lauer RM. Left ventricular hypertrophy in children with blood pressures in the upper quintile of the distribution. The Muscatine Study. Hypertension 1981;3:669–675.
52. Culpepper WS. Cardiac anatomy and function in juvenile hypertension. Current understanding and future concerns. Am J Med 1983;75:57–61.
53. Richter R. [Echocardiography studies of children and adolescents with primary hypertension] Echokardiographische Untersuchungen von Kindern und Jugendlichen mit primarer Hypertonie. Kinderarztl Prax 1993;61: 279–284.

54. Belsha CW, Wells TG, McNiece KL, et al. Influence of diurnal blood pressure variations on target organ abnormalities in adolescents with mild essential hypertension. Am J Hypertens 1998;11:410–417.
55. Johnson MC, Bergersen LJ, Beck A, et al. Diastolic function and tachycardia in hypertensive children. Am J Hypertens 1999;12:1009–1014.
56. Sorof JM, Hanevold C, Portman RJ, Daniels SR. Left ventricular hypertrophy in hypertensive children: a report from the international pediatric hypertension association. Am J Hypertens 2002;15:31A–31A. Abstract.
57. White WB. Hypertensive target organ involvement and 24-hour ambulatory blood pressure measurement. In: Waeber B, O'Brien E, O'Malley K, Brunner H, eds. Ambulatory Blood Pressure Monitoring. New York: Raven, 1994;47–60.
58. The Fourth Report on the Diagnosis, Evaluation and Treatment of High Blood Pressure in Children and Adolescents. Pediatrics, in press.
59. Sorof JM, Cargo P, Graepel J, et al. Beta-blocker/thiazide combination for treatment of hypertensive children: a randomized double-blind, placebo-controlled trial. Pediatr Nephrol 2002;17(5):345–350.
60. Sorof JM, Poffenbarger T, Franco K, Portman R. Evaluation of white coat hypertension in children: importance of the definitions of normal ambulatory blood pressure and the severity of casual hypertension. Am J Hypertens 2001;14(9 Pt 1):855–860.
61. Soergel M, Kirschstein M, Busch C, Danne T, Gellerman J, Holl R, Krull F, Reichert H, Reusz GS, Rascher W. Oscillometric twenty-four-hour ambulatory blood pressure values in healthy children and adolescents: a multicenter trial including 1141 subjects. J Pediatr 1997;130(2):178–184.

# 9 Secondary Forms of Hypertension in Children

*Michael J. Dillon*, MD

***Contents***



## INTRODUCTION

Secondary hypertension (HTN) is HTN for which an underlying cause can be identified. In childhood, this constitutes a significant proportion of HTN requiring treatment. This is in marked contrast to the situation applicable to adults, where primary or essential HTN predominates. Current evidence suggests that 80–90% of children with severe HTN have an identifiable cause and some form of predominating renal disease. In adults the reverse applies. Normally, over 90% of adults with significantly increased blood pressure (BP) have essential HTN, with much smaller groups affected by secondary causes. However, the changing pattern in childhood, primarily owing to increasing childhood obesity, is modifying these findings, the cause of which is primary HTN in an increasing proportion of children requiring antihypertensive medication.

In considering secondary HTN it is helpful, if possible, to categorize the increase in BP as acute and transient, or chronic and sustained. There is considerable overlap between the two groups. Short-lived causes of increased BP can become chronic if the underlying causal condition is not resolved. Likewise, sustained HTN can resolve over a period of time with a return to normotension.

From: *Clinical Hypertension and Vascular Disease: Pediatric Hypertension*
Edited by: R. J. Portman, J. M. Sorof, and J. R. Ingelfinger © Humana Press Inc., Totowa, NJ

This chapter emphasizes the chronic and sustained causes of childhood HTN. In addition, I will briefly discuss the transient causes in order to present a more complete picture of childhood HTN.

## ACUTE "TRANSIENT" CAUSES OF HYPERTENSION

There are many causes of transiently increased BP in children. The most common are depicted in Table 1. Table 1 shows us that renal disease is the most common etiological factor in "acute" causes of HTN. HTN associated with some form of postinfectious glomerulonephritis (GN), or the nephritis of Henoch-Schönlein purpura (HSP), are the most frequently-encountered renal disorders; the next frequent are hemolytic-uremic syndromes and other causes of acute renal functional deterioration. The mechanisms for HTN in acute GN, and in nephritis of HSP, are somewhat similar, in that salt retention and water retention play an important role. In some postinfectious GN cases, however, renin is increased, as opposed to being suppressed, and in HSP the vasculitic process may also contribute to a hyperreninemic hypertensive situation. In hemolytic uremic syndrome (HUS) hyperreninemia is an important contributor to increased BP, but fluid overload owing to acute renal failure is also a factor, as it is in other causes of acute renal impairment.

The hypertensive states seen in some acutely salt- and water-depleted individuals, or in the course of nephrotic relapse, is interesting and important. It is a profound hyperreninemic state, in spite of incipient or established circulatory volume depletion, that produces intense vasospasm via angiotensin II (ANG II). The resulting HTN is responsive to volume repletion.

It must also be remembered that acute urinary tract obstruction may be associated with HTN that settles after drainage or relief of the obstruction. Compression of the kidneys (e.g., a tight abdominal wall surgical closure in infants) may be associated with HTN that settles with the release of tension.

When considering the neurological causes of HTN, it is important to remember the causes associated with disturbances of the autonomic nervous system. The increased BP levels associated with Guillain-Barré syndrome are linked to autonomic dysfunction. Increased BP levels in patients with genetically determined dysautonomic states, such as the Riley-Day syndrome, are also linked to autonomic dysfunction.

The often unrecognized relationship between HTN and leg fractures requiring traction for treatment is also a largely neurologically determined phenomenon, subsequent to the occurrence of reflex-mediated alteration in a patient's vasculature.

## CHRONIC "SUSTAINED" CAUSES OF SECONDARY HYPERTENSION

The main causes of sustained HTN, as well as acute, transiently increased BP, are renal. Renal parenchymal disease occurs most frequently. The most common cause of significant HTN in childhood is coarsely scarred kidneys, the result of reflux nephropathy or the nephropathy associated with obstructive uropathy. This type of coarse scarring contributes 30–40% of the hypertensive patients seen in major childhood hypertensive services, with some form of chronic GN being the next most common at 23–28%. Renovascular disease, although critically important as a potentially curable form of HTN, occurs in approximately 10% of tertiary referral centre patients with HTN, with approximately the same incidence as coarctation of the aorta. Table 2 outlines the main categories of secondary HTN in children, and although other important causes are recorded, such as pheochromocytoma and various low renin hypertensive states, these are rare, contributing 4–5% and <1% respectively to most large series. The experience of one large tertiary referral service is outlined in Table 3.

**Table 1**
**Causes of Acute (Transient) HTN**

| |
|---|
| *Renal parenchymal disease* |
| Postinfectious glomerulonephritis |
| Henoch–Schönlein glomerulonephritis |
| Acute relapses of systemic disease, e.g., SLE, vasculitis, etc. |
| Hemolytic uremic syndromes |
| Acute tubulointerstitial nephritis |
| Nephrotic syndrome (in certain circumstances) |
| *Associated with acute renal failure* |
| Acute tubular necrosis |
| Rapidly progressive glomerulonephritis of various etiologies |
| Renal vein thrombosis |
| Drug induced, e.g., nephrotoxins, and NSAIDS |
| Any of the renal parenchymal causes if acute renal failure ensues |
| *Renal trauma* and other trauma, e.g., lower limb fractures requiring traction |
| *Acute urinary tract obstruction* |
| *Salt and water overload* |
| Iatrogenic—saline, plasma, etc. |
| Associated with acute renal failure |
| Associated with salt-retaining hormone administration |
| *Salt and water depletion and nephrotic relapse* |
| Secondary HTN owing to circulatory volume depletion |
| *Vascular causes* |
| Renal vein and renal artery thrombosis |
| Vascular occlusions from emboli, e.g., subacute bacterial endocarditis |
| Vascular compromise owing to vasculitis including hypertensive damage |
| Trauma |
| Iatrogenic, e.g., following surgery or angioplasty |
| Renal compression |
| Arterio-venous fistulae |
| *Neurological causes* |
| Associated with raised intracranial pressure from many causes, e.g., tumor, hydrocephalus |
| Seizures |
| Gullain–Barré syndrome |
| Poliomyelitis |
| Spinal cord injury |
| Dysautonomia |
| *Drug-mediated causes (partial list)* |
| Oral contraceptives |
| NSAIDS |
| Sympathomimetic drugs |
| Cocaine |
| Erythropoietin |
| *Diet-mediated causes (partial list)* |
| Alcohol |
| Caffeine |
| Tyramines |
| Licorice |

**Table 2**
**Causes of Chronic (Sustained) HTN**

| |
|---|
| *Coarctation of aorta* |
| *Associated with chronic renal failure and end-stage renal failure* |
| *Parenchymal renal disease* |
| Reflux nephropathy |
| Chronic glomerulonephritis of various sorts |
| Congenital renal anomalies, e.g., dysplasia |
| Inherited parenchymal disease of kidney, e.g., ADPKD, ARPKD, etc. |
| Other acquired disease, e.g., post hemolytic-uremic syndrome |
| *Renovascular HTN* |
| Renal artery stenosis |
| Renal artery stenosis and mid-aortic syndrome |
| Renal artery stenosis and intracranial arterial disease |
| Renal artery stenosis and inherited syndromes, e.g., neurofibromatosis |
| *Renal tumor associated* |
| Wilms |
| Hemangiopericytoma |
| Hamartomas |
| *Catecholamine excess* |
| Pheochromocytoma |
| Neuroblastoma |
| Paraganglioma |
| Iatrogenic |
| *Corticosteroid excess states/low-renin HTN* |
| Iatrogenic |
| Cushings disease and syndrome |
| Conn's syndrome—hyperplasia/tumor |
| Glucocorticoid-remediable aldosteronism (GRA) |
| Apparent mineralocorticoid excess |
| Liddle's syndrome |
| Gordon's syndrome |

These secondary causes of HTN will be described in further detail in the following pages. This chapter might mention or purposefully exclude material covered in detail in other chapters, such as the HTN associated with chronic kidney disease, end-stage renal disease (ESRD), the neonate, and monogenic hypertensive disorders, the diagnostic evaluation of pediatric HTN, or pharmacological treatment except where necessary.

## COARCTATION OF THE AORTA

Coarctation of the aorta is the cause of severe HTN in approx 9–10% of children with HTN in major childhood referral centers *(1)*. This incidence is similar to that of renovascular disease. Interestingly, in some series coaractation of the aorta accounts for far fewer cases of severe HTN, even as low as 2% *(2)*. In infancy, this cause of severe HTN figures more prominently (in up to one-third of patients) *(3)*.

The cause of the increased BP in patients with coarctation of the aorta is complex. From experimental animal data there is evidence that the kidneys have an important role similar to that seen in the 2-clip model of renal artery stenosis *(4)*. This would be associated, in experi-

Table 3
**Causes of Sustained HTN at Great Ormond Street Hospital for Children**

| | |
|---|---|
| Renal scarring | |
| (Reflux nephropathy and obstructive uropathy) | 36% |
| Glomerulonephritis | 23.3% |
| Renovascular disease | 9.5% |
| Coarctation of the aorta | 8.9% |
| Renal polycystic kidney disease | 5.5% |
| Post hemolytic-uremic syndrome | 4.0% |
| Idiopathic (? Essential) | 3.4% |
| Catecholamine excess states | 2.8% |
| Wilms tumour | 2.4% |
| Miscellaneous other causes | 4.6% |

mental circumstances, with an initial increase in plasma renin levels. The plasma renin levels would return to normal within several days, although still inappropriately elevated, since there would be expansion of extracellular fluid at this time *(5)*. The latter would be owing to sodium retention because of renal hypoperfusion.

In addition, it would seem that neural factors also contribute with resetting of barcoceptors and increased sympathetic activity on top of the purely mechanical contribution that increases peripheral resistance *(6)*.

The most common anatomical lesion in patients with coarctation of the aorta is narrowing in the thorax, with over 90% of cases occurring just below the origin of the left subclavian artery. This type of coarctation is twice as common in males as in females but is also well recognized in Turner's syndrome *(7)*. It is important to be aware that coarctation can occur at other sites. Of particular importance is the so-called mid-aortic syndrome, where variably extensive abdominal aortic narrowing occurs, often associated with bilateral renal artery stenosis and abnormalities of other abdominal arteries (for example, the celiac axis and the mesenteric vessels) *(8–10)*. The mid-aortic syndrome may be caused by to fibromuscular dysplasia, either in isolation or as part of the arterial pathology seen in neurofibromatosis *(1)*. Similar appearances can be found in Takayasu disease *(11)* and occasionally in William's syndrome *(12)*.

The clinical manifestations classically involve disparity in pulsation and BP between the arms and legs. A systolic ejection murmur may be heard over the base of the heart and precordium, and in the interscapular region. Occasionally, murmurs may be heard over collateral vessels in long-standing cases.

Chest x-rays may reveal notching of ribs owing to the collaterals. An electrocardiogram (ECG) will reveal left ventricular hypertrophy (LVH) and an echocardiogram with color Doppler mapping the site and severity of the lesion *(13)*. At times, magnetic resonance imaging (MRI) scanning is used to delineate the lesion in more detail *(14)*.

Most patients will require surgical treatment. The procedure of choice is excision of the area of coarctation and a primary anastomosis. If the length of the constriction will not allow this, then an arterial graft is necessary. Mid-aortic stenosis may be amenable to transluminal angioplasty but surgery in the form of bypass grafting or aortic replacement may be necessary. The development of extensive collateral circulation may obviate the need for surgery or other forms of intervention in childhood.

Following surgical repair, persistent or paradoxical HTN might occur. The mechanism of paradoxical HTN remains obscure, but may be linked to activation of the sympathetic nervous system or the development of gradients across the renal arteries giving rise to relative renal ischaemia *(15,16)*. This HTN may well require antihypertensive therapy but often settles with time.

Most patients do well after coarctation repair, but long-term observation is essential owing to the risk of re-coarctation caused by scar tissue. Re-coarctation or a residual gradient at the site of repair may prove amenable to angioplasty dilatation *(17)*.

## HYPERTENSION ASSOCIATED WITH CHRONIC AND END-STAGE RENAL FAILURE

The cause of HTN associated with chronic and end-stage renal failure is multifactorial. Sodium and water retention is the predominant factor, but increased activity of the renin-angiotensin system (RAS), sympathic nervous system activity, and increased circulating nitric oxide (NO) inhibitors contribute *(18)*. The nature of the underlying disorder that has caused the renal impairment is also relevant since HTN is much more likely in glomerulonephritides, reflux nephropathy, and polycystic kidney disease than in some other causes of renal failure. In the HTN seen posttransplantation, a number of factors play a part, including rejection, volume expansion, anti-rejection drug therapy (such as cyclosporin A or FK506 as well as steroids), and vascular compromise *(19,20)*. This and the broader topic of HTN in chronic and end-stage renal failure will be dealt with elsewhere in this book.

## PARENCHYMAL RENAL DISEASE

Table 2 shows that there are many parenchymal renal causes of HTN in childhood. Two categories predominate: the coarse renal scarring of reflux nephropathy or obstructive uropathy, and the various forms of chronic glomerulonephritis (GN) *(9,21,22)*. Other causes, such as the various forms of polycystic kidney disease *(23–25)* and damaged kidneys as a result of HUS *(26)*, are important but much less common. Furthermore, because HTN associated with chronic GN is essentially managed along the lines of the underlying condition, or as part of renal failure, this section will emphasize the association of HTN with reflux nephropathy.

Reflux nephropathy can be defined as the coarse renal scarring associated with vesico-ureteric reflux and previous urinary tract infection (Fig. 1). Reflux nephropathy might occur as a sequel to acute episodes of pyelonephritis or be linked to damage associated with varying degrees of obstructive uropathy plus or minus infection.

In childhood, approx 10% of children with reflux nephropathy will develop HTN *(27)*, and by late adolescence the prevalence will be of the order of 18–20% *(28)*. Long-term follow shows between 30 and 40% of subjects will become hypertensive *(29)*, emphasizing the importance of HTN in this group of patients.

The pathogenesis of the increased BP remains controversial. There is no doubt that the RAS has a role *(28,30–32)*, but other factors contribute. Chronic renal impairment contributes. Loss of renal medullary vasodilator substances *(33)* and increased circulating NO inhibitors might also contribute *(34)*. With age, there is an increasing tendency to develop primary HTN in vulnerable families, another possible contributor *(35)*.

What is clear is that untreated HTN in these individuals carries serious sequelae in terms of morbidity and mortality. It is also well known that a period of uncontrolled HTN can seriously and permanently affect renal function *(36)*.

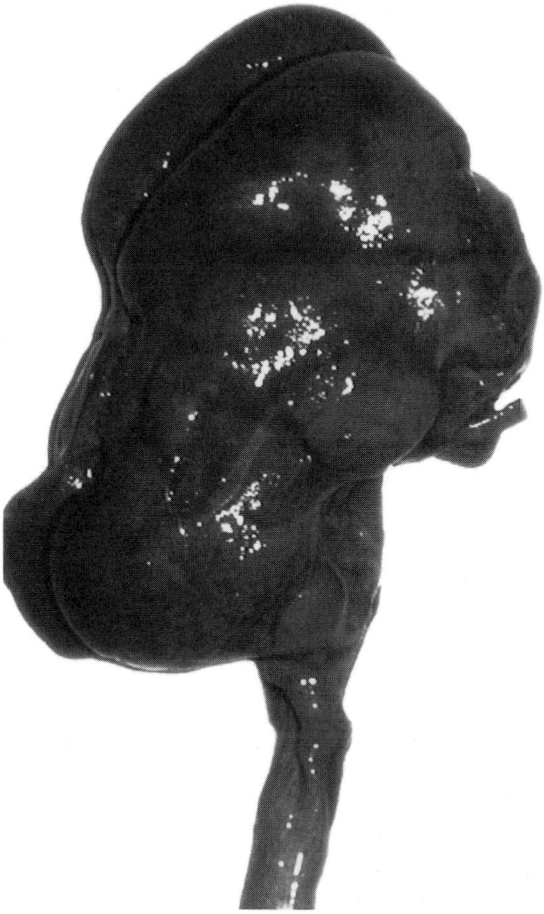

Fig. 1. Coarsely scarred kidney associated with vesico-ureteric reflux and previous urinary tract infection.

The evaluation of such patients essentially focuses on demonstrating that there is renal scarring of a characteristic appearance and that there is no other obvious cause for the increased BP. Ultrasonography may reveal typical parenchymal loss, and isotope scanning (e.g., Tc99DMSA) may well reveal typical areas of decreased isotope uptake *(37)*. The demonstration of vesico-ureteric reflux will be helpful, if present, and may additionally reveal clubbed calyces. The absence of reflux does not exclude the diagnosis because it may have already resolved with time. An intravenous urogram may well be helpful in these circumstances showing the characteristic decrease in cortical thickness at sites of scarring served by clubbed calyces. An increased plasma renin level for age is often a feature *(38)*, but it does not predict those patients destined to develop HTN in the long term *(28)*.

Treatment is essentially medical with standard antihypertensive agents. The role of surgery is not clear. However, nephrectomy can be considered, especially with unilateral disease and markedly diminished renal function on the affected side—e.g., <10% with a normal kidney contralaterally. In an attempt to predict the success of surgical intervention, renal vein renin studies have been conducted to localize renin release to the affected kidney with suppression of renin from the opposite kidney. Such findings might predict success in curing the HTN by removing the high-renin-release kidney *(39)*. There are, unfortunately, problems in utilizing this technique for this purpose. First, the contralateral kidney may be suppressed in terms of renin release but may not be "normal" and, if scarring were to be present, it could well contribute to maintaining HTN once the more severely affected kidney were to be removed. Utilizing segmental renal vein renin sampling may help to obviate this by detecting localized areas that might be missed by main renal vein renin sampling alone. In a large study *(40)*, although renal vein renin sampling was helpful in identifying localized areas of renin release in reflux nephropathy; unlike the situation in renovascular disease the technique was not reliable in predicting surgical cure.

In the long term, patients affected by reflux nephropathy with HTN require, in general, indefinite antihypertensive therapy. Angiotensin-converting enzyme (ACE) inhibitors are not usually contraindicated, and may also have a protective role in individuals with considerable renal damage. However, there are some patients who, after a protracted period of antihypertensive medication, find that the elevated BP becomes less of an issue with time. Ischemic areas within the scarred segments of kidney may necrose and cease to be a source of renin release, normalizing BP. However, individuals with extensive scarring are at greater risk of developing HTN, and of progressing to chronic renal failure, with its own contribution to maintaining HTN *(41)*.

## RENOVASCULAR HYPERTENSION

Renovascular HTN can be defined as HTN resulting from a lesion (or lesions) that impairs blood flow to a part, or all, of one or both kidneys. It constitutes between 5 and 25% of cases of secondary HTN in children *(42)*, in contrast to the prevalence of renovascular disease in hypertensive adults, which is less than 1% *(43)*. It is more common in younger children and it contributes 8–10% of patients with HTN seen at major pediatric hypertensive centers *(9,44)*. It is potentially curable, second only to coarctation of the aorta as a cause of surgically treatable HTN in children *(45,46)*. The most common abnormality is some form of renal artery stenosis, but other forms of renal vascular pathology occur. The first published case of renovascular HTN treated surgically was a 5-yr-old boy whose BP was cured by nephrectomy *(47)*.

The most common form of renal artery stenosis causing renovascular disease in children is fibromuscular dysplasia *(45,46,48–52)* (Fig. 2), in contrast to adults, where atherosclerosis is the most common finding *(51)*. The lesions of fibromuscular dysplasia often cause areas of arterial narrowing, and alternating with aneurysmal sections, give rise to a "string of beads" appearance on angiography. The intima and/or the media of the vessel walls are affected, and it seems likely that uncontrolled release of growth factors probably play a role in the development of the lesions during angiogenesis.

Intimal hyperplasia occurs in association with neurofibromatosis *(1,53–57)*, however, there are familial cases of fibromuscular dysplasia without this association *(58)*. Renal artery stenosis is also seen in association with idiopathic hypercalcemia *(12)*, Marfan's syndrome *(59)*, the rubella syndrome *(60)*, Takayasu disease *(11)*, the Klippel-Trenaunay-Weber syndrome *(61)*, and the Feuerstein-Mims syndrome *(9)*. Renal artery stenosis can also be found following systemic vasculitis *(62)*, renal artery trauma *(45)*, neonatal renal artery thrombosis associated with umbilical artery cathetization *(63)*, abdominal radiation *(64,65)*, or external compression due to tumors *(66)* or glands *(9)*. Renovascular HTN can also be seen with arteriovenous fistulae *(67)* and in children with renal artery aneurysms *(58)*.

The anatomical presentations vary. One main renal artery may be affected (Fig. 3). In childhood, however, it is common to see bilateral disease (Fig. 4), and intrarenal artery pathol-

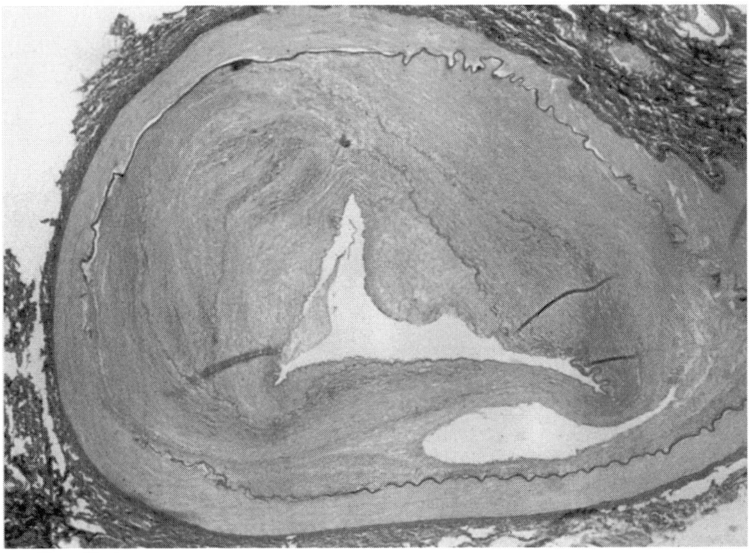

Fig. 2. Fibromuscular dysplasia in renal artery affected by renal artery stenosis.

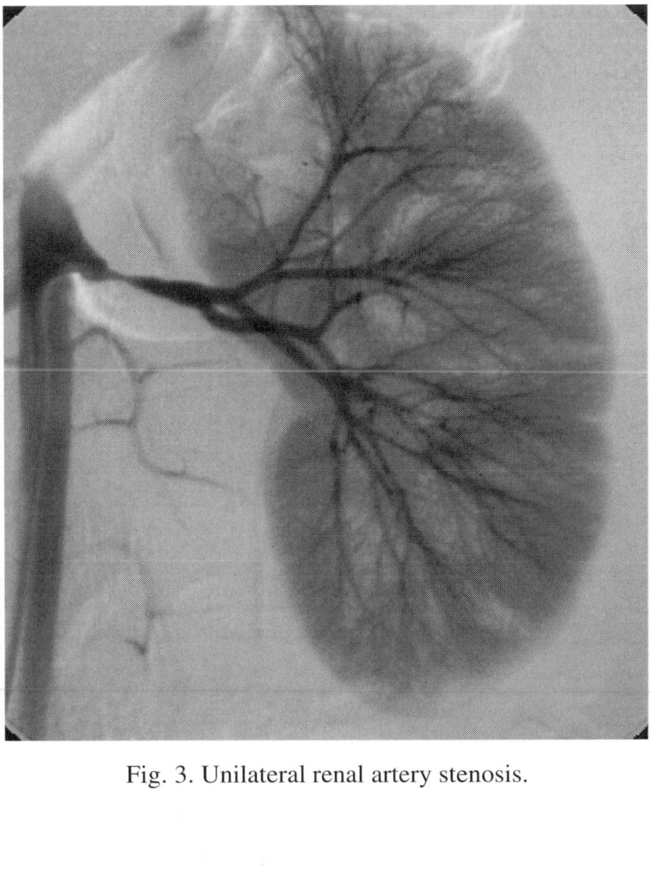

Fig. 3. Unilateral renal artery stenosis.

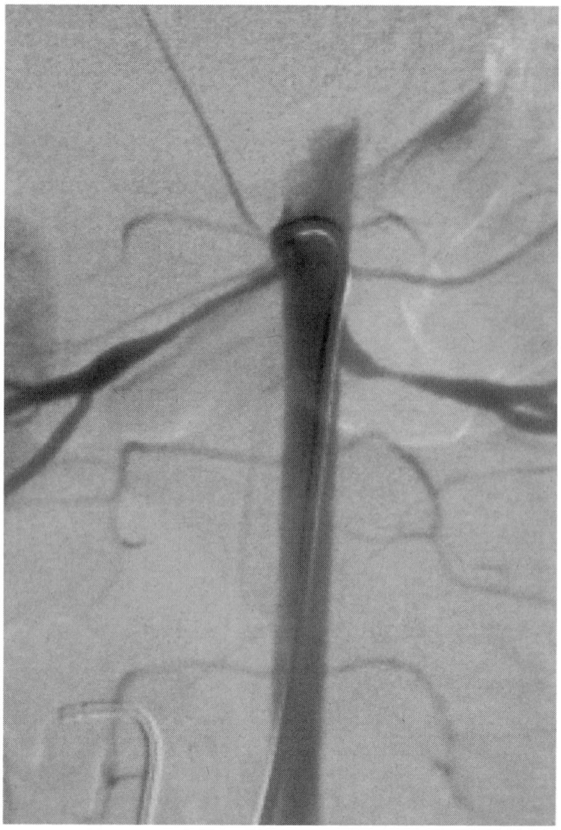

Fig. 4. Bilateral renal artery stenosis.

ogy (Fig. 5) with or without main artery abnormalities. In addition, it is well-recognized that other non-renal arteries are affected, including the mesenteric, splenic, and hepatic arteries in the abdomen, and the intracranial vessels *(9,68)*. It is also well-recognized that the aorta is involved with the middle aortic syndrome (Fig. 6) associated with renal artery disease *(8,10)*.

The clinical presentation of children with renovascular disease is variable. Some are entirely asymptomatic *(42,69)*, while others present with more characteristic features, including headache (in older children) or failure to thrive (in younger patients) *(9)*. Unfortunately the first sign of HTN might be the development of an accelerated hypertensive state with, for example, fits, hemiplegia, visual symptoms or facial palsy. There may be evidence of a syndrome associated with renovascular disease and there maybe bruits over the abdomen, flanks, neck, or head indicating underlying vascular pathology. However, physical examination may be particularly unhelpful and the diagnosis might only be revealed by further investigation.

Standard investigative approaches to the child with HTN will need to be implemented *(70)*; these are covered in detail in a subsequent chapter. There may be evidence of end-organ effects on the heart or kidneys, and evidence of hypokalemia, seen in individuals with secondary hyperaldosteronism as a sequel to excess renin release. Abdominal ultrasonography may reveal asymmetric kidney size but may be entirely normal. Doppler ultrasonography might show changes in flow over stenotic renovascular lesions *(71,72)* that may be emphasized using the color Doppler technique *(73)*. However, Doppler ultrasound may be entirely normal in the presence of significant renal artery narrowing and it is unhelpful in detecting intrarenal pathol-

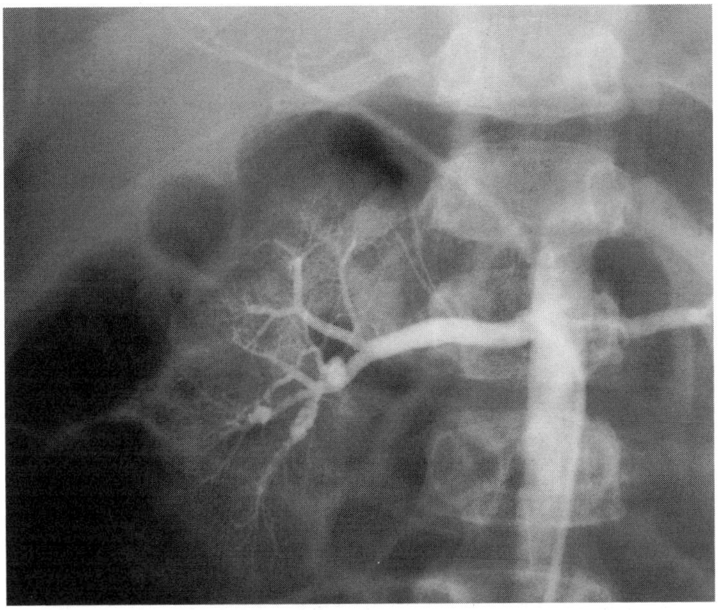

Fig. 5. Renovascular disease showing intrarenal "string of beads" appearances owing to fibromuscular dysplasia.

ogy. Isotopic scanning (Tc99 DMSA, Tc99 DTPA or MAG 3) may help identify a renovascular cause especially if the captopril priming technique is utilized *(74–76)*. Unfortunately, the sensitivity and specificity of these sophisticated investigative modalities still remain unacceptable in terms of definitive diagnostic security. Despite the sensitivity and specificity issues, when the results of these investigative procedures are abnormal, they can be helpful in defining the next stage of investigation as well as in monitoring the effectiveness of treatment *(77)*.

The gold standard investigative tool for childhood renovascular disease is contrast digital subtraction angiography *(78,79)*, usually associated with a renal vein renin study *(39,40)*. The angiography must involve bilateral selective renal angiograms as well as an aortogram (Figs. 3–6). The renal vein renin study must involve the main renal veins and low inferior vena cava (IVC) plus segmental sampling from the upper, middle, and lower pole veins to detect local sources of renin release *(40)*.

Magnetic resonance angiography awaits validation in the evaluation of childhood renovascular disease. It is currently unable to detect intrarenal arterial pathology, a frequent feature of childhood renovascular HTN *(79,80)*. Computed tomography (CT) angiography is even less securely established in evaluation of childhood renovascular disease, because it fails to pick up small vessel abnormalities and subjects the child to both a radiation and contrast medium burden *(81)*.

Because of the recognized association of intracranial arterial disease in subjects with renovascular pathology, cerebral angiography may be indicated in patients with renovascular HTN *(68)*. This would be mandatory in patients with neurological complications or cerebral or carotid bruits, but may also be justified in those subjects in whom a defect in cerebral perfusion was co-identified with renovascular disease *(82)*.

Treatment for renovascular disease would initially involve antihypertensive drugs to stabilize the BP. ACE inhibitors or ANG II antagonists would be contraindicated until it was clear

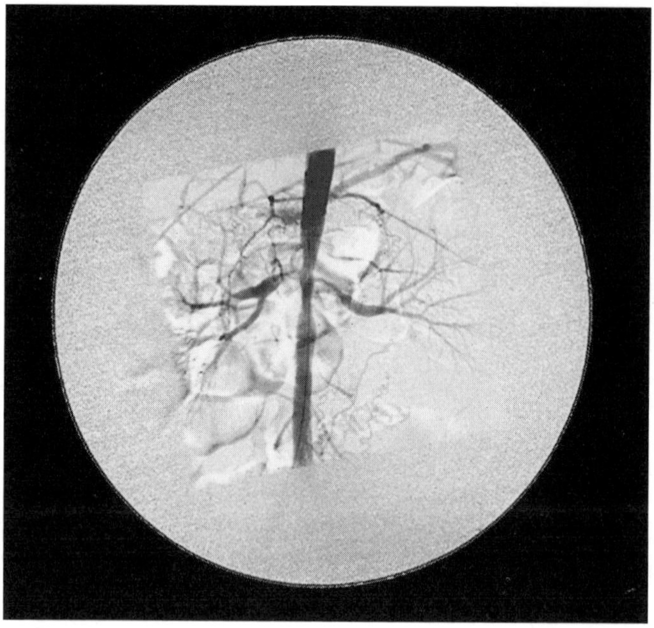

Fig. 6. Mid-aortic syndrome plus bilateral renal artery stenosis.

that the patient did not have major or critical main artery stenosis and, particularly, bilateral disease of this severity. However, if there were to be no significant reduction of renal perfusion on captopril primed isotope scans, or if the renal artery pathology affected more peripheral vessels, then such therapeutic agents might be considered if the BP was not controlled adequately on other therapy *(83)*. In children with significant intracranial arterial pathology, it must also be remembered that a substantial reduction of BP may be contraindicated because of risks of severe cerebral ischemia *(68,83)*. In fact some children require a degree of HTN that in other circumstances would be contraindicated to keep their brain perfusion adequate.

Once the BP is adequately controlled, even if not normal, decisions then need to be made as to whether the underlying renovascular pathology is amenable to intervention. The intervention may be transluminal angioplasty or revascularization surgery or a combination of both. Occasionally, embolization might be considered if no other option is available. Nephrectomy or partial nephrectomy may be indicated for lateralized or localized disease in certain circumstances.

The ideal lesion for transluminal angioplasty would be a non-ostial short segment main renal artery stenosis with no intrarenal or contralateral disease along with clear lateralization of renin release to the affected side and suppression of renin release contralaterally *(84–88)*. However, modern transluminal angioplasty techniques allow for more complex lesions to be treated including, at times, ostial sites of stenosis, bilateral disease, and intrarenal branch artery stenosis *(89)*. Very tight stenotic lesions or those that recur after apparently successful previous dilatation may be amenable to stenting *(90–92)*.

Results vary in terms of success of transluminal angioplasty in children, but the experience of Great Ormond Street Hospital for Children was that 21% of patients were cured in terms of HTN, 50% were normotensive yet still required antihypertensive therapy in reduced dosages, 17% were normotensive on the same drugs, and 12% failed to show benefit *(89)*. These data are not dissimilar to the findings of other series.

Some patients are not amenable to angioplasty treatment. Others, who have undergone angioplasty treatment, failed to achieve its objective. Such children may benefit from surgery either in the form of some type of revascularization procedure (e.g., direct reanastomosis, spleno-renal, hepato-renal, or internal iliac renal anastomosis) or the use of some Dacron/ Gortex grafting procedure with or without auto-transplantation, or a combination of these *(9,45,46,48,58,93–96)*. Nephrectomy or partial nephrectomy might be considered if revascularization is inappropriate or attempted and failed. Decisions concerning which kidney to revascularize would be taken on the basis of the anatomical abnormalities, the renal functional status, and the renal vein renin data. Results of surgical intervention, particularly the data from Stanley and colleagues of Michigan *(97)*, show that it can be very successful with a number of large series. The Great Ormond Street Hospital data show that 45% of patients were cured, 50% were normotensive but still needed some antihypertensive therapy, and in only 5% did the procedure fail *(9)*. It is to be remembered, however, that a large number of patients had lesions of such complexity that they were deemed unsuitable for surgical intervention and were treated medically.

## RENAL TUMOR-ASSOCIATED HYPERTENSION

HTN can be associated with a variety of renal tumors. More than 50% of Wilms tumor patients are hypertensive either owing to renin production by the tumor or to intrarenal artery compression *(98)*. In addition, there are tumors of the juxtaglomerular cells that produce HTN because of excess renin release. These are known as hemangiopericytomas and are often less than 1 cm in diameter and difficult to identify *(99,100)*. CT scanning usually reveals the lesion but arteriography often fails to locate it *(101)*. Renal vein renin studies may prove helpful in localizing the sites of such tumors in the renal parenchyma. Treatment is surgical, ideally by heminephrectomy, if the tumor site is identified, but at times, even if suspected, the lesion is not found and pharmacological treatment with ACE inhibitors or ANG II receptor antagonists may be preferable to full nephrectomy. Hamartomas that behave in a similar fashion to the hemangiopericytoma are occasionally reported *(102)*.

## CATECHOLAMINE EXCESS STATES

Catecholamine excess HTN is rare but important in childhood *(103,104)*. It is secondary to excess catecholamine release from some form of neural crest tumor (pheochromocytoma, paraganglioma, or possibly neuroblastoma). Pheochromocytomas arise from the adrenal medulla. Paragangliomas arise from adrenal sites anywhere in the sympathetic chain. It is unclear whether neuroblastomas cause HTN as a result of excess catecholamine release or by impingement of the kidney adjacent to the tumor, resulting in hyperreninemic HTN.

In children, pheochromocytomas and paragangliomas are often multiple and are known to be associated with neurofibromatosis *(105,106)*, von Hippel-Lindau disease *(107)*, and multiple endocrine neoplasia (MEN) syndromes *(108–110)*. Molecular genetic advances have allowed precise identification of these syndromes which may not have been so readily recognized in the past in patients with catecholamine excess HTN *(111)*.

Symptoms of catecholamine excess are quite variable, but include headache, sweating, nausea and vomiting, visual disturbances, abdominal pain, polydipsia and polyuria, and fits and peripheral circulatory disturbances akin to acrocyanosis *(103,104)*. The increased BP maybe episodic, but, contrary to popular belief, is more often sustained *(103)*.

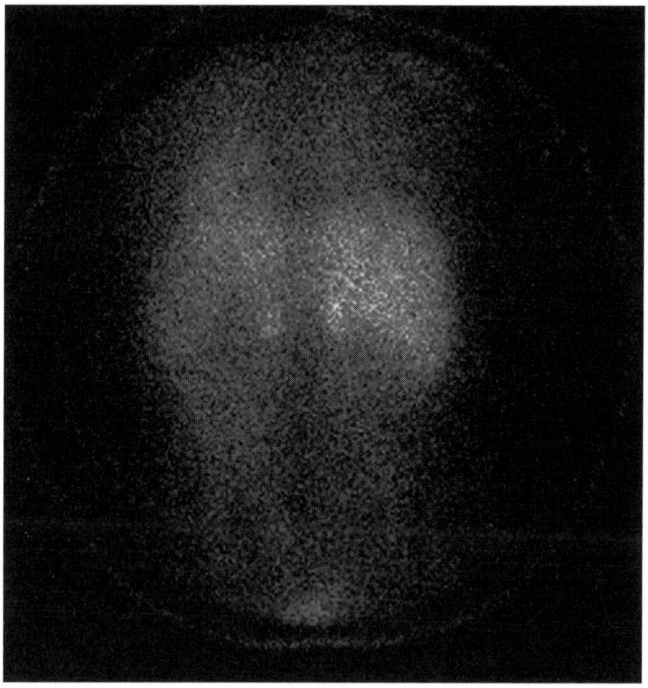

Fig. 7. $I^{123}$ MIBG scan showing bilateral adrenal pheochromocytomata

The presence of such a tumor should be suspected when excess catecholamine production is identified either via urine catecholamine analysis or by the detection of increased plasma catecholamines *(112)*.

A tumor might be identified in the abdomen by means of abdominal ultrasonography, but often this is not possible *(104)*. Usually an $I^{131}$ or $I^{123}$ meta-iodo-benzyl-guanidine ($I^{131}$ or $I^{123}$ MIBG) scan is the next investigative procedure (Fig. 7) *(113,114)*. MIBG is taken up by active neural crest tissue and can detect pheochromocytomata and paragangliomata in the abdomen. MIBG is not so effective in detecting pheochromocytomata and paragangliomata in the thorax. It is important to note that a substantial lesion can be missed using MIBG, and, currently, an adjunct to MIBG scanning is to utilize labelled somatostatin. Labelled somtatostatin is an alternative scanning technique that has the ability to identify tumors missed by MIBG *(115)*.

CT scanning and MRI imaging have roles in localizing tumors *(104,116)*, but the most effective means, and certainly the approach necessary if other tests are negative, is venous catecholamine sampling *(104)*. Venous catecholamine sampling assesses venous blood for a localized increase in catecholamine production. The sample sources may be taken from the jugular veins, superior vena cava (SVC), high IVC, renal veins, adrenal veins if possible, low IVC, and the iliac veins. Angiography is also indicated at times and, it, as well as the catecholamine sampling, should only be undertaken after appropriate pharmacological sympathetic blockade has been introduced *(104)*.

Treatment consists of $\alpha$ and usually $\beta$-sympathetic blockade ideally utilizing phenoxybenzamine and propranolol or another form of $\beta$-blocking agent. Calcium channel blockers, such as nifidipine, have some roles, but phenoxybenzamine is undoubtedly superior *(104)*. Preoperatively, the patient needs to be adequately hydrated to fill the increasingly dilated vascular compartment owing to α-blockade and to minimize the severe hypotension that can result when the tumor is removed surgically *(104)*. The procedure should only be undertaken in centers with considerable experience. Perioperatively, there is a need for adequate rapid acting antihypertensive agents such as sodium nitroprusside, phentolamine with or without labetalol, as well as substantial quantities of blood, plasma, and saline to compensate for the sudden expansion of the vascular volume when the tumor is removed (or its venous drainage occluded) in the presence of massive α-blockade *(104,117)*. Postoperatively, care is required to manage the fluid balance as the α-blockers wear off and the vasculature constricts; many children run the risk of acute volume overload at this stage and need aggressive diuresis.

After removal of a pheochromocytoma or paraganglioma, the patient needs long-term monitoring to detect the emergence of subsequent lesions. Usually, regular BP checks suffice, but for completeness and security regular catecholamine measurements might be appropriate for a year or two. The risk of malignancy with childhood catecholamine producing tumors is low but it can and does occur occasionally *(104)*.

## CORTICOSTEROID EXCESS STATES

Corticosteroid excess from endogenous production of glucocorticoids or mineralocorticoids is a rare cause of HTN in children. In contrast, exogenous administration of glucocorticoids often leads to an increased BP.

Cushing's syndrome caused by adrenal tumor or Cushing's disease caused by hypersecretion of adrenocorticotropic hormone (ACTH) are uncommon *(118)*. The cause of the HTN seen in these disorders is a combination of mineralocorticoid effect produced by cortisol, increased renin substrate, and, possibly, increased vascular responsiveness to vasoconstrictors *(119)*. Diagnosis is based on demonstrating excess cortisol and cortisol-metabolite excretion in urine, as well as evidence of increased plasma cortisol with loss of diurnal rhythm *(120)*. Dexamethasone suppression testing may distinguish between Cushing's syndrome and Cushing's disease with suppression of cortisol levels in the latter with high dosage. Some obese children have excess excretion of urinary 17-hydroxycorticoids, but these levels can be suppressed by a low dose dexamethasone suppression test, thus distinguishing these patients from those with frank hypercorticalism *(121)*.

Other investigative procedures might be indicated, including a corticotrophin-releasing hormone (CRH) stimulation test to distinguish between a pituitary-mediated Cushing's disease and an ectopic ACTH secretion state. Additionally, ultrasonographic, CT, and MRI studies of the abdomen with or without arteriography and venography may assist in making the correct diagnosis if an adrenal tumor is suspected. Cranial MRI and occasionally sampling of petrosal blood may be necessary for localizing a pituitary adenoma.

Treatment of adrenal tumor is surgical, but preoperatively there may be a need to reduce hypercorticism with the adrenocorticolytic drug o,pDDD, or consideration given to other appropriate therapy for adrenal carcinoma, if present *(122)*. Removal of a pituitary adenoma can cure Cushing's disease *(123)*, but alternative approaches include bilateral adrenalectomy *(124)* or treatment with drugs such as cyproheptadine *(125)*.

Congenital adrenal hyperplasia is sometimes associated with HTN. 11-β-hydroxylase and 17-α-hydroxylase deficiencies, in particular, fit into this category *(126,127)*. In 11-β-hydroxylase, DOC (deoxycorticosterone) and compound S (11-deoxycortisol) accumulate, and in 17-α-hydroxylase deficiency 17-desoxysteroids accumulate. Patients with 11-β-hydroxylase deficiency are virilized, but this is not a feature of 17-α-hydroxylase deficiency.

Twenty-four hour steroid determinations, plasma levels of DOC and compound S, as well as the finding of a suppressed plasma renin are helpful diagnostically. Treatment consists of replacing cortisol, which suppresses ACTH and hence reduces mineralocorticoid secretion.

Both of these disorders are recessively inherited; the genes have been identified *(128)* and are covered in more detail in the section on monogenic hypertensive disorders later in this volume.

Isolated overproduction of aldosterone (Conn's syndrome) is extremely unusual in childhood *(129)*. It may be caused by adrenal hyperplasia or tumor. Hyperplasia is the more common cause of Conn's syndrome. Investigation reveals evidence of potassium wasting in a sodium replete state with a high plasma aldosterone and a suppressed plasma renin. The distinction between tumor and bilateral adrenal hyperplasia is complicated, and probably beyond the scope of this volume. However, tests include imaging studies such as ultrasound, CT and MRI scanning, adrenal venous aldosterone and cortisol sampling, plus a number of functional studies (including aldosterone responses to posture, saline infusion, and ACE inhibition). Medical treatment with spironolactone is indicated for hyperplasia and surgery for tumors.

Other forms of HTN associated with mineralocorticoid excess, or what appears to be mineralocorticoid excess, include glucocorticoid-remediable aldosteronism and apparent mineralocorticoid excess (AME). Both these are monogenic forms of HTN caused by specific genetic defects *(130,131)*.

The major differential diagnosis for AME is Liddle's syndrome, also a cause of hypokalemic low renin HTN owing to inherited defects of the sodium channel *(132)*. This, and the other forms associated with mineralocorticoid excess, are covered in the monogenic hypertensive section of this book and will not be described in further detail here.

Finally, Gordon's syndrome, another low-renin hypertensive disorder which is unusually associated with hyperkalemic hyperchloremic acidosis and normal renal function, is likely to be caused by a single gene defect *(133)* and will be described further in the monogenic HTN section.

## REFERENCES

1. Leumann EP. Blood pressure and hypertension in childhood and adolescence. Ergsb Inn Med Kinderheilk 1979;43:109–183.
2. Londe S. Causes of hypertension in the young. Pediatr Clin North Am 1978;25:55–58.
3. Cobanoglu A, Teply TF, Grunkemeir GL. Coarctation of the aorta in patients younger than 3 months. J Thorac Cardiovasc Surg 1985;89:128–135.
4. Bagby SP. Dissection of pathogenetic factors in coarctation hypertension. In: Loggie JMH, Horan MJ, Gruskin AB, eds. NHLBI Workshop on Juvenile Hypertension. New York: Biomedical Information Corporation, 1984;253–266.
5. Yagi S, Kramsch DM, Madoff IM, Hollander W. Plasma renin activity in hypertension associated with coarctation of the aorta. Am J Physiol 1968;215:605–610.
6. Matsuyama K, Sonoda E, Nakao K, Horio Y, Yasue H. Baroceptor reflex in a patient with coarctation. Clin Cardiol 1987;10:535–536.
7. Flynn MT, Ekstrom L, De Arce M, Costigan C, Hoey HM. Prevalence of renal malformations in Turner syndrome. Pediatr Nephrol 1996;10:498–500.
8. Sumboonanonda A, Robinson BL, Gedroyc WMW, Saxton HM, Reidy JF, Haycock GB. Middle aortic syndrome: clinical and radiological findings. Arch Dis Child 1992;67:501–505.
9. Deal JE, Snell ME, Barratt TM, Dillon MJ. Renovascular disease in childhood. J Pediatr 1992;121:378–384.
10. O'Neill JA, Berkowitz H, Fellows KJ, Harmon CM. Mid aortic syndromes and hypertension in childhood. J Pediatr Surg 1995;30:164–171.

11. Wiggelinkhuizen J, Cremin BJ. Takayasu arteritis and renovascular hypertension in childhood. Pediatrics 1978;62:209–217.
12. Wiltse HE, Goldbloom RB, Antia AU, Otteson DE, Rowe RD, Cooke RE. Infantile hypercalcaemia syndrome in twins. N Engl J Med 1996;275:1157–1160.
13. Shaddy RE, Snider AR, Silverman NH, Lutin W. Pulsed Doppler findings in patients with coarctation of the aorta. Circulation 1986;73:82–88.
14. Boxer RA, La Corte MA, Singh S, et al. Nuclear magnetic resonance imaging in evaluation and follow up of children treated for coarctation of the aorta. J Am Coll Cardiol 1986;7:1095–1098.
15. Rocchini AP, Rosenthal A, Barger AC, Castaneda AR, Nadas AS. Pathogenesis of paradoxical hypertension after coarctation resection. Circulation 1976;54:382–387.
16. Leenen FHH, Balfe JA, Pelech AN, Barker GA, Balfe JW, Olley PM. Post operative hypertension after repair of coarctation of the aorta in children: protective effect of propranolol. Am Heart J 1987;5:1164–1173.
17. Wu JL, Leung MP, Karlberg J, Chiu C, Lee M, Mok CK. Surgical repair of coarctation of the aorta in neonates: factors affecting early mortality and recoarctation. Cardiovasc Surg 1995;3:573–578.
18. Kari JA, Donald AE, Vallance DT, et al. Physiology and biochemistry of endothelial function in children with chronic renal failure. Kidney Int 1997;52:468–472.
19. Broyer M, Guest G, Gagnadoux MF, Beurton D. Hypertension following renal transplantation in children. Pediatr Nephrol 1987;1:16–21.
20. Baluarte HJ, Gruskin AB, Ingelfinger JR, Stablein D, Tejani A. Analysis of hypertension in children post renal transplantation—a report of the North American Pediatric Renal Transplant Cooperative Study (NAPRTCS). Pediatr Nephrol 1994;8:570–573.
21. Still J L, Cottom D. Severe hypertension in childhood. Arch Dis Child 1967;42:34–39.
22. Gill DG, Mendes da Costa B, Cameron JS, Joseph MC, Ogg CS, Chantler C. Analysis of 100 children with severe and persistent hypertension. Arch Dis Child 1976;51:951–956.
23. Rahill WJ, Rubin MI. Hypertension in infantile polycystic renal disease. The importance of early recognition and treatment of severe HTN in polycystic renal disease. Clin Pediatr 1971;11:232–235.
24. Nash DA. Hypertension in polycystic kidney disease without renal failure. Arch Intern Med 1977;137:1571–1575.
25. Kaplan BS, Fay J, Shah V, Dillon MJ, Barratt TM. Autosomal recessive polycystic kidney disease. Pediatr Nephrol 1989;3:43–49.
26. Grunfeld B, Gimenez M, Liapchuc S, Mendilaharzu J, Gianantonio C. Systemic hypertension and plasma renin activity in children with the hemolytic-uremic syndrome. Int J Pediatr Nephrol 1982;3:211–214.
27. Wallace DMH, Rothwell DL, Williams DI. Long term follow up of surgically treated vesico ureteric reflux. Br J Urol 1978;50:479–484.
28. Goonasekera CDA, Shah V, Wade AM, Barratt TM, Dillon MJ. 15-year follow-up of renin and blood pressure in reflux nephropathy. Lancet 1996;347:640–643.
29. Zhang Y, Bailey RR. A long term follow up of adults with reflux nephropathy. NZ Med J 1995;108:142–144.
30. Savage JM, Dillon MJ, Shah V, Barratt TM, Williams DI. Renin and blood pressure in children with renal scarring and vesico ureteric reflux. Lancet 1978;ii:441–444.
31. Savage JM, Koh CT, Shah V, Barratt TM, Dillon MJ. Five year prospective study of plasma renin activity and blood pressure in patients with long standing reflux nephropathy. Arch Dis Child 1987;62:678–682.
32. Jardim H, Shah V, Savage JM, Barratt TM, Dillon MJ. Prediction of blood pressure from plasma renin activity in reflux nephropathy. Arch Dis Child 1991;66:1213–1216.
33. Taverner D, Fletcher A, Russel GI, Bing RF, Jackson J, Swales JD, Thurston H. Chemical renal medullectomy: effect on blood pressure in normal rats. J Hypertens 1983;1(Suppl 2):43–45.
34. Goonasekera CDA, Rees DD, Woolard P, Freud A, Shah V, Dillon MJ. Nitric oxide synthase inhibitors and hypertension in children and adolescents. J Hypertens 1997;15:901–909.
35. Goonasekera CDA, Jardim H, Shah V, Dillon MJ. Abnormalities of erythrocyte sodium transport in reflux nephropathy. J Hum Hypertens 1996;10:473–476.
36. Heale WF. Hypertension and reflux nephropathy. Aust Paediatr J 1997;13:56.
37. Merrick MV, Uttley WS, Wild SR. The detection of pyelonephritic scarring in children with radioisotope imaging. Brit J Radiol 1980;53:544–556.
38. Dillon MJ, Smellie JM. Peripheral plasma renin activity, hypertension and renal scarring in children. In: Hodson CJ, Heptinstall RH, Winberg J, eds. Contributions to Nephrology. Reflux Nephropathy Update: 1983. Basel: Karger, 1984; 68–80.

39. Dillon MJ, Shah V, Barratt TM. Renal vein renin measurements in children with hypertension. Brit Med J 1978;11:168–170.
40. Goonasekera CDA, Shah V, Wade AM, Dillon MJ. The usefulness of renal vein renin studies in hypertensive children: a 25 year experience. Pediatr Nephrol 2002;17:943–949.
41. Jacobson SH, Eklof O, Lins LE, Wikstad I, Winberg J. Long term prognosis of post infectious scarring in relation to radiological findings in childhood—a 27 year follow up. Pediatr Nephrol 1992;6:19–24.
42. Watson AR, Balfe JW, Hardy BW. Renovascular hypertension in childhood: a changing perspective in management. J Pediatr 1985;106:366–378.
43. Berglund G, Andersson O, Wilhelmson L. Prevalence of primary and secondary hypertension: studies in a random population sample. Br Med J 1976;2:554–556.
44. Loirat C, Pillion G, Blum C. Hypertension in children: present data and problems. Adv. Nephrol 1982;11:65–98.
45. Fry WJ, Ernst CB, Stanley JC, Brinnk B. Renovascular hypertension in the pediatric patient. Arch Surg 1973;107:692–698.
46. Stanley JC. Surgical intervention in pediatric renovascular hypertension. Child Nephrol Urol 1992;12: 167–176.
47. Leadbetter WF, Burkland CE. Hypertension in unilateral renal disease. J Urol 1938;39:611–626.
48. Lawson JB, Boerth R, Foster JH, Dean RH. Diagnosis and management of renovascular hypertension in children. Arch Surg 1977;122:1307–1316.
49. Stanley P, Gyepes MT, Olsen DL, Gates FG. Renovascular hypertension in children and adolescents. Radiology 1978;129:123–131.
50. Makkar SP, Moorthy B. Fibromuscular dysplasia of renal arteries. An important cause of renovascular hypertension in children. J Pediatr 1979;95:940–945.
51. Wise KL, McCann RL, Dunnick NR, Paulson DF. Renovascular hypertension. J Urol 1988;140:911–924.
52. Wells TG, Belsha CW. Pediatric renovascular hypertension. Curr Opinion Ped 1996;8:128–134.
53. Halpern M, Currarino G. Vascular lesions causing hypertension in neurofibromatosis. N Engl J Med 1965;273:248–252.
54. Mena E, Bookstein JJ, Holt JF, Fry WJ. Neurofibromatosis and renovascular hypertension in children. Am J Roentgenol 1973;118:39–45.
55. Green JF, Fitzwater JE, Burgess J. Arterial lesions associated with neurofibromatosis. Am J Clin Pathol 1974;62:481–487.
56. Muller-Wiefel DE. Renovascular hypertension bei neurofibromatose von Recklinghausen. Monatsschr Kinderheilk 1978;126:113–118.
57. Fossalli E , Signorini E, Intermite RC, et al. Renovascular disease and hypertension in children with neurofibromatosis. Pediatr Nephrol 2000;14:806–810.
58. Kaufmann JJ, Goodwin WE, Waisman J, Gyepes MT. Renovascular hypertension in children. Report of seven cases treated surgically including two cases of renal auto transplantation. Am J Surg 1972;124:149–157.
59. Loughridge LW. Renal abnormalities in the Marfan syndrome. Quart J Med 1959;28:531–544.
60. Menser MA, Dorman DC, Reye RDK, Reid RR. Renal artery stenosis in the rubella syndrome. Lancet 1966;i:790–797.
61. Proesmans W. Syndrome de Kleppel-Trenaunay avec hypertension arterielle et insuffisance renale chronique. Ann Pediatr 1982;29:671–674.
62. Leenhardt A, Guillevin L, Bletry O, Godean P. Arterial hypertension in periarteritis nodosa. 37 case reports. Arch Mal Coeur Vas 1984;77:197–202.
63. Adelman RD. Neonatal hypertension. Pediatr Clin North Am 1978;25:99–110.
64. O'Malley B, D'Angio GJ, Vawter GF. Late effects of roentgen therapy given in infancy. Am J Roentgenol 1963;89:1067–1074.
65. Koskimies O. Arterial hypertension developing 10 years after radiotherapy for Wilms' tumour. Brit Med J 1988;285:996–998.
66. Alvestrand A, Bergstroem J, Wehle B. Phaeochromocytoma and renovascular hypertension. A case report and review of the literature. Acta Med Scand 1977;202:231–236.
67. Palmer JM, Connelly JE. Intrarenal arterio venous fistula: surgical excision under selective renal hypothermia with kidney survival. J Urol 1966;96:599–605.
68. Daman Willems CD, Salisbury DM, Lumley JSP, Dillon MJ. Brain revascularisation in hypertension. Arch Dis Child 1985;60:1177–1179.

69. Daniels SR, Loggie JMH, McEnery PT, Towbin RB. Clinical spectrum of intrinsic renovascular hypertension in children. Pediatrics 1986;80:698–704.
70. Dillon MJ. Investigation and management of hypertensive children. Pediatr Nephrol 1987;1:59–68.
71. Rosendahl W, Grunert D, Schoning M. Duplex sonography of renal arteries as a diagnostic tool in hypertensive children. Eur J Pediatr 1994;153:588–593.
72. Brun P, Kchouk H, Mouchet B. Value of Doppler ultrasound for the diagnosis of renal artery stenosis in children. Pediatr Nephrol 1997;11:27–30.
73. Riehl J, Schmitt H, Bongartz D, Bergmann D, Sieberth HG. Renal artery stenosis: evaluation with color duplex ultra-sonography. Nephrol Dial Transplant 1997;12:1608–1614.
74. Rosen PR, Treves S, Ingelfinger JR. Hypertension in children. Increased efficacy of Tc-99 m succinate in screening for renal disease. Am J Dis Child 1985;139:173–177.
75. Taylor A, Nally J, Aurell M, et al. Consensus report on ACE inhibitor renography for detecting hypertension. J Nucl Med 1996;37:1876–1882.
76. Chandar JJ, Sfakianakis GN, Zilleruelo GE, et al. ACE inhibition scintigraphy in the management of hypertension in children. Pediatr Nephrol 1999;13:493–500.
77. Ng CS, de Bruyn R, Gordon I. Investigation of renovascular hypertension in children: the accuracy of radisotopes in detecting renovascular disease. Nucl Med Commun 1997;18:1017–1028.
78. Dillon MJ. The diagnosis of renovascular disease. Pediatr Nephrol 1997;11:366–372.
79. Shahdadpuri J, Frank R, Gauthier BG, Siegel DN, Trachtman H. Yield of renal arteriography in the evaluation of pediatric hypertension. Pediatr Nephrol 2000;14:816–819.
80. Maier SE, Scheidegger MB, Liu K, Schneider E, Bollinger A, Boesiger P. Renal artery velocity mapping with MR imaging. J Magn Reson Imaging 1995;5:669–676.
81. Olbricht CJ, Galanski M, Chavan A, Prokop M. Spiral CT angiography: can we forget about arteriography to diagnose renal artery stenosis? Nephrol Dial Transplant 1996;11:1227–1231.
82. Dillon MJ, Deal JE. Renovascular hypertension in children. In: Novick A, Scoble J, Hamilton G, eds. Renal Vascular Disease. London: WB Saunders, 1996;235–244.
83. Dillon MJ. Therapeutic strategies in renovascular hypertension. Baillières Clinical Paediatrics 1997;5:675–686.
84. Sos TA, Seddekni S. Pediatric renovascular hypertension: the role of renal angioplasty. Dialog Ped Urol 1985;8:7–9.
85. Chevalier RL, Tegtmeyer CJ, Gomez RA. Percutaneous transluminal angioplasty for renovascular hypertension in children. Pediatr Nephrol 1987;1:89–98.
86. Norling LL, Chevalier RL, Gomez RA, Tegtmeyer CJ. Use of interventional radiology for hypertension due to renal artery stenosis in children. Child Nephrol Urol 1992;12:162–166.
87. Tegtmeyer CJ, Matsumoto AH, Angle JF. Percutaneous transluminal angioplasty in fibrous dysplasia in children. In: Novick A, Scoble J, Hamilton G, eds. Renal Vascular Disease. London: WB Saunders, 1996; 363–383.
88. Tyagi S, Kaul UA, Satsangi DK, Arora R. Percutaneous transluminal angioplasty for renovascular hypertension in children: Initial and long term results. Pediatrics 1997;99:44–49.
89. Davies R, Barkovics M, Gordon I, Shah V, Chan M, Dillon MJ. Percutaneous transluminal angioplasty for renovascular hypertension in children. Pediatr Nephrol 1999;13:C53.
90. Dorros G, Prince C, Mathiak L. Stenting of a renal artery stenosis achieves better relief of the obstructive lesion than balloon angioplasty. Cath Cardiovasc Diagn 1993;29:191–198.
91. Trost D, Sos TA. Endovascular Stents. In: Novick A, Scoble J, Hamilton G, eds. Renal Vascular Disease. London: WB Saunders, 1996;363–383.
92. Isles CG, Robertson S, Hill D. Management of renovascular disease: a review of renal artery stenting in ten studies. Quart J Med 1999;92:159–167.
93. Stoney RJ, Cooke PA, Stoney ST. Surgical treatment of renovascular hypertension in children. J Pediatr Surg 1975;10:631–639.
94. Novick AC, Straffon RA, Stewart BH, Benjamin S. Surgical treatment of renovascular hypertension in the pediatric patient. J Urol 1978;119:794–805.
95. Berkowitz HD, O'Neill JA. Renovascular hypertension in children. Surgical repair with special reference to the use of reinforced grafts. J Vasc Surg 1989;9:46–55.
96. Sinaiko A, Najarian J, Michael AF, Mirkin BL. Renal auto transplantation in the treatment of bilateral renal artery stenosis. Relief of hypertension in an eight year old boy. J Pediatr 1973;83:409–413.

97. Stanley JC, Zelenock GB, Messina LM, Wakefield TW. Pediatric renovascular hypertension: a thirty year experience of operative treatment. J Vasc Surg 1995;21:212–226.
98. Steinbrecher HA, Malone PS. Wilms' tumour and hypertension: incidence and outcome. Br J Urol 1995;76: 241–243.
99. Robertson PW, Klidjian A, Harding LK, Walters G, Lee MR, Robb-Smith AH. Hypertension due to a renin-secreting tumour. Am J Med 1967;43:963–976.
100. Warshaw BL, Anand SK, Olsen DL, Gruskin CM, Heuser ET, Liebermann E. Hypertension secondary to a renin producing juxta glomerular cell tumour. J Pediatr 1979;94:247–250.
101. Haab F, Duclos JM, Guyenne T, Plouin PF, Corvol P. Renin secreting tumours: diagnosis, conservative surgical approach and long term results. J Urol 1995;153:1781–1784.
102. Hirose M, Arakawa K, Kikuchi M, Kawasaki T, Omoto T. Primary reninism with renal hamartomatous alteration. JAMA 1974;230:1288–1292.
103. Stackpole RH, Melicow MM, Uson AC. Pheochromocytoma in children. J Pediatr 1963;63:315–330.
104. Deal JE, Sever PS, Barratt TM, Dillon MJ. Phaechromocytoma—investigation and management of 10 cases. Arch Dis Child 1990;65:269–274.
105. Glushien AS, Mansuy MM, Littman DS. Pheochromocytoma: its relationships to neurocutaneous syndromes. Am J Med 1953;14:318–327.
106. Chapman RC, Kemp VA, Taliaferro I. Pheochromocytoma associated with multiple neurofibromatosis and intracranial hemangioma. Am J Med 1959;26:883–890.
107. Sever PS, Roberts JC, Snell ME. Phaeochromocytoma. Clin Endocrinol Metab 1980;9:543–568.
108. Sipple JH. The association of pheochromocytoma with carcinoma of the thyroid gland. Am J Med 1961;31:163–166.
109. Keiser HR, Beaven MA, Doppman J, Wells S, Buja LM. Sipple's syndrome, medullary thyroid carcinoma, pheochromocytoma and parathyroid disease. Studies in a large family. NIH conference. Ann Intern Med 1973;78:561–579.
110. Lips KJ, Van der Sluys Veer L, Struyvanberg A, et al. Bilateral occurrence of pheochromocytoma in patients with multiple endocrine neoplasia syndrome Type 2A (Sipple's syndrome). Am J Med 1981;70:1051–1060.
111. Koch CA, Vortmeyer AO, Huang SC, Alesci S, Zhuang Z, Pacak K. Genetic aspects of pheochromocytoma. Endocr Regul 2001;35:43–52.
112. Bravo EL, Gifford RW. Pheochromocytoma: diagnosis, evaluation and management. N Engl J Med 1984;311:1298–1303.
113. Shapiro B, Copp JE, Sisson JC, Eyre PL, Wallis J, Beierwaltes WH. Iodine-131 meta iodobenzylguanidine for the locating of suspected pheochromocytoma: experience in 400 cases. J Nucl Med 1985;26:576–585.
114. Shulkin B, Shapiro B, Francis IR, Dorr R, Shen SW, Sisson JC. Primary extra-adrenal pheochromocytoma: positive I-123 MIBG imaging with negative I-131 MIBG imaging. Clin Nucl Med 1986;11:851–854.
115. Van der Harst E, de Herder WW, Bruining HA, et al. 123I metaiodobenzylguanidine and III In octreotide uptake in benign and malignant pheochromocytomas. J Clin Endocrinol Metab 2001;86:685–693.
116. Schmedtje JF, Sax S, Pool JL, Goldfarb RA, Nelson EB. Localization of ectopic pheochromocytoma by magnetic resonance imaging. Am J Med 1987;83:770–772.
117. Ellis D, Gartner JC. The intraoperative medical management of childhood pheochromocytoma. J Pediatr Surg 1980;15:655–659.
118. Loriden L, Senior E. Cushing's syndrome in infancy. J Pediatr 1969;75:349–359.
119. Krakoff LR, Garbowit D. Hypertension of Cushing's syndrome. In: Biglieri EG, Melby JC eds. Endocrine hypertension. New York: Raven, 1990;113–123.
120. Margioris AN, Chrousos GP. Cushing's syndrome: diagnostic evaluation. In: Biglieri EG, Melby JC, eds. Endocrine hypertension. New York: Raven, 1990:99–111.
121. Migeon CJ, Green OC, Eckert JP. Study of adrenocortical function in obesity. Metabolism 1963;12:718–739.
122. Schteingart DE. Cushing's syndrome. Endocrinol Clin North Am 1989;18:311–338.
123. Styne DM, Grumbach MM, Kaplan SL, Wilson CB, Conte FA. Treatment of Cushing's disease in childhood and adolescence by transphenoidal microadenectomy. N Engl J Med 1984;310:889–893.
124. McArthur RG, Hayles AB, Salassa RM. Childhood Cushing's disease: results of bilateral adrenalectomy. J Pediatr 1979;95:214–219.
125. Wiesen M, Ross F, Krieger DT. Prolonged remission in a case of Cushing's disease following cessation of cyproheptadine therapy. Acta Endocrinol 1983;102:436–438.

126. De Santo NG, Anastasio P, Spitali L, et al. Endocrine-metabolic hypertension. Child Nephrol Urol 1992;12: 147–153.
127. New MI, Levine LS. Adreno cortical hypertension. Pediatr Clin North Am 1978;25:67–81.
128. Dacon-Voutetakis C, Maniati-Christidi M, Dracopoulou-Vabouli M. Genetic aspects of congenital adrenal hyperplasia. J Pediatr Endocrinol Metal 2001;14(Suppl 5):1303–1308.
129. Rauh W, Oberfeld SF. The adrenal cortex in childhood hypertension. Paediatr Adolesc Endocrinol 1984;13:210–230.
130. Jackson RV, Lafferty A, Torpy DJ, Stratakis C. New genetic insights in familial hyperaldosteronism. Ann NY Acad Sci 2002;970:77–88.
131. Whorwood CB, Stewart PM. Human hypertension caused by mutations in the 11 beta-hydnoxy steroid dehydrogenase gene: a molecular analysis of apparent mineralocorticoid excess. J Hypertens Suppl 1996;14: S19–S24.
132. Hansson JH, Nelson-Williams C, Suzuki K, et al. Hypertension caused by a truncated epithelial sodium channel gamma sub unit: genetic heterogeneity in Liddle's syndrome. Nat Genet 1995;11:76–82.
133. Archard JM, Disse-Nicodeme S, Fiquet-Kempf B, Jeunemaitre X. Phenotypic and genetic heterogeneity of familial hyperkalaemic hypertension (Gordon syndrome). Clin Exp Pharmacol Physiol 2001;28:1048–1052.

# 10 Essential Hypertension in Children

*Tej K. Mattoo,* MD, DCH, FRCP (UK)
*and Alan B. Gruskin,*[*] MD

*CONTENTS*



## INTRODUCTION

Pickering stated, "The relationship between arterial pressure and mortality is quantitative, the higher the pressure the worse the prognosis."*(1)* Hypertension (HTN) detection and follow up programs have inferred that mild HTN is also associated with an increased mortality *(2)*. Essential HTN, which affects almost 20% of adults and is a major public health issue, is increasingly thought to have its antecedents during childhood. It is important that those providing care to children approach the issue of HTN both as a societal challenge as well as a disease affecting discrete individuals. This chapter provides a general overview of the significant progress made over the past half century in understanding the many issues concerning essential HTN, including the diagnosis, risk factors involved, pathogenesis, etiology, and treatment, as well as the tracking of blood pressure (BP).

## DEFINITIONS AND TECHNIQUES

HTN is defined by an arbitrary division in the continuum of BP, concurrent with an increased risk of recognizable morbidity and mortality that becomes increasingly prevalent as BP increases. A pragmatic definition of HTN would be the level of systolic BP and/or diastolic BP

*Deceased

From: *Clinical Hypertension and Vascular Disease: Pediatric Hypertension*
Edited by: R. J. Portman, J. M. Sorof, and J. R. Ingelfinger © Humana Press Inc., Totowa, NJ

Table 1
Criteria to Use in Diagnosing Essential HTN in Children

*Primary criteria*
* An average of two to three readings of systolic BP and/or diastolic BP exceeding the 95th percentile for age, gender and height repeated three times over a 2–3 mo period and/or
* Ambulatory blood pressure measurements over a 24-h period that exceed the 95th percentile for age matched controls and/or a failure to find a nocturnal dip
* Unable to identify a known secondary cause of HTN

*Supportive criteria*
* Abnormal response to mental stress
* Idiopathic hypertension associated with high, normal, or low PRA
* Evidence of end-organ effect; fundoscopic changes, cardiac hypertrophy/enlargement by electrocardiogram and/or echocardiogram
* Family history of HTN

above which recognizable morbidity occurs. As of this writing, there are no data that adequately define HTN in children.

The ideal BP for any individual can be viewed as the pressure that is needed to propel blood from the bottom of the left ventricle to the top of the brain. Height should be taken into account when interpreting BP values. BP in shorter people ought to be lower than in taller people. A few studies have documented that BP remains constant throughout childhood when corrected for the height between the tip of the heart and the top of the skull.

HTN can manifest as an isolated elevation in systolic BP, diastolic BP, or both. In adults, HTN is generally defined as BP greater than 140/90 mmHg. In children, it is defined as BP exceeding the 95th percentile for age, gender, and height. Not everyone agrees with the definition because only the first BP reading was used to define normal values in the report of the 1987 Second Task Force on Blood Pressure in Children and Adolescents, which included more than 70,000 black, Latino, and white children from nine sources in the United States *(3)*. Borderline HTN (prehypertension) is defined as BP between the 90th and 95th percentile, and severe HTN is defined by systolic BP and/or diastolic BP exceeding the 99th percentile for age, sex, and height. Criteria for making a diagnosis of essential HTN are summarized in Table 1. It is currently recommended that two or more BP readings be averaged at each visit. Abnormally high BP readings should be classified as labile or fixed based on follow up studies. A diagnosis of persistent HTN is made when elevated values are documented on three visits over a period of 4-8 wk. The most widely used normograms for BP in children are those reported by the Second Task Force on Blood Pressure in Children and Adolescents. It is noteworthy that a comparison of normal BP readings reported by 10 different investigators reveals that the highest and lowest (50th and 95th) percentile values for boys differ by 20 mmHg *(4)*. Confounding factors include the cuff size, number of measure-ments made, type of instruments used, patient position (supine or sitting) and the choice of sound (Korotkoff [K]4 vs K5) used for defining diastolic BP.

The bladder of the BP cuff should completely encircle the arm. Another important issue in children is that of cuff size width. It is generally recommended that the bladder width be about two-thirds to three-fourths of the olecranon-acromion distance *(3)*.

Too wide a cuff may give inappropriately low readings, whereas too narrow a cuff overestimates it. Working groups including the American Heart Association, the National High Blood Pressure Education Program, and the 1996 Working Group on Childhood Hypertension *(4)* recommend that the cuff width equal 40% of the circumference of the upper arm. Two recent pediatric studies have documented inconsistencies in criteria on cuff selection with anatomical measurements of arm size in children *(5)* and differences in actual BP measurements obtained in children intra-arterially when compared to those obtained with the recommended size bladder width cuffs. Using the 40% upper arm criterion gave comparable readings for systolic BP but not for diastolic BP *(6)*. When a cuff two-thirds to three-fourths of the upper arm length was used, significantly lower values for both systolic BP and diastolic BP were found.

BP should be taken with the arm cuff at the level of the heart. Since anxiety acutely raises pulse rate and BP, the most reproducible readings are obtained when the pulse rate is both steady and within the normal range. Repeating the pulse rate a number of times until the rate is normal and/or reproducible avoids obtaining falsely elevated readings. It is recommended that the first and fifth Korotkoff sounds (onset and disappearance of a tapping sound) be recorded. Despite the fact that the mercury sphygmomanometer is the most accurate instrument for measuring BP, its future availability may be restricted because of its potential for introducing mercury poisoning in patients. Automated oscillometric devices, on the other hand, require maintenance and repeated calibration procedures that are rarely followed in routine clinical settings.

Automated ambulatory blood pressure monitoring (ABPM) has been used increasingly over the past decade as a technique to diagnose HTN, to define diurnal variability of BP measurements in normal and hypertensive populations (including children) *(7)*, and to evaluate therapy. Normally, BP readings follow a circadian pattern, highest late in the day and lowest during nighttime sleeping hours. Typically, readings using oscillometric methodology are taken every 20 min during awake and every 30–60 min during sleep periods. The percentage of BP readings above the 95th percentile (BP load), peak values, sleep values, pulse rate, and nocturnal dipping, (e.g., a fall in systolic BP of < 10%) are believed to better represent the systemic arterial pressure that individuals confront over the course of their routine activities including work, play, emotional stress, etc. Nocturnal dipping is believed to reflect decreased sympathetic nervous system activity. BP load and nondipping have been associated with end organ changes. Problems associated with ABPM include inconsistent readings that range from about 15% to 25% of cuff size, limited but increasing data on normal values *(8,9)*, correlation with readings obtained with other instruments, the need to hold the arm steady during BP reading, problems with using equipment on young children, and stress associated with wearing the instrument *(10)*.

Studies which used ABPM have shown that hypertensive adolescents are less likely to display nocturnal dipping, more likely to be African-Americans, and have lower excretory rates of catecholamines and heightened $\alpha$- and $\beta$-adrenergic responses *(11,12)*. Sleep systolic BP in adolescents correlates with left ventricular (LV) mass *(13)*.

Even though much of the ABPM methodology has been automated, it remains time consuming and expensive. Additional studies over the next decade should define its role and value. Also, home BP measurements are used increasingly for diagnostic and therapeutic purposes in children. Yet, standards for the taking and interpretation of home BP vary considerably *(14)*. The use of ABPM offers standardization.

There are no agreed-upon criteria for defining the severity of increases in BP in children as an indicator of the rapidity with which diagnosis and therapy ought to be pursued. Increases in BP may be defined as mild, moderate, severe, and an impending hypertensive crisis when

Table 2
The Basic Blood Pressure Formula and Its Physiologic Transformation to HTN

1. Pressure equals flow times resistance.
2. BP = volume times resistance.
3. BP = CO times total peripheral resistance.
4. BP = flow (preload + contractility) × resistance (arteriolar functional contraction + vessel anatomical changes), e.g., BP = Flow × Resistance
5. HTN = a net increase in CO and/or increased peripheral resistance.

diastolic BP levels in children exceed the 95th percentile by up to 15%, 30%, 45% and greater than 45% respectively. These incremental increases were derived from recommendations made in adult populations.

## PATHOGENESIS OF HYPERTENSION

Because BP readings are the result of a complex interaction of many factors, it is not surprising that many different mechanisms play a role in essential HTN. An overview of the many steps involved in the generation and persistent phases of HTN (Tables 2 and 3) serves as a basis upon which risk factors, clinical evaluation, and treatment of essential HTN in children are better understood. The physiologic transformation of the basic pressure formula states that the observed BP equals cardiac output (CO) (preload volume times rate) times total peripheral resistance (TPR) (vasoconstriction). HTN occurs when the sum of CO and TPR increases. Each parameter, in turn, is influenced by a large number of factors, some of which are capable of increasing or decreasing the relative contribution of volume and/or vasoconstrictor components of the BP formula.

The factors involved in increasing BP during the generation and maintenance phases of essential HTN are often different. In one form of essential HTN, the increase in CO during its early stages has been attributed to a hyperkinetic circulation characterized by increased heart rate (HR), cardiac index, and increased forearm blood flow secondary to increases in sympathetic tone and cardiac contractility *(15)*. Fixed persistent essential HTN is characterized by an increase in TPR and a return to a normal CO.

A large number of individuals with early HTN have been observed to have increased left ventricular (LV) mass, as have normotensive offspring of hypertensive parents. These observations raise the possibility that repeated neural stimulation and upregulation of cardiac receptors may be the primary events in the onset of essential HTN *(16)*. Some adolescents with labile HTN have hyperkinetic circulation. Others have increased peripheral resistance and a normal cardiac output (CO) *(17)*.

The observed changes, from that of an increased to normal CO, and an increased TPR over time, enable a constant blood flow to organs in experimental animals and humans. There is controversy over which of two mechanisms is primarily involved *(18)*. The first is auto regulation, an intrinsic feature of vasculature characterized by increased flow-induced vasoconstriction. The second involves structural changes, hypertrophy, and eventually fibrosis. These mechanisms may operate alone or together. The presence of functional vs irreversible structural changes helps explain the ease of response to therapy and the potential reversibility of the hypertensive process aggravated by obesity, stress, and/or excessive salt intake.

Abundant evidence exists to support a major role for sodium intake in the etiology of essential HTN (Table 4). A significant fraction of the adult population is salt-sensitive. BP changes

**Table 3**
**Factors Involved in the Generation and/or Persistence of HTN**

*Cardiac output*
Preload
Increased fluid volume
* Renal Sodium Retention: genetic factors, decreased glomerular filtration surface, and renin-aldosterone effect
* Excess Sodium Intake
Volume redistribution
* Sympathetic nervous system overactivity: genetic factors, stress (personal, environmental), and renin angiotensin excess
Contractility
* Sympathetic nervous system overactivity, and genetic factors

*Total peripheral resistance*
Functional vasoconstriction
* Renin angiotensin excess, sympathetic nervous system overactivity, genetic influence on cell membrane function, and endothelins
Structural constriction
* Renin angiotensin excess, sympathetic nervous system overactivity, endothelins, hyperinsulinemia

correlate with an increase or decrease in salt intake in such populations. Defects in the renal sodium handling resulting in increased sodium reabsorption cause HTN. In HTN, the normal relationship between BP and natriuresis is reset at a higher level. The defect leading to the right shift of the pressure natriuresis curve may be inherited. It can be corrected by transplanting a kidney from a normotensive to a hypertensive rat and vice versa *(19)*.

Genetic renal defects known to be involved in the abnormal sodium homeostasis in essential HTN include an increase in efferent arteriolar tone that in turn increases filtration fraction and sodium reabsorption, a congenital reduction in the number of nephrons and filtering surface *(20)*, nephron heterogeneity (a subpopulation of ischemic nephrons) *(21)*, and nonmodulation that involves abnormal adrenal and renal responses to angiotensin II (ANG II) infusions *(22)*.

Blood volume and total exchangeable sodium are generally normal or low in patients with essential HTN compared to to those with normal BP levels. These observations, however, do not rule out the possibility of a role for sodium and circulatory volume in the hypertensive process. When total blood volume is compared to diastolic BP, a negative correlation is found in normotensive but not in hypertensive adults. This indicates that hypertensive individuals have an increase in blood volume per unit of BP and/or resistance *(23)*. The reported increase in interstitial and intracellular volume in HTN is also supportive of an effect of increased intra-arterial pressure *(24)*.

Salts, other than sodium chloride, also influence BP regulation. Chloride, potassium, and calcium affect BP regulation independent of sodium. In animal models, sodium chloride, but not sodium bicarbonate, causes HTN and chloride without sodium fails to increase BP. In humans, NaCl increases BP more than nonchloride salts. Since most of the chloride ingested is in the form of sodium salts, the issue of chloride is not clinically relevant. An increase in sodium-to-potassium ratio (high sodium or low potassium intake) is associated with HTN. Changes in calcium and phosphorous metabolism may contribute to the HTN process *(25)*. Increased renal calcium excretion, either intrinsic or secondary to volume expansion and/or

Table 4
Role of Sodium in Essential HTN

*Experimental evidence*
* High salt intake increases renal vascular vasoconstriction, catecholamine release, and Na-K-ATPase inhibitor oubain, which in turn leads to increase in intracellular calcium and sodium.
* In salt-sensitive patients with essential HTN, BP varies directly with changes in sodium intake.
* Decreases in salt intake in people with borderline high BP may prevent the onset of HTN.
* The time and the quantity of sodium administration to rats genetically predisposed to HTN determine the onset and the level of BP.
* Similar mother and offspring BP response to sodium restriction supports a genetic predisposition to salt sensitivity.

*Epidemiologic evidence*
* Significant correlations between salt intake and BP have been demonstrated in large population studies.
* Primitive isolated societies which naturally ingest low sodium diets do not develop HTN, nor does BP rise with age.
* Primitive isolated societies increase their BP after being exposed to environments where excess sodium is ingested.

increased sodium excretion, can lead to a decreased serum level of ionized calcium and hyperparathyroidism, which in turn causes HTN presumably by altering vascular contractility in vascular smooth muscle.

A number of factors acting independently or collectively influence the degree of vasoconstriction (i.e., TPR). The renin-angiotensin system (RAS) influences both limbs of the BP formula. ANG II binding to angiotensin II Type 1 ($AT_1$) receptors in vascular smooth muscle increase contractility as well as sensitivity to catecholamines. Binding within the adrenal gland leads to increased aldosterone production, sodium retention by the kidney, and volume expansion. The $AT_2$ receptor, which is not involved in the vascular/smooth muscle contraction, is known to play a role in cell differentiation and hypertrophy.

Sympathetic nervous system activity can function as an initiator and as a secondary contributing factor. Stress and/or a primary catecholamine regulation defect in the brain may directly cause vascular vasoconstriction. Sympathetic nervous system stimuli from the vasomotor center activates efferent pathways that ultimately cause norepinephrine release at peripheral nerve endings and in turn stimulate adrenergic receptors. Circulating epinephrine derived from the adrenal medulla can stimulate norepinephrine release through stimulation of presynaptic β-2 receptors. The catecholamines can also enter nerve endings at the sympathetic cleft and function as a co-transmitter when sympathetic nerves are stimulated. Excessive circulating of catecholamines increases the BP response to a sodium load. Baroreceptor dysfunction, a reflex arc within the sympathetic nervous system, occurs in some patients with essential HTN. When BP is elevated, this arc, which is activated by either an increase in central venous pressure, or by an increase in BP, lowers BP by reducing sympathetic outflow from vasomotor centers and by increasing the vagal tone. The responsiveness of this system rapidly resets itself to a higher level when BP elevations persists and plays a role in the persistence phase of the hypertensive process *(26)*.

Stress of all types can increase BP. When compared to those with normal BP levels, greater increases in sympathetic nervous system and cardiovascular activity occur in offspring of hypertensive parents and in hypertensive individuals.

A number of factors influence arteriolar and capillary contractibility. Endothelial cell function influences the underlying smooth muscle contractility. Endothelial relaxation factor (nitric oxide, NO) release is modified by pressure, sheer force, circulating hormones, platelet function, hypercholesterolemia, and hyperlipidemia. A reduction in endothelial relaxation factors, and excessive exposure to prostaglandin $H_2$ and other endothelins, result in vasoconstriction.

A number of cell membrane abnormalities involving the transmembrane movement of ions, which in turn are thought to be related to cardiac hypertrophy and/or contractility, have been described in patients with essential HTN. Defects have been described in a number of different cell types including smooth muscle, red blood cells (RBCs), white blood cells (WBCs), and platelets. Genetic abnormalities described include defects in $Na^+$ $K^+$ pump and the $Na^+$ $K^+$ $Cl^-$ cotransport. These abnormalities affect the ability of cells to extrude excess $Na^+$. Defects in sodium channel leakage, $Na^+$ $Li^-$ countertransport, and the maximum rate of cotransport increase intracellular $Na^+$. Available evidence also supports a role for an acquired increase in a circulating inhibitor, perhaps ouabain, of the sodium pump $Na^+/K^+$ ATPase *(27)*. Patients with essential HTN are also known to have defects in calcium binding to cell membranes (destabilization of the membrane increases $Ca^{++}$ entry) and a reduced ability of the $Ca^{++}$ pump and $Na^{++}$ - $Ca^{++}$ exchanger to extrude intracellular accumulated $Ca^{++}$ *(28)*. The increased intracellular $Ca^{++}$ in turn increases vascular smooth muscle contraction. A 50% increase in vascular smooth muscle tone occurs when inhibition of the sodium pump increases intracellular $Na^+$ by 5% and $Na^{++}$ - $Ca^{++}$ exchange is inhibited *(29)*.

Hyperinsulinism associated with obesity increases renal sodium reabsorption and extracellular volume, which in turn leads to an increase in CO and HTN. It also stimulates sympathetic nervous system activity. Insulin resistance may contribute to HTN by impairing vasodilation, enhancing renal sodium and $H_2O$ retention, altering transmembrane electrolyte transport of $Na^+$ and $Ca^{++}$, increasing growth factor activity, increasing secretion of endothelin, and augmenting responses to ANG II. Whether insulin is a primary or secondary factor in the hypertensive process remains unclear.

Obesity may lead to HTN by mechanisms other than impaired glucose metabolism *(30)*. One interesting hypothesis is that, in obesity, fatty deposits within the kidney compress the renal parenchyma, stimulate tubular changes in sodium handling, and increase renin release. Another hypothesis is that this augmented tubuloglomerular feedback leads to renal ischemia, tubulointerstitial disease, and salt-sensitive HTN.

The major factors involved in the persistence of HTN are the persistence of the factors discussed above, HTN-induced changes in vessel compliance, endothelial dysfunction, vessel wall hypertrophy, remodeling (a normal amount of tissue surrounding a smaller lumen), and, ultimately, intimal fibrosis and athersosclerotic changes. Reversibility depends on the degree of permanent change that has occurred in response to the increase in BP.

A number of observations support the belief that many of the postulated mechanisms leading to HTN involve a fetal event that influences BP later in life. A syndrome of impaired genetic homeostasis has been suggested to explain the recent increase in cases with documented HTN *(31)*. The theory postulates that there is a mismatch between genes involved in the regulation of BP and the acculturated changes in the society in which we live. Low birth weight, increased placenta weight, and HTN *(32)* result in a phenotype that is insulin-resistant and hypertensive. This phenotype is perhaps associated with abnormalities in 11 β-hydroxysteroid dehydrogenese activity *(33)*. Synchronicity, a process by which growth spurts are associated with increases in BP, may be accelerated in genetically prone hypertensive individuals *(34)*. Allometric

Table 5
Percentage of 650 Adolescent Males Having High BP Readings

The second and third readings were obtained 1 and 12 mo after the initial reading. Adapted from ref. *155*.

| *BP Reading* | *Freshman* | *Sophomores* | *Juniors* | *Urban adolescents*[a] |
|---|---|---|---|---|
| First | 7.7 | 11.0 | 15.5 | 10.2 |
| Second | 3.4 | 4.7 | 5.8 | 3.9 |
| Third | 1.8 | 4.2 | 7.9 | 1.8 |

[a]Adapted from ref. *156*.

dysfunction, a process by which somatic and renal growth fail to match each other, might lead to HTN if environmental factors enable excessive nongenetically determined growth to occur *(35)*. The failure of renal vascular remodeling to occur during fetal and postnatal life might alter the expected decreases in the activity of RAS and/or sodium regulatory mechanisms. Premature telomere shortening, a process associated with normal aging, may lead to HTN *(36)*. Finally, perturbation in neural development of the sympathetic nervous system and/or cardiac $\beta_1$-receptors may predispose newborns to develop a hyperkinetic circulation and therefore, HTN *(37)*.

## PREDICTORS OF ESSENTIAL HYPERTENSION

### *Tracking*

Tracking refers to the pattern of repeated BP measurements over a period of time. The importance of tracking is its ability to identify children at risk for developing essential HTN later in life and to implement strategies that could prevent or slow down the onset of persistent HTN and its cardiovascular complications. Tracking, which is greater for systolic BP than diastolic BP, is less consistent in children prior to puberty than after puberty. Tracking shows a better correlation in children whose BP exceeds the 94th percentile, particularly in the presence of a family history for HTN, obesity, increased LV mass, or adolescent age *(38,39)*. A larger body size during adolescence is associated with increased BP. The earlier rise in BP correlates with an earlier onset of maturation *(40)*. Tracking studies have been used to document the persistence of elevated BP and the onset of HTN. Repeated measurements, over time, in adolescents involved in screening programs (Table 5) are often lower, and the prevalence of HTN decreases.

BP during adolescence is highly predictive of BP in adult life. In a group of 50 adolescents whose BPs were between the 90th and 95th percentile, 28 (56%) developed fixed essential HTN during the follow up period of 5–41 mo *(41)*. Those developing fixed essential HTN had a strong family history of HTN, were heavier, had higher resting pulse rates, and exhibited a greater response to mental stress. Data obtained during the Muscatine, Iowa longitudinal BP study conclusively demonstrated that essential HTN in young adults has much of its origin during the childhood years *(42)*. Follow up data in 1276 males and 2445 females aged 20–30 yr who had BPs taken one to three times between the ages of 7 and 18 yr revealed that there is a relationship among the frequency and level of both systolic and diastolic BP, Quetelet index, body size, and change in ponderosity (Table 6). An isolated systolic but not diastolic BP reading correlated with adult BP readings. Two or more high readings of both systolic and diastolic BP during childhood clearly correlated with adult BP readings.

Table 6
Relationship Between Childhood BP and Repeat Measurements as Young Adult Values (80% and 90% refer to the percentile BP value)

| *Childhood BP readings* | *Percentage of adults with high readings* |
|---|---|
| BP ever > 90% | 25% > 90% |
| Systolic BP ever >80% | 39% > 80% |
| Diastolic BP ever >90% | 17% > 90% |
| Diastolic BP ever >80% | 32% > 80% |
| Three normal systolic BP <90% | 6% > 90% |
| Only one systolic BP >90% | 17% > 90 % |
| Two or more >90% systolic BP | 24% > 90% |
| Three normal diastolic BP <90% | 7% > 90% |
| Only one diastolic BP <90% | 9% > 90% |
| Two or more diastolic BP >90% | 24% > 90% |

Adapted from ref. *157*.

## RISK FACTORS INVOLVED IN CHILDHOOD ESSENTIAL HYPERTENSION

A number of factors independently influence BP regulation and more than one factor is often present in a hypertensive individual.

### *Race and Ethnicity*

The prevalence of essential HTN is clearly influenced by race and ethnicity *(43)*. Sex does not seem to play a role. Native Americans have the same or higher rate of essential HTN compared to Hispanics who have the same or lower BP than Caucasians. The prevalence of HTN in blacks is twice that of whites; it also has an earlier onset and more end organ damage. These differences are most likely quantitative *(44)* for the characteristics of the hypertensive process are remarkably similar in blacks and whites when corrected for age, cardiovascular and renal damage, and level of BP *(45)*. Blacks have higher sleep and less dipping in their nighttime ABPM values than age matched whites *(46)*. Blacks experience a greater degree of renal global, segmental, and interstitial sclerosis than whites at an earlier age, despite having similar BP and degrees of proteinuria *(47)*. Possible factors include increased activity of the RAS (greater ACE/ID deletion polymorphism) and transforming growth factor-β.

Blacks are more likely to be salt-sensitive, and to have a higher rate of low renin essential HTN. Several studies have reported that blacks have a poorer response to both angiotensin-converting enzyme (ACE) inhibitors and calcium channel blockers. The addition of a diuretic to these agents improves the response. Decreased activity of the renal kallikrein system with associated salt sensitivity also occurs more frequently in African-American populations *(48)*. Adult blacks in the USA have a higher prevalence of HTN than blacks in the UK *(49)*. Possible reasons include selective migration of the survival of salt-sensitive individuals in the US, and a different socioeconomic milieu.

### *Renin Profiling*

One of the controversial issues in the field of HTN is the volume vasoconstrictor hypothesis of Laragh and co-workers. This hypothesis divides those with essential HTN into three groups, normo, hyper, and hypo reninemia based on renin profiling, e.g., the comparison of plasma renin activity (PRA) to sodium excretion. (Some use upright PRA alone.) This group concluded that high renin essential HTN patients are at greater risk for vasoocclusive events such as stroke, infarction, and renal failure *(50),* whereas those with low renin essential HTN are volume over expanded and less likely to experience the aforementioned end organ damage. Moreover, these investigators suggest that drug therapy should be targeted at the underlying primary pathophysiology involved in generating HTN. They suggest that renin inhibitors and diuretics be used initially to treat patients with high and low renin essential HTN, respectively.

Only a few studies included renin profiling in children with essential HTN. Clearly, the RAS functions differently in children with essential HTN. The earliest study included 16 adolescents aged 14–19 yr, and documented for the first time in children normal, high and low PRA in 50%, 25%, and 19% of the individuals, respectively *(51)*. A subsequent report compared 34 normotensive age-matched black controls to 32 hypertensive adolescent blacks *(52)*. High renin essential HTN was found in 14% of the test subjects. Suppressed PRA activity (failure to increase PRA activity) was found in 19% ($N = 5$) of 27 hypertensives whose urine sodium excretion decreased to less than 50 mEq/d/1.73 $m^2$ after ingesting a low sodium diet for 3 d. Two of these five also exhibited suppressed PRA activity after being given furosemide 1.0 mg/kg orally while on a normal sodium diet, indicating that suppressed PRA may be more easily identified by means of a low sodium diet. An increased response in PRA (increase by >350%) occurred in 11% of the children with essential HTN after furosemide administration. There are currently no long-term data on the outcome of children with essential HTN who were renin profiled at the time of diagnosis.

PRA was higher in those with high uric acid levels. Fractional excretion of uric acid was inversely related to serum uric acid levels and PRA, suggesting the presence of altered glomerulo tubular balance in the hypertensive group. Hyperuricemic hypertensive patients, when compared to normouricemic hypertensive patients, also had a less severe diuretic response to oral furosemide challenge. In a group of 31 children, including 26 adolescents, uric acid levels were above age-matched controls in 42% of the children *(53)*. The importance of using hyperuricemia as a screening test for increased PRA in hypertensive children needs future study. Hyperuricemia itself may be a risk factor. Serum calcium and phosphorous was higher in the hypertensive group, but calcium excretion was similar to that of the control group *(54)*.

### *White Coat Hypertension*

White coat hypertension (WCH) refers to elevated BP readings in an office setting prior to or during antihypertensive therapy when actual BP is normal. In adults, the prevalence of WCH ranges from 16 to 60% when ABPM criteria was used for normal BP ranges from 131/80 to 150/90 mmHg *(55)*. It has been estimated that the recognition of WCH may enable up to 25% of patients with essential HTN to discontinue antihypertensive medication *(56)*. The primary postulated mechanisms, which remain unproven, include nervous system reactions to exposure or conditioned responses to medical personnel. The critical issue is whether WCH is a precursor to the onset of essential HTN, and remains controversial. Two studies, utilizing ABPM in adults, concluded that the long-term risk of WCH does not exceed that observed in normotensive people *(57,58)*. Others have reported abnormalities in renin, aldosterone, renal sodium handling, catecholamines, and insulin *(59)*. Serious cardiovascular outcomes in affected adults have also been reported *(60)*. Compared to those with renal related HTN, patients with WCH have the same or increased LV mass, similar myocardial function, similar numbers of central nervous system (CNS) lacunae on magnetic resonance imaging (MRI), less vascular compliance, and similar increased microalbumin excretory rates *(55)*.

In children whose casual BP readings in-office exceeds the 95th percentile *(61)*, the prevalence of WCH is as high as 35%–44%. A high prevalence (76%) of WCH has been observed utilizing ABPM in children with mild to moderate BP elevation *(62)*. The observation that adolescents with WCH have increased urinary excretion of cortisol and endothelin identifies a group with distinct metabolic abnormalities *(63)*. Since urinary endothelin is derived from the kidney, these findings support a dysregulation of renal function. It is possible that WCH in children represents two overlapping populations, one destined to develop essential HTN and the other to remain with isolated WCH or revert to normotension.

### *Fetal Development*

The origin of HTN may begin during fetal development. An association between the development of cardiovascular disease in adults and prenatal growth was first reported in 1989 *(64)*. An inverse relationship between birth weight and HTN has been described in a number of epidemiologic studies. One study reported a decrease in systolic BP at ages 64–71 yr of 5.2 mmHg for each kg increase in birth weight *(65)*. Postulated mechanisms include insulin resistance, exposure of a malnourished fetus to maternal glucocorticoids that alter subsequent steroid sensitivity, as well as the metabolism of placenta cortisol *(66)*, and the presence of a reduced number of glomeruli.

A number of studies support the hypothesis that maternal malnutrition combined with excessive glucocorticoid activity suppresses the fetal RAS. Other studies have shown that the decreased activity of 11β-hydroxysteroid dehydrogenase and the placenta enzyme that inactivates cortisol in humans is reduced when the mother is protein-restricted. Excessive fetal glucocorticoids may suppress nephrogenesis by reducing renin and $AT_1$ receptor gene activity. The net result is a reduced number of glomeruli (as much as 25% in experimental animals), a decreased glomerular surface area, and a reduction in glomerular filtration rate (GFR) per nephron *(67)*.

The impaired nephron function eventually leads to HTN. A similar outcome occurs if the RAS is blocked with losartan immediately after birth. Moreover, the HTN produced is salt-sensitive. A recent case control prospective study found that ABPM at age twelve was similar in full term normals and small for gestational age *(68)*. Differences in BP could be explained by differences in body mass.

### *Obesity*

The relationship between weight and BP was reported as long ago as 1924. Obesity, which is found in 35–50% of hypertensive adolescents, is one of the most important factors involved in both the generation and persistence of childhood essential HTN. A direct relationship between obesity and HTN has been reported to occur as early as 5 yr of age *(69)*. The Muscatine Study showed that changes in ponderosity over 11 yr correlated directly with changes in BP *(70)*. A number of prevalence studies, including tracking studies of weight change and BP in young adults *(71)*, have reported an increase in HTN in obese subjects. The quantity of central vs peripheral body fat correlates positively with BP *(72)*. In a study of 314 children (essential HTN in 218), body mass index (BMI) was clearly greater in children with essential HTN than in those with secondary HTN and correlated with the age of onset of HTN *(73)*.

Seventy-five percent of obese children aged 9–13 yr do not change their habits and become obese adults *(74)*. Contributing factors in the United States include a lack of exercise and a sedentary lifestyle. Approximately 25% of children spend 4 or more hours a day watching TV, and 27% of high school children spend less than 30 min a day in moderate activity at least five times a week. In a group of 2460 students (mean age 15.1 yr), the prevalence of HTN and obesity were 16.8% and 23%, respectively *(75)*. HTN was three times more common in obese children (33% vs 11%). Obese children were also found to have hyperkinetic cardiovascular systems, manifested by increased HR and increased variability in their ABPM profiles, including both daytime and nighttime systolic BP and diastolic BP.

According to the National Health and Nutrition Examination Survey III (NHANES) document, 13% and 14% of children aged 6–14 and 12–19 yr, respectively, are overweight *(76)*. This is triple the number reported prior to 1976 and double the number reported by NHANES in 1976. A major source of additional calories during childhood has been the substitution of inexpensive corn-based sweeteners in the 1980s—the period of onset of a marked increase in obesity and type II diabetes *(77)*. Concomitantly, many new sweetened snack foods also became available. As much as 10–20% of ingested calories during childhood years come from corn sweeteners. The substitution of fructose for other carbohydrates elevates triglycerides shortly after eating, a factor that is felt to increase the risk of obesity and heart disease.

Obesity has recently been shown to be an independent factor in the development of heart failure in adults *(78)*, and in progressive renal failure in children *(79)*. Others have not found this association in children *(80)*. Left ventricular hypertrophy (LVH), utilizing adult as well as pediatric criteria, was found in 15.8 and 38.3%, respectively, of 133 children whose mean age was 13.6 ± 3.6 yrs and whose BMI was 27.5 ± 7.4 kg/m$^2$.

Glucose intolerance occurs in 20–25% of severely obese adolescents. Obesity is associated with the so-called "metabolic syndrome," which is characterized by insulin resistance, an atherogenic dyslipidemia, activation of the sympathetic nervous system, and an increased tendency for thrombosis. Other suggested mechanisms of obesity-related HTN include hyperinsulinemia, hyperproinsulinemia, renal sodium retention, increased sympathetic activity, increased plasma volume, increased levels of dehydroepiandrosterone *(81)*, and increased CO. Increased plasma aldosterone activity in obese adolescents correlates with increases in their mean BP; the BP level falls when weight loss occurs *(82)*. Even though a direct relationship between PRA and plasma aldosterone levels does not exist, incremental increase of PRA seem to result in a greater increment of plasma aldosterone. It may be that adrenal glands in obese individuals have increased sensitivity to ANG II. An increase in ACTH activity, which also occurs in obesity, may contribute to the increase in aldosterone secretion. Any increase in aldosterone production will, secondarily, increase renal sodium retention.

Of interest is the observation that child abuse is also associated with excessive weight gain *(83)*. In summary, the perturbations that occur in obesity influence both the volume and vasoconstrictive components of the BP formula. Its growing prevalence has made it one of our principle public health issues.

### *Salt Intake*

Sodium intake influences BP. Estimates of salt sensitivity in the western world range from 25 to 50% of the adult population. It is estimated that, since the Paleolithic period, the average sodium intake in an American diet has increased almost fivefold to approx 3400 mg/d, a level sufficiently high enough to enable high-BP expression in salt-sensitive individuals *(84)*. During the same period, potassium intake has fallen by almost 75%, and the sodium-to-potassium ratio has markedly increased. Processed foods, the mainstay of many diets, often contain high levels of sodium and relatively low levels of potassium.

Of note, formula-fed neonates for a number of decades were fed formula in which sodium content was based on the fourfold greater sodium content of cow milk (16 mEq/L), rather than human milk (4 mEq/L). If the BP response in humans to the timing and quantity of sodium exposure is similar to that observed in genetically prone essential HTN experimental animals, a large fraction of the current adult population may be at risk. Experimental studies have shown that the amount and time of introduction of sodium in the diet of newborn rats influences the onset and persistence of HTN. In human neonates, the ingestion of the lower sodium (4 mEq/L) containing formula after birth was associated with a 2.1 mm/Hg lower BP after 6 mo *(85)*. Even though this difference did not persist a few years later, it is still possible that a life-long effect may be seen.

Potassium intake influences BP. Increased potassium intake by Dutch children over a 7-yr period was associated with a mean yearly increase in systolic BP of 1.4 mmHg, while children ingesting a low potassium intake experienced a systolic BP raise of 2.4 mmHg per year *(86)*. An inverse relationship is reported between BP and the urinary sodium/potassium ratio in adolescent females *(87)*.

Divalent ions are also known to influence BP. Low calcium intake has been reported to be associated with HTN *(88)*.

### *Exercise*

Exercise, both aerobic and static, transiently increases BP. Exercise provides a number of benefits: increased caloric expenditure, appetite suppression, and improved exercise tolerance. Exercise levels are inversely related to cholesterol and triglyceride levels. Increasingly, children are leading a more sedentary life. The BP response of hypertensive adolescents is similar to that of normotensive adolescents, but starts and finishes at higher levels *(89)*. Peak systolic BP in an adolescent, exceeding 210 mmHg, and a rise in diastolic BP with dynamic exercise, is used by some to determine if antihypertensive drug therapy should be initiated *(90)*.

### *Hyperkinetic Cardiovascular State*

An impaired neurogenic state, characterized by an increased sensitivity to adrenergic input and/or a decrease in parasympathetic activity, exists in borderline hypertensive as well as in those who later develop fixed essential HTN. An elevated HR has been associated with borderline BP and the eventual development of HTN in young adults *(91)*. In response to mental stress stimuli, adolescents with essential HTN have greater BP and pulse rate responses, as well as a dampened reduction phase in their BP and pulse rate *(41)*. Postulated mechanisms include gene effects and chronic exposure to stress.

### *Cigarette Smoking*

Cigarette smoking indirectly, but acutely, increases BP. Chronic smoking itself doesn't increase BP; it is associated with increased cholesterol levels and lower levels of high density lipoprotein (HDL), which increase the risk of atherogenesis.

### *Lipids*

Prolonged elevation of cholesterol is strongly associated with an increased risk of coronary artery disease Evaluations of the coronary arteries and aorta of 35 children and young adults dying from noncoronary artery disease events revealed fatty aortic streaks in 61%, coronary artery fibrous streaks and/or plaques in 85%, and raised plaques in 25% of the late adolescent males *(92)*. Fibrous plaques were limited to males. The fatty streaks were more extensive in blacks than in whites. The extent of involvement correlated directly with total cholesterol and low density lipoprotein (LDL) and, inversely, with the ratio of HDL to LDL cholesterol. Obesity is the most common cause of hypertriglyceridemia, often associated with a low HDL in adolescents. It is well known that a number of inherited disorders of lipid metabolism markedly increase the risk of early cardiovascular disease.

### *Genetics*

There is an accumulating body of evidence that describes a major role for genes in influencing normal and abnormal BP regulation. Studies of families and twins provide clear documentation of the role of genetics in essential HTN. Approximately 60–70% of HTN in families can be attributed to genetic factors. The remainder can be attributed to environmental factors *(93)*. Most twin studies have shown evidence for a genetic component of BP. Comparison of dizygotic with monozygotic twins supports a hereditary estimate of 0.72 and 0.28 for diastolic BP and systolic BP, respectively *(94)*. The observations that dizygotic correlations are higher than other first degree relatives support a role for a nongenetic, shared environmental cause *(95)*.

The Montreal twin adoption study on normal BP defined the relative influence of shared genes (33%), across a generation-shared environment (24%), and the environment shared within generations (43%) *(96,97)*. A family history of HTN can be found in 50% of hypertensive children *(90)*. The percentage of hypertensive children reflects the presence or absence in their parents of normotension (N) and HTN (H). N × N matings give rise to 4.2–17.6% hypertensive children, which is less than N × H matings (15.9–56.8%), which in turn is less than H × H matings (44.0–73.3%) *(98)*. When examined in the reverse order, a greater prevalence of HTN is found in the parents and grandparents of hypertensive children *(99)*. Additional evidence supporting genetic predisposition to BP regulation is provided by a number of studies involving normotensive and hypertensive offspring of one or both parents with essential HTN (Table 7).

Attempts to identify specific candidate genes causally involved in essential HTN have yielded inconsistent results. Such differences may reflect environmental factors, the influence of other genes, evolutionary diversion (race and ethnicity), and study design and/or technical issues. The processes involved in identifying candidate genes include genetic linkage and association methods. The former evaluates (lod score) a quantitative, or discrete, trait for cosegregation (linkage) to polymorphic DNA markers (often microsatellite) in related individuals (usually sibling pairs or offspring).

Association studies (usually case controlled) are directed toward the detection of an association between specific alleles and disease (essential HTN). At least 25–30 genes have been suggested as contributors to the hypertensive process by affecting critical factors involved in the vasoconstriction and/or volume limbs of the BP formula (Table 8). No single gene seems to be reproducibly involved across various subpopulations of humans, supporting the conclusion that a number of different genes and their alleles, when summated, each contributes to the generation and/or persistence phases of the essential HTN process. Racial and ethnic differences in genes involved have been documented. The development of microarray technology has allowed for the identification of single nucleotide polymorphisms, genomic mismatches, and microsatellite mapping to identify and understand the role of genes in hypertensive populations and individuals.

Table 7
Findings in Normotensive Offspring of Hypertensive Parents

* Increased urinary excretion of calcium *(158)*
* Less nocturnal dipping, lower rates of catecholamine excretion and increased response to sympathetic nervous system stimulation previously used
* Office BP and ABPM are higher LV mass index is greater and pressor response is similar. Less significant abnormalities occurred in FH ± *(159)*
* Mean ABPM values are higher in children with a positive family history *(160)*
* Male adolescents with at least one hypertensive parent had thickened interventricular septum and posterior wall, LV mass, and cross sectional area *(161)*
* In Japanese children, plasma renin activity and systolic BP was higher in offspring of hypertensive parents *(162)*
* Normotensive offspring have a reduced renal functional reserve and increased microalbuminuria *(i)* Offspring of hypertensive parents are 30% more likely to track in the upper quartile of systolic BP over an 8-yr period of age, starting at ages 2–14 *(164)*
* Offspring of hypertensive parents have a greater degree of natriuresis *(165)*
* Offspring of hypertensive parents have a higher rate of red cell sodium lithium countertransportation *(166)*. Offspring have an increased number of platelet adrenoceptors
* Normotensive offspring of hypertensive parents have higher BP and forearm vascular resistance responses to mental stress (even greater after ingesting a high sodium diet).
* Offspring of hypertensive parents have exaggerated BP responses to both isometric and static exercise *(167)*

A number of studies support a role for the genes involved in the control of the renin angiotensin system (RAS). ACE/ID polymorphisms are believed to play a major role in both the onset of essential HTN and its treatment. Individuals homozygotic for the D allele have higher levels of ACE. The DD genotype has been associated in some, but not all, studies with a reduced antiproteinuric effect to ACE inhibitor antihypertensive agents. In such patients, $AT_1$ receptor blockades may improve BP response and retard progression of renal disease *(100)*. The $C^{1166}$ variant of the $AT_1$ receptor is also associated with BP vasoregulatory dysfunction and low BP in adults *(101)*. Animal experiments clearly demonstrate a relationship between the number of copies of genes involved in the regulation of the RAS and natriuretic peptides. The genes controlling plasma angiotensinogen (AGT) clearly influence BP while those involved in ACE production do not *(102)*. In experimental animals and human HTN, the steady state concentration of AGT is directly related to the number of copies of the ACT genes, increases in ANG II, and the observed BP. Similar changes in the expression of ACE genes are not always expressed by changes in angiotensin II levels. When AGT decreases, ANG I decreases and, if ACE is constant, ANG II production will fall. Conversely, if ACE expression is reduced, the conversion of ANG I to ANG II falls, but because AGT is unaffected, ANG I production increases and more ANG II can be made, although there is less ACE present. These studies help explain the variability reported in the study of RAS genes in human HTN.

A number of genes have been implicated in salt-sensitive HTN and are more prevalent in blacks. A genetic component of salt sensitivity has been described in adults with the haptoglobin 1-1 phenotype *(103)*. The Gly-460Trp variant of the α-adducin gene has been associated with HTN more in blacks *(104)* than in whites *(105)*. Similarly, increased renal sodium reabsorption, an increased BP response to saline infusion, a greater drop in BP, and reduction in stroke and MI after diuretic therapy *(106)* are all more prevalent in blacks than in whites.

Table 8
Partial Listing of Chromosomes, Genes, and Flanking Markers Involved in HTN

*Chromosome 5q31-q34 (marker bordering region D5S2093), ADRB2 allele Arg16Gly*
- * β-adenoceptor-G protein system: chromosome 20q13.2, gene GNAS1 exon 5, allele Fok1. chromosome 12p13, gene GNB3, exon 10. allele C825T

*α-adducin*
- * Chromosome 4p, gene α adducin. Allele Gly460Trp
- * Catecholamine synthetic enzymes
  - Dopamine-β-hydroxylase gene
  - Phenylethanolamine *N*-methyltransferase gene
  - Tyrosine hydroxylase gene
- * Chromosome 18q *(168)*
- * Genomic Array Identified Genes
  - 2p22.1-2p21, 5p33.3-5q34, 6q23.1-6q24.1, 15q23.1-15q26.1
  - Chromosome 11q, marker D11S934
  - Chromosome 15q, marker D158203
- * Lipoprotein metabolism

*Chromosome 8p22, gene lipoprotein lipase*
- * Chromosome 2p24, gene apolipoprotein, allele β 3' promoter hypervariable region
- * Miscellaneous Genes
  - Glucagon receptor
  - Glucocorticoid receptor
  - Prostacyclin synthase
  - Transforming growth factor-β (TGF-β) 1 gene
- * Renal kallikrein-kinin system
  - Chromosome 19q13, gene tissue kallikrein (KLK1) 5' proximal promotor
- * Renin Angiotensin System
  - Angiotensinogen gene alleles M235T, A-6G, A-20C
  - ACE locus deletion/insertion (D/I) polymorphism intron 16
- * Aldosterone synthase (CYP11B2 on chromosome 8p21) alleles -344T
- * Epithelial sodium channel (ENaC)
  - Subunit β T594M mutation (nearby β gene 16p12.3) *(110)*

Adapted unless otherwise stated from ref. *169.*

Despite the clear-cut association of genes involved in the regulation of sodium channels in Lodd's syndrome, their involvement in the essential HTN process has not yet been proven. Genes involved in the B-subunit of the epithelial sodium channel have been associated with HTN in blacks *(107)*. Genes involved in the renin angiotensin aldosterone system also influence salt sensitivity. The I allele of the ACE I/D and alleles of the 11β-hydroxysteroid dehydrogenase type 2 polymorphisms are associated with salt-sensitive HTN *(108)*, and may be markers of salt-sensitive HTN. The response to ANG I is enhanced in those with a DD genotype and who are on a liberal salt intake, but not on a low salt diet *(109)*.

Gene abnormalities have been found in other systems whose dysfunction contributes to HTN. Genes involved in the endothelin system seem to participate in the hypertensive process in some cases. Genes specifically involved in NO regulation, missense alteration Glu298Asp, and a point mutation T-7860.C (C/C genotype) have been associated with HTN *(110)*. The roles of genes involved in the natriuretic peptide system, whose effects are opposite those of the RAS system, have not yet been clarified.

A number of renal transplantation experiments, between genetic strains of essential HTN and normotensive rats, as well as human transplantation *(111)*, supports the concept that the genetic composition of the kidney plays a dominant role in determining HTN. The chromosome responsible for causing HTN has been shown to regulate BP when transplanted either inside or outside of the kidney *(112)*. The mechanisms and specific genes involved have not yet been determined.

### *Alcohol*

Proposed mechanisms that explain increased BP with chronic alcohol ingestion include an increase in HR, increased sensitivity to circulating catecholamines, increased activity of the RAS, enhanced cortisol production, and changes in calcium related vasoconstriction *(113)*.

### *Stress*

Environmental stress clearly influences BP. Following the 1994 earthquake in Los Angeles, the number of sudden deaths on that day attributed to cardiovascular causes was significantly high *(114)*. A 30-yr follow-up of 144 nuns in Italy, compared to 138 laywomen, documented significantly lower BP and fewer strokes and myocardial infarctions in the cloistered group. Except for environmental factors, no differences in baseline BP, salt excretion, family history, or body mass could be identified *(115)*. Poverty, sociocultural factors, racial issues, and migration are also known to increase BP. Both systolic BP and diastolic BP can be correlated with chronic hostility, tenseness, and the demanding perception of environment in adolescents *(116)*. Stress increases CNS sympathetic outflow and the adrenal outflow of catecholamines. Type A behavior is associated with increases in systolic BP, but not diastolic BP *(117)*. Mental stress is believed by some to be the primary determinant of essential HTN. Three models of psychosocial stress that might explain the genesis of essential HTN are the Defense Defeat Model, Demand Control, and Lifestyle Incongruity Index *(118)*. These models deal with issues such as fight flight, control, aggression, depression, subordination, the relationship between psychologic demand factored by the available latitude of decisionmaking, and differences between occupational and social class and achievement vs accomplishment.

## CLINICAL EVALUATION OF HYPERTENSIVE CHILDREN

All children presenting with HTN need an assessment for etiology and the severity of HTN. This should include a detailed history and physical exam, as well as a set of laboratory and, if indicated, imaging studies to enable a presumptive and definitive diagnosis. Once the evaluation is completed, consideration can be given to management. Components of the assessment are outlined in Table 9. The diagnosis of essential HTN remains a diagnosis of exclusion. Criteria for its diagnosis have been previously considered. Its presence is more likely if the child is older than 10 yr of age, is an African-American, has a positive family history, is obese, and has minimally increased levels of BP. Essential HTN is rarely diagnosed in children less than 10 yr of age. Unless history, physical examination, and screening laboratory tests (urinalysis, electrolytes creatinine glucose) indicate the presence of a secondary form of HTN, the so-called "mega workup" is unlikely to identify the cause of HTN, particularly if the child fits the profile above.

**Table 9**
**Assessment of a Child With Elevated Blood Pressure**

*History*
* CNS: headache (continuous, paroxysmal), visual disturbance; seizures, tremors
* Hearing: deafness
* Cardiovascular: palpations, irregular pulse
* Renal: edema (peripheral, eyelid, swollen abdomen), unexplained fever, abnormal urine color, enuresis, flank pain, dysuria,
* Skin: rash, sweating, pallor
* Respiratory: epistaxis, difficulty in breathing
* Past medical history: previous surgery, and hospitalizations
* Drug usage (therapeutic, contraceptives, and illicit): alcohol, caffeine, and tobacco usage
* Family history: hypertension, early myocardial infarction, diabetes, stroke
* Sexual history: pregnancy
* Neonatal history: use of umbilical artery catheters
* Growth history: excessive weight gain/loss, growth percentile, and change in percentiles over time

*Dietary history*
* Types and amounts of foods ingested; quantity of fluid ingested, salt craving

*Social history*
* Stress factors at home (parental discordance, etc.) and work (school performance, interactions with peers, child abuse)

*Physical examination*
* General: height, weight (changes over time)
* Vital signs: pulse presence (femoral), rate and rhythm, BP in all extremities
* Skull: elfin facies
* Eyes: fundoscopic arterial/venous abnormalities, papilledema
* Neck: thyroid enlargement, webbing
* Cardiovascular: pulses in all four extremities, bruits
* Cardiac: murmur, autonomic dysfunction, heart size
* Abdomen: unilateral and/or bilateral masses, bruits
* Genitalia: appearance, tanner staging
* Extremities: casts, edema, traction, unilateral limb enlargement, wide carrying angle
* Skin: rashes, striae, neurofibroma, café au lait spots, widely spaced nipples
* Joints: arthritis
* CNS: ascending paralysis, cranial nerve dysfunction (hemiparesis)

*Laboratory studies*
CBC, urinalysis (dipstix and if indicated microscopy) electrolytes, BUN, creatinine, glucose, uric acid, plasma renin (renin profiling), plasma and urinary aldosterone, TSH, T3,T4 if indicated, ECG, urinary and blood catecholamines, free cortisol, 18-hydroxycorticosterone

*Imaging studies*
ECHO, chest film if indicated; abdominal and renal ultrasound (CAT, MRI if indicated); Doppler Flow Study; VCUG and radionuclide studies if indicated.

A detailed dietary history of caloric and sodium intake of the affected individual and the family is important. BMI (weight in kilograms divided by height in meters squared) can be used to estimate the degree of obesity. Values less than 24.9, 25–29.9, 30–39.9 and above 40 are considered normal, overweight, obese, and markedly obese, respectively.

Renin profiling is useful to screen for secondary forms of HTN, and as a means of classifying the type of essential HTN. Recently, an automated test for measuring direct renin (DR), which is easier to measure than PRA, has become available. The ratio of DR to PRA is 8 to 1.

## TREATMENT OF CHILDHOOD HYPERTENSION

There are a number of reasons to treat and, if possible, prevent HTN. Higher BP is associated with the increased risk of strokes, renal failure, and heart disease. Successful antihypertensive treatment reduces cardiovascular morbidity and mortality. Higher pressures are associated with even greater increase in pressure over time. Lowering BP by even a small degree can result in positive outcomes. It has been suggested that a decrease in diastolic BP of 2.0 mmHg decreases the incidence of HTN by 17%, coronary heart disease by 6%, and stroke and/or CNS ischemia by 15% *(119)*. Moreover, treatment considerations need to address both public health issues and individual needs.

### *Nonpharmacologic Therapy*

Nonpharmacologic therapy (weight reduction, lowered salt intake, exercise, and stress reduction) produces variable results. Yet, it is worth considering, especially in those with borderline HTN. Attempts to modify these factors may be more successful when families and peer groups can be involved. The National High Blood Pressure Committee has recently published its recommendations for the primary prevention of HTN. The committee states that the strategies of approaching, preventing and/or controlling HTN from the perspective of an individual, as well as society at large, are complementary. It further states that the same lifestyle approaches recommended for adults are applicable to childhood populations *(120)*.

### *Altering Dietary Salt Intake*

Lowering dietary sodium in adults (adolescents) to less than 125 mmol per day generally results in a decrease in BP in salt-sensitive individuals, children with borderline high BP, and offspring of hypertensive parents. A 50% reduction in the average dietary intake of salt, which in North America averages 8–10 g/d, will lower BP by about 2 mmHg *(121)*. The addition of diuretics to a low salt diet does not seem to improve BP control *(122)*. Obese adolescents also ingest more salt than the nonobese. Diets rich in vegetables and fruits and low in fat are generally also low in sodium. Reductions or elimination of foods containing large amounts of salt (e.g., potato chips, pretzels, processed foods, etc.) are required in order to achieve a positive outcome.

Initially, one can recommend a no added salt diet. Involving the entire family is generally helpful. Altering the sodium contained in a school lunch program can lower sodium excretion and BP *(123)*. In this study, the monitoring of urinary sodium excretion documented the effect of the reduced salt intake. Overnight urine collections, e.g., first morning urine in these adolescents, was utilized to document that sodium excretion, which averaged 70–110 mEq per g creatinine, fell to less than 50 mEq per g of creatinine and a mean drop in both systolic and diastolic BP of 1.5–2.0 mmHg. An increase of calcium intake in a group of girls aged 3–6 yr was also shown to lower systolic BP by 2.27 mmHg without affecting diastolic BP *(124)*. It has also been suggested that lowering the salt content of processed foods could result in a positive public health benefit for the 25% of the population that is salt-sensitive.

Currently, there are no agreed-upon recommendations for using other salts such as potassium, calcium, or magnesium to treat persistent HTN in children. Attempts to lower BP in children by adding potassium to their diets has not worked uniformly *(87)*. Adult data clearly support increasing potassium intake as a means of lowering BP, while increasing calcium intake remains more problematic.

### *Diet Modification*

A number of studies, including a 6-mo randomized controlled study in adults, have shown that increasing the intake of fruits and vegetables to five portions daily lowers BP (systolic BP/diastolic BP decrease of 4.0/1.5 mmHg, respectively) and increases levels of some antioxidants *(125)*. Weight did not change significantly. Encouragement to reduce intake and anticipatory guidance about the role of alcohol in the hypertensive process should contribute to a positive outcome.

### *Weight Loss*

The sheer magnitude of the problem of obesity requires that it be addressed at both the individual and the national level. Weight reduction in obese adolescents, which, during its early phases is also associated with a sodium diuresis, leads to normalization of BP *(126)*. It is also associated with increases in lean body mass and HDL, and decreases in triglycerides and body fat *(127)*. At the office level, primary care physicians make recommendations for weight control in 49%, 82%, and 88% of preschool children, school-age children, and adolescents, respectively *(128)*. Interventions based on improving eating and activity in children have been shown to have positive long-term outcomes that are superior to those obtained in adults *(129)*. Specific dietary recommendations currently used by primary care physicians include changes in eating patterns, limitation of specific foods, low fat diets, modest to marked caloric restriction, and commercial diets.

Barriers in implementing treatment for obesity in children include lack of parental interest, motivation, and involvement, as well as inavailability of support services. Obese children also have low self-esteem, an increased incidence of depression, and an increased number of psychiatric problems. Successful outcome depends on the development and implementation of parenting techniques, parental involvement *(130)*, resolving family conflict, behavior management strategies, and individual/family counseling. Strategies helpful in assisting children to lose weight include a personal diet history kept by the child with periodic reviews of sweets, fats, snacks, and "good foodstuffs," nutritional education, contracts, and behavior modification, including more exercise and fewer "couch potato" activities. A reasonable weight loss goal is 1–2 lbs/wk in adolescents. Limiting TV time can also lead to weight loss *(131)*.

The observation that neonates whose parents are obese have a reduced energy expenditure of 21% at 3 mo of age, when compared to offspring of lean mothers, supports the need to institute weight control measures very early in life *(132)*. It is noteworthy that young obese children are more likely to outgrow their obesity than older children *(133)*, which supports the belief that the weight control programs that are most likely to be successful over time will be those directed toward younger children and, perhaps, even infants. Clearly there exists a public health need to develop, implement, and evaluate school classroom programs that teach and reinforce the importance of a positive lifelong outcome involving weight control, a healthy diet, and routine exercise.

### *Exercise*

A sustained increase in aerobic exercise in sedentary individuals clearly lowers BP and weight. Exercise in obese adolescents lowers BP, in part by its effect on lowering plasma insulin *(134)*. Activity interventions to consider include reductions in sedentary activity, increases in routine, and either unstructured or organized physical activities. Exercise prescriptions should define the type, frequency, intensity, and duration of exercise required. A reasonable ultimate goal should be 30–60 min of aerobic exercise three to four times a week. Warm up and cool down periods that involve stretching or walking should be included. Treatment effect can be monitored by measuring the pulse rate. The goal should be to reach an HR of 70–80% of one's age-related maximal HR. It is noteworthy that a recent study in obese adolescents failed to document improvement in LV function despite 8 mo of physical training that resulted in an improvement in overall cardiac function and adiposity *(135)*.

At the public health level in the US, VERB, which started in July 2002, is a national campaign aimed at children 9–13 yr of age. Its message is to pick one's favorite action verb and do it—swim, run, bike, etc. In addition to such programs, pediatricians can also work to influence school boards to modify current practices. Efforts are needed to enhance physical activity programs at all levels of education and to offer healthier lunches while limiting access to high-calorie snacks and beverages in vending machines and cafeterias.

### *Guidelines for Participation in Sports*

Definitive long-term data on participation in athletics by children with high, normal and/or mildly elevated BP are lacking. In the absence of any organ effects, e.g., ECHO, etc., these children should be allowed to participate in dynamic exercise. Reevaluation is indicated should they become symptomatic. Despite the fact that isometric exercise and weight training have been shown to lower BP as long as the activities were continued, many still recommend that children with essential HTN avoid weightlifting. Once children with persistently elevated BP are on antihypertensives and have been documented to have normal BP and myocardial function, participation in aerobic exercise with ongoing monitoring can be permitted.

### *Stress Reduction*

When compared to an outpatient group of placebo-treated adolescents with essential HTN, hospitalization of a similar group was associated with a drop in both systolic BP and diastolic BP and HR, which returned to pretreatment levels within a few weeks *(136)*. In adults, hospitalization is associated with a decrease in urinary catecholamine excretion but not with plasma norepinephrine levels, which is indicative of decreased sympathetic nervous system activity. Stress-reduction techniques can be taught to children as young as 8 yr of age. Success with relaxation, biofeedback, and meditation programs has been demonstrated to lower BP.

### *Prenatal Interventions*

Prenatal interventions, which can influence maternal and fetal nutrition and fetal development, can potentially reduce the development of essential HTN.

**Table 10**
**Selected Antihypertensive Agents and Class That Have Been Used in Children With Essential HTN**

| *Agent* | *Class* |
|---|---|
| Amlodipine | calcium channel blocker |
| Bisoprolol fumarate | calcium channel blocker, in combination with hydrochlorothiazide, thiazide diuretic |
| Clonidine | central nervous system inhibitor |
| Enalapril | ACE inhibitor |
| Felodipine | calcium channel blocker |
| Guanabenz | central nervous system inhibitor |
| Isradipine | calcium channel blocker |
| Hydrochlorothiazide | thiazide diuretic |
| Lisinopril | ACE inhibitor |
| Metoprolol | β-blocker *(170)* |
| Nifedipine | calcium channel blocker |
| Nitrendipine | calcium channel blocker *(171)* |
| Propranolol | β-blocker |

## PHARMACOLOGIC THERAPY

Most agree that antihypertensive drug therapy is indicated when children have persistently elevated BP and are at increased risk of developing long-term consequences. Because oral contraceptives may increase BP, their use should be avoided in hypertensive sexually active adolescents. Despite the increased emphasis on evaluating antihypertensive agents in children, FDA approval for using these agents in children, particularly those less than 12 yr of age, is limited. Between 1980 and 1993, fewer than five studies directed toward the use of antihypertensive agents to treat essential HTN became available *(137)*. The Food and Drug Modernization Act of 1997 has been the motivation for a considerable number of industry-sponsored pediatric drug trials; a number of clinical trials involving large numbers of hypertensive children have been completed. A smaller number of retrospective and/or single-center safety and efficacy studies involving antihypertensive drug usage in children have also been published. Finally, a number of studies that have evaluated antihypertensive agents in the treatment of secondary forms of HTN are available. Antihypertensive agents that have been studied in children (some with very few patients) with essential HTN are listed in Table 10.

Only one drug, Enalapril, has received FDA approval as an antihypertensive drug for children. Approval followed the completion of both a pharmacokinetic *(138)* and a dose-dependent trial *(139)*. The former demonstrated similar pharmacokinetics in infants and children when compared to adults, while the latter reported a dose-dependent response, together with a low incidence of side effects. Lisinopril has also been shown to have similar pharmacokinetic parameters in children at all ages *(140)*.

A randomized controlled trial of the selective B1-adrenergic blocking agent bisoprolol fumarate, in combination with hydrochlorothiazide ($N = 62$) vs placebo ($N = 32$), reduced systolic BP by a mean of 9.3 vs 4.9 mmHg and diastolic BP by 7.2 vs 2.7 mm Hg in the treatment and placebo groups, respectively *(141)*. Because the placebo-subtracted BP reductions were greater in those with higher BP and in younger children, the number of children whose BP fell to values less than the 90% did not differ significantly. Also, fewer than 50%

of treated children attained the targeted BP of more than 90%. Another study, comparing a combination of propranolol and chlorthalidone to placebo, reported significant reductions in both systolic BP and diastolic BP over a 30-mo period *(142)*. Metoprolol at a dose of 100–200 mg/d for 3–12 mo lowered systolic BP, diastolic BP, and HR in a group of adolescents, including some with essential HTN *(143)*.

### *Calcium Channel Blocking Agents*

A prospective safety and efficacy study, utilizing ABPM to evaluate amlodipine once daily to treat essential HTN in 16 children, found that 0.23 ± 0.14 (maximum 0.5) mg/kg/d was effective in 14 of the 16 children *(144)*. In another study involving 55 children, 43 of whom had essential HTN, monotherapy with amlodipine started at a mean dose of 0.13 mg/kg/d and increased to 0.15 mg/kg/d, effectively lowering BP *(145)*. Children <12 and >12 yr of age required a mean dose of 0.14 and 0.10 mg/kg/d, respectively. Thirteen children needed more than one group of antihypertensive drugs, but it was not clear whether they had essential HTN or secondary HTN. Noncompliance may have occurred. In a multi-center randomized, placebo-controlled trial of amlodipine at a dose of 2.5 or 5.0 mg/d, in which 102 of 268 enrolled children (mean age 11.9 ±3.3 yr) had essential HTN, mean BPs fell from 138/74 to 129/70 mm/Hg, $p = <0.001$ *(146,147)*. The mean systolic BP decrease in both the essential HTN and the secondary high BP group was similar and dose dependent. Children <12 and >12 yr of age required a mean dose of 0.14 and 0.10 mg/kg/d, respectively. Isradipine, as a dose of 0.46 ± 0.28 mg/kg/d, divided into two doses, has also been shown to lower BP in children with essential HTN *(148)*. In another study, isradipine, at a dose of 36 ± 0.17 mg/kg/d, given three to four times a day, has been shown to lower systolic, but not diastolic, BP in a few children with essential HTN *(149,150)* .

### *α-2 Receptor Blocking Antihypertensive Agents*

A study was conducted using 29 adolescent subjects with essential HTN. Given a treatment objective of lowering the diastolic BP to less than 90%, clonidine (0.1–0.2 mg twice daily) and hydrochlorothiazide (25–50 mg twice daily) were administered *(143)*. Clonidine lowered both systolic and diastolic BP. Hydrochlorothiazide lowered only the systolic BP. It is noteworthy that neither agent altered the systolic response, while clonidine was associated with a significant reduction in the diastolic BP response to mental stress. Guanabenz, in an open-labeled study of 14 adolescents given a dose of 0.08–0.20 mg/kg twice daily, lowered systolic and diastolic BP from 138/92 to 129/72 mmHg *(151)*.

### *Other Medications*

Yet to be studied in children are aldosterone-blockers, such as eplerenone. Preliminary studies suggest that these agents may be particularly effective in treating African-Americans with essential HTN *(152)*.

There are a number of issues to consider when selecting antihypertensive agents to treat HTN in children (Table 11). Currently, there is no agreement on which antihypertensive drug to use first. It makes sense to choose an agent that affects the basic pathophysiology involved. Available adult data support the use of ACE inhibitors in patients with renal dysfunction. Mechanisms other than the lowering of BP may retard the progression of renal disease *(153)*. Also, ACE inhibitor usage may be associated with increases in serum creatinine, and may need to be discontined when the increase in serum creatinine exceeds 20–30%, or the serum potas-

Table 11
Questions to Consider When Prescribing Antihypertensive Agents in Children

- * Do children respond differently than adults?
- * Is the drug a tetratogen?
- * What electrolyte abnormalities may occur?
- * Is GFR lowered when using the drug?
- * Do the side effects of the agent increase the risk of atherosclerosis?
- * What drug interactions may occur?
- * Are the side effects of the drug physiologic or idiosyncratic?
- * Does the drug specifically target a step in the pathogenesis of the hypertensive process?
- * Does the drug nonspecifically lower the blood pressure?
- * How frequently must the drug be administered?
- * What formulations are available, iv, tablets, capsules, liquid?
- * Has the agent received FDA approval?
- * Are combination agents available?

sium remains elevated, despite utilizing maneuvers to lower it *(154)*. The small decrease in GFR after starting ace inhibitors may be, over a period of years, associated with improved renal function. In addition, the recommendation that blacks should initially be treated with either diuretics or calcium channel blockers may not be correct for two reasons: first, many hypertensive blacks have normal or high PRA activity and second, recent therapeutic trials report beneficial effects when ACE inhibitors are used alone or in combination with calcium channel blockers *(44)*. There is an ongoing controversy about the predictability of the antihypertensive response to ACE inhibitors when PRA is normal or high in blacks.

### *General Approach*

The starting dose of antihypertensive agents should be the lowest known effective dose. It can be increased stepwise every few weeks. In adult HTN, the controversy concerning the administration of the maximum dose or initiating treatment with a second agent continues, although there are some data that suggest that better outcomes when two agents are used instead of higher doses of a single agent. No data are available in children. Because most children with essential HTN experience only a mild to moderate increase in their BP, the likelihood of responding to a single agent is considerable. In adults, it has been shown that the higher the initial BP, the more drugs are necessary to achieve effective BP control. The target BP goal when treating children with essential HTN remains unstudied. Available data obtained in adults support a therapeutic BP goal that, if translated to children, would be close to the mean of 75% for age- and size-related normal BP values, not just lowering the BP to the 90–95th percentile. Also, there are almost no data in children with essential HTN defining and approaching therapeutic refractiveness. Since there have been no long-term studies of the efficacy of antihypertensive agents started during childhood, it remains unclear as to how long they should be treated. There are data to suggest that, after 6–12 mo of antihypertensive therapy in adults, the BP homeostatic set point may return to normal. Tapering of antihypertensive agents over a period of weeks to months, particularly in those with mild elevations in their BP, should be considered. It is unusual to find evidence of renal dysfunction in children with essential HTN. Major confounding factors in treating children with essential HTN include liability in their baseline BP, compliance issues, and the fact that they feel well. Advances in the understanding of genetic mechanisms hold the yet unfulfilled but likely promise of gene therapy, designer drug therapy, modification of behavioral traits, and improved interpretation of gene expression involved in the genesis and persistence of HTN.

## REFERENCES


1. Pickering G. Mechanisms, methods, management in hypertension: definitions, natural histories and consequences. In: Laragh J, ed. Hypertension Manual. New York: York Medical Books, 1973;3–10.
2. Taylor J. The hypertension detection and follow-up program: a progress report. Circ Res 1977;40:I109.
3. Report of the Second Task Force on Blood Pressure Control in Children—1987. Pediatrics 1987;79:1–25.
4. Park MK, Troxler RG. Systemic hypertension. In: Park MK, Troxler RG, eds. Pediatric Cardiology for Practitioners, Fourth ed. St. Louis: Mosby, 2002;408–416.
5. Arafat M, Mattoo TK. Measurement of blood pressure in children: recommendations and perceptions. Pediatrics 1999;104:e30,1–5.
6. Clark JA, Lieh-Lai MW, Sarnaik A, Mattoo TK. Discrepancies between direct and indirect blood pressure measurements using various recommendations for arm cuff selection. Pediatrics 2002;110(5)920–923.
7. Sorof JM, Portman RJ. Ambulatory blood pressure monitoring in the pediatric patient. J Pediatr 2000;136:578–586.
8. Soergel M, Kirschstein M, Busch C, et al. Oscillometric twenty-four-hour ambulatory blood pressure values in healthy children and adolescents: a multicenter trail including 1141 subjects. J Pediatr 1997;130:178–184.
9. O'Sullivan JJ, Derrick G, Griggs P, et al. Ambulatory blood pressure in school children. Arch Dis Child 1999;80:529–532.
10. Daniels SR, Loggie JM, Burton, T, Kaplan S. Difficulties with ambulatory blood pressure monitoring in children and adolescents. J Pediatr 1987;111:397–400.
11. Sherwood A, Steffen PR, Bumenthal JA, et al. Nighttime blood pressure dipping: the role of the sympathetic nervous system. Am J Hypertension 2002;15:111–118.
12. Meiniger JC, Liehr P, Mueller WH, Chan W, Smith GL, Portman RJ. Stress-induced alterations of blood pressure and 24 h ambulatory blood. Blood Press Monit 1999;4:115–120.
13. Belsha CW, Wells TG, McNiece KL, et al. Influence of diurnal blood pressure variations on target organ abnormalities in adolescents with mild essential hypertension. Am J Hypertens 1998;11:410–417.
14. Bald M, Hoyer PF. Measurement of blood pressure at home: survey among pediatric nephrologists. Pediatr Nephrol 2001;16:1058–1062.
15. Julius S, Krause L, Schork NJ, et al. Hyperkinetic borderline hypertension in Tecumseh, Michigan. J Hypertens 1991b;9:77–84.
16. Korner PI, Bobik A, Angus JJ. Are cardiac and vascular "amplifiers" both necessary for the development of hypertension? Kidney Int 1992;41(Suppl 37):S38–S44.
17. Gavignon A, Rey C, Payot M, et al. Hemodynamic studies of labile essential hypertension in adolescents. In: New MI, Levine LS, eds. Juvenile Hypertension. New York: Raven, 1977;189–193.
18. Ledingham JM. Autoegulation in hypertension: a review. J Hypertens 1989;7(Suppl 4):S97–S104.
19. Dahl LK, Heine M. Primary role of renal homografts in setting chronic blood pressure levels in rats. Circ Res 1975;36:692–696.
20. Brenner BM, Garcia DL, Anderson S. Glomeruli and blood pressure. Less of one, more the other? Am J Hypertens 1988;1:335–347.
21. Sealey JE, Blumenfeld JD, Bell GM, et al. On the renal basis for essential hypertension: nephron heterogeneity with discordant renin secretion and sodium excretion causing a hypertensive vasoconstriction-volume relationship. J Hypertens 1988;6:763–777.
22. Hollenberg NK, Adams DF, Soloman H, et al. Renal vascular tone in essential and secondary hypertension: hemodynamic and angiographic responses to vasodilators. Medicine 1975;54:29–41.
23. London GM, Safer ME, Weiss YA, et al. Volume dependent parameters in essential hypertension. Kidney Int 1977;11:204–208.
24. Bauer JH, Brooks CS. Volume studies in men with mild to moderate hypertension. Am J Cardiol 1979;44:1163–1170.
25. Staessen J, Sartor F, Roels H, et al. The association between blood pressure, calcium and other divalent cations: a population study. J Hum Hypertens 1991b;5:485–494.

26. Gruskin AB, Dabbagh S, Fleischmann, et al. Mechanisms of hypertension in childhood diseases. In: Barratt TM, Avner ED, Harmon WE, eds. Pediatric Nephrology, Fourth ed. Baltimore: Lippincott Williams & Williams, 1999;992.
27. Ludens JH, Clark MA, Robinson FG, DuCharme DW. Rat adrenal cortex is a source of circulating ouabain like compound. Hypertension 1992;19:721–724.
28. Postnov YV. An approach to the explanation of cell membrane alteration in primary hypertension. Hypertension 1990;15:332–337.
29. Blaustein MP. Sodium/calcium exchange and the control of contractility in cardiac muscle and vascular smooth muscle. J Cardiovasc Pharmacol 1988;12(Suppl 5):S56–S68.
30. Flack JS. Hypertension in blacks. In: Oparil S, Weber MA, eds. Hypertension: A Companion to Brenner & Rector's The Kidney. Philadelphia: WB Saunders, 2000;558–563.
31. Neel JV, Weder AB, Julius S. Type II diabetes, essential hypertension, and obesity as "syndromes of impaired genetic homeostasis": the "thrifty genotype" hypothesis enters the 21st century. Perspect Biol Med 1998;42: 44–74.
32. Baker DJP, ed. Fetal and Infant Origins of Adult Disease. London: BMJ, 1993.
33. Seckl JR. Glucocorticoids, feto-placental 11β-hydroxysteroid dehydrogenase type 2, and the early life origins of adult disease. Steroids 1997;62:89–94.
34. Akahoshi M, Soda M, Carter R, et al. Correlation between systolic blood pressure and physical development in adolescents. Am J Epidemiol 1996;144:51–58.
35. Weder AB, Schork NJ. Adaptation, allometry and hypertension. Hypertension 1994;24:145–156.
36. Aviv A, Aviv H. Reflections on telomeres, growth, aging, and essential hypertension. Hypertension 1997;29:1067–1072.
37. Julius S, Quadir H, Gajendragadkar S, Hyperkinetic state: a precursor of hypertension? A longitudinal study of borderline hypertension. In: Gross F, Strasser T, eds. Mild Hypertension: Natural History and Management. London: Pittman, 1979;116–126.
38. Falkner B. Vascular reactivity and hypertension in childhood. Semin Nephrol 1989;9:247–252.
39. Hasen HS, Nielsen JR, Froberg K, Hyldebrandt N. LV hypertrophy in children from the upper five percent of the BP distribution. The Odense school child study. J Hum Hypertens 1992;10:677–682.
40. Katz S, Hediger ML, Schall JI, et al. Blood pressure growth and maturation through adolescence: mixed longitudinal analyses of the Philadelphia blood pressure project. Hypertension 1980;2(Suppl 1):I-55–I-69.
41. Falkner B, Kushner H, Onesti G, Angelakos ET. Cardiovascular characteristics in adolescents who develop essential hypertension. Hypertens 1981;3:521–527.
42. Lauer RM, Clarke WR. Childhood risk factors for high adult blood pressure: the Muscatine Study. Pediatrs 1989;84:633–641.
43. Cornoni-Huntley J, Lacroix AZ, Havlik RJ. Race and sex differentials in the impact of hypertension in the United States. The National Health and Nutrition Examination Survey I Epidemiologic Follow-up Study. Arch Intern Med 1989;149:780–788.
44. Flack JM, Peters R, Hehra VM, Nasar S. Hypertension in special populations. Cardiology Clinics 2002;20: 303–319.
45. Flack JM, Gardin JM, Yunis C, et al. Static and pulsatile blood pressure correlates of left ventricular structure and function in black and white young adults: the CARDIA study. Am Heart J 1999;138:856–864.
46. Harshfield GA, Alpert BS, Pulliam DA, et al. Ambulatory blood pressure recordings in children and adolescents. Pediatrics 1994:94:180–184.
47. Marcantoni C, Li-Jun M, Federspiel C, Fogo AB. Hypertensive nephrosclerosis in African Americans versus Caucasians. Kidney International 2002;62:172–180.
48. Parmer RJ, Song Q, Kailasam MT, et al. Renal kallikrein excretion is associated with allelic variations in the human tissue kallikren promoter on chromosome 19q families with essential hypertension. Hypertension 1999;34:29A.
49. Cruickshank JK, Jackson SH, Beevers DG, Bannan LT, Beevers M, Stewart VL. Similarity of blood pressure in blacks, whites and Asians in England: the Birmingham Factory Study. J Hypertens 1985;3:365–371.
50. Brunner HR, Laragh JH, Baer L, et al. Essential hypertension: renin and aldosterone, heart attack and stroke. N Engl J Med 1972;286:441–449.
51. Kilcoyne MM. Adolescent hypertension: II. Characteristics and response to treatment. Circulation 1974;50:1014–1019.

52. Gruskin AB, Perlman S, Prebis J, et al. Primary hypertension in the adolescent: facts and unresolved issues. In: Loggie JMH, Hohn AR, Gruskin AB, Dunbar JB, Havlik RJ, eds. Proceedings of the NHLBI Workshop on Juvenile Hypertension. New York: Biomedical Information Corporation, 1984;305–333.
53. Prebis JW, Gruskin AB, Polinsky MS, et al. Uric acid in childhood essential hypertension. J Pediatr 1981;98:702–707.
54. Perlman SA, Prebis JW, Gruskin AB, et al. Calcium homeostasis in adolescents with essential hypertension. Semin Nephrol 1983;3:149–158.
55. Mansoor GA, White WB. White-Coat Hypertension. In: Oparil S, Weber MA, eds. Hypertension: A Companion to Brenner & Rector's The Kidney. Philadelphia: WB Saunders, 2000;314–321.
56. Staessen JA, Byttebier G, Buntinx F, et al. Anthihypertensive treatment based on conventional or ambulatory blood pressure measurement: a randomized controlled trial. JAMA 1997;278:1065–1072.
57. Perloff D, Sokolow M, Cowan RM, Juster RP. Prognostic value of ambulatory blood pressure measurements: further analyses. J Hypertens 1989;7(Suppl 3):S3–S10.
58. Verdecchia P, Porcellati C, Schillaci G, et al. Ambulatory blood pressure: an independent predictor of prognosis in essential hypertension. Hypertension 1994;24:793–801.
59. Weber MA, Neutel JM, Smith DHG, Graettinger WF. Diagnosis of mild hypertension by ambulatory blood pressure monitoring. Circulation 1994;90:2291–2298.
60. Nalbantgil I, Onder R, Nalbantgil S, et al. The prevalence of silent myocardial ischaemia in patients with white-coat hypertension. J Hum Hypertens 1998;12:337–341.
61. Hornsby JL, Mongan PF, Taylor AT, Treiber FA. "White coat" hypertension in children. J Fam Pract 1991:33:617–623.
62. Sorof JM, Poffenbarger T, Franco K, Portman R. Evaluation of white coat hypertension in children: importance of the definitions of normal ambulatory blood pressure and the severity of casual hypertension. Am J Hypertens 2001;14:855–860.
63. Vaindirlis I, Peppa-Patrikiou M, Dracopoulou M, et al. "White coat hypertension" in adolescents: increased of urinary cortisol and endothelin. J Pediatr 2000;136:359–364.
64. Baker DJP, Winter PD, Osmond C, et al. Weight in infancy and death from ischemic heart disease. Lancet 1989;2:577–580.
65. Law CM, deSwiet M, Osmond C, et al. Initiation of hypertension in utero and its amplification throughout life. Br Med J 1993;306:24–27.
66. Benediktsson R, Lindsay RS, Noble J, et al. Glucocorticoid exposure in utero: new model for adult hypertension. Lancet 1993;341:339–341.
67. Woods LL. Fetal origins of adult hypertension: a renal mechanism? Curr Opin Nephrol Hy 2000;9:419–425.
68. Rahiala E, Sirpa T, Vanninine E. Ambulatory blood pressure in 12 year old children born small for gestational age. Hypertension 2002;39:909–913.
69. Gutin B, Basch C, Shea S, et al. Blood pressure, fitness and fatness in 5 and 6 year old children. JAMA. 1990;264:1123–1127.
70. Clark W, Woolson R, Lauer R. Changes in ponderosity and blood pressure in childhood: the Muscatine Study. Am J Epidemiol 1986;124:195–206.
71. Khoury P, Morrison JA, Mellies MJ, Glueck CJ. Weight change since age 18 years in 30- to 55-year whites and blacks: associations with lipid values, lipoprotein levels and blood pressure. JAMA 1983;250:3179–3187.
72. Shear CL, Freedman DS, Burke GL, et al. Body fat patterning and blood pressure in children and young adults. the Bogalusa heart study. Hypertension 1987;9:236–244.
73. Batisky DL, Robinson RF, Nahata MC, et al. Significance of body mass index in primary and secondary pediatric hypertension. Pediatr Res 2002;21:431A.
74. Hellmich N. Sedentary kids called to action. USA Today 7/17/2002;p6D.
75. Sorof JM, Bernard L, Franco K, Portman RJ. The relationship between hypertension and obesity in children is characterized by a hyperkinetic hemodynamic state. Pediatr Res 2002;21:431A.
76. National Health and Nutrition Examination Survey (NHANES) III (2001). Prevalence of overweight among children and adolescents: United States, 1999. Retrieved July 18, 2001 from the Centers for Disease Control website: http:/www.cdc.gov/nchs/products/pubs/pubd/hestats/overwght99.htm.
77. Pollan M. When a crop becomes king. New York Times Editorial/Op-Ed July 19, 2002.
78. Kenchaiah S, Evans JC, Levy D, et al. Obesity and the risk of heart failure. N Engl J Med 2002;347:305–312.
79. Adelman RD, Restaino IG, Alon US, Blowey DL. Proteinuria and focal segmental glomerulosclerosis in severely obese adolescents. J Pediatr 2001;138:481–485.

80. Gipson D, Szuch CL, Moore C, et al. Obesity and focal segmental glomerulosclerosis in children. Pediatr Res 2002;21:429A.
81. Katz SH, Soffer B, Hediger ML, Zemel BS, Parks JS. Blood pressure, body fat, and dehydroepiandrosterone sulfate variation in adolescence. Hypertension 1986;8:277–284.
82. Rocchini AP, Katch VL, Grekin R, Moorehead C, Anderson J. Role for aldosterone in blood pressure regulation of obese adolescents. Am J Cardiol 1986;57:613–618.
83. Felitti VJ. Childhood sexual abuse, depression, and family dysfunction in adult obese patients: a case control study. South Med J 1993;86:732–736.
84. Eaton SB, Konner M, Shostak M. Stone agers in the fast lane-chronic degenerative diseases in evolutionary perspective. Amer J Med 1988;84:739–749.
85. Hofman A, Hazebroek A, Valkenburg HA. A randomized trial of sodium intake and blood pressure in newborn infants. JAMA 1983;250:370–373.
86. Gelenijnse JM, Grobbee DE, Hofman A. Sodium and potassium intake and blood pressure change in childhood. Br Med J 1990;300:899–902.
87. Sinaiko AR, Gomez-Marin O, Prineus RJ. Effect of low sodium diet or potassium supplementation on adolescent blood pressure. Hypertens 1993;21:989–994.
88. McCarron DA, Morris DA, Cole C. Dietary calcium in human hypertension. Science 1982;217:267–269.
89. Wilson SL, Gaffney FA, Laird WP, Fixler DE. Body size, composition, and fitness in adolescents. Hypertension 1985;7:417–422.
90. Jung FF, Ingelfinger JR. Hypertension in childhood and adolescence. Pediatrics in Review 1993;14:169–179.
91. Levy RL, Hillman CC, Stroud WD, White PD. Transient hypertension; its significance in terms of later development of sustained hypertension and cardiovascular disease. JAMA 1944;126:829–833.
92. Berenson GS, Mcmann CA, Voors AW, et al. Cardiovascular Risk Factors in Children: The Early Natural History of Atherosclerosis and Essential Hypertension. New York: Oxford University Press, 1990.
93. Ward R. Familial aggregation and genetic epidemiology of blood pressure. In: Laragh J, Brenner B, eds. Hypertension-Pathophysiology, Diagnosis and Management. New York: Raven, 1990;81–100.
94. Christian JC. Twin Studies of Blood Pressure in Children's Blood Pressure 1985. Report of the 85th Ross Conference on Pediatric Research 1985;51–55.
95. Feinleib M, Garrison R, Borhani N, et al. Studies of hypertension in twins, In: Paul O, ed. Epidemiology and Control of Hypertension. New York: Stratton Intercontinental Medical Book Corp, 1975;3–20.
96. Mongeau JG, Biron P, Sing CF. The influence of genetics and household environment on the variability of normal blood pressure: The Montreal Adoption Survey. In: Children's Blood Pressure. Report of the 85th Ross Conference on Pediatric Research. 1985;55–62.
97. Annest JL, Sing CF, Biron P, Mongeau JG. Familial aggregation of blood pressure and weight in adoptive families. II Estimation of the relative contributions of genetic and common environmental factors to blood pressure correlations between family members. Am J Epidemiol 1979;110:492–503.
98. Miyao S, Furusho T. Genetic study of essential hypertension. Jpn Circ J 1978;42:1161–1186.
99. Cassimos CHR, Aivazis V, Karamperis S, et al. Aterial blood pressure lipids and cardiovascular complications in families of hypertensive children. Acta Páediatr Scand 1982;71:235–238.
100. van Essen GG, Rensma PL, de Zeeuw D, et al. Association between angiotensin-converting-enzyme gene polymorphism and failure of renoprotective therapy. Lancet 1996;347;94–95.
101. Castellano M, Muiesan ML, Beschi M, et al. Angiotensin II type 1 receptor A/C-1166 polymorphism—relationship with blood pressure and cardiovascular structure. Hypertension 1996;28:1076–1080.
102. Smithies O, Hyung-Suk K, Nobuyuki T, Edgell, MH. Importance of quantitative genetic variations in the etiology of hypertension. Kidney Int 2000;58:2265–2280.
103. Weinberger MH, Miller JZ, Fineberg NS, Luft FC, Grim CE, Christian JC. Association of haptoglobin with sodium sensitivity and resistance of blood pressure. Hypertension 1987;10:443–446.
104. Barlassina C, Norton GR, Samani NJ, et al. Alpha-adducin polymorphism in hypertensives of South African ancestry. Am J Hypertens 2000;13:719–723.
105. Bray MS, Li L, Turner ST, Kardia SL, Boerwinkle E. Association and linkage analysis of the alpha-adducin gene and blood pressure. Am J Hypertens 2000;13:699–703.
106. Psaty BM, Smith NL, Heckbert SR, et al. Diuretic therapy, the α-adducin gene variant, and the risk of myocardial infarction or stroke in persons with treated hypertension. JAMA 2002:287;1680–1689.
107. Baker FH, Dong YB, Sagnella GA, et al. Association of hypertension with T594M mutation in β subunit of epithelial sodium channels in black people resident in London. Lancet 1998;351:1388–1392.

108. Poch E, Gonzalez D, Giner V, et al. Molecular basis of salt sensitivity in human hypertension: evaluation of renin-angiotensin-aldosterone system gene polymorphisms. Hypertension 2001;38:1204–1209.
109. Frank GH, Frohlich ED, Grim C, et al. Recommendations for human blood pressure determination by sphygmomanometers: report of a special task force appointed by the Steering Committee, American Heart Association. Hypertension 1988;11:210A–222A.
110. Hyndman ME, Parson HG, Verma S, et al. Mutation in endothelial nitric oxide synthase is associated with hypertension. Hypertension 2002;39:919–922.
111. Curtis JJ, Luke RG, Dustan HP, et al. Remission of essential hypertension after renal transplantation. N Engl J Med 1983;309:1009–1015.
112. Churchill PC, Churchill MC, Bidani AK, Kurtz TW. Kidney specific chromosome transfer in genetic hypertension: the Dahl hypothesis revisited. Kidney Int 2001;60:705–714.
113. Potter JF, Beevers DG. The possible mechanisms of alcohol associated hypertension. Ann Clin Res 1985;27:97–102.
114. Leor J, Poole WK, Kloner RA. Sudden cardiac death triggered by an earthquake. N Eng J Med 1996;334:413–419.
115. Timio M, Lippi G, Venanzi S, et al. Blood pressure trend and cardiovascular events in nuns in a secluded order: a 30-year follow up study. Blood Pressure 1997;6:81–87.
116. Southard DR, Coates TJ. Kolodner relationship between mood and blood pressure in natural environment: andolescent population. Health Psychol 1986;5:469–480.
117. Siegel J, Matthews KA, Leitch CJ. Blood pressure variability and the type A behavior pattern in adolescence. J Psychosom Res 1983;27:265–272.
118. Pickering TG. Psychosocial stress and hypertension: clinical and experimental evidence. In: Swales JD ed. Textbook of Hypertension. Oxford: Blackwell Scientific, 1994;640–654.
119. Cook NB, Cohen J, Herbert J, et al. Implications of small reductions in diastolic blood pressure for primary prevention. Arch Intern Med 1995;155:701–709.
120. Whelton PK, He J, Appel L, et al. Primary prevention of hypertension: clinical and public health advisory from the national high blood pressure education program. JAMA 2002:288:1882–1888.
121. Cutler JA, Follman D, Allender PS. Randomized trials of sodium reduction: an overview. Am J Clin Nutri 1997:65(Suppl 2):643S–651S.
122. Van Brummelen P, Schalekamp M, Graeff J. Influence of sodium intake on hydrochlorothiazide-induced charges in blood pressure serum electrolytes, rennin and aldosterone in essential hypertension. Acta Med Scand 1978;204:151–157.
123. Ellison RC, Capper AL, Goldberg RJ, et al. The environmental component: changing school food service to promote cardiovascular health. Health Educ Q 1989;16:285–297.
124. Gillman MW, Oliveria SA, Moore LL, Ellison RC. Inverse association of dietary calcium with systolic blood pressure. JAMA 1992;267:2340–2343.
125. John JH, Ziebland S, Yudkin P, et al. Effects of fruit and vegetable consumption on plasma antioxidant concentrations and blood pressure: a randomized controlled study. Lancet 2002;359:1969–1974.
126. Rocchini AP. Adolescent obesity and hypertension. Pediatr Clin North Am 1993;40:81–92.
127. Rocchini AP, Katch VK, Anderson JA, et al. Blood pressure in obese adolescents: effects of weight loss. Pediatrics 1988;82:16–23.
128. Barlow SE, Trowbridge FL, Klish WJ, Dietz WH. Treatment of child and adolescent obesity: reports from pediatricians, pediatric nurse practitioners, and registered dietitians. Pediatrics 2002;110:229–235.
129. Epstein LH, Valoski A, Wing RR, McCurley J. Ten-year outcomes of behavioral family-based treatment for childhood obesity. Health Pyschol 1994;13:373–383.
130. Israel AC, Stolmaker L, Andrian CAG. The effects of training parents in general child management skills on a behavioral weight loss program for children. Behav Ther 1985;16:169–180.
131. Robinson TN. Reducing children's television viewing to prevent obesity: a randomized controlled trial. JAMA 1999;282:1561–1567.
132. Roberts SB, Savage J, Coward WA, et al. Energy expenditure and intake in infants born to lean and overweight mothers. N Engl J Med 1988;318:461–466.
133. Whitaker RC, Wright JA, Pepe MS, et al. Predicting obesity in young adulthood from childhood and parental obesity. N Engl J Med 1997;337:869–873.
134. Rocchini AP, Katch V, Schork, A, Kelch RP. Insulin and blood pressure during weight loss in obese adolescents. Hypertension 1987;10:267–273.

135. Mitchell BM, Gutin B, Kapuku G, et al. Left ventricular structure and function in obese adolescents: relations to cardiovascular fitness, percent body fat, and visceral adiposity, and effects of physical training. Pediatrics 2002;109(5):E73.
136. Falkner B, Thanki BH. Effect of hospitalization versus placebo in hypertensive adolescents. J Adoles Health Care 1982;3:173–176.
137. Gruskin A, Dabbagh S, Fleischmann LE, Bassam AA. Application since 1980 of anti-hypertensive agents to treat pediatric disease. J Hum Hypertens 1984;8:381–388.
138. Shahinfar S, Rippley R, Hogg RJ, et al. Multicenter study of enalapril pharmacokinetics in hypertensive children and infants. Pediatr Res 2000;47:473A.
139. Wells T, Frame V, Soffer B, et al. (Enalapril Pediatric Hypertension Collaborative Study Group). A double-blind, placebo-controlled, dose–response study of the effectiveness and safety of enalapril for children with hypertension. J Clin Pharmacol 2002;42(8):870–880.
140. Shaw W, Hogg R, Delucchi A, et al. Multicenter study of lisinopril (L) pharmacokinetics (PK) in hypertensive children and infants. Pediatr Res 2002;215:431A.
141. Sorof JM, Cargo P, Graepel J, et al. β-Blocker/thiazide combination for treatment of hypertensive children: a randomized double-blind, placebo-controlled trail. Pediatr Nephrol 2002;17:345–350.
142. Berenson GS, Shear CL, Chiang YK et al. Combined low dose medication and primary intervention over a 30 month period for sustained high blood pressure in childhood. Am J Med Sci 1990;299:79–86.
143. Falkner B, Onesti G, Affrime MB, Lowenthal DT. Effects of clonidine and hydrochlorothiazide on the cardiovascular response to mental stress in adolescent hypertension. Clin Sci 1982;63:455–458.
144. Tallian KB, Nahata MC, Turman MA, et al. Efficacy of amlodipine in pediatric patients with hypertension. Pediatr Nephrol 1999;13:304–310.
145. Robinson RF, Parker M, Nahata MC, et al. The role of amlodipine in primary and secondary hypertension. Pediatr Res 2001;49:426A.
146. Flynn JT, Hogg RJ, Portman RJ, et al. Multicenter trials of amlodipine (AML) in children with hypertension (HTN). Pediatr Res 2002;21:430A.
147. Flynn JT, Smoyer WE, Bunchman TE. Treatment of hypertension children with amlodipine. Am J Hypertens 2000;13:1061–1066.
148. Johnson CE, Jacobson PA, Song MH. Isradipine therapy in hypertensive pediatric patients. Ann Pharmacother 1997;31:704–707.
149. Flynn JT, Kershaw DB, Sedman AB, et al. Efficacy of isradipine as an anti-hypertensive agent in children. Pediatr Res 1998;43:307A.
150. Flynn JT, Warnick SJ. Isradipine treatment of hypertension: a single center experience. Pediatr Neph 2002;17:748–753.
151. Walson PD, Graves P, Rath A, et al. Effects of guanabenz in adolescent hypertension. J Cardiovasc Pharmacol 1984;6:S814–S817.
152. Stier CT, Jr. Eplerenone, a selective aldosterone blocker. Cardiovascular Drug Rev 2003;21(3):169–184.
153. Bakris GL, Weir MR. Angiotensin-converting enzyme inhibitor-associated elevations in serum creatinine: is this cause for concern? Arch Int Med 2001;160:685–693.
154. Palmer BF. Current concepts: renal dysfunction complicating anti-hypertensive thereapy. N Eng J Med 2002;347:1256–1261.
155. Falkner B, Hamstra B, Lombardo R, et al. Blood pressure variability in adolescent males. Int J Ped Neph 1981;2:177.
156. Katz SH, Heidiger ML, Schall JI, et al. Blood pressure, growth and maturation from childhood through adolescence. Hypertension 1980;2:55–69.
157. Lauer RM, Clarke WR. Childhood risk factors for high adult blood pressure: the Muscatine Study. Pediatrics 1989;84:633–641.
158. van Hoft IMS, Grobbee DE, Frolich M, et al. Alterations in calcium metabolism in young people at risk for primary hypertension. The Dutch Hypertension and Offspring Study. Hypertension 1993;21:267–272.
159. Ravogli A, Trazzi S, Villani A, et al. Early 24-hour blood pressure elevation in normotensive subjects with parental hypertension. Hypertension 1990;16:491–497.
160. van Hooft IM, Grobbee DE, Waal Manning HJ, Hofman A. Twenty-four-hour ambulatory blood pressure pattern in youngsters with a different family history of hypertension: the Dutch Hypertension and Offspring Study. J Hypertens Suppl 1989;7:66–67.

161. Radice M, Alli C, Avanzini F, et al. Left ventricular structure and function in normotensive adolescents with a genetic predisposition to hypertension. Am Heart J 1986;111:115–120.
162. Shibutani Y, Sakamoto K, Katsuno S, et al. An epidemiological study of plasma rennin activity in schoolchildren in Japan: distribution and its relation with family history of hypertension. J Hypertens 1988;6:489–493.
163. Grunfeld B, Perelstein E, Simsolo R, et al. Renal functional reserve and microalbuminuria in offspring of hypertensive parents. Hypertension 1990;15:257–261.
164. Shear CL, Burke GL, Freedman DS, Berenson G. Value of childhood blood pressure measurements and family history in predicting future blood pressure status: results from 8 years of follow-up in the Bogalusa heart study. Pediatrics 1986;77:862–869.
165. Bianchi G, Cusi D, Guidi E, Renal hemodynamics in human subjects and in animals with genetic hypertension during the prehypertensive stage. Am J Nephrol 1983;3:73–79.
166. Canessa M, Adragna N, Solomon HS, et al. Increased sodium lithium countertransport in red cells of patients with essential hypertension. N Engl J Med 1980;302:772–776.
167. Liberman E. Hypertension in childhood and adolescence. In: Kaplan NM, Lieberman E, eds. Clinical Hypertension. Baltimore: Williams and Wilkins, 1994;437–462.
168. Kristjansson K, Manolescu A, Kristinsson A. Linkage of essential hypertension to chromosome 18q. Hypertens 2002;39:1044–1049.
169. Timberlake DS, O'Connor DT, Palmer RJ. Molecular genetics of essential hypertension: recent results and emerging strategies. Current Opin Nephrol Hy 2001;10:713–779.
170. Falkner B, Lowenthal DT, Affrime MB. The pharmacodynamic effectiveness of metoprolol in adolescent hypertension. Pediatr Pharmacol 1982;2:49–55.
171. Wells TG, Sinaiko AR. Anti-hypertensive effect and pharmacokinetics of nitrendipine in children. J Pediatr 1991;118:638–643.

# 11 Sequelae of Hypertension in Children and Adolescents

*Stephen R. Daniels*, MD, PhD

*CONTENTS*



## INTRODUCTION

Blood pressure (BP) elevation is one of the most important risk factors for cardiovascular disease in adults. It has been estimated that the adverse effects of hypertension (HTN) result in a cost of more than $14 billion for the US health care system annually *(1)*. In adults, the outcomes associated with HTN include cerebrovascular disease, atherosclerotic coronary heart disease, renal failure, and congestive heart failure. All of these could result in substantial morbidity and, ultimately, mortality *(2)*.

Treatment of BP elevation in adults has been clearly shown to reduce the risk of adverse outcomes. The first study to demonstrate this was the Veterans Administration Cooperatives Study *(3)*. More recently, the Treatment of Mild Hypertension Study (TOMHS) showed a 33% reduction of cardiovascular events in subjects treated over 4 yr with a combination of lifestyle modification and pharmacologic treatment, compared to those treated with lifestyle modification alone *(4)*.

## ADVERSE OUTCOMES IN CHILDREN AND ADOLESCENTS

### *Severe Hypertension*

It has long been known that acute severe HTN in children is associated with important morbidity and mortality. The sequelae of severe HTN in pediatric patients includes hyperten-

From: *Clinical Hypertension and Vascular Disease: Pediatric Hypertension*
Edited by: R. J. Portman, J. M. Sorof, and J. R. Ingelfinger © Humana Press Inc., Totowa, NJ

sive encephalopathy, cerebrovascular accident, seizures, and hemiplegia. In 1967, Still and Cottom reported that 18% of children who presented with severe HTN had neurologic complications *(5)*. In 1976, Gill et al. reported that 11% of children with severe HTN had seizures *(6)*. Although these children are candidates for serious problems, prompt recognition and treatment of severe HTN can result in a good outcome. Trompeter et al. reported that the prognosis for children with a single episode of hypertensive encephalopathy was quite good. Long-term follow up showed no significant differences in neurocognitive testing when compared to a control group of children with chronic renal disease *(7)*.

Most severe HTN in children and adolescents results from secondary forms of HTN, such as glomerulonephritis and renal artery stenosis. These forms of HTN are relatively uncommon, particularly for older children and adolescents. Although these are severe forms of HTN, complications at presentation are not uniform. Watson et al. found 9 of 17 patients with renovascular HTN to be asymptomatic at presentation *(8)*, whereas Daniels et al. found 22 of 27 patients had no symptoms *(9)*. In addition to the more severe complications of severe HTN, children may have milder symptoms, such as headaches, anorexia, and transient growth failure.

## HYPERTENSION AND ADVERSE OUTCOMES IN END-STAGE RENAL DISEASE

Blood pressure elevation may also contribute to adverse outcomes in the presence of other chronic diseases. One example of this is end-stage renal disease (ESRD). Cardiac complications are common in adults with chronic renal disease, on dialysis, or after renal transplantation. Cardiovascular disease has become the most common cause of mortality in this population *(10,11)*.

More recent studies have also demonstrated that cardiac abnormalities occur frequently in children with chronic renal insufficiency. Children with chronic renal disease have been shown to have abnormalities of both left ventricular (LV) structure and function, including a high prevalence of left ventricular hypertrophy (LVH) *(12,13)*. While there are numerous potential mechanisms for the development of LVH, it is likely that chronic volume and pressure overload are important factors. In adults, Levin et al. showed that anemia and HTN were independent predictors of increased LV mass for individuals with renal insufficiency prior to dialysis *(14)*. In a study of children, Johnstone et al. evaluated 32 patients aged 1.5–17 yr with chronic renal insufficiency *(15)*. LV mass was significantly correlated with the level of serum creatinine and systolic BP.

Increased LV mass may be adaptive in the short term. However, Mitsnefes et al. have shown that pediatric patients on dialysis have blunted contractile reserve demonstrated on exercise testing *(15a)*. This suggests that the LVH may be beneficial at rest as it normalizes LV performance. However, the ability to adapt to exercise is limited. Similar results have also been found in adults. Fontanet et al. showed that hypertensive adults with LVH had limited myocardial contractile reserve when tested with dobutamine stress echocardiography *(16)*.

As a result, BP elevation appears to contribute to the physiologic processes by which renal insufficiency may result in cardiovascular abnormalities and, ultimately, morbidity and mortality. Future studies focused on aggressive control of BP elevation are needed to determine if these processes can be interrupted and the prognosis improved.

## LESS-SEVERE HYPERTENSION

The most prevalent form of BP elevation in children and adolescents is primary HTN. Primary HTN in childhood is often associated with obesity and a family history of HTN. In this population, BP elevation may occur in combination with other abnormalities, such as insulin resistance and lipid and lipoprotein abnormalities *(17)*. BP levels in pediatric primary HTN are often mildly to moderately elevated, but are not markedly elevated. In addition, the BP elevation in primary HTN is more chronic than acute.

Clearly, primary HTN in young individuals is usually not associated with a risk of immediate and clinically apparent adverse outcomes. However, it is known that BP elevation that begins in childhood is likely to result in ongoing BP elevation into adulthood. As we learn more about the adverse effects of primary HTN in children, it is becoming clearer that it is not a benign condition, even in the short term. Primary HTN may affect the heart, kidney, retinal vasculature, and other target organs. Subsequent sections will deal with abnormalities in these organ systems related to BP elevation.

### *Blood Vessels*

Abnormalities in arterial structure and function related to HTN are important because they underlie many of the adverse effects of HTN in a variety of organ systems. HTN may result in abnormalities to blood vessels in a number of ways. Elevated BP may result in increased wall tension. This may cause endothelial dysfunction. It may also result in arterial smooth muscle hyperplasia and hypertrophy. This process involves increased synthesis of protein, collagen, and elastin. It can result in increased fibromuscular thickening of the intima and media of small, medium, and large sized arteries *(18,19)*.

Vascular ultrasound has provided a way to noninvasively study vascular changes in children and adolescents. Ultrasound can be used to evaluate the carotid artery's intimal-medial thickness (IMT). In adults, this method has gained acceptance as a way to evaluate the degree of development of atherosclerosis. For example, carotid IMT has been shown to be associated with incident myocardial infarction and stroke *(20–22)*. The association persists after adjustment for other cardiovascular risk factors. This has led to the use of carotid IMT as an endpoint in clinical trials aimed at preventing cardiovascular disease *(23)*. The ability of carotid IMT to predict cardiovascular events later in life has not been demonstrated in younger adults.

Three case-control studies of young adults with HTN have demonstrated increased carotid IMT, compared to controls, after statistical adjustment for other risk factors *(24–26)*. Other risk factors for cardiovascular disease have also been shown to be associated with increased carotid artery IMT.

There are few data concerning the measurement of IMT of the carotid artery in children and adolescents. In one cross-sectional study of subjects aged 10–24 yr, the mean carotid IMT was $0.50 \pm 0.04$ mm for boys and $0.48 \pm 0.03$ mm for girls *(27)*. Carotid IMT was associated with systolic BP in boys, but there was no association with risk factor levels in girls. In a study of children with type 1 diabetes and hypercholesterolemia, they had increased carotid IMT compared to controls *(28)*. In these patients, diastolic BP was also significantly associated with increased carotid IMT. However, in the Muscatine Study, childhood cholesterol levels were found to be a risk factor for increased carotid IMT measured in young adulthood, but childhood BP levels were not *(29)*.

In a study of young patients with BP elevation, Sorof et al. measured carotid IMT *(30)*. They found that carotid IMT was associated with weight, body mass index (BMI), and LV mass index, but not with weight or age.

Another method used to evaluate vascular abnormalities specifically in the coronary arteries is the measurement of calcium using computed tomography (CT). The deposition of calcium in the coronary arteries is thought to be an important part of the process of atherosclerosis. The presence of calcified lesions in the coronary artery occurs almost exclusively when an atherosclerotic lesion is present. Research evaluating the use of CT to evaluate coronary artery calcium in the clinical setting in adults has shown that it is a reasonably accurate test with good sensitivity and moderate specificity *(31,32)*.

Few studies using CT to evaluate coronary artery calcium have been done in pediatric populations. Gidding et al. studied 29 patients aged 11–23 yr with heterozygous familial hypercholesterolemia *(33)*. Deposits of calcium in the coronary artery were found in 7 of 29 subjects. The presence of calcium deposits was associated with higher BMI, but not with BP elevation. The Muscatine Heart Study evaluated the relationship of risk factor levels in childhood to the presence of coronary artery calcium in young adulthood *(34,35)*. The prevalence of coronary artery calcium in this group of subjects aged 29–37 yr was 30% for males and 13% for females. In young adult males, childhood values for weight, BMI, and triceps skinfold thickness were significantly higher in those with detectable coronary artery calcium. For females, the childhood measures of weight, BMI, and triceps skinfold thickness, as well as systolic and diastolic BP, were higher in those with coronary artery calcium.

These results from studies using noninvasive methodology support the view that elevated BP in childhood is associated with the development of vascular abnormalities. The ideal method to evaluate vascular change is direct pathologic inspection. However, this sort of evaluation can only occur at autopsy. Two studies provide such data—the Bogalusa Heart Study and the Pathobiological Determinants of Atherosclerosis in Youth (PDAY) Study. In the Bogalusa study, autopsies were performed on 204 individuals aged 2–39 yr who died of accidental causes. Of those subjects, 93 had previously participated in epidemiologic studies to assess cardio-vascular risk factors in childhood *(36,37)*. They found that BMI, lipid and lipoprotein concentrations, as well as systolic and diastolic BP, were associated with the presence of fatty streaks and fibrous plaques in the aorta and coronary arteries. Furthermore, the presence of multiple risk factors was associated with even more extensive atherosclerosis.

The PDAY study investigators also evaluated the relationships of risk factors to the extent of development of atherosclerosis in young accident victims who underwent autopsy *(58,59)*. They did not have data on antemortem risk factor levels. Therefore, the PDAY investigators had to estimate BP indirectly from the vascular intimal thickness of renal arteries. When individuals with normal lipids and lipoproteins were studied, hypertensive African-American subjects had more extensive raised lesions in both the coronary arteries and the aorta than African-American subjects without evidence of BP elevation. However, they did not find an association between HTN and raised lesions in white subjects and they did not find an association between HTN and fatty streaks in either African-American or white subjects. It may be that their indirect evaluation of BP produced an imprecise measure, making it more difficult to demonstrate a statistically significant association.

Studies of young subjects using several different methods to assess vascular outcomes have generally shown a direct relationship between BP elevation and vascular abnormalities. The results of the PDAY study may indicate that BP elevation has more of a role in the progression from fatty streaks to raised plaque lesions. However, the results of the Bogalusa study implicate BP elevation in the entire process of atherosclerosis development.

## RETINAL VASCULATURE

Observation of abnormalities in the blood vessels of the retina has been a method by which the effect of HTN on the vasculature has been judged. In adults with HTN, abnormalities of the retinal vasculature have been reported, with severe and acute BP elevation, and with more moderate and chronic BP elevation. It has been observed that, in adults, changes in retinal arteries may reflect both atherosclerotic abnormalities and hypertensive retinopathy. In 1934, Keith, Wagener, and Barker published a method of classifying retinal vascular changes related to the severity of BP elevation *(40)*. Subsequent studies have demonstrated that the grade of abnormality in the retinal vessels is also predictive of mortality *(41)*.

There have been few studies of retinal abnormalities in children and adolescents with BP elevation. Skalina et al. studied newborn infants with HTN *(42)*. They found that approximately one-half of the patients had retinal vascular abnormalities. These abnormalities were similar to those observed in adults with HTN. It is also of interest that most infants were given repeat examinations, and those whose BP elevations were resolved, experienced normalization of retinal vascular abnormalities.

## THE KIDNEYS

The kidney is thought to play a central role in the development of many forms of HTN. For this reason, it has often been difficult to determine the cause and effect relationships between BP elevation and renal abnormalities. An example of this is the approach used to evaluate the effect of HTN on the formation of atherosclerotic disease in the PDAY study *(38,39)*. Because these subjects, who died prematurely, did not have premortem evaluation of cardiovascular risk factors, surrogate markers of risk were developed. To evaluate the presence of elevated BP, an algorithm was used to estimate the mean arterial pressure from the intimal thickness of the renal arteries. This raises the important question of whether these renal arterial lesions developed in response to elevated BP, whether they can be implicated in the pathogenesis of BP elevation, or both.

As early as 1925, Fishberg described a pathologic pattern of renal vascular abnormalities in patients with HTN *(43)*. Subsequently, Tracy confirmed that renal arteriolar lesions are associated with both the duration and severity of HTN *(44)*. It appears that structural changes in the renal vasculature may play a role in the development of HTN, and almost certainly play a role in the maintenance and progression of HTN.

The prevalence of ESRD secondary to HTN in adults appears to be increasing and may account for 25% or more of new patients requiring dialysis in the US. This means that diabetes and HTN are now the two most common courses of ESRD *(45)*. However, the extent to which mild to moderate BP elevation leads to progression of renal abnormalities and ESRD is not known *(46)*. This issue is difficult to resolve because there are no sensitive noninvasive methods available to detect subtle and progressive changes in renal function.

The mechanisms by which mild to moderate HTN might produce clinically important changes in renal function are also not well understood. Possible mechanisms include loss of glomeruli with hyperfiltration in the remaining glomeruli interstitial damage, renal hypertrophy and hyperplasia, and metabolic stress from free radical formation or inflammation *(47)*.

Data from animal studies support these mechanisms, but the relevance to human HTN is not known. Studies of human childhood and adolescent populations are more difficult to conduct than studies of human adults.

Schmieder et al. have suggested that glomerular hyperfiltration is an indicator of the effects of HTN on the kidney *(48)*. They found that a subset of adults with HTN and LVH also had elevation in their glomerular filtration rate, suggesting a more generalized adverse impact of HTN.

Children and adolescents usually do not develop clinically apparent renal abnormalities in response to BP elevation. It remains to be determined, however, if less apparent, but important, renal changes are occurring in children with mild to moderate HTN.

## THE HEART

HTN is an important contributor to the leading causes of death in the US. In adults, a 10 mmHg increase in systolic BP increases the age-adjusted risk of cardiovascular events by 20% at ages 35–64 yr. A 10 mmHg increase in diastolic BP increases risk of cardiovascular events by 13% in this age group *(49)*. In adults, HTN is a risk factor for coronary artery disease, congestive heart failure, and sudden cardiac death. In the Framingham study, the level of BP elevation was associated with increased risk over a follow-up period of 18 yr for coronary heart disease, ischemic stroke, congestive heart failure, and peripheral vascular disease *(50)*. From a cardiac standpoint, the greatest risk, compared to other adverse outcomes, is that of congestive heart failure associated with HTN.

Some cardiovascular endpoints related to HTN appear to be mediated by the development of LVH. HTN in adults has been associated with increased LV mass *(51–53)*. LVH is an end organ effect of high BP. However, a constellation of risk factors including obesity and BP elevation contribute to LVH. In turn, LVH is an independent risk factor for the development of cardiovascular disease *(53)*.

Normally, the left ventricle of the heart grows from birth into adulthood. Cellular hypertrophy, rather than hyperplasia, is the major mechanism in this growth stage *(54)*. Abnormal increases in LV mass may occur in response to pathologic changes in hemodynamics. The left ventricle may be affected by both changes in volume and pressure. Alterations in volume affect the cardiac output (CO) and stroke volume through the increased size of the LV chamber *(55,56)*. Two factors in the pathogenesis of essential HTN, obesity and increased dietary intake of sodium, affect the stroke volume. Conversely, increased afterload results in increased pressure through increased peripheral vascular resistance. These changes may result in increased wall stress of the left ventricle and, ultimately, increased thickness of the LV myocardium, as well as increased LV mass *(57)*. Relative changes in volume and pressure status produce an alteration of LV geometry. The geometry of the left ventricle is usually divided into four categories: normal, concentric remodeling (normal LV mass, increased relative wall thickness), concentric hypertrophy (increased LV mass and relative wall thickness), and eccentric hypertrophy (increased LV mass, normal relative wall thickness) *(58)*. Of these geometric patterns, concentric hypertrophy is associated with the highest risk of cardiovascular disease in adults *(58)*.

In adults with HTN, LVH has been found to be present in 20%–60% of patients *(59,60)*. In severe HTN, the prevalence of LVH may be as high as 90% *(55)*. LVH is well known to predict morbidity and mortality in adults with HTN. DeSimone et al. have shown that a LV mass index greater than 51 $g/m^{2.7}$ is associated with a fourfold increase in risk of adverse cardiovascular events in adults with HTN *(61)*. In the Framingham heart study, LV mass and age were strong and consistent predictors of all cause mortality, cardiac death, and coronary heart disease events in adults over age 40 yr *(53)*.

The mechanism by which LVH increases the risk of cardiovascular disease is not specifically known. We know, however, that LVH increases the myocardial oxygen requirement, which may make the heart more vulnerable to ischemia *(62)*. A second mechanism by which LVH may be problematic is the development of abnormalities of diastolic function. When the left ventricle is hypertrophied it may not fill as effectively because the ventricle becomes stiffer and less compliant. Diastolic functional abnormalities may develop into systolic functional problems *(63)*. A third mechanism by which LVH may increase the risk of cardiovascular disease is by induction of electrophysiologic abnormalities *(64)*. Consequently, patients with LVH may be at higher risk for arrhythmias and sudden death.

A number of studies have investigated the relationship of BP and LV mass in children and adolescents. Burke et al. reported data from the Bogalusa Heart Study *(65)*. They found that LV wall thickness was associated with the level of systolic BP. Malcolm et al. also found a strong direct association between LV mass and both systolic and diastolic BP in the Muscatine Study *(66)*. Daniels et al. evaluated correlates of LV mass in a group of 201 normotensive subjects aged 6–17 yr *(67)*. They reported that both systolic and diastolic BP were univariate correlates of LV mass. In a multiple regression analysis, lean body mass, fat mass, and systolic BP were significant independent correlates of LV mass.

The previous studies evaluated relationships in normal children. Treiber et al. studied children with a family history of HTN *(68)*. They found that significant correlates of LV mass index included systolic, but not diastolic, BP.

Other pediatric investigations have focused on the prevalence and correlates of LVH in children and adolescents with BP elevation. Belsha et al. found a prevalence of LVH of 34% in 29 untreated adolescents with mild BP elevation *(69)*. Significant correlates of LV mass index were casual systolic and diastolic BP, 24 h, daytime, and sleep systolic BP. Sorof et al. found a prevalence of 38% of LVH in 115 children undergoing evaluation for HTN *(70)*. This is striking because it indicated that LVH may occur early in the course of HTN in young individuals. In this study patients with LVH were more overweight than those without hypertrophy. Chamontin et al. studied 49 young adults with a history of childhood HTN *(71)*. They found that daytime systolic BP was associated with LV mass index. Daniels et al. studied 130 young patients with persistent elevation of BP *(72)*. They found that 55% of the patients with chronic elevation of BP had a LV mass index above the 90th percentile, while 14% had LV mass above the cutpoint of 51 $g/m^{2.7}$, which is associated with a fourfold increased risk of cardiovascular outcomes in adults with HTN *(61)*. They found that of the 61 patients with LV mass greater than the 95th percentile, 22 had concentric hypertrophy and 39 had eccentric hypertrophy. An additional 12 patients had concentric remodeling *(72)*.

In adults, left atrial enlargement has also been associated with cardiovascular disease. In the Framingham study, Benjamin et al. found that left atrial enlargement was associated with an increased risk of stroke in men, and in mortality in both sexes after multivariable adjustment *(73)*. Daniels et al. evaluated children and adolescents with an average age of 14.2 yr and with essential HTN *(74)*. They found that approximately half of the patients had left atrial size greater than the 95th percentile. In multiple regression analysis, weight, BMI, systolic BP, and LV geometry were significant independent predictors of left atrial size. These results indicate that left atrial enlargement is prevalent in children and adolescents with essential HTN.

## SUMMARY

It is clear that BP elevation has a major impact on a variety of organ systems in young patients. Previously, much of the rationale for aggressively treating BP elevation in children was based on the concept that children with high BP were likely to become adults with high BP. While the concept of tracking remains important, it is also significant that early abnormalities in the cardiovascular system and the kidneys can be attributed to BP elevation. This further strengthens the position that BP elevation in children and adolescents is not innocuous. Children with elevated BP must be identified early in the course of the disease and treated appropriately.

Further studies are needed to document the specific effects of treatment of BP on various outcomes. This will strengthen the base of evidence and provide important information about the best timing of treatment and the levels of BP necessary to achieve to ameliorate target organ abnormalities.

## REFERENCES

1. Fernandes E, McCrindle BW. Diagnosis and treatment of hypertension in children and adolescents. Can J Cardiol 2000;16:801–811.
2. MacMahon S, Peto R, Cutler J, et al. Blood pressure, stroke and coronary heart disease. I. Prolonged differences in blood pressure—prospective observational studies corrected for the regression dilution bias. Lancet 1990;335:764–774.
3. Veterans Administration Cooperative Study Group on Antihypertensive Agents: effects of treatment on morbidity in hypertension. Results in patients with diastolic blood pressures averaging 115 through 129 mmHg. JAMA 1967;202:116–122.
4. Neaton JD, Grimm RH Jr, Prineas RJ, et al. Treatment of mind hypertension study. Final results. JAMA 1993;270:713–724.
5. Still JL, Cottom DG. Severe hypertension in childhood. Arch Dis Child 1967;42:34–39.
6. Gill DG, Mendes da Costa B, Cameron JS, Joseph MC, Ogg CS, Chantler C. Analysis of 100 children with severe and persistent hypertension. Arch Dis Child 1976;51:951–956.
7. Trompeter RS, Smith RL, Hoare RD, Neville BGR, Chantler C. Neurological complications of arterial hypertension. Arch Dis Child 1982;57:913–917.
8. Watson AR, Balfe JW, Hardy BE. Renovascular hypertension in childhood: a changing perspective in management. J Ped 1985;106:366–372.
9. Daniels SR, Loggie JMH, McEnery PT, Towbin RB. Clinical spectrum of intrinsic renovascular hypertension in children. Pediatrics 1987;80:698–704.
10. The USRD 1998 Annual Report. Causes of death. Am J Kidney Dis Suppl 1998;1:S81–S88.
11. Foley RN, Palfrey PS, Sarnak MJ. Clinical epidemilogy of cardiovascular disease in chronic renal disease. Am J Kidney Dis Suppl 1998;3:S112–S119.
12. Mitsnefes MM, Daniels SR, Schwartz SM, Meyer RA, Khoury P, Strife CE. Severe left ventricular hypertrophy in pediatric dialysis: prevalence and predictors. Pediatr Nephrol 2000;14:898–902.
13. Mitsnefes, MM, Daniels SR, Schwartz SM, Khoury P, Strife CF. Changes in left ventricular mass in children and adolescents during chronic dialysis. Pediatr Nephrol 200;16:318–323.
14. Levin A, Singer J, Thompson CR, Ross H, Lewis M. Prevalent left ventricular hypertrophy in the predialysis population: identifying opportunities for intervention. Am J Kidney Dis 1996;27:347–354.
15. Johnstone LM, Jones CL, Grigg LE, Wilkinson JL, Walker RG, Powell HR. Left ventricular abnormalities in children, adolescents and young adults with renal disease. Kidney Int 1996;50:998–1006.
15a. Mitsnefes MM, Kimball TR, Witt SA, Glascock BJ, Khoury PR, Daniels SR. Left ventricular mass and systolic performance in pediatric patients with chronic renal failure. Circulation 2003;107(6):864–868.
16. Fontanet HL, Perez JE, Davila-Roman VG. Diminished contractile reserve in patients with left ventricular hypertrophy and increased end-systolic stress during dobutamine stress echocardiography. Am J Cardiol 1996;78:1029–1035.
17. Sorof JM, Daniels SR. Obesity hypertension in children: a problem of epidemic proportions. Hypertension 2002;40:441–447.

18. Hollander W. Role of hypertension in atherosclerosis and cardiovascular disease. Am J Cardiol 1976;28:786–800.
19. Blackburn WR. Vascular pathology in hypertensive children. In: Loggie JMH, Horan MJ, Gruskin AB, Hohn AR, Dunbar JB, Havlik RJ, eds. NHLBI Workshop on Juvenile Hypertension. New York, NY: Biomedical Information, 1984, 335–364.
20. O'Leary DH, Polak JF, Kronmal RA, Manolio TA, Burke GL, Wolfeson SK. Carotid-artery intima and media thickness as a risk factor for myocardial infarction and stroke in older adults. N Engl J Med 1999;340:14–22.
21. Chambless LE, Heiss G, Folsom AR, et al. Association of coronary heart disease incidence with carotid arterial wall thickness and major risk factors: the Atherosclerosis Risk in Communities (ARIC) Study, 1987–1993. Am J Epidemiol 146:483–494.
22. Chambless LE, Folsom AR, Clegg LX, et al. Carotid wall thickness is predictive of incident clinical stroke. Am J Epidemiol 2000;151:478–487.
23. Lonn EM, Yusuf S, Dzavik V, et al. Effects of ramipril and vitamin E on atherosclerosis. Circulation 2001;103:919–925.
24. Lemne C, Jogestrand T, de Faire U. Carotid intima-media thickness and plaque in borderline hypertension. Stroke 1995;26:34–39.
25. Pauletto P, Palatini P, DaRos S, et al. Factors underlying the increase in carotid intima-media thickness in borderline hypertensives. Arterioscler Thromb Vasc Biol 1999;19:1231–1237.
26. Lonati L, Cuspidi C, Sampieri L, et al. Ultrasonographic evaluation of cardiac and vascular changes in young borderline hypertensives. Cardiology 1993;83:298–303.
27. Sass C, Herbeth B, Chapet O, Siset G, Visvikis S, Zannad F. Intima-media thickness and diameter of carotid and femoral arteries in children, adolescents and adults from the Stanislas cohort. J Hypertens 1998;16:1593–1603.
28. Jarvisalo MJ, Jartti L, Nanto-Salonen K, et al. Increased aortic intima-media thickness: a marker of preclinical atherosclerosis in high risk children. Circulation 2001;104:2943–2947.
29. Davis PH, Dawson JD, Riley WA, Lauer RM. Carotid intimal-medial thickness is related to cardiovascular risk factors measured from childhood through middle age. Circulation 2001;104:2815–2819.
30. Sorof JM, Alexandrov AV, Cardwell G, Portman RJ. Carotid artery intimal-medial thickness and left ventricular hypertrophy in children with elevated blood pressure. Pediatrics 2003;111:61–66.
31. Mautner GC, Mautner SL, Froehlich J, et al. Coronary artery calcification: assessment with electron beam CT and histomorphometric correlation. Radiology 1994;192:619–623.
32. Nallamothu BK, Saint S, Bielak LF, et al. Electron-beam computed tomography in the diagnosis of coronary artery disease. Arch Intern Med 2001;161:833–838.
33. Gidding SS, Bookstein LC, Chomka, EV. Usefulness of electron beam tomography in adolescents and young adults with heterozygous familial hypercholesterolemia. Circulation 1998;98:2580–2583.
34. Mahoney LT, Burns TL, Stanford W, et al. Usefulness of the Framingham Risk Score and Body Mass Index to predict early coronary artery calcium in young adults (Muscatine Study). Am J Cardiol 2001;88:509–15.
35. Mahoney LT, Burns TL, Stanford W, et al. Coronary risk factors measured in childhood and young adult life are associated with coronary artery calcification in young adults: the Muscatine Study. JACC 1996;27: 277–284.
36. Newman WP III, Freedman DS, Voors AW, et al. Relation of serum lipoprotein levels and systolic blood pressure to early atherosclerosis: the Bogalusa Heart Study. N Engl J Med 1986;314:138–144.
37. Berenson GS, Srinivasan SR, Bao W, Newman WP 3rd, Tracy RE, Wattigney WA. Association between multiple cardiovascular risk factors and atherosclerosis in children and young adults. The Bogalusa Heart Study. N Engl J Med 1998;335:1650–1656.
38. McGill HC Jr, McMahan CA, Tracy RE, et al. Relation of a postmortem renal index of hypertension to atherosclerosis and coronary artery size in young men and women. Arterioscler Thromb Vase Biol 1998;18: 1108–1118.
39. McGill HC Jr, McMahan CA, Zieske AW, Malcom GT, Tracy RE, Strong JP. Effects of nonlipid risk factors on atherosclerosis in youth with a favorable lipoprotein profile. Circulation 2001;103:1546–1550.
40. Keith NM, Wagener HP, Barker NW. Some different types of essential hypertension, their course and prognosis. Am J Med Sci 1939;197:332–343.
41. Svardsudd K, Wedel H, Aurell E, Tibblin G. Hypertensive eye ground changes. Acta Med Scand 1978;204:159–167.
42. Skalina MEL, Annable WL, Kleigman RM, Fanaroff AA. Hypertensive retinopathy in the newborn infant. J Pediatr 1983;103:781–786.

43. Fishberg AM. Anatomic findings in essential hypertension. Arch Intern Med 1925;35:650–668.
44. Tracy RE. Hypertension and arteriolar sclerosis of the kidney, pancreas, adrenal gland and liver. Virchows Arch 1981;391:91–106.
45. U.S. Renal Data System. In: USRDS 1989 Annual Data Report. Bethesda: The National Institutes of Health, National Institute of Diabetes and Digestive and Kidney Diseases, 1989.
46. Weisstuch JM, Dworkin LD. Does essential hypertension cause end-stage renal disease? Kidney Int 1992;41(Suppl 36):S-33–S-37.
47. El Nahas AM. Glomerulosclerosis: are we any wiser? Klin Wochenschr 1989;67:876–881.
48. Schmieder RE, Messerli FH, Garavaglia GE, Nunez BD. Glomerular hyperfiltration indicates target organ disease in essential hypertension. Circulation 1987;76:III-273.
49. Kannel WB. Hypertension: epidemiological appraisal. In: Robinson K, ed. Preventive Cardiology: A Guide for Clinical Practice. Armonk, NY: Futura Publishing, 1998;1–14.
50. Kannel WB. Role of blood pressure in cardiovascular disease. The Framingham Study. Angiology 1975;26:1.
51. Levy D, Salomon M, D'Agostino RB, Belanger AJ, Kannel WB. Prognostic implications of baseline electrocardiographic features and their serial changes in subjects with left ventricular hypertrophy. Circulation 1994; 90:1780–1793.
52. Kannel WB, Dannenberg AL, Levy D. Population implications of electrocardiographic left ventricular hypertrophy. Am J Cardiol 1987;60:851–931.
53. Levy D, Garrison RJ, Savage DD, Kannel WB, Castelli WP. Prognostic implications of echocardiographically determined left ventricular mass in the Framingham Heart Study. N Engl J Med 1990;322:1561–1566.
54. Linzbach AJ. Hypertrophy, hyperplasia and structural dilatation of the human heart. Adv Cardiol 1976;18:1–13.
55. Messerli FH, Sundgaard-Riise K, Reisen ED, et al. Dimorphic cardiac adaptation to obesity and arterial hypertension. Ann Intern Med 1983;99:757–761.
56. Khaw KT, Barrett-Connor E. The association between blood pressure, age, and dietary sodium and potassium: a population study. Circulation 1988;77:53–61.
57. Blake J, Devereux RB, Herrold EM, et al. Relation of concentric left ventricular hypertrophy and extracardiac target organ damage to supranormal left ventricular performance in established essential hypertension. Am J Cardiol 1988;62:246–252.
58. Ganau A, Devereux RB, Roman MJ, et al. Patterns of left ventricular hypertrophy and geometric remodeling in essential hypertension. J Am Coll Cardiol 1992;19:1550–1558.
59. Devereux RB, Pickering TG, Harshfield GA, et al. Left ventricular hypertrophy in patients with hypertension: importance of blood pressure responses to regularly recurring stress. Circulation 1983;68:470–476.
60. Abi-Samra F, Fouad RM, Tarazi RC. Determinants of left ventricular hypertrophy and function in hypertensive patients. Am J Med 1983;75(Suppl 3A):26–33.
61. deSimone G, Devereux RG, Daniels SR, Koren MJ, Meyer RA, Laragh JI-L. Effect of growth on variability of left ventricular mass: assessment of allometric signals in adults and children and their capacity to predict cardiovascular risk. J Am Coll Cardiol 1995;25:1056–1062.
62. Inou T, Lambeth WC Jr, Koyanagi S, Harrison DG, Eastham CL, Marcus ML. Relative importance of hypertension after coronary occlusion in chronic hypertensive dogs with LVH. Am J Physiol 1987;253:H1148–H1158.
63. Snider AR, Gidding SS, Rocchini AP, et al. Doppler evaluation of left ventricular diastolic filling in children with systemic HTN. Am J Cardiol 1985;56:921–926.
64. Zehender M, Meinertz T, Hohnloser S, et al. Prevalence of circadian variations and spontaneous variability of cardiac disorders and ECG changes suggestive of myocardial ischemia in systemic arterial hypertension. Circulation 1992;85:1808–1815.
65. Burke GL, Arcilla RA, Culpepper WS, Webber LS, Chiang YK, Berenson GS. Blood pressure and echocardiographic measures in children: the Bogalusa Heart Study. Circulation 1987;75:106–114.
66. Malcolm DD, Burns TL, Mahoney LT, Lauer RM. Factors affecting left ventricular mass in childhood: the Muscatine study. Pediatrics 1993;92:703–709.
67. Daniels SR, Kimball TR, Morrison JA, Khoury P, Witt S, Meyer RA. Effect of lean body mass, fat mass, blood pressure, and sexual maturation on left ventricular mass in children and adolescents. Statistical, biological, and clinical significance. Circulation 1995;92:3249–3254.
68. Treiber FA, McCaffrey F, Pflieger K, Raunikar RA, Strong WB, Davis H. Determinants of left ventricular mass in normotensive children. Am J Hypertens 1993;6:505–513.

69. Belsha CW, Wells TG, McNiece KL, Seib PM, Plummer JK, Berry PL. Influence of diurnal blood pressure variations on target organ abnormalities in adolescents with mild essential hypertension. Am J Hypertens 1998;11:410–417.
70. Hanevold C, Waller J, Daniels S, Portman R, Sorof J; International Pediatric Hypertension Association. The effects of obesity, gender, and ethnic group on left ventricular hypertrophy and geometry in hypertensive children: a collaborative study of the International Pediatric Hypertension Association. Pediatrics 2004;113(2):328–333.
71. Chamontin B, Amar J, Barthe P, Salvador M. Blood pressure measurements and left ventricular mass in young adults with arterial hypertension screened at high school check-up. J Hum Hypertens 1994;8:357–361.
72. Daniels SR, Loggie JMH, Khoury P, Kimball TR. Left ventricular geometry and severe left ventricular hypertrophy in children and adolescents with essential hypertension. Circulation 1998;97:1907–1911.
73. Benjamin EJ, D'Agostino RB, Belanger AJ, Wolf PA, Levy D. Left atrial size and the risk of stroke death. The Framingham Heart Study. Circulation 1995;92:835–841.
74. Daniels SR, Witt SA, Glascock B, Khoury P, Kimball TR. Left atrial size in children with hypertension: the influence of obesity, blood pressure and left ventricular mass. J Pediatr 2002;141:186–190.

# 12 Monogenic and Polygenic Genetic Contributions to Hypertension

*Julie R. Ingelfinger,* MD

***Contents***



## INTRODUCTION

More than 3 yr have elapsed since the publication in February 2001 of the first map of the human genome *(1,2)*. In the present postgenomic era, the identification of a specific gene, or genes, as the cause of a given disease would seem feasible. Indeed, genes that lead to a few rare forms of familial hypertension (HTN) have now been identified. However, although the identification of a gene associated with a Mendelian HTN is approachable using positional cloning, such an approach does not work as effectively for non-Mendelian forms of high blood pressure (BP), which have multiple genetic determinants (*see* Table 1). This chapter discusses both monogenic and polygenic aspects of HTN.

## MONOGENIC FORMS OF HUMAN HYPERTENSION

Genes for a number of monogenic forms of human HTN have been identified, via positional cloning (in the past called "reverse genetics"), with the following approach *(3–5)*:

From: *Clinical Hypertension and Vascular Disease: Pediatric Hypertension*
Edited by: R. J. Portman, J. M. Sorof, and J. R. Ingelfinger © Humana Press Inc., Totowa, NJ

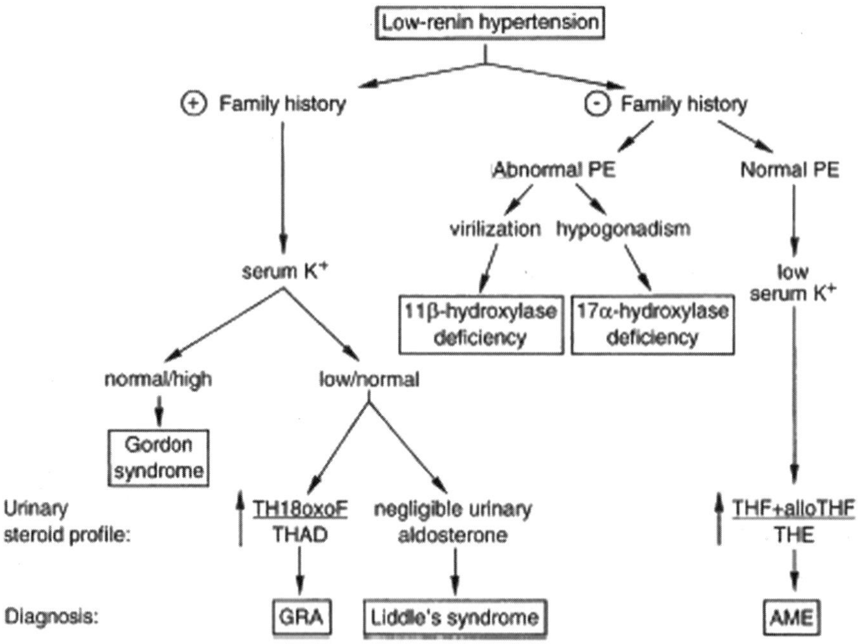


Fig. 1. Algorithm for evaluating pediatric patients with low-renin hyportension. Several hypertensive syndromes share as a common feature very low plasma renin activity (PRA). These disorders are inherited as either an autosomal dominant (positive family history) or autosomal recessive (negative family history) trait. Children with any if three syndromes, GRA, Liddle's syndrome, an apparent mineralocorticoid excess (AME), share a clinical phenotype characterized by normal physical examinations (PE), low PRA, and hypokalemia. Those disorders are distinguishable from one another on the basis of characteristic urinary steroid profiles and genetic testing. *$K^+$*, Potassium; *TH18oxoF/THAD* ratio of urinary 18-ototetrahydrocortisol (Th18oxoF) to urinary tetrahydroaldosterone (THAD) (normal 0–0.4, GRA patients > 1); *THF+ alloTHF/THE* ratio of the combined urinary tetrahydrocortisol (THF) and allotetrahydrocortisol (alloTHF) to urinary tetrahydrocortisone (THE) (normal < 1.3, AME patients 5- to 10-fold higher) *(6,18,19)*.

Large kindreds with many affected family members are phenotyped, followed by an analysis to determine how the disease is inherited (autosomal recessive, dominant, sex-linked, co-dominant, etc.). Subsequently, linkage analysis is carried out using highly polymorphic genetic markers, such as microsatellite markers that occur widely throughout the genome and that are evenly spaced at approx 10-centimorgan (cM) intervals. Since most people (about 70%) are heterozygous, the inheritance of alleles can be traced through large pedigrees. In a successful linkage analysis, a specific chromosomal region in the genome linked to the trait is identified. A logarithm of the odds (LOD) score describes the presence of such a region. The generally accepted LOD score indicating linkage is greater than 3.3, corresponding to a genome-wide significance level of $4.5 \times 10^{-5}$ *(4)*. Once linkage is found, a search commences for known genes in the area that might be involved. A search using additional highly polymorphic markers may also narrow the area of interest, leading to sequences of possible genes within the area.

Most monogenic forms of HTN identified to date are owing to gain-of-function mutations *(6–7)*, most of which result in overproduction of mineralocorticoids or increased mineralocorticoid activity. Severe HTN, often from early life (even infancy), is not unusual. Clinical hallmarks include apparent volume expansion and suppressed plasma renin activity with variable hypokalemia. A paradigm for evaluation of those forms associated with hypokalemia and suppressed renin activity is shown in Fig. 1 *(8)*.

Table 1
When to Suspect a Hypertensive Genetic Disorder

| |
|---|
| At-risk members of kindreds with a known monogenic hypertensive disorder (e.g., multiple endocrine neoplasia, syndromes) |
| Hypokalemia in hypertensive children and their first-degree relatives |
| Juvenile onset of HTN, particularly if plasma renin is suppressed |
| Physical findings suggestive of syndromes or hypertensive disorders (e.g., retinal angiomas, neck mass, or hyperparathyroidism in patient with a pheochromocytoma) |

Adapted from ref. *7*.

Gain-of-function mutations in transporters in the distal nephrons of the renal tubules result in HTN via salt and water retention by the kidney *(9)*. (While mutations and polymorphisms in the genes of various components of the renin-angiotensin-aldosterone system [RAS] may lead to excessive renal sodium retention, no single RAS polymorphism causes monogenic HTN.) Clinically, most monogenic HTN can be divided into those mutations that lead to overproduction of mineralocorticoids or increased mineralocorticoid activity, and those that result in abnormalities of electrolyte transport (Tables 1 and 2) *(7)*. Additionally, some mutations in proto-oncogenes and genes that involve response to hypoxia have been linked to chromaffin tumors *(10)*.

## *Glucocorticoid-Remediable Aldosteronism (OMIM #103900)*

Glucocorticoid-remediable aldosteronism (GRA), an autosomal dominant disorder, is considered the most common type of monogenic HTN and presents in early infancy in some patients *(11–15)*. GRA has been recognized since the 1960s, when Sutherland et al. *(16)* and New et al. *(17)* reported on patients in whom severe HTN was accompanied by suppressed renin and increased aldosterone secretion, and who were found to be treatable with dexamethasone. GRA is listed in the Online Mendelian Inheritance in Man index (OMIM) as #103900 (OMIM can be accessed at http://www.ncbi.nlm.nih.gov/Omim ). HTN in GRA is moderate to severe, owing to increased aldosterone secretion driven by adrenocorticotropic hormone (ACTH).

A chimeric gene (Fig. 2) containing the 5' regulatory sequences of 11-β-hydroxylase (which confers ACTH responsiveness), fused with the distal coding sequences of aldosterone synthase, is responsible for ACTH (rather than angiotensin II [ANG II] or potassium) serving as the main controller of aldosterone secretion *(18,19)*. Both serum and urine aldosterone levels tend to be elevated, though not invariably. The chimeric gene product converts cortisol to 18-hydroxy and 18-oxo metabolites *(20–22)*, which can be detected in urine, and which are pathognomonic. The elevations of urinary cortisol metabolites TH18oxoF and 18-hydroxycortisol, and an elevated ratio of TH18oxoF/THAD metabolites, can be measured with a commercially available urinary steroid profile (Nichols Institute, San Juan Capistrano, CA), and will distinguish GRA patients from others with apparent mineralocorticoid excess (AME) or Liddle's syndrome *(23)*. However, specific genetic testing, which is both sensitive and specific, has largely supplanted the urinary testing when the condition is suspected.

Not all affected members of GRA families develop HTN in childhood *(24)*. In a recent paper assessing 20 children in 10 unrelated GRA pedigrees, 16 of the 20 developed HTN as early as 1 mo of age. However, four children were normotensive. Monotherapy, using glucocorticoid suppression, or aldosterone receptor and epithelial sodium cotransporter (ENaC) antagonists, was sufficient to control BP in half of the hypertensive children. The other patients required polypharmacy. Three had uncontrollable HTN *(24)*.

**Table 2**

| *Disorder* | *Hormonal findings* | *Source* | *Genetics* | *Comment* |
|---|---|---|---|---|
| *Steroidogenic enzyme defects* | | | | |
| Steroid 11β-hydroxylase deficiency | ⇓ PRA and aldo; high serum androgens/ urine 17 keto-steroids; elevated DOC and 11-deoxycortisol | Adrenal: Zona fasciculata | CYP11B1 mutation (encodes cytochrome $P_{450}$11β/18 of ZF); impairs synthesis of cortisol and ZF 17-deoxysteroids | Hypertensive virilizing CAH; most patients identified by time they are hypertensive. Increased BP may also occur from medication side effects |
| Steroid 11α-hydroxylase/ 17,20-lyase deficiency | ⇓ PRA and aldo; low serum/ urinary 17-hydroxysteroids; decreased cortisol, ⇑ corticosterone (B), and DOC in plasma; serum androgens and estrogens very low; serum gonadotrophins very high | Adrenal: Zona fasciculata; Gonadal: interstitial cells (Leydig in testi; theca in ovary) | CYP17 mutation (encodes cytochrom $P_{450}$C17) impairs cortisol and sex steroid production | CAH with male pseudoher-maphroditism; female external genital phenotype in males; primary amenorrhea in females |
| *Hyperaldosteronism* | | | | |
| Primary aldosteronism | ⇓ PRA; ⇑plasma aldosterone, 18-OH- and 18 oxoF; normal 18-OH/aldo ratio | Adrenal adenoma: clear cell tumor with suppression of ipsilateral ZG | Unknown; very rare in children; female:male ratio is 2.5–3/1 | Conn syndrome with aldo producing adenoma; muscle weakness and low K+ in sodium-replete state |
| Adrenocortical hyperplasia | As above; source of hormone established by radiology or scans | Adrenal: Focal or diffuse adrenal cortical hyperplasia | Unknown | As above |
| Idiopathic primary aldosteronism | High plasma aldo; elevated 18-OHF/aldo ratio | Adrenal: Hyper-activity of ZG of adrenal cortex | Unknown | As above |

(continued)

**Table 2 (continued)**

| *Disorder* | *Hormonal findings* | *Source* | *Genetics* | *Comment* |
|---|---|---|---|---|
| Glucocorticoid-remediable aldosteronism (GRA) | Plasma and urinary aldo responsive to ACTH; dexamethasone suppressible within 48h; ⇑ urine and plasma 18OHS, 18-OHF, and 18 oxoF | Adrenal: abnormal presence of enzymatic activity in adrenal ZF, allowing completion of aldo synthesis from 7-deoxy steroids | Chimeric gene that is expressed level in ZF [regulated like CYP11B1] and has 18-oxidaseactivity [CYP11B2 functionality] | Hypokalemia in sodium-replete state |
| *Apparent mineralocorticoid excess (AME)* | ⇑ plasma ACTH and secretory rates of all corticosteroids; nl serum F [delayed plasma clearance] | ⇑ plasma F bioact. in periphery [F→E] of bi-dir. 11βOHSD or slow clearance by 5 α/β reduction to allo dihydro-F | Type 2 11βOHSD mutations | Cardiac conduction changes; LVH, vessel remodeling; some calcium abnormalities; nephrocalcinosis; rickets |
| *Nonsteroidal defects* | | | | |
| Liddle's Syndrome | Low plasma renin, low or normal K+; negligible urinary aldosterone | Not a disorder of steroidogenesis, but of transport | Autosomal dominant abnormality in epithelial sodium transporter, EnaC, in which channel is constitutively active | Responds to triamterene |
| Pseudohypoaldosteronism II-Gordon's Syndrome | Low plasma renin, normal or elevated K+ | Not a disorder of steroidogenesis, but of transport | Autosomal dominant abnormality in WNK1 or WNK4 | Responds to thiazides |

Adapted and expanded from ref. *92*.

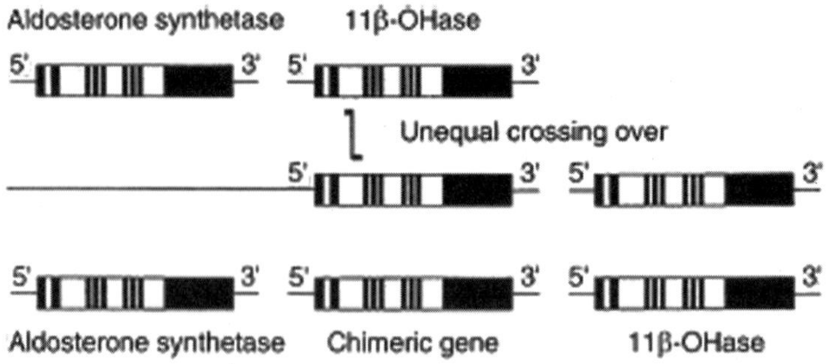


Fig. 2. Chimeric gene duplication in glucocorticoid remediable aldosteronism (*GRA*). The genes encoding aldosterone synthetase and 11β-hydroylase (*11β-OHase*) are represented by *wide bars*, and the locations of the exons in each are indicated by *bands*. These highly homologous genes are tightly linked on chromosome 8 and lie in the orientation shown. An unequal crossing over event between these genes produces as one of its products a chimeric gene duplication that fuses the regulatory sequences of 11β-OHase with the coding sequences of aldosterone synthetase. Reprinted from ref. *18* with permission.

Cerebral hemorrhage at an early age (mean age 32 yr) is common in GRA pedigrees. And almost half of reported pedigrees (48%), and 18% of individual GRA patients, have been noted to develop cerebrovascular complications *(6,7,18)*.

### *Apparent Mineralocorticoid Excess (OMIM #218030 and #207765)*

Low-renin HTN, often severe and accompanied by hypokalemia and metabolic alkalosis *(25)*, is the hallmark of apparent mineralcorticoid excess (AME), first described in 1977 by New et al. *(26,27)*. Spironolactone is often effective initially, but patients on this drug often become refractory. In AME 11-β-hydroxysteroid dehydrogenase (11-β-HSD) is absent, resulting in HTN in which cortisol acts as if it were a potent mineralocorticoid. The microsomal enzyme 11-β-hydroxysteroid dehydrogenase interconverts active 11-hydroxyglucocorticoids to inactive keto-metabolites. Cortisol and aldosterone have an affinity for the mineralocorticoid receptor. Normally, 11-β-HSD is protective, preventing binding of cortisol to the mineralocorticoid receptor, but in AME, the slower-than-normal metabolism of cortisol to cortisone results in cortisol acting as a potent mineralocorticoid *(26,27)*, while metabolism of cortisone to cortisol is normal.

Persons with classic AME usually become symptomatic in early childhood, often presenting with failure to thrive, severe HTN, and persistent polydipsia. Affected patients appear volume-expanded and respond to dietary sodium restriction. Plasma renin activity is very low. A high cortisol:cortisone ratio in plasma, or an abnormal urinary ratio of tetrahydrocortisol/tetrahydrocortisone (THF/THE) in which THF predominates, makes the diagnosis.

Affected children are at high risk for cardiovascular complications, and some develop nephrocalcinosis and renal failure *(28)*; early therapy may lead to better outcome.

Several variants of AME have been reported, including a mild form in a Mennonite kindred in which there is a P227L mutation in the HSD11B2 gene *(29,30)*, a coactivator defect with resistance to multiple steroids *(31)*, and HTN without the characteristic findings of AME in a heterozygous father and homozygous daughter who have mutations in 11-β-HSD2 *(32)*.

## STEROIDOGENIC ENZYME DEFECTS LEADING TO HYPERTENSION

Rare autosomal recessive defects in steroidogenesis associated with HTN were well recognized before the genomic era. Cortisol is normally synthesized under the control of ACTH in the zona fasciculata, while aldosterone is synthesized largely under the influence of ANG II and potassium in the zona glomerulosa. Aldosterone synthesis is not normally controlled by ACTH, but if any of the several enzymes that are involved in cortisol biosynthesis acts abnormally or is defective, the usual feedback is interrupted. Consequently, plasma ACTH will increase, and aberrant products—some of which lead to HTN—will accumulate.

Together, inherited defects of steroid biosynthesis (all autosomal recessive) are termed congenital adrenal hyperplasia (CAH). Each defect results in a characteristic clinical and biochemical profile *(7,33,34)*. Any enzyme in the pathways of steroidogenesis may contain a mutation, most commonly 21-hydroxylase, which is not generally associated with HTN. Enzyme mutations that are associated with HTN include (in order of frequency) 11-β-hydroxylase, 3-β-hydroxysteroid dehydrogenase, 17-α-hydroxylase, and cholesterol desmolase. Patients with the 11-β-hydroxylase and 3-β-hydroxysteroid dehydrogenase defects have a tendency to retain salt and, subsequently, become hypertensive. It is also important to remember that any person with CAH may develop HTN owing to overzealous replacement therapy.

### *Steroid 11-β-Hydroxylase Deficiency*

The mineralocorticoid excess in 11-β-hydroxylase deficiency *(33–38)*, a form of CAH accompanied by virilization, leads to decreased excretion with volume expansion, renin suppression, and HTN. Elevated BP is not invariant in 11-β-hydroxylase deficiency, and is most often discovered in late childhood or adolescence, frequently with an inconsistent correlation to the biochemical profile *(33,34)*. Hypokalemia is variable, but total body potassium may be markedly depleted in the face of normal serum or plasma potassium. Renin is generally decreased, but aldosterone is increased.

Therapy of 11-β-hydroxylase deficiency should focus on normalizing steroids. Administered glucocorticoids should normalize cortisol and reduce ACTH secretion and levels to normal, thus stopping oversecretion of deoxycorticosterone (DOC). HTN generally resolves with such therapy *(34)*. When HTN is severe, antihypertensive therapy should be instituted until the BP is controlled; the therapy can be tapered later.

Additional mutations can cause this syndrome—for example, a patient with 11-β-hydroxylation inhibition for 17-α-hydroxylated steroids, but with intact 17-deoxysteroid hydroxylation *(38)*. Multiple mutations affecting the CYP11B1 gene have been described; these include frameshifts, point mutations, extra triplet repeats, and stop mutations *(25,39–42)*.

### *Steroid 17-α-Hydroxylase Deficiency*

Abnormalities in 17-α-hydroxylase affect both the adrenals and gonads, since a dysfunctional 17-α-hydroxylase enzyme results in decreased synthesis of both cortisol and sex steroids *(33,34,43–45)*. Affected persons appear phenotypically female (or occasionally have ambiguous genitalia), regardless of their genetic sex, and puberty does not occur. Consequently, most cases are discovered after a girl fails to enter puberty *(33,34,43–45)*. An inguinal hernia is another mode of presentation. HTN and hypokalemia are characteristic, owing to notable overproduction of corticosterone (compound B).

Glucocorticoid replacement is effective therapy. However, should replacement therapy fail to control the HTN, appropriate pharmacotherapy should be instituted to restore BP to within the normal range.

## MUTATIONS IN RENAL TRANSPORTERS CAUSING LOW-RENIN HYPERTENSION

### *Pseudohypoaldosteronism Type II—Gordon Syndrome (OMIM #145260)*

Pseudohypoaldosteronism type II, known as Gordon's syndrome, or familial hyperkalemia (OMIM #145260), is an autosomal dominant form of HTN associated with hyperkalemia, acidemia and increased salt reabsorption by the kidney *(8,46–48)*. It is caused by mutations in the WNK1 and WNK4 kinase family. Though the physiology and response to diuretics suggested a defect in renal ion transport in the presence of normal glomerular filtration rate, the genetics have only recently been delineated. Affected persons have low-renin HTN and improve with thiazide diuretics or with triamterene. Aldosterone receptor antagonists do not correct the observed abnormalities.

PHAII genes were mapped to chromosomes 17, 1, or 12 *(46–48)*. One kindred was found to have abnormalities in WNK1, large intronic deletions that increase WNK1 expression. Another kindred with missense mutations in WNK4, which is on chromosome 17, has been described. Whereas WNK1 is widely expressed, WNK4 is expressed primarily in the kidney, localized to tight junctions. WNKs alter the handling of potassium and hydrogen in the collecting duct, leading to increased salt reabsorption and increased intravascular volume by as yet unknown means.

### *Liddle's Syndrome (OMIM #177200)*

In 1963, Liddle *(49)* described early onset of autosomal dominant HTN in a family in whom hypokalemia, low renin, and aldosterone concentrations were noted in affected members. Inhibitors of renal epithelial sodium transport, such as triamterene, worked well in controlling HTN, but inhibitors of the mineralocorticoid receptor did not. A general abnormality in sodium transport seemed apparent, because the red blood cell transport systems were not normal *(50)*. A major abnormality in renal salt handling seemed likely when a patient with Liddle's syndrome underwent a renal transplant. Subsequently, HTN and hypokalemia were resolved posttransplant *(51)*.

While the clinical picture of Liddle's syndrome is one of aldosterone excess, aldosterone levels, as well as renin levels, are very low *(8)*. Hypokalemia is not invariably present. A defect in renal sodium transport is now known to cause Liddle's syndrome. The mineralocorticoid-dependent sodium transport within the renal epithelia requires activation of the epithelial sodium channel (ENaC), which is composed of at least three subunits normally regulated by aldosterone. Mutations in the $\beta$ and $\gamma$ subunits of the ENaC have been identified (both lie on chromosome 16) *(52,53)*. Subsequently, the defect in Liddle's syndrome leads to constitutive activation of amiloride-sensitive ENaCs in distal renal tubules, causing excess sodium reabsorption. Additionally, these gain-in-function mutations prolong the half-life of ENaCs at the renal distal tubule apical cell surface, resulting in increased channel number *(54)*.

## PHEOCHROMOCYTOMA-PREDISPOSING SYNDROMES

A variety of RET protooncogene mutations and abnormalities in tumor suppressor genes are associated with autosomal dominant inheritance of pheochromocytomas, summarized in Table 3 *(10,55–60)*. A number of paraganglioma and pheochromocytoma susceptibility genes inherited in an autosomal dominant pattern appear to convey a propensity toward developing such tumors *(10)*. Both glomus tumors and pheochromocytomas derive from neural-crest tissues,

Table 3. Hereditary Syndromes Associated With Pheochromocytoma[a]

| *Syndrome* | *Clinical phenotype* | *% Risk of pheochromocytoma* | *Mutated germ-line gene* |
|---|---|---|---|
| MEN-2A | Medullary carcinoma of the thyroid, hyperparathyroidism | 50 | *RET* (proto-oncogene) |
| MEN-2B | Medullary carcinoma of the thyroid, multiple mucosal neuromas, marfanoid habitus, hyperparathyroidism | 50 | *RET* (proto-oncogene) |
| Neurofibromatosis type 1 | Neurofibromas of peripheral nerves, café-au-lait spots | 1 | *NF1* |
| Von Hippel-Lindau disease (retinal cerebellar hemangioblastosis) | Retinal angioma, CNS hemangioblastoma, renal-cell carcinoma, pancreatic and renal cysts | 10–20 | *VHL* |
| Familial paraganglioma syndrome | Carotid-body tumor (chemodectoma) | 20 (estimated) | *SDHD, SDHB* |

[a]MEN-2A denotes multiple endocrine neoplasia type 2A, MEN-2B multiple endocrine neoplasia type 2B; CNS, central nervous system; *SDHD*, the gene for succinate dehydrogenase subunit D; and *SDHB*, the gene for succinate dehydrogenase subunit B. From ref. *10*.

and the genes identified in one type of tumor may appear in the other *(61)*. For instance, germ line mutations have been reported in families with autosomal-dominant glomus tumors, and in registries with sporadic cases of pheochromocytoma *(62)*. In addition, other pheochromocytoma-susceptibility genes include the proto-oncogene *RET* (multiple endocrine neoplasia syndrome type 2 [MEN-2]), the tumor-suppressor gene *VHL* seen in families with von Hippel-Lindau syndrome, and the gene that encodes succinate dehydrogenase subunit B *(SDHB)*.

The genes involved in some of these tumors appear to encode proteins with a common link involving tissue oxygen metabolism *(63–65)*. In von Hippel-Lindau disease, there are inactivating (loss-of-function) mutations in the VHL suppressor gene, which encodes a protein integral to the degradation of other proteins, some of which, such as hypoxia-inducible factor, are involved in responding to low oxygen tension. Interestingly, the mitochondrial complex II, important in $O_2$ sensing and signaling, contains both SDHB and succinate dehydrogenase subunit D (SDHD). Thus, mutations in the VHL gene, and SDHB, and SDHD might lead to increased activation of hypoxic signaling pathways leading to abnormal proliferation.

In multiple endocrinopathy-2 (MEN-2) syndromes, mutations in the *RET* proto-oncogene lead to constitutive activation (activating mutations) of the receptor tyrosine kinase. The end result is hyperplasia of adrenomedullary chromaffin cells (and in the parathyroid, calcitonin-producing parafollicular cells). In time, these cells undergo a high rate of neoplastic transformation. It now appears that apparently sporadic chromaffin tumors may contain mutations in these genes, as well.

## WHEN TO SUSPECT MONOGENIC HYPERTENSION

Table 1 lists situations in which the astute clinician should consider monogenic HTN *(7)*. These include clinical and laboratory findings that should point toward further evaluation. Important findings are a strong family history of HTN, particularly when BP is difficult to control within the family. Low plasma renin activity should also point towards the possibility that a defined form of HTN may be present.

## POLYGENIC HYPERTENSION

Cardiovascular risk factors such as HTN are common. The genetic contribution to a highly prevalent condition such as HTN is generally thought to involve multiple genes, and is termed polygenic. The possibility for determining which genes are involved seems far more feasible in the current genomic era, yet clear identification has proved elusive. Relevant background for considering the genetic factors predisposing one towards HTN follow.

## EXPERIMENTAL HYPERTENSION AS A TOOL TO INVESTIGATE POLYGENIC HYPERTENSION

A large number of studies in inbred experimental animals, mainly rats and mice, have aimed to identify genes controlling BP. In the 1980s, it was estimated that 5 to10 genes control BP *(66)*. More recently, it was reported that 24 chromosomal regions in 19 chromosomes were associated with HTN in various rat strains *(67)*. That being said, studies using inbred rat strains have still not identified polygenes and their associated alleles *(67)*. A large number of chromosomal regions, and some candidate genes, have also been suggested from experimental studies in mice. For example, targeted gene deletion studies have shown an effect on BP in more than a dozen genes, among them endothelial nitric oxide synthase, insulin receptor substrate, the dopamine receptor, apolipoprotein E, the bradykinin receptor, the angiotensin type 2 receptor, and other members of the RAS *(68)*.

Genetic manipulation in mice has been successful in exploring contributions of various candidate genes (reviewed in *69*), most notably those of the RAS, through two approaches, over-expression of a given gene (with "transgenic" and "knock-in" animals) and deleting gene function (with "knockouts"). Transgenic animals are created by injecting naked DNA containing the regulatory and coding regions of a gene of interest into the pronucleus of fertilized eggs *(70)*. These pieces of DNA then integrate randomly into the mouse genome (in concatemers of variable copy number). Depending on the location and copy number, effects can vary. Deletion of a gene is also informative, because the phenotypic change may help determine the gene's significance. An additional approach is to use gene targeting in embryonic stem (ES) cell cultures *(71,72)*.

Inbred strains, rather than transgenic or knockouts, have led to important findings *(73–75)*. Certain studies, notably those of Jacob et al. *(73)* and Hilbert et al. *(74)*, found linkage in rat models of HTN that pointed to the angiotensin-converting enzyme (ACE) gene's importance in determining HTN. Since those reports of more than a decade ago, a large number of clinical studies have suggested a link between ACE polymorphisms in humans and HTN.

## HUMAN HYPERTENSION

A variety of studies have pointed to a link between human HTN and genes of the RAS (summarized in *76,77*). However, it is important to note that people with common diseases such as HTN do not have disease alleles *per se*, but should be considered to have susceptibility alleles. Furthermore, some people who have a particular susceptibility allele do not have the disease, either because they don't have the environmental exposure that brings on the condition, or because they lack another allele (or alleles) necessary to cause a given clinical problem.

Table 4
**Genome-Wide Linkage Surveys for BP Loci in Human Populations: Chromosomes With Identified Linkage**

| *Chromosome* | *Population(s)* | *Reference* |
|---|---|---|
| 1 | Quebec | *78* |
| 2 | Amish, Quebec, Finnish, US white | *78,79*; Pankow et al.; Krushkal et al. |
| 3 | Chinese | *84* |
| 5 | Quebec, US white | *78,81* |
| 6 | US African-American and US white; UK | *80,81*; Caulfield |
| 7 | Quebec | *78* |
| 8 | Quebec | *78* |
| 11 | Chinese, unspecified | *83,84* |
| 15 | Chinese, US white | *80,84* |
| 16 | Chinese | *84* |
| 17 | US white | *82* |
| 18 | US white | *80,82* |
| 19 | Quebec | *78* |
| 22 | Finnish | *79* |
| X | Finnish | *79* |

Adapted from refs. *68* and *89*.

Because there are multiple potential interactions, and susceptibility alleles are generally common, following a given allele through pedigrees is difficult. In such a circumstance segregation analysis is difficult, particularly if a given susceptibility allele has a small effect. Indeed, to date, linkage has been reported to 15 chromosomes in humans, noted in Table 4 *(68,78–84)*.

Linkage analysis is the initial step *(3–5)*, but it is not as powerful a tool as it is in Mendelian diseases, because many people without the disease may carry the susceptibility allele. Using affected siblings (sib pairs) may be helpful to gain a better understanding of the possible genetics. Siblings who are both affected with a given problem, such as HTN, would be anticipated to share more than half their alleles near or at the susceptibility locus; then the chance of this occurrence is calculated *(3–5)*. A LOD score of greater than 3.6 is taken as evidence of a linked locus, which is often very large (in the range of 20–40 cM). Once a putative linkage is confirmed in a replicate study, finer mapping can be performed to home in on the genetic region that contains the putative gene. This is done via linkage disequilibrium, or association testing between disease and genetic markers, often with single nucleotide polymorphisms (SNPs). SNPs occur roughly every 1000 base pairs and lend themselves to automated testing. Using SNPs, a broad region (10–40 cM) can be narrowed to a far smaller region of roughly $1 \times 10^6$ base pairs (BPs) *(85,86)*.

At least 20 genome-wide screens of the human genome have been carried out to discover and report HTN genes *(87)*. In total, these suggested at least 27 loci of interest. These genome-wide screens have included subjects of diverse phenotypes, ethnicity, and selection criteria. The numbers and composition of families have ranged from single, large pedigrees to more than 2000 sib pairs from approx1500 families *(88)*. Using genomic scan data from four partner networks, the US Family Blood Pressure Program (FBPP) *(89)* sought to use phenotypic strategies that reflect the ethnic demography of the US. To date, no genome-wide significance has been attained in any of the reports from the USFBP Program. A 140–170 cM region of chromosome 2 has been linked to HTN in several populations—Chinese sibling pairs *(84)*, Finnish twins *(79)*, and a discordant sibling-pair screen . Recently, Caulfield et al. phenotyped 2010 sib pairs drawn from 1599 families with severe HTN as part of the BRIGHT study (Medical Research Council **BRI**tish **G**enetics of **H**yper**T**ension), and performed a 10-cM genome-wide scan *(89)*. Their linkage analysis identified a locus on chromosome 6q with a LOD score of 3.21 and genome-wide significance of 0.042. However, the end of a chromosome may generate errors, and this locus is at the end of chromosome 6. Caution is required in drawing conclusions from these findings. The Caulfield group found three other loci with LOD scores above 1.57 *(89)*. One of these loci was the same as that found in the Chinese and Finnish studies *(89)*.

## CANDIDATE GENES

Another approach in assessing polygenic HTN is to use *candidate genes* near the peak of observed genetic linkage. A gene is a good candidate if it has a known or suspected role in the condition being studied. It is easier to proceed if one knows the full sequence of the candidate.

In the Caulfield study *(89)*, for example, there are a number of candidate genes that are within the linkage analysis-identified areas on chromosomes 2 and 9. Genes that encode serine-threonine kinases, STK39 and STK17B, are on chromosome 2q; PKNBETA, a protein kinase, is on chromosome 9q; G protein-coupled receptors on chromosome 9 (GPR107 9q and GPR21 on 9q33); and a potassium channel, KCNJ3, on 2q24.1.

The study used microarrays to identify differential expression of expressed sequences in tissues from affected and unaffected persons. These are available as full-length cDNAs, or as expressed sequence tags (ESTs).

## CANDIDATE SUSCEPTIBILITY GENES

A number of genes have become candidate susceptibility genes, particularly those of the RAS. A number of these genes were associated with HTN and cardiovascular regulation in the pregenomic era. Many associations have been described or imputed, including not only members of the RAS, but many other genes as well. Recently, Izawa et al. *(90)* chose 27 candidate genes based on reviews of physiology and genetic data that looked at vascular biology, leukocyte and platelet biology, glucose, and lipid metabolism. Then, they selected 33 SNPs of these genes—largely related in promoter regions, exons, or spliced donor or acceptor sites in introns—and looked at their relationship to HTN in a cohort of 1940 persons. They found that polymorphisms in the CC chemokine receptor 2 gene was associated with HTN in men, and that the TNF-$\alpha$ gene was associated with HTN in women *(90)*.

## VARIANTS OR SUBPHENOTYPES

Analysis of so-called subphenotypes via positional cloning may illuminate the discussion *(3–5,91)* if a particular variant of a complex disease is clinically distinct. In this instance, there may be fewer susceptibility genes involved. However, subphenotypes, most likely involving an intricate physiology, may be difficult to study. An example of this situation is salt-sensitive HTN *(91)*. In order to study subjects, it is necessary to perform careful metabolic studies that confirm the subphenotype (HTN with salt sensitivity) and that is also standard during testing.

## PRESENT IMPLICATIONS FOR PEDIATRIC HYPERTENSION

A search for monogenic forms of HTN is clearly indicated in an infant, child, or teenager with elevated BP and history or signs compatible with one of these diagnoses. There will be specific therapy if a child is found to have one of the rare forms of monogenic HTN. However, as of this writing, few data exist to guide the clinician in undersanding the role of polygenic HTN in children.

## REFERENCES


1. Venter JC, Adams MD, Myers EW, et al. The sequence of the human genome. Science 2001; 291:1304–1351.
2. International Human Genome Sequencing Consortium. Initial sequencing and analysis of the human genome. Nature 2001;409:860–921.
3. Bogardus C, Baier L, Permana P, Prochazka M, Wolford J, Hanson R. Identification of susceptibility genes for complex metabolic diseases. Ann NY Acad Sci 2002;967:1–6.
4. Lander E, Kruglyak L. Genetic dissection of complex traits: guidelines for interpreting and reporting linkage results. Nat Genet 1995;11:241–247.
5. Wang DG, Fan J-B, Siao CJ, et al. Large-scale identification, mapping and genotyping of single-nucleotide polymorphisms in the human genome. Science 1998;280:1077–1082.
6. Lifton RP, Gharavi AG, Geller DS. Molecular mechanisms of human hypertension. Cell 2001;104:545–556.
7. Dluhy RG. Screening for genetic causes of hypertension. Curr Hypertension Rep 2002;4:439–444.
8. Yiu VW, Dluhy RG, Lifton RP, Guay-Woodford LM. Low peripheral plasma renin activity as a critical marker in pediatric hypertension. Pediatr Nephrol 1997;11:343–346.
9. Wilson H, Disse-Nicodeme S, Choate K, et al. Human hypertension caused by mutations in WNK knases. Science 2001;293:1107–1111.
10. Dluhy RG. Pheochromocytoma: the death of an axiom. N Engl J Med 2002;346:1486–1488.
11. Miura K, Yoshinaga K, Goto K, et al. A case of glucocorticoid-responsive hyperaldosteronism. J Clin Endocrinol Metab 1968;28:1807.
12. New MI, Siegal EJ, Peterson RE. Dexamethasone-suppressible hyperaldosteronism. J Clin Endocrinol Metab 1973;37:93.
13. Biebink GS, Gotlin RW, Biglieri EG, Katz FH. A kindred with familial glucocorticoid-suppressible aldosteronism. J Clin Endocrinol Metab 1973;36:715.
14. Grim CE, Weinberger MH. Familial dexamethasone-suppressible hyperaldosteronism. Pediatrics 1980: 65:597.
15. Oberfield SE, Levine LS, Stoner E, et al. Adrenal glomerulosa function in patients with dexamethasone-suppressible normokalemic hyperaldosteronism. J Clin Endocrinol Metabl 1981;53:158.
16. Sutherland DJA, Ruse JL, Laidlaw JC. Hypertension, increased aldosterone secretion and low plasma renin activity relieved by dexamethasone. Can Med Assoc J 1966;95:1109.
17. New MI, Peterson RE. A new form of congenital adrenal hyperplasia J Clin Endocrinol Metab 1967;27:300.
18. Lifton RP, Dluhy RG, Powers M, et al. Chimeric 11b-hydroxylase/aldosterone synthase gene causes GRA and human hypertension. Nature 1992;355:262–265.
19. Lifton RP, Dluhy RG, Powers M, et al. Hereditary hypertension caused by chimeric gene duplications and ectopic expression of aldosterone synthetase. Nature Genet 1992;2:66–74.
20. Ulick S, Chu MD. Hypersecretion of a new cortico-steroid, 18-hydroxycortisol in two types of adrenocortical hypertension. Clin Exp Hypertens 1982;4(9–10):1771–1777.
21. Ulick S, Chu MD, Land M. Biosynthesis of 18-oxocortisol by aldosterone-producing adrenal tissue. J Biol Chem 1983;258:5498–5502.
22. Gomez-Sanchez CE, Montgomery M, Ganguly A, et al. Elevated urinary excretion of 18-oxocortisol in glucocorticoid-suppressible aldosteronism. J Clin Endocrinol Metab 1984;59:1022–1024.
23. Shackleton CH. Mass specrometry in the diagnosis of steroid-related disorders and in hypertension research. J Steroid Biochem Mol Biol 1993;45:127–140.
24. Dluhy RG, Anderson B, Harlin B, Ingelfinger J, Lifton R. Glucocorticoid-remediable aldosteronism is associated with severe hypertension in early childhood. Pediatr 2001;138:715–720.
25. Cerame BI, New MI. Hormonal hypertension in children: 11-β-hydroxylase deficiency and apparent mineralocorticoid excess. J Pediatr Endocrinol 2000;13:1537–1547.

26. New MI, Levine LS, Biglieri EG, Pareira J, Ulick S. Evidence for an unidentified ACTH-induced steroid hormone causing hypertension. J Clin Endocrinol Metab 1977;44:924–933.
27. New MI, Oberfield SE, Carey RM, Greig F, Ulick S, Levine LS. A genetic defect in cortisol metabolism as the basis for the syndrome of apparent mineralocorticoid excess. In: Mnatero F, Biglieri EG, Edwards CRW, eds. Endocrinology of Hypertension. Serono Symposia No. 50. New York: Academic, 1982:85–101.
28. Moudgil A, Rodich G, Jordan SC, Kamil ES. Nephrocalcinosis and renal cysts associated with apparent mineralocorticoid excess syndrome. Pediatr Nephrol 2000;15:60–62.
29. Mercado AB, Wilson RC, Cheng KC, Wei JQ, New MI. Prenatal treatment and diagnosis of congenital adrenal hyperplasia owing to steroid 21-hydroxylase deficiency. J Clin Endocrinol Metab 1995;80:2014–2020.
30. Ugrasbul F, Wiens T, Rubinstein P, New MI, Wilson RC. Prevalence of mild apparent mineralocorticoid excess in Mennonites. J Clin Endocrinol Metab 1999;84:4735–4738.
31. New MI, Nimkarn S, Brandon DD. Resistance to multiple steroids in two sisters. J Ster Biochem Molec Biol 2001;76:161–166.
32. Li A, Li KXZ, Marui S, et al. Apparent mineralocorticoid excess in a Brazilian kindred: hypertension in the heterozygote state. J Hypertens 1997;15:1397–1402.
33. New MI, Wilson RC. Steroid disorders in children: congenital adrenal hyperplasia and apparent mineralocorticoid excess. PNAS 1999;96:12,790–12,797.
34. New MI, Seaman MP. Secretion rates of cortisol and aldosterone precursors in various forms of congenital adrenal hyperplasia. J Clin Endocrinol Metab 1970;30:361.
35. New MI, Levine LS. Hypertension of childhood with suppressed renin. Endocrinol Rev 1980;1:421–430
36. New MI, Levine LS. Congenital adrenal hyperplasia. Adv Hum Genet 1973;4:251–326.
37. Mimouni M, Kaufman H, Roitman A, Morag C, Sadan N. Hypertension in a neonate with 11 beta-hydroxylase deficiency. Eur J Pediatr 1985;143:231–233.
38. Zachmann M, Vollmin JA, New MI, Curtius C-C, Prader A. Congenital adrenal hyperplasia due to deficiency of 11-hydroxylation of 17α-hydroxylated steroids. J Clin Endocrinol Metab 1971;33:501.
39. White PC, Dupont J, New MI, Lieberman E, Hochberg Z, Rosler A. A mutation in CYP11B1 [Arg448His] associated with steroid 22-β-hydroxylase deficiency in Jews of Moroccan origin. J Clin Invest 1991;87: 1664–1667,
40. Curnow KM, Slutker L, Vitek J, et al. Mutations in the CYP11B1 gene causing congenital adrenal hyperplasia and hypertension cluster in exons 6,7 and 8. Proc Natl Acad Sci USA 1993;90:4552–4556.
41. Skinner CA, Rumsby G. Steroid 11-β-hydroxylase deficiency caused by a 5-base pair duplication in the CYP11B1 gene. Hum Mol Genet 1994;3:377–378.
42. Helmberg A, Ausserer B, Kofler R. Frameshift by insertion of 2 basepairs in codon 394 of CYP11B1 causes congenital adrenal hyperplasia due to steroid 11-β-hydroxylase deficiency. J Clin Endocrinol Metab 1992;75:1278–1281.
43. Biglieri EG, Herron MA, Brust N. 17-hydroxylation deficiency. J Clin Invest 1966;45:1946.
44. New MI. Male pseudohermaphroditism due to 17-α-hydroxylase deficiency . J Clin Invest 1970;49:1930.
45. Mantero F, Scaroni C. Enzymatic defects of steroidogenesis: 17α-hydroxylase deficiency. Pediatr Adol Endocrinol 1984;13:83–94.
46. Mansfield TA, Simon DB, Farfel Z. Multilocus linkage of familial hyperkalaemia and hypertension, pseudohypoaldosteronism type II, to chromosomes 1q31-42 and 17p11-q21. Nat Genet 1997;16:202–205.
47. Wilson FH, Disse-Nicodeme S, Choate KA. Human hypertension caused by mutations in WNK kinases. Science 2001;293:1107–1112.
48. Erdogan G, Corapciolgu D, Erdogan MF, Hallioglu J, Uysal AR. Furosemide and dDAVP for the treatment of pseudohypoaldosteronism type II. J Endocrinol Invest 1997;20:681–684.
49. Liddle GW, Bledsoe T, Coppage WS. A familial renal disorder simulating primary aldosteronism with negligible aldosterone secretion. Trans Assoc Phys 1963;76:199–213.
50. Wang C, Chan TK, Yeung RT, Coghlan JP, Scoggins BA, Stockigt JR. The effect of triamterene and sodium intake on renin, aldosterone, and erythrocyte sodium transport in Liddle's syndrome. J Clin Endocrinol Metabol 1981;52:1027–1032.
51. Botero-Velez M, Curtis JJ, Warnock DG. Brief report: Liddle's syndrome revisited—a disorder of sodium reabsorption in the distal tubule. N Engl J Med 1994;330:178–181.
52. Shimkets RA, Warnock DG, Bositis CM, et al. Liddle's syndrome: heritable human hypertension caused by mutations in the beta subunit of the epithelial sodium channel. Cell 1994;79:407–414.

53. Hansson JH, Nelson-Williams C, Suzuki H, et al. Hypertension caused by a truncated epithelial sodium channel gamma subunit: genetic heterogeneity of Liddle syndrome. Nat Genet 1995;11:76–82.
54. Rossier BC. 1996 Homer Smith Award Lecture: cum grano salis: the epithelial sodium channel and the control of blood pressure. J Am Soc Nephrol 1997;8:980–992.
55. Eng C, Crossey PA, Milligan LM, et al. Mutations in the RET proto-oncogene and the von Hippel-Lindau disease tumour suppressor gene in sporadic and syndromic phaeochromocytomas. J Med Genet 1995;32:934–937.
56. Erickson D, Kudva YC, Ebersold MJ, et al. Benign paragangliomas: clinical presentation and treatment outcomes in 236 patients. J Clin Endocrinol Metab 2001;86:5210–5216.
57. Baysal BE, Ferrell RE, Willett-Brozick JE, et al. Mutations in SDHD, a mitochondrial complex II gene, in hereditary paraganglioma. Science 2000;287:848–851.
58. Gimm O, Armanios M, Dziema H, Neumann HPH, Eng C. Somatic and occult germ-line mutations in SDHD, a mitochondrial complex II gene, in nonfamilial pheochromocytoma. Cancer Res 2000;60:6822–6825.
59. Aguiar RC, Cox G, Pomeroy SL, Dahia PL. Analysis of the SDHD gene, the susceptibility gene for familial paraganglioma syndrome (PGL1), in pheochromocytomas. J Clin Endocrinol Metab 2001;86:2890–2894.
60. Santoro M, Carlomagno F, Romano A, et al. Activation of RET as a dominant transforming gene by germline mutations of MEN2A and MEN2B. Science 1995;267:381–383.
61. Neumann HPH, Berger DP, Sigmund G, et al. Pheochromocytomas, multiple endocrine neoplasia type 2, and von Hippel-Lindau disease. N Engl J Med 1993;329:1531–1538.
62. Neumann HPH, Bausch B, McWhinney SR, et al. Germ-line mutations in nonsyndromic pheochromocytoma. N Engl J Med 2002;346:1459–1466.
63. Maxwell PH, Wiesener MS, Chang GW, et al. The tumour suppressor protein VHL targets hypoxia-inducible factors for oxygen-dependent proteolysis. Nature 1999;399:2713–275.
64. Scheffler IE. Molecular genetics of succinate: quinone oxidoreductase in eukaryotes. Prog Nucleic Acid Res Mol Biol 1998;60:267–315.
65. Ackrell BA. Progress in understanding structure-function relationships in respiratory chain complex II. FEBS Lett 2000;466:1–5.
66. Harrap SB. Genetic analysis of blood pressure and sodium balance in the spontaneously hypertensive rat. Hypertension 1986;8:572–582.
67. Rapp JP. Genetic analysis of inherited hypertension in the rat. Physiol Rev 2000;80:135–172.
68. Doris PA. Hypertension genetics, SNPs, and the common disease: common variant hypothesis. Hypertension 2002;39:323–331.
69. Cvetkovic B, Sigmund CD. Understanding hypertension through genetic manipulation in mice. Kidney Int 2000;57:863–874.
70. Gordon JW, Ruddle FH. Gene transfers into mouse embryos: production of transgenic mice by pronuclear integration. Methods Enzymol 1983;101:411–433.
71. Evans MJ, Kaufman MH. Establishment in culture of pluripotential cells from mouse embryos. Nature 1981;292:154–156.
72. Capecchi MR. Altering the genome by homologous recombination. Science 1989;244:1288–1292.
73. Jacob HJ, Lindpaintner K, Lincoln SE, et al. Genetic mapping of a gene causing hypertension in the stroke-prone spontaneously hypertensive rat. Cell 1991:67:213–224.
74. Hilbert P, Lindpaintner K, Beckmann JS, et al. Chromosomal mapping of two genetic loci associated with blood-pressure regulation in hereditary hypertensive rats. Nature 1991;353:521–529.
75. Stoll M, Kwitek-Black AE, Cowley AW, et al. New target regions for human hypertension via comparative genomics. Genome Research 2000;10:473–482.
76. Lalouel J-M, Rohrwasser A, Terreros D, Morgan T, Ward K. Angiotensinogen in essential hypertension: from genetics to nephrology. J Amer Soc Nephrol 2001;12:606–615.
77. Zhu X, Yen-Pei CC, Yan D, et al. Associations between hypertension and genes in the renin-angiotensin system. Hypertension 2003;41:1027–1034.
78. Rice T, Rankinen T, Province MA, et al. Genome-wide linkage analysis of systolic and diastolic blood pressure: the Quebec family study. Circulation 2000;102:1956–1963.
79. Perola M, Kainulainen K, Pajukanta P, et al. Genome-wide scan of predisposing loci for increased diastolic blood pressure in Finnish siblings. J Hypertens 2000;18:1579–1585.
80. Pankow JS, Rose KM, Oberman A, et al. Possible locus on chromosome 18q influencing postural systolic blood pressure changes. Hypertension 2000;36:471–476.

81. Krushkal J, Ferrell R, Mockrin SC, Turner ST, Sing CF, Boerwinkle E. Genome-wide linkage analyses of systolic blood pressure using highly discordant siblings. Circulation 1999;99:1407–1410.
82. Levy D, DeStefano AL, Larson MG, et al. Evidence for a gene influencing blood pressure on chromosome 17: genome scan linkage results for longitudinal blood pressure phenotypes in subjects from the Framingham Heart Study. Hypertension 2000;36:477–483.
83. Sharma P, Fatibene J, Ferraro F, et al. A genome-wide search for susceptibility loci to human essential hypertension. Hypertension 2000;35:1291–1296.
84. Xu X, Rogus JJ, Terwedow HA, et al. An extreme-sib-pair genome scan for genes regulating blood pressure. Am J Hum Genet 1999;64:1694–1701.
85. Wang DG, Fan J-B, Siao C-J, et al. Large-scale identification, mapping and genotyping of single-nucleotide polymorphisms in the human genome. Science 1998;280:1077–1082.
86. The International SNP Map Working Group. A map of human genome sequence variation containing 1.42 million single nucleotide polymorphisms. Nature 2001;409:928–933.
87. Harrap SB. Where are all the blood pressure genes? Lancet 2003;361:2149–2151.
88. Province MA, Kardia SLR, Ranade K, et al. A meta-analysis of genome-wide linkage scans for hypertension: the National Heart Lung and Blood Institute Family Blood Pressure Program. Am J Hypertens 2003;16: 144–147.
89. Caulfield M, Munroe P, Pembroke J, et al. Genome-wide mapping of human loci for essential hypertension. Lancet 2003;361:2118–2123.
90. Izawa H, Yamada Y, Okada T, Tanaka M, Hirayama H, Yokota M. Prediction of genetic risk for hypertension. Hypertension 2003;41:1035–1040.
91. Reudelhuber TL. Salt-sensitive hypertension: if only it were as simple as rocket science. J Clin Invest 2003;111:1115–1116.
92. New MI, Crawford C, Virdis R. Low renin hypertension in childhood. In: Lifshitz F, ed. Pediatric Endocrinology, Third ed. New York: Marcel Dekker, 1995;775–789.

# 13 Perinatal Programming and Blood Pressure

*Julie R. Ingelfinger,* MD

*CONTENTS*



## INTRODUCTION

Epidemiological studies published in the late 1980s by Barker and his group *(1,2)* and since replicated in a number of populations provide evidence of an inverse relationship between birthweight and the risk of cardiovascular disease (CVD), hypertension (HTN), and renal dysfunction in adult life. Clinical studies and a number of animal models have been used to investigate mechanisms underlying these observations (as cited in recent reviews *[3–6]*). The concept that changes in the intrauterine milieu affect the growing fetus, resulting in alterations in physiology and general health in later life, has been termed perinatal programming. Yet, despite a large and burgeoning body of literature about this phenomenon and its relationship to CVD, the involved mechanisms remain elusive.

For a number of years it has been hypothesized that nephron number may strongly influence blood pressure (BP) and susceptibility to renal disease in later life. Brenner, Garcia and Anderson *(7)* were among the first to hypothesize that nephron number influenced the propensity to develop HTN. Recent clinicopathologic observations suggest the existence of a more direct relationship. For example, Keller et al. *(8)* reported fewer nephrons in a small cohort of hypertensive adults who had died in accidents as compared to normotensive persons who succumbed to the same fate. The nephrons among hypertensive subjects were also larger than those in the normotensive group.

Nephron number is not only related to HTN, but also to the tendency to develop chronic kidney disease. For example, Cass et al. *(9)* reported an association between low birthweight, HTN, and later renal disease.

From: *Clinical Hypertension and Vascular Disease: Pediatric Hypertension*
Edited by: R. J. Portman, J. M. Sorof, and J. R. Ingelfinger © Humana Press Inc., Totowa, NJ

A growing body of laboratory work supports the concept that perinatal programming is linked to maternal malnutrition or maternal exposure to certain substances during gestation (e.g., glucocorticoids). The result is subtle alterations that cause offspring to have a propensity to develop high BP or renal dysfunction when they become adults *(10–14)*. For example, numerous studies indicate that pregnant rats or guinea pigs that were administered low protein diets during gestation produce offspring with relatively low birthweights and a propensity for elevated BP at maturity *(10–17)*. The HTN in experimental models is often detected early in life, and appears to persist, unless treated, throughout life *(10–17)*. The kidney, obviously involved in BP control, appears to have undergone deficient nephrogenesis when maternal protein intake is decreased during pregnancy *(12,16)*.

## CLINICAL OBSERVATIONS ON PROGRAMMING AND BLOOD PRESSURE IN CHILDREN

In an early study of this phenomenon, Barker et al. examined BP in 9921 10-yr-old children in whom birthweight was available. They found that systolic blood pressure was inversely related to birthweight *(18)*. Law et al. *(19)* and Whincup et al. *(20)* also reported a direct relationship between birthweight and BP in children, an effect that seems definite, although small *(21–23)*. For example, Seidman et al. *(21)* noted that birthweight had a less significant effect than present weight. Siewert-Delle and Ljungman *(24)* reported that gestational age, rather than birthweight itself, appeared associated with both systolic and diastolic BP in middle-aged men. Their study *(24)* also suggested that middle-aged men who had been term infants had BP that related only to their adult body mass index (BMI), not to birthweight *per se*. Evaluating the weight of the evidence has not been feasible in prospective studies. However, in a systematic review of more than 444,000 male and female subjects ranging in age from infancy to 84 yr of age published in 2000, Huxley and her colleagues *(25)* reviewed 80 studies and drew the conclusion, based on their analysis, that birthweight is inversely related to later systolic BP levels. However, they also concluded that other factors, particularly the rate of postnatal growth, are influential in determining BP *(25)*.

Consequently, as variables other than birthweight exert major influences on BP in children, adolescents, and adults, the inverse relationship between birthweight and the later BP level is not evident in all studies. The effect of current weight may outstrip the effects of birthweight. In data from the Bogalusa Heart Study, children with birthweights less than 2.5 kg were compared to those weighing more than 2.5 kg at birth; no association with birthweight and later blood pressure was discerned, likely owing to the effect of present weight *(26)*. In a study involving 7-yr-old children, Yiu et al. *(27)* found a positive effect of birthweight on HTN after an adjustment for present weight was used in the analysis at the time of follow-up.

## OBSERVATIONAL STUDIES IN EXPERIMENTAL MODELS

A number of investigators *(12,14,15,28–30)* studying models of perinatal programming have demonstrated that low protein diets administered to pregnant rats during gestation can lead to HTN and renal dysfunction in their offspring after the pups mature. Recent publications have elaborated on these observations, citing studies based on the premise that adaptations are necessary to maintain renal hemodynamics if structural impairment of the kidney occurs during organogenesis in fetal life *(28–30)*.

A multideficient diet in a laboratory model reproduces the malnutrition seen in people during famine, war, and in circumstances of severe deprivation. The point in gestation during which the dietary deficiency is experienced makes a large impact. For example, Paixao *(31)* examined two different multideficient diets as compared to a normal diet in Wistar rats. Control mothers ingested a standard diet, while a second group was administered a multideficient diet during both mating and pregnancy, but a normal diet during lactation. A third group was administered a multideficient diet throughout mating, pregnancy, and lactation. Adult offspring of mothers who had been fed a multideficient diet throughout pregnancy *and* lactation had higher mean arterial BP, a decreased number of nephrons, glomerular hypertrophy, and renal arterial vasoconstriction. Adult offspring whose mothers had been fed a multideficient diet only during pregnancy, but not during lactation, had a decreased nephron number and elevated BP, yet did not develop glomerular hypertrophy. Thus, the timing and degree of the insult determines the impact of the given exposures on organogenesis.

Kwong et al. *(32)* showed that a low-protein diet administered solely during the preimplantation period of gestation (from mating to 4.25 d postmating) is sufficient to cause lower birthweight and altered organ/body weight ratios at birth, and subsequently to cause elevated BP and altered rates of postnatal growth by three months after birth. Embryos exposed to this pre-implantation low-protein milieu collected prior to implantation showed a decrease in the numbers of cells in the inner cell mass of the early blastocyst, and a decreased number of cells in the inner cell mass and trophoectoderm of the mid-to-late blastocyst. Cellular proliferation was apparently slower in these fetuses, but apoptosis did not appear to be accelerated. The pregnant mothers subjected to this low-protein diet showed significant decreases in circulating insulin and essential amino acid levels, as well as mildly increased plasma glucose levels, which might have influenced early fetal maldevelopment in that the requisite stem cell lineages failed to reach sufficient size.

Initially, animals born with smaller kidneys may exhibit catch-up growth in measured kidney size, although hyperfiltration may occur if nephrogenesis is inadequate. Nwagwu et al. *(33)* examined the effect of a gestational low-protein diet (90g casein/kg) as compared to a normal protein (180 g casein/kg) diet in offspring in which BP, creatinine clearance, blood urea nitrogen, plasma and urinary albumin, renal morphometry, and metabolic activity were determined. Those mothers exposed to low protein had offspring with higher BP at 4, 12, and 20 wk of age, even when kidney size appeared to "catch up." At 4 wk of age, the low-protein (LP) offspring had smaller kidneys and decreased creatinine clearance compared to the normal-diet offspring. These relative differences were no longer present in 12- and 20-wk-old animals. Nevertheless, low protein-exposed animals in the older age groups had higher blood urea nitrogen levels and more albumin excretion than the control animals. These findings suggest that alterations in postnatal renal hemodynamics render low protein-exposed animals more prone to progressive renal function loss.

In addition to low protein, other maternal exposures can lead to similar phenomena. For example, Lewis et al. *(34)* showed that restricting iron intake in the pregnant rat led to decreased birthweight in the pups and subsequent HTN in adult life. Iron-restricted mothers were anemic at delivery, and their pups had lower hemoglobin levels as compared to normal offspring. At three months of age, offspring remained anemic, and their systolic BP was elevated as compared to BP in offspring of mothers that had not been iron-restricted. Iron-restricted offspring had decreased fasting serum triglyceride, though fasting serum cholesterol and free fatty acid concentrations were similar in both groups. Insulin levels were no different. Maternal iron restriction seemed to "program" offspring for future HTN, with certain findings reminiscent of the maternal protein-restriction model.

Large animal models that produce decreases in fetal growth have also been used to investigate the phenomenon of perinatal programming—maternal undernutrition *(35)*, restriction of iron intake *(36)*, and brief exposure to dexamethasone in utero *(37)*. For example, Dodic et al. *(37)* reported that adult offspring of pregnant ewes exposed to dexamethasone in early pregnancy (e.g., d 26–28 [ovine pregnancy is 145–150 d]), presented with higher BP levels than adult offspring not exposed. The exposed offspring exhibited an elevated cardiac output, reset heart rate, and mean arterial pressure reflexes. At the sheep's midlife (7 yr of age), investigators observed left ventricular hypertrophy and reduced cardiac functional capacity *(38–41)*. The peripheral renin-angiotensin system (RAS) is not activated in adult offspring exposed to dexamethasone *in utero*, although several lines of evidence indicate perinatal RAS activation in the kidney and brain. In this model, for instance, mRNA for $AT_1$ and $AT_2$ receptors in the kidney is increased late in gestation (130 d) *(41)*.

## MECHANISMS

What are the underlying mechanisms responsible for the clinical and laboratory observations? The coordinated developmental events involved in organogenesis are extremely complex *(6)*. It has been recognized for many years that toxic events that interrupt gestation can lead to such disordered development that a fetus does not survive *(42,43)*. For decades, toxicological studies have constituted a major portion of new drug development, as well as a major medicolegal focus when a medication produces serious fetal abnormalities. In contrast to the effects of known toxins, the insults incurred by the fetus owing to malnutrition do not generally produce clearly visible or identifiable abnormalities at birth. Several approaches have been used to find the mechanisms responsible for perinatal programming. The first approach is to examine candidate genes and systems. The idea here is to search for changes in steroid metabolism and feedback in vasoactive systems such as the RAS (these changes are known to affect organogenesis and repair), and in biological systems that might lead to fibrogenesis.

A number of observations support the idea that alterations in steroid metabolism can be caused by maternal diet and medication that can lead to changes in renal structure and function *(44)*. For example, protein restriction decreases the amount of 11-β-hydroxysteroid dehydrogenase (HSD) in the placenta. Decreases in this enzyme, which inactivates maternal cortisol or corticosterone, lead to increased fetal exposure to glucocorticoids from the mother *(45)*. This increased exposure may lead to steroid actions on nuclear receptors, which may influence the development of the kidney and vasculature. Infants with lower birthweight have been found to have placentas with relatively low 11-β hydroxysteroid dehydrogenase activity, supporting the idea of an increased glucocorticoid exposure *(46)*. This basic observation has led to the hypothesis that, in conditions of low protein intake, placental 11-βHSD is decreased, with a subsequent increase in the amount of maternal steroids reaching the fetus, and the attendant changes in nephrogenesis. Indeed, dexamethasone administered to pregnant rats crosses the placenta but is not metabolized by 11-βHSD, resulting in low-birthweight pups with hypertensive tendencies in adulthood *(47,48)*. Carbenoxolone (an inhibitor of 11βHSD) has also resulted in low-birthweight animals with hypertensive tendencies in one study *(49)*, but not in another *(50)*.

Since dexamethasone is often clinically prescribed to accelerate fetal pulmonary development, Ortiz et al. *(44)* examined the impact of prenatal dexamethasone on renal development, reasoning that dexamethasone would predispose rats toward renal disease and HTN later in life. Beginning at mid-gestation, pregnant rats received vehicle or intraperitoneal injections of dexamethasone (0.2 mg/kg body weight) on just 2 d (gestation days: 11 and 12, 13 and 14, 15 and 16, 17 and 18, 19 and 20, or 20 and 21). On d 60 and 90 of postnatal life, tail cuff BP, glomerular number, and insulin clearance were measured in offspring. The prenatal dexamethasone exposure had no effect on the length of gestation, litter size, total body weight, or kidney weight measured on d 1 of life. Offspring of mothers that had received dexamethasone on gestation days 15 and 16 had a 30% reduction in glomerular number relative to controls determined at 60–70 d of age; and on d 17 and 18, 20% fewer glomeruli ($p < 0.01$). However, glomerular filtration was similar in all groups. At 60 to 90 d BP in offspring whose mothers had received dexamethasone on d 15 and 16 of gestation had systolic BP higher than any other group of rats ($p < 0.05$). So whereas the two daily doses of prenatal dexamethasone (0.2 mg/kg body weight) in pregnant rats did not lead to intrauterine growth retardation, the adult progeny had a reduced number of nephrons and HTN, depending on when the dexamethasone was administered.

Manning et al. *(51)* hypothesized that changes in the fetal kidney would program inappropriate sodium retention in later life as one explanation for the HTN observed. They subsequently examined the role of sodium transporters, speculating that at least one would demonstrate increased activity. They fed timed-pregnant Sprague Dawley rats a 6% protein diet or an isocaloric 20% protein diet (normal protein) from d 12 of gestation until delivery, after which mothers nursed pups while receiving a normal-protein diet. As anticipated, pups had a decrease in body and kidney weight at birth; at 8 wk of age (but not at 4 wk), LP offspring had developed HTN. LP offspring showed evidence of upregulation of mRNA for two transporters, Renal BSC1 and TSC, at 4 wk of age, prior to the development of HTN.

Lucas et al. *(52)* reproduced the undernutrition model and examined in some detail what happens within hypertrophic glomeruli. In their model, 50% food restriction involving the mothers led to offspring with a decreased number of glomeruli that exhibited increased glomerular diameter, suggesting compensatory hypertrophy and hyperfiltration. They posited that glomerular hypertrophy would ultimately lead to renal damage, and have now carried out morphological, immunohistochemical, and functional studies in offspring exposed to this energy restriction in utero. Both control and intrauterine food-restricted animals were examined at 3 and 18 mo of age. The glomerular filtration rate (GFR) was significantly diminished in 18-mo-old offspring of restricted rats compared to control rats (2.42 ± 0.15 mL/min/kg; $n = 28$; $p < 0.05$ as compared to 4.19 ± 0.10 mL/min/kg; $p < 0.05$). Furthermore, the percentage of glomeruli with sclerosis was greater in restricted rats than with controls at 18 mo (13.01% ± 2.95%; $n = 9$; $p < 0.01$ cf. 2.71% ± 0.35%; $n = 6$). The offspring of restricted rats exhibited intense tubulointerstitial lesions and immunohistochemical alterations in the renal cortex-increased fibronectin and desmin expression in glomeruli and tubulointerstitium and increased vimentin and α-smooth muscle actin in the tubulointerstitial area from the renal cortex. Furthermore, desmin was increased at the periphery of glomeruli, which implies likely podocyte injury. The authors suggest that the aberrant glomerulogenesis in the malnourished dams leads to hyperfiltration and ensuing renal damage. Of course, these observations are not specific and might well occur in any model of hyperfiltration.

The intrarenal RAS generally demonstrates altered expression in the offspring of mothers who have been subjected to protein restriction during gestation. The kidneys of rat pups born to protein-restricted mothers show a dramatic decrease in renin mRNA, protein, immunostaining, and angiotensin II (ANG II) levels *(16,30,53)*. The decrease in intrarenal ANG II is of particular interest, since that octapeptide is critical to normal growth and remodeling, and therefore important in nephrogenesis *(54)*. Finding alterations in the RAS is consistent with prior reports that manipulations that alter the production of ANG II, or block ANG II receptors, will result in changes in normal renal development. Woods et al. have performed careful morphometry, and demonstrated association of decreased glomerular number with early suppression of the intrarenal RAS *(28)*. Other groups have examined the circulating RAS and its relation to perinatal programming. For example, Langley-Evans *(39)* determined the levels of circulating renin in offspring of protein-restricted mothers, and observed decreased plasma renin activity. Vehaskari et al. *(30)* found similar results, although differences between the reports may reflect that different groups utilized different degrees of protein deprivation and timed their measurements accordingly. However, the data taken together suggest that restriction of maternal dietary protein suppresses the perinatal RAS. On the other hand, Peers et al. *(38)* did not observe changes in the fetal RAS. However, the data taken together suggest that interruption of normal functions of the RAS could result in fewer nephrons, ultimately predisposing one to HTN in adult life *(55)*.

Many distinct and separate studies have shown that the RAS is critical to normal renal development. For example, some transgenic animals with altered RAS genes develop severe HTN, but others do not; in still others, HTN can be induced, which lends emphasis to the critical nature of the RAS in controlling blood pressure level *(56)*. Additionally, "knockout" animals that lack RAS genes may demonstrate renal maldevelopment *(57–59)*. Pharmacologic agents, such as angiotensin-converting enzyme (ACE) inhibitors, if given to experimental animals or to humans during gestation, can result in extreme fetopathy *(60–61)*. Similarly, angiotensin receptor blockers can also lead to renal maldevelopment. The $AT_1$ receptor antagonist losartan, when given to rat pups during postnatal day 1–12 (during which nephrogenesis continues), diminishes the nephron number and results in subsequent HTN in adult life *(55)*.

Increasing maternal salt intake can result in changes in renal structure and function quite similar to those produced by protein restriction. Since increased salt intake in itself decreases fetal RAS expression, it would appear that a similar mechanism is operative *(16)*. Programming exhibits sexual dimorphism, given that males and females are not similarly prone to experience perinatal programming given the same exposures *(62)*. For example, Holemans et al. *(63)* showed that male offspring of mothers who had been given low-protein diets in the latter half of pregnancy were far more susceptible to low birthweights as compared to their female littermates. The female littermates then appeared to be resistant to elevated BP as adults. Woods et al. have also noted that male pups were more susceptible to decreases of intrarenal renin and ANG II; males, but not females, later became hypertensive *(51)*.

Vickers et al. *(64–65)* have induced maternal undernutrition throughout pregnancy, followed by postnatal hypercaloric nutrition in offspring to produce a rat model of syndrome X. They observed the development of hyperphagia, obesity, HTN, hyperinsulinemia, and hyperleptinemia in offspring whose mothers had been subjected to undernutrition in pregnancy. This model has also been used to study the influence of insulin-like growth factor 1 (IGF-1) administration. Pregnant Wistar rats were fed either *ad libitum* or with a diet that contained only 30% of the *ad libitum* intake throughout gestation. Once weaned, female offspring were placed on a control diet or a hypercaloric (30% fat) diet and observed. At d 175 of life, systolic BP was measured in these female offspring, and measured again after recombinant human IGF-1 infusion (3 μg/g/d via osmotic minipump for 2 wk). Prior to the IGF-1 therapy, the offspring of mothers that had received a deficient diet during pregnancy, and that were placed on a hypercaloric diet were hypertensive, hyperphagic, and obese, exhibiting hyperinsulinemia and hyperleptinemia. IGF-I therapy was still associated with weight gain when added to the hypercaloric diet, but BP, as well as plasma leptin and insulin concentrations, fell dramatically. IGF binding proteins (38–44 kDa and 28–30 kDa) increased 300–500% when the animals received IGF-1. The conclusion was that it appeared that IGF-1 treatment ameliorated hyperphagia, obesity, hyperinsulinemia, hyperleptinemia, and HTN in a model of metabolic syndrome X.

## GROWTH FACTORS

Growth factors are important in nephrogenesis, and their alterations may lead to aberrant renal morphogenesis *(67–68)*. Rees et al. *(69)* have demonstrated that maternal protein deficiency leads maternal decrease in circulating threonine, and is associated with hepatic hypermethylation of DNA. They fed pregnant rats with diets that contained 18% casein, 9% casein, or 8% casein supplemented with threonine. Then, they examined the hypothesis that added threonine would correct diminished circulating threonine concentrations in the pregnant rats receiving protein-deficient diets. The fetuses of the mothers that received the low-protein diet and the low-protein diet supplemented with threonine were similarly and significantly smaller than the control fetuses. Liver homogenates prepared from mothers fed the diet containing 9% casein-oxidized threonine at approx twice the rate of those homogenates prepared from mothers fed the normal diet. Therefore, it is likely that maternal levels of threonine diminish from an increase in the activity of the metabolic pathway in which homocysteine is produced by the transulfuration of methionine. These findings suggest that alterations in methionine metabolism lead to an increased homocysteine production, which might alter fetal DNA methylation. The altered DNA methylation might account for differences that affect organogenesis, and much later, increase the offspring's chances of developing several diseases in adult life.

The coordinated program necessary for kidney formation requires the development and regression of the pronephros and mesonephros, and the interaction of the mesonephros with the metanephros *(70)*. The changes brought about by perinatal programming would more than likely be reflected by subtle alterations in the process of nephrogenesis.

The hypothesis and observation that adult HTN is associated with fewer nephrons has been well-documented by Brenner et al. *(71)*. Fewer glomeruli have been reported in autopsies of human infants with intrauterine growth retardation, which is consistent with the hypothesis *(72)*. Kwong *(32)* observed increased apoptosis in blastocysts of rats exposed to a low protein diet in the preimplantation stage of gestation. Welham et al. *(73)* noted that protein restriction during gestation in rats appears to be associated with increased apoptosis in mesenchymal cells. Welham et al. *(73)* point out that the metanephric mesenchyme, a subset of which is induced to form nephrons, is derived from the intermediate mesoderm. The intermediate mesoderm is also the source of the pronephros and mesonephros, which eventually become residual structures, such as the wolffian duct. Metanephric mesenchyme recruited via factors emanating from the ureteric bud to form the final kidney will undergo apoptosis unless rescued. Increased apoptosis would presumably result in fewer generations of nephrons. Welham et al. have observed increased apoptosis in metanephroi dissected from the embryos of pregnant rats subjected to low protein intake *(73)*. Though this study showed substantial overlap in observed apoptotic and mitotic cells, it may also provide an important link to observed association between a low nephron number and HTN in adult life.

What do these observations tell us? Basic studies provide substantial evidence that intrauterine events affect nephrogenesis, perhaps in subtle ways, and induce effects that can be observed only later in life. The propensity to develop HTN, renal disease, and CVD may well be initiated, at least in some persons, by intrauterine and perinatal events that impact organogenesis in subtle ways.

## REFERENCES


1. Barker D, Bull A, Osmond C, Simmonds S. Fetal and placental size and risk of hypertension in adult life. BMJ 1990;301:259–262.
2. Barker D, Godfrey K, Osmond C, Bull A. The relation of fetal length, ponderal index and head circumference to blood pressure and the risk of hypertension in adult life. Paed Perinatal Epidemiol 1992;6:35–44.
3. Langley-Evans SC, Gardner DS, Welham SJM. Intrauterine programming of cardiovascular disease by maternal nutritional status. Nutrition 1998;14:39–47.
4. Woods LL. Fetal origins of adult hypertension: a renal mechanism? Curr Opin Nephrol Hypertens 2000; 9(4):419–425.
5. Barker DJP. Mothers, Babies and Health in Later Life. 2nd ed. Edinburgh: Churchill Livingstone, 1998.
6. Godfrey KM, Barker DJ. Fetal programming and adult health. Public Health Nutr 2001;4(2B):611–624.
7. Brenner BM, Garcia DL, Anderson S. Glomeruli and blood pressure. Less of one, more the other? Am J Hypertens 1988;1:335–347.
8. Keller G, Zimmer G, Mall G, Ritz E, Amann K. Nephron number in patients with primary hypertension. New Engl J Med 2003;348(2):101–108.
9. Cass A, Cunningham J, Snelling P, Wang Z, Hoy W. End-stage renal disease in indigenous Australians: a disease of disadvantage. Ethnicity & Disease 2002;12(3):373–378.
10. Langley-Evans SC, Phillips GJ, Jackson AA. In utero exposure to maternal low protein diets induces hypertension in weanling rats, independently of maternal blood pressure changes. Clin Nutr 1994;13:319.
11. Persson E, Jansson T. Low birth weight is associated with elevated adult blood pressure in the chronically catheterized guinea pig. Acta Physiol Scand 1995;115:195.
12. Merlet-Benichou C, Gilbert T, Muffat-Joly M, Lelievre-Pegorier M, Leroy B. Intrauterine growth retardation leads to a permanent nephron deficit in the rat. Ped Nephrol 1994;8:175–180.
13. Timofeeva NM, Egorova VV, Nikitina AA. Metabolic/food programming of enzyme systems in digestive and nondigestive organs of rats. Doklady Biological Sciences 2000;375:587–589.
14. Langley-Evans SC. Critical differences between two low protein diet protocols in the programming of hypertension in the rat. Int J Food Sci Nutr 2000;51(1):11–17.
15. Langley-Evans SC, Welham SJM, Jackson AA. Fetal exposure to a maternal low protein diet impairs nephrogenesis and promotes hypertension in the rat. Life Sci 1999;64:965–974.
16. Ingelfinger JR, Haveran L, Hsu C-Y, Woods LL. Maternal low protein or high salt diet in the perinatal period suppresses newborn intrarenal renin-angiotensin system (RAS) and programs for hypertension in adult offspring. Ped Res 1998;43:309A.
17. Manning J, Vehaskari VM. Low birth weight-associated adult hypertension in the rat. Pediatr Nephrol 2001; 16(5):417–422.
18. Barker DJ, Osmond C, Golding J, Kuh D, Wadsworth ME. Growth in utero, blood pressure in childhood and adult life, and mortality from cardiovascular disease. BMJ 1989;298(6673):564–567.
19. Law C, de Swiet M, Osmond C, Fayers PM, Barker DJP, Cruddas AM. Initiation of hypertension in utero and its amplification throughout life. BPJ 1993;306:24–27.
20. Whincup PH, Cook DG, Shaper AG. Early influences on blood pressure: a study of children aged 5–7 years. BMJ 1989;299:587–591.
21. Seidman D, Laor A, Gale R, Stevenson D, Mashiach S, Danon Y. Birth weight, current body weight and blood pressure in late adolescence. BMJ 1991;302:1235–1237.
22. Whincup P, Cook D, Papacosta O, Walker M. Birth weight and blood pressure: cross sectional and longitudinal relations in childhood BMJ 1995;311:773–776.
23. Taylor SJ, Whincup PH, Cook DG, Papacosta O, Walker M. Size at birth and blood pressure: cross sectional study in 8–11 year old children. BMJ 1997;314:475.

24. Siewert-Delle A, Ljungman S. The impact of birth weight and gestational age on blood pressure in adult life: a population based study of 49-year old men. Am J Hypertens 1998;II:946–953.
25. Huxley RR, Shiell AW, Law CM. The role of size at birth and postnatal catch-up growth in determining systolic blood pressure: a systematic review of the literature. J Hypertension 2000;18:815–831.
26. Donker G, Labarthe DR, Harriat RB, Selwyn BJ, Wattigney W, Berenson GS. Low birth weight and blood pressure at age 7–11 years in a biracial sample. Am J Epidemiol 1997;147:87–88.
27. Yiu V, Buka S, Zurakowski D, McCormick M, Brenner B, Jabs K. Relationship between birthweight and blood pressure in childhood. Am J Kidney Dis 1999;33(2):253–260.
28. Woods LL, Ingelfinger JR, Nyengaard JR, Rasch R. Maternal protein restriction suppresses the newborn renin-angiotensin system and programs adult hypertension in the rat. Pediatr Res 2001;49:460–467.
29. Sahajpal V, Ashton N. Renal function and angiotensin AT1 receptor expression in young rats following intrauterine exposure to a maternal low-protein diet. Clinical Science 2003;104(6):607–614.
30. Vehaskari VM, Aviles DH, Manning J. Prenatal programming of adult hypertension in the rat. Kidney Int 2001; 59:238–245.
31. Paixao AD, Maciel CR, Teles MB, Figueiredo-Silva J. Regional Brazilian diet-induced low birth weight is correlated with changes in renal hemodynamics and glomerular morphometry in adult age. Biol Neonate 2001;80(3):239–246.
32. Kwong WY, Wild AE, Roberts P, Willis AC, Fleming TP. Maternal undernutrition during the preimplantation period of rat development causes blastocyst abnormalities and programming of postnatal hypertension. Dev Suppl 2000;127(19):4195–4202.
33. Nwagwu MO, Cook A, Langley-Evans SC. Evidence of progressive deterioration of renal function in rats exposed to a maternal low-protein diet in utero. Br J Nutr. 2000;83(1):79–85.
34. Lewis RM, Petry CJ, Ozanne SE, Hales CN. Effects of maternal iron restriction in the rat on blood pressure, glucose tolerance, and serum lipids in the 3-month-old offspring. Metabolism 2001;50(5):562–567.
35. Gallaher BW, Breier BH, Keven CL, Harding JE, Gluckman PD. Fetal programming of insulin-like growth factor (IGF)-I and IGF-binding protein-3: evidence for an altered response to undernutrition in late gestation following exposure to periconceptual undernutrition in the sheep. J Endocrinol 1998;159(3):501–508.
36. Mostello D, Chalk C, Khoury J, Mack CE, Siddiqi TA, Clark KE. Chronic anemia in pregnant ewes: maternal and fetal effects. Am J Physiol 1991;261:R1075–R1083.
37. Dodic M, May CN, Wintou EM, Coghlan JP. An early prenatal exposure to excess glucocorticoid leads to hypertensive offspring in sheep. Clin Sci (Colch) 1998;94:103–109.
38. Peers A, Campbell DJ, Wintour EM, Dodic M. The peripheral renin-angiotensin system is not involved in the hypertension of sheep exposed to prenatal dexamethasone. Clin Exp Pharmacol Physiol 2001;28:306–311.
39. Gatford KL, Wintour EM, De Blasio MJ, Owens JA, Dodic M. Differential timing for programming of glucose homoeostasis, sensitivity to insulin and blood pressure by in utero exposure to dexamethasone in sheep. Clin Sci (Colch) 2000;98:553–560.
40. Dodic M, Baird R, Hantzis V, et al. Organs/systems potentially involved in one model of programmed hypertension in sheep. Clin Exp Pharmacol Physiol 2001;28:952–956.
41. Moritz KM, Johnson K, Douglas-Denton R, Wintour EM, Dodic M. Maternal glucocorticoid treatment programs alterations in the renin-angiotensin system of the ovine fetal kidney. Endocrinol 2002;143:4455–4463.
42. Mantovani A, Calamandrei G. Delayed developmental effects following prenatal exposure to drugs. Curr Pharm Des 2001;7:859–880.
43. Nagao T, Wada K, Marumo H, Yoshimura S, Ono H. Reproductive effects of nonylphenol in rats after gavage administration: a two-generation study. Reprod Toxicol 2001;15:293–315.
44. Ortiz LA, Quan A, Weinberg A, Baum M. Effect of prenatal dexamethasone on rat renal development. Kidney Int 2001;59:1663–1669.
45. Edwards LJ, Simonetta G, Owens JA, Robinson JS, McMillen IC. Restriction of the placental and fetal growth in sheep alters fetal blood pressure responses to angiotensin II and captopril. J Physiol (Lond) 1999;515:897–904.
46. Seckl JR, Benediktsson R, Lindsay RS, Brown RW. Placental 11 beta-hydroxysteroid dehydrogenase and the programming of hypertension. J Steroid Biochem Molec Biol 1995;55:447–455.
47. Celsi G, Kistner A, Aizman R, et al. Prenatal dexamethasone causes oligonephronia, sodium retention and higher blood pressure in the offspring. Pediatr Res 1998;44:317–322.
48. Benediktsson R, Lindsay RS, Noble J, Seckl JR, Edwards CRW. Glucocorticoid exposure in utero: a new model for adult hypertension. Lancet 1993;341:339–341.

49. Langley-Evans SC. Maternal carbenoxolone treatment lowers birthweight and induces hypertension in the offspring of rats fed a protein-replete diet. Clin Sci 1997;93:423–429.
50. Gomez-Sanchez, Elise P, Gomez-Sanchez CE. Maternal hypertension and progeny blood pressure: role of aldosterone and 11 beta-HSD. Hypertension 1999;33:1369–1373.
51. Manning J, Beutler K, Knepper MA, Vehaskari VM. Upregulation of renal BSC1 and TSC in prenatally programmed hypertension. Am J Physiol 2002;283(1):F202–F206.
52. Lucas A. Programming by nutrition in man. In: Conning D, ed. Early Diet, Later Consequences. London: British Nutrition Federation, 1992;24.
53. Langley-Evans SC. Fetal programming of cardiovascular function through exposure to maternal undernutrition. Proceedings of the Nutrition Society 2001;60:505–513.
54. Tufro-McReddie A, Romano LM, Harris JM, Ferber L, Gomez RA. Angiotensin II regulates nephrogenesis and renal vascular development. Am J Physiol 1995;269:F110–F115.
55. Woods LL, Rasch R. Perinatal Ang II programs adult blood pressure, glomerular number, and renal function in rats. Am J Physiol 1998;275:R1593–R1599.
56. Mullins JJ, Peters J, Ganten D. Fulminant hypertension in transgenic rats harbouring the mouse Ren-2 gene. Nature 1990;344(6266):541–544.
57. Nishimura H, Yerkes E, Hohenfellner K, et al. Role of the angiotensin type 2 receptor gene in congenital anomalies of the kidney and urinary tract. CAKUT, of mice and men. Mol Cell 1999;3:1–10.
58. Okubo S, Niimura F, Matsusaka T, Fogo A, Hogan BL, Ichikawa I. Angiotensinogen gene null-mutant mice lack homeostatic regulation of glomerular filtration and tubular reabsorption. Kidney Int 1998;53:617–625.
59. Tsuchida S, Matsusaka T, Chen X, et al. Murine double nullizygotes of the angiotensin type 1A and 1B receptor genes duplicate severe abnormal phenotypes of angiotensinogen nullizygotes. J Clin Invest 1998;101:755–760.
60. Sedman AB, Kershaw DB, Bunchman TE. Recognition and management of angiotensin converting enzyme inhibitor fetopathy. Pediatric Nephrology 1995;9(3):382–385.
61. Barr M. Teratogen update: angiotensin-converting enzyme inhibitors. Teratology 1994;50:399–409.
62. Ingelfinger JR, Rasch R, Shih S, Woods LL. Sexual dimorphism in perinatal programming: effect of maternal protein restriction on the renin-angiotensin system and renal development. Pediatr Res 2000;47:71A.
63. Holemans K, Gerber R, Meurrens K, DeClerck F, Poston L, Van Assche F. Maternal food restriction in the second half of pregnancy affects vascular function but not blood pressure of rat female offspring. Br J Nutr 1999;81:73–79.
64. Vickers MH, Ikenasio BA, Breier BH. IGF-I treatment reduces hyperphagia, obesity, and hypertension in metabolic disorders induced by fetal programming. Endocrinology 2001;142(9):3964–3973.
65. Vickers MH, Reddy S, Ikenasio BA, Breier BH. Dysregulation of the adipoinsular axis — a mechanism for the pathogenesis of hyperleptinemia and adipogenic diabetes induced by fetal programming. J Endocrinol 2001;170(2):323–332.
66. Green LR. Programming of endocrine mechanisms of cardiovascular control and growth. J Soc Gynecol Invest 2001;8:57–68.
67. Muaku SM, Beauloye V, Thissen JP, et al. Long-term effects of gestational protein malnutrition on postnatal growth, insulin-like growth factor and IGF-binding proteins in rat progeny. Pediatr Res 1996;39:649–655.
68. Tufro A, Norwood VF, Carey RM, Gomez RA. Vascular endothelial growth factor induces nephrogenesis and vasculogenesis. J Am Soc Nephrol1999;10(10):2125–2134.
69. Rees WD, Hay SM, Buchan V, Antipatis C, Palmer RM. The effects of maternal protein restriction on the growth of the rat fetus and its amino acid supply. Br J Nutr 1999;81:243–250.
70. Kuure S, Vuolteenaho R, Vainio S. Kidney morphogenesis: cellular and molecular regulation. Mech Develop 2000;92(1):31–45.
71. Brenner BM, Mackenzie HS. Nephron mass as a risk factor for progression of renal disease. Kidney International-Supplement 1997;63:S124–S127.
72. Abitbol CL, Bauer CR, Montane B, Chandar J, Duara S, Zilleruelo G. Long-term follow-up of extremely low birth weight infants with neonatal renal failure. Pediatr Nephrol. 2003;18(9):887–893.
73. Welham SJ, Wade A, Woolf AS. Protein restriction in pregnancy is associated with increased apoptosis of mesenchymal cells at the start of rat metanephrogenesis. Kidney International 2002;61(4):1231–1242.

# 14 Cardiovascular Reactivity in Youth

## *Toward a Gene-Environment Model of Stress-Induced Cardiovascular Disease*

*Frank A. Treiber, PhD and Harold Snieder, PhD*

**CONTENTS**



## INTRODUCTION

Although the incidence rate of coronary heart disease (CHD) has declined over the past several decades, it continues to be the leading cause of death in adults in the US *(1)*. Essential hypertension (HTN), a primary risk factor for CHD, is the most common cardiovascular disease (CVD), affecting approximately 50 million Americans *(1,2)*. Necropsy studies have clearly established that the pathogenesis of CVD has its origins in childhood *(3–5)*. Consequently, primary prevention efforts may prove more beneficial if initiated during childhood, rather than in early to middle adulthood, by which time many pathophysiologic alterations related to CVD have already occurred *(6–8)*. Although overt manifestations of CVD often do not occur until middle adulthood, recent advances in noninvasive medical technology permit us to evaluate preclinical manifestations of CVD, allowing researchers to examine correlates of CVD prior to the development of overt disease.

Only about 50% of the variance of new CVD cases can be attributed to classic risk factors, such as family history, obesity, smoking, diabetes mellitus, and hypercholesteremia *(9)*. As a result, much effort has been devoted to the identification of other potential risk factors. Cardio-

From: *Clinical Hypertension and Vascular Disease: Pediatric Hypertension*
Edited by: R. J. Portman, J. M. Sorof, and J. R. Ingelfinger © Humana Press Inc., Totowa, NJ

vascular reactivity (CVR), defined as the magnitude or pattern of an individual's hemodynamic responses to behavioral stressors, has been identified as a potential risk factor for the development of CVD. The "reactivity hypothesis" posits that CVR may play a role as a marker or mechanism in the pathogenesis of CVD *(10)*. A number of review articles, monographs, and books have been written about CVR in animals, adults, and youth *(e.g., 10–15)*. This chapter is not meant to be a review of the entire field. The purpose is to provide an overview of CVR in youth. The emphasis is on prospective work which has examined the relationship of CVR to behavioral/psychological stressors in the prediction of preclinical markers of CVD risk. Included among these preclinical markers are: (1), sustained increases in blood pressure (BP) and/or development of essential HTN, and (2), increased left ventricular (LV) mass. We then propose a gene-environment model of stress-induced CVD that depicts several pathways by which exaggerated CVR, in combination with genetic susceptibility and unfavorable environmental factors, may eventually lead to such overt manifestations of CVD such as essential HTN.

## STABILITY OF CARDIOVASCULAR REACTIVITY

A crucial assumption of the reactivity hypothesis is that CVR is a stable individual difference characteristic, consistent across time (i.e., temporal stability) and stressors (i.e., intertask consistency) *(11,15–17)*. If the relationship of CVR to stress plays a role in the prediction of CVD, this consistency must be seen as a prerequisite and is most likely established relatively early in life *(12)*.

### *Temporal Stability of Cardiovascular Reactivity*

The longest time interval studied to date (in adults or youth) is 28 yr. Cold pressor reactivity was assessed on 151 subjects from a cohort initially 6–19 yr old *(18)*. All 31 subjects in the follow-up sample who had originally been classified as hyperreactive (systolic BP increase >20 mmHg) were still classified as hyperreactive at follow-up, and 99 of the 120 normoreactive subjects retained their initial classification.

Since that time a number of pediatric studies have evaluated the stability of BP, heart rate (HR), and most recently, cardiac output (CO) and total peripheral resistance (TPR) (the underlying hemodynamic regulators of BP control) across time periods ranging from one week to 6 yr *(19–29)*. In general, these findings have indicated that, regardless of sex and ethnicity, CVR is stable in youth for a variety of stressors, including video game challenge, postural change, cold pressor, isometric handgrip, mirror image tracing, and mental arithmetic. Stability coefficients are similar to those observed for resting BP and HR, particularly when absolute stressor response levels are used ($r$ range = 0.40–0.70) *(22,23)*. When change scores are used, there tends to be a decrease in the correlation coefficients comparable to adult findings (for reviews, *see 15,30*). Lower stability coefficients for change scores are expected, since change scores contain potential measurement error of both the baseline measure and of the response measure. It should be noted that Kamarck and colleagues *(31–33)* have shown that aggregating adults' cardiovascular (CV) responses to comparable behavioral stressors increase the temporal stability coefficients of change scores ($r$ range = 0.85–0.96). Such approaches may prove beneficial in CVR studies involving youth.

### *Intertask Consistency of Cardiovascular Reactivity*

Another underlying assumption of the reactivity hypothesis is that an individual who is hyperreactive to one stressor (e.g., mental arithmetic) is likely to exhibit similar hemodynamic response changes to other stressors (e.g., video game challenge). Similarly to adult studies, of the few studies conducted with youth, the majority have evaluated BP and HR responses, and observed moderate consistency across a variety of stressor comparisons *(20,34,35)*. For instance, Parker et al. *(36)* observed intertask correlations of peak BP responses from 0.53 to 0.84 to hand cold pressor, isometric handgrip exercise, and postural change. Matthews et al. *(23)* observed consistency in BP and HR change scores to mental arithmetic, mirror image tracing, and isometric handgrip exercise (r range = 0.30–0.60). Musante et al. *(37)* examined the consistency of children's BP, CO, and TPR change scores to postural change, forehead cold, and a challenging video game (Atari(r) "Breakout"). The highest coefficients across stressors were noted for CO and TPR (r range = .32–.68). These findings, along with those of McGrath and O'Brien *(19)*, indicate that intertask consistency is comparable or may be higher for the underlying hemodynamic regulators of BP control (i.e., CO and TPR) compared to BP responses, particularly diastolic responses, and are consistent with findings in adults *(30,38)*.

## CARDIOVASCULAR REACTIVITY IN THE LABORATORY VS THE FIELD

Another assumption of the reactivity hypothesis is that individuals who are hyperresponsive in the lab will also be hyperresponsive to naturally-occurring stressors in the free-living environment. Although ambulatory BP monitoring (ABPM) has permitted such evaluations to be conducted, relatively few studies have been conducted in youth. Findings have indicated low to moderate relationships between CVR to laboratory stressors and ambulatory BP measurements in various field settings *(39–41)*. For example, Matthews, Manuck, and Saab *(42)* found that teenagers classified as being hyperreactive to serial subtraction, isometric handgrip exercise, and star tracing also exhibited elevated CV responses while giving a speech at school. Twenty-four hour ambulatory BP in youth was found to correlate significantly with BP responses to a variety of stressors (i.e., postural change, video game, forehead cold, and dynamic exercise) *(43)*. In a longitudinal study, Rosario et al. *(44)* found that in addition to the contributions of anthropometrics, demographics, and resting BP, BP and/or TPR responses to a behavioral challenge (i.e., video game) and to postural change (supine to standing position) were predictive of 24-h ambulatory BP two years later in children with family histories of essential HTN. Collectively, these findings are promising with regard to the potential value of laboratory-based CVR studies in predicting CV functioning in the free-living environment, particularly given the lack of control over various moderating influences upon BP (e.g., posture, physical activity, affective state, etc.) *(16)*. Recent advances in monitoring such influences via electronic diaries should prove beneficial in linking lab-based CVR to behavioral stressors with CV variations related to behavioral stress in the natural environment.

In summary, CVR to behavioral challenges in the laboratory is a stable individual difference dimension in childhood, as noted by its relative stability over time and across challenges. There is an indication that CVR in the lab may be representative of CVR in the natural setting. However, further research is needed, particularly with regard to lab to field generalization of CVR to behavioral stress.

## PREDICTION OF PRECLINICAL CARDIOVASCULAR DISEASE STATES IN YOUTH

The pathogenesis of CVD follows a relatively consistent progression *(45–47)*. Devereux and colleagues have coined the term "preclinical disease states" to describe pathogenic changes in CV structure or function that, if uninterrupted, will often progress to overt manifestations of CVD, including myocardial infarction (MI), stroke, and essential HTN *(48–50)*. Over the past decade, a number of pediatric studies have examined the relationship between acute CVR to laboratory stimuli and longitudinal changes in noninvasive measures of preclinical CVD.

Below we examine pediatric CVR studies that have included two types of preclinical measures: increased resting BP and left ventricular (LV) mass. Essential HTN in adulthood, typically defined as systolic BP exceeding 140 mmHg and/or diastolic BP exceeding 90 mmHg *(51)*, is the typical target of treatment. However, even within the normotensive range, increased resting BP is a major independent risk factor for future essential HTN and CHD *(52–54)*. Importantly, BP tracks from late childhood into adulthood *(55)*. Increases in resting BP over time, then, constitute an important preclinical measure of CVD risk for the purpose of this review. The processes by which exaggerated CVR has been posited to contribute to essential HTN (for example, vascular remodeling and autoregulatory processes) *(56,57)* should also be expected to affect resting BP in the normotensive range.

The second preclinical measure that will be covered is LV mass. Left ventricular hypertrophy (LVH) has been identified as a significant independent risk factor for CV morbidity (including MI, arrhythmia, congestive heart failure) and mortality *(58–64)*. The risk conferred by increased LV mass is independent of traditional CV risk factors *(65)*, as well as other measures of CVD, such as number of diseased vessels, or ventricular function *(66)*. Although this condition is important prognostically, its determinants are only beginning to be understood. In addition to the effects of resting BP and anthropometric factors (e.g., height and body mass), a variety of hemodynamic and neuroendocrine factors that may be influenced by behavioral stress have been shown to alter the development of LV mass. These types of influences might be expected to be more prevalent among individuals who exhibit exaggerated CVR during behavioral stress.

## PREDICTION OF FUTURE BLOOD PRESSURE LEVELS

To date, only one study has evaluated relationships between CVR in healthy, normotensive youth and the clinical endpoint of essential HTN in adulthood. Wood et al. *(67)* conducted a 45-yr follow-up using cold pressor BP reactivity data collected in the 1930s *(68,69)* Findings indicated that 71% of subjects classified as hyperreactive in childhood (6–19 yr of age) had developed essential HTN in adulthood.

Eleven additional studies have assessed relationships between BP reactivity to acute laboratory stressors and subsequent BP levels in normotensive children and adolescents. A variety of stressors were used, including cold stimulation *(29,70,71)* and more purely psychological challenges (e.g., video games, serial subtraction, mirror-tracing, reaction time) *(29,44,72–77)*. In brief, all 11 studies reported positive results. For example, Murphy et al. *(76)* measured BP reactivity to a video game challenge in 292 European-American (EA) and 46 African-American (AA) third graders to predict resting BP levels 5 yr later. Regression analyses indicated that diastolic BP and systolic BP reactivity to the video game were stronger predictors of BP levels 5 yr later than resting BP at study entry among AA children. In contrast, among EA children, resting BP at study entry was the best predictor of BP level 5 yr later. Video game BP reactivity enhanced the prediction of subsequent systolic BP but not diastolic BP. In summary, when resting BP, resting HR, obesity, and age were entered as the first four variables in regression models, the video game BP responses continued to be significant predictors of subsequent BP in both EA and AA children.

More recently, Treiber et al. *(29,71,74,75,77)* reported a series of findings on a longitudinal study of AA and EA children (6–16 yr old at study onset) having family histories of essential HTN. After controlling for contributions of ethnicity, sex, anthropometrics (e.g., height, weight, adiposity) and initial resting BP levels, systolic BP and diastolic BP responses to a video game challenge, and forehead stimulation, each predicted resting systolic BP and diastolic BP at both the 1- and 5-yr follow-ups. The most comprehensive study in this series examined 385 normotensive youth (mean age 12.7 yr at baseline) who had been evaluated annually on four occasions following the initial baseline visit *(75)*. Aggregated measures of systolic BP and diastolic BP reactivity to a battery of stressors (i.e., video game, social competence interview, parent-child conflict discussion, postural change) were assessed at baseline. Separate prediction models for each year were derived from stepwise hierarchical block regressions and applied to all other years. The most generalizable model revealed that systolic BP and diastolic BP reactivity accounted for 2–6% and 1–4% additional variance respectively, after accounting for significant contributions of traditional risk factors, including ethnicity (AAs > EAs), sex (males > females), family history of CVD, anthropometrics (increased waist-to-hip ratio, height, weight, body mass index [BMI]), and initial baseline BP levels. In summary, evidence indicates that CVR is a consistent independent predictor of future BP levels 1–6 yr later in youth, but its independent predictive value is diminished somewhat when adjustments are made for variables known to be related to BP (e.g., initial BP, weight, adiposity, gender, ethnicity).

## PREDICTION OF LEFT VENTRICULAR MASS

Although increased LV mass is the strongest predictor of CVD morbidity and mortality other than advancing age, relatively few pediatric studies have been conducted using CVR to predict cardiac structure. Murdison et al. *(78)* examined a comprehensive set of demographic, anthropometric, and CV predictors of LV mass, with data collected an average of 2.6 yr earlier in a sample of 30 EA and 56 AA normotensive youth with family histories of essential HTN (mean age = 12.6 ± 2.3 yr at initial visit). An aggregate index of BP reactivity to a battery of laboratory stressors (i.e., parent-child conflict discussion, social stressor interview, video game challenge and postural change) was a significant predictor of LV mass/height$^{2.7}$ and LVH at follow up. These findings held after adjusting for a variety of significant covariates including initial LV mass/height$^{2.7}$, weight, and ethnicity (AAs > EAs).

Papavassiliou et al. *(79)* utilized a battery of stressors (i.e., postural change, treadmill exercise, forehead cold stimulation) in the prediction of LV mass 3.6 yr later in a sample of 46 EA and 22 AA children (7.9 ± 0.7 yr at baseline). Controlling for significant contributions of baseline adiposity (i.e., BMI), CO, and systolic BP reactivity to postural change accounted for 18% additional variance in LV mass/height$^{2.7}$.

Recently, Kapuku et al. *(80)* evaluated predictors of future LVmass in a cohort of 71 EA and 75 AA normotensive adolescents who were initially an average of 14.2 ± 1.8 yr of age. They were evaluated on two occasions, which were separated by an average of 2.3 yr. After adjustment for the significant contributions of initial LV mass/body surface area, weight, gender (males > females), and baseline resting TPR, systolic BP reactivity to a virtual reality car driving simulation was a significant independent predictor of LV mass/body surface area at follow-up (3% additional variance). However, this association was not consistent when LV mass was indexed by height$^{2.7}$. Although systolic BP reactivity was significantly related to follow-up LV mass/height$^{2.7}$ at the univariate level, it did not add significantly to a multiple regression model in which initial LV mass/height$^{2.7}$, BMI, gender, and supine resting TPR were already included.

In summary, CVR is an independent predictor of increased LV mass in youth. However, the clinical significance of these findings and implications for improved prevention of CVD are yet to be determined. Long term follow-up studies are clearly needed to determine whether these CVR-related findings are stable with respect to further increased risk of development of LVH and, ultimately, manifestation of essential HTN and/or CHD.

## TOWARD A GENE-ENVIRONMENT MODEL OF STRESS-INDUCED CARDIOVASCULAR DISEASE

Our overview of the available pediatric studies suggests that there is reasonable evidence that CVR can predict the development of some preclinical CVD states (e.g., increased LV mass and BP). However, some prospective investigations of the reactivity hypothesis have shown disappointing results in terms of CVR serving as a significant predictor of CVD endpoints. Light (2001) noted that this could be partially attributed to lack of evaluation of partially moderating effects, particularly genetic susceptibility and chronic stress *(82)*. Light and colleagues *(81,82)* proposed a "Gene and Environmental Modulated Reactivity Hypothesis." Her model proposes that individuals who exhibit high cardiovascular reactivity will be more likely to develop essential HTN and/or CHD if they also display a high genetic susceptibility (e.g., a positive family history of essential HTN) and/or are exposed to chronic stress (e.g., high job demand, low socioeconomic status, lack of social support), i.e., a high environmental susceptibility.

## ANIMAL MODEL STUDIES

Animal models have provided support for a gene by the environment interaction model of stress-induced essential HTN. Examples include Henry's animal paradigm in mice of psychosocial essential HTN, achieved through designing social environments that enhance confrontations regarding dominance *(83)*, and the borderline hypertensive rat (BHR) that develops sustained essential HTN after weeks of daily exposure to shock-avoidance tasks *(84)*. Friedman and Iwai *(85)* reported that chronic exposure to environmental stress (foot shock) resulted in persistent elevations in systolic BP in the hypertension-prone Dahl Salt-Sensitive (SS) but not the Dahl Salt-Resistant (SR) rats. These models establish that stress exposure leading to regular periods of high BP reactivity can be a critical causal factor in the development of esssential HTN. However, stress exposure only seems to lead to essential HTN in genetically susceptible animals *(81,82,86)*. For example, extensions of Henry's work from mice to rats have shown that essential HTN in his model only develops in the most susceptible rat strains. Many strains do not develop essential HTN, including strains that show large BP reactivity to acute dominance confrontations *(87–89)*.

## PROPOSED MODEL OF STRESS-INDUCED HYPERTENSION

Animal models of stress-induced essential HTN therefore highlight the important contributions of genetic susceptibility in combination with stressful environmental exposure in the reactivity hypothesis and support Light's *(82)* "Gene and Environmental Modulated Reactivity Hypothesis." Not only is the susceptibility to the development of essential HTN and CHD

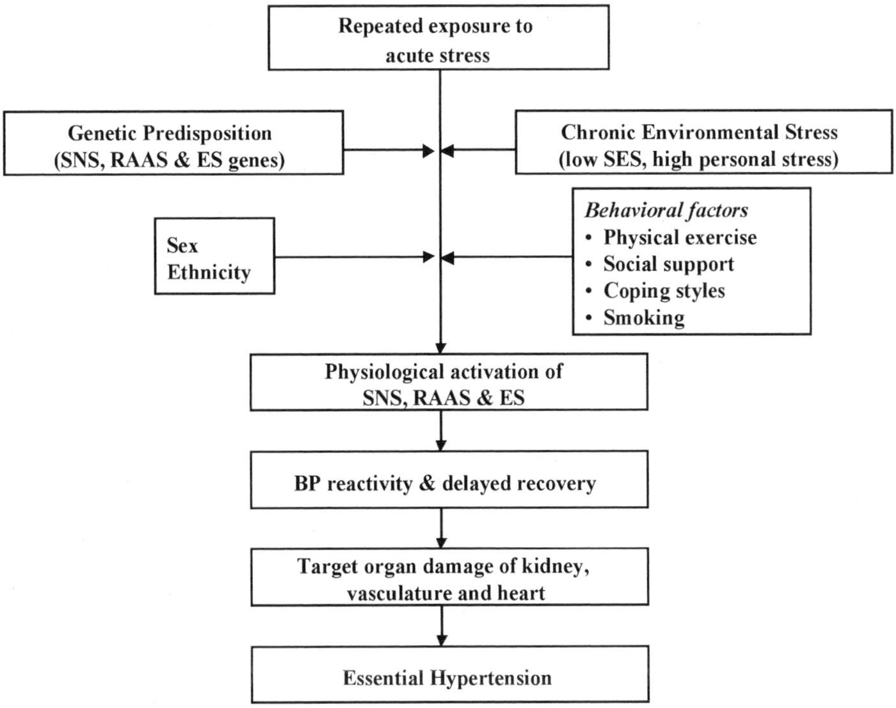


Fig. 1. Bio-behavioral model of stress-induced essential hypertension. SNS = sympathetic nervous system; RAAS = Renin-angiotensin-aldosterone system; ES = endothelial system; SES = socioeconomic status. Figure adapted from Snieder et al. *(99)*.

influenced by genetic factors, as indicated by reviews of twin studies, but individual differences in CVR appear to have genetic underpinnings as well *(90,91)*. Indeed, the same genes that underlie CVR may also confer susceptibility to essential HTN and/or CHD.

Guided by evidence from these animal models in combination with our recent findings *(80,92–96)* and those of others *(81,97,98)* in humans, we have proposed a bio-behavioral model of stress-induced essential HTN *(99)*. Our model outlines that genetic predisposition (e.g., genetic variation in the sympathetic nervous system [SNS], the renin-angiotensin-aldosterone system [RAAS] and/or the endothelial system [ES] function), in concert with chronic stress exposure (e.g., low socioeconomic status [SES], high personal life stress), adversely affects BP reactivity to, and BP recovery from, exposure to repeated acute stress, both of which affect the progression of the development of preclinical measures of essential HTN in youth, and culminate in essential HTN (Fig. 1).

We propose that three pathways play a central role in stress-induced EH, namely SNS, RAAS, and ES. Several lines of evidence point to a genetic basis of the two major intermediate phenotypes of our model: CVR to behavioral stress and stress-induced $Na^+$ retention, representing the CV and renal stress response, respectively. We propose that polymorphic variation in candidate genes underlying the SNS, RAAS, ES, and $Na^+$ reabsorption in the kidney are at least partly responsible for these genetic influences.

Genetic susceptibility has often been defined in terms of a positive family history of essential HTN and CVD. However, given the recent completion of the human genome, an increasing number of candidate genes will become available *(100)*. We therefore argue that common variation in these genes (polymorphisms) can, and should be, directly measured to improve

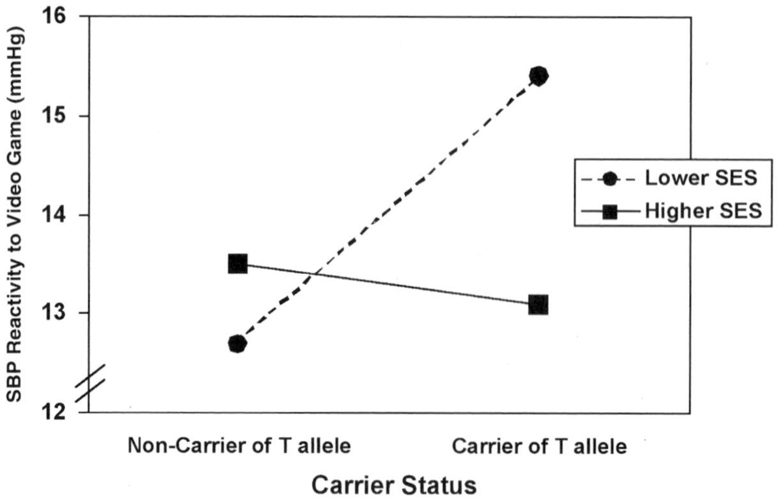


Fig. 2. Interaction of T allele carrier status of Endothelin-1 gene Lys198Asn polymorphism with SES for video game SBP reactivity.

insight into the regulation of physiological pathways leading to susceptibility for stress-induced essential HTN.

Recent findings from our laboratory provide tentative support for this model *(101)*. Among a cohort of 374 youth (mean age = 18.5 ± 2.7 yr), we examined the influence of the ET1 298Lys/Asn polymorphism on BP at rest and in response to acute stress. This polymorphism has been associated with hypertension and increased BP levels in several adult studies *(102,103)*. As depicted in Fig. 2, an interaction effect was observed; carriers of the T allele who came from lower SES backgrounds exhibited the greatest increases in systolic BP in response to a video game challenge.

Our model is by no means comprehensive. Other biological systems and risk factors could mediate the influence of stress on the development of essential HTN, such as the hypothalamic pituitary adrenal axis, parasympathetic autonomic reactivity, and serotonin function in the central nervous system. Studies that have measured indices of these systems (corticosteroid levels, respiratory sinus arrythmia, and serotonin metabolites, respectively) indicate the importance of genetic variation in these systems as well *(104–107)*. Others emphasize the effect of the early environment in the vulnerability to stress *(108)*.

In summary, three physiological systems that mediate the stress response of the heart, vasculature, and kidney play a central role in our proposed model. Future studies testing the reactivity hypothesis should measure not only hemodynamics, but also hormones representing one or more of these systems, as well as measures of chronic environmental stress. These factors should also be evaluated within the context of single nucleotide polymorphisms within candidate genes related to these physiological systems, which collectively increase one's susceptibility to the development of stress-induced essential HTN and its sequelae. The result will be a better understanding of the genetic and environmental contributions to stress-induced CVD.

## SUMMARY AND CLINICAL CARE IMPLICATIONS

CVD remains the leading cause of death of American adults; almost 1 million per year die from the various forms of CVD. The origins of CVD occur in the childhood years. Identification of the disease process at an early stage offers the chance for more successful primary prevention interventions, which would be beneficial not only to the individual, but also to society, given that preventive costs are likely to be much lower than treatment costs. Given the present levels of CVD in adults, the potential CVD-related health care costs faced by future generations is considerable. Research has enabled the identification of preclinical markers of future CVD. These markers include changes in CV structure and/or function, in addition to changes in BP that are not in themselves clinical symptoms, but which could be if the etiologic process is not halted. The current literature suggests that excessive CVR to stress is an independent contributor to the development of these markers (i.e., increased BP and LV mass/height$^{2.7}$). If further research supports this notion, psychological/behavioral stress testing might contribute useful diagnostic information (along with traditional CVD risk factors) when deciding whether intervention is warranted.

The significance of this work is particularly relevant for pediatric populations. The sooner primary prevention intervention efforts can be initiated with at-risk individuals, the greater the chances of ameliorating disease progression. The studies reviewed in this chapter suggest that preclinical markers of CVD can be identified in youths, and that CVR likely plays a contributing role. Collectively, these findings point to the need for development of effective CVD primary prevention approaches in youth, which include efforts to decrease CVR.

A variety of nonpharmacologic approaches have been used in efforts to lower BP in youth. Electrolyte control/supplementation, diet, and/or physical exercise interventions over 1-mo to 3-yr intervals have met with mixed results, with most studies finding minimal to no effect on resting BP in normotensive youth *(6,109)*. Given the inconsistency in electrolyte control/supplementation, diet, and/or exercise interventions upon BP control and the potential role of psychosocial stress in the development of essential HTN, stress reduction approaches may prove to be more beneficial in the reduction of BP in youth. To date, only a few stress reduction interventions in youth have been conducted. However, initial findings are promising; significant reductions in resting BP and/or BP reactivity to acute laboratory stressors in youth with high normal BP levels have been observed as a result of progressive muscle relaxation *(110)* or transcendental meditation *(111)*.

## ACKNOWLEDGMENT

Support for this work was provided in part by National Heart Lung and Blood Institute Grants HL56622 and HL69999.

## REFERENCES

1. American Heart Association. 2001 Heart and Stroke Statistical Update. Dallas, Texas. 2000.
2. Stamler J, Stamler R, Neaton JD. Blood pressure, systolic, diastolic, and cardiovascular risks: US population data. Arch Intern Med 1993;153:598–615.
3. Berenson GS, Wattigney WA, Tracy RE, et al. Atherosclerosis of the aorta and coronary arteries and cardiovascular risk factors in persons aged 6 to 30 years and studied at necropsy (The Bogalusa Heart Study). Am J Cardiol 1992;70:851–858.
4. Newman WP, Freedman DS, Voors AW, et al. Relation of serum lipoprotein levels and systolic blood pressure to early atherosclerosis: The Bogalusa Heart Study. N Engl J Med 1986;314:138–144.
5. PDAY Research Group. Relationships of atherosclerosis in young men to serum lipoprotein cholesterol concentrations and smoking: a preliminary report from the Pathobiological Determinants of Atherosclerosis in Youth (PDAY) Research Group. JAMA 1990;264:3018–3024.
6. Alpert BS, Murphy JK, Treiber FA. Essential hypertension: approaches to prevention in children. Medical Exercise Nutrition of Health 1994;3:296–307.

7. Strong WB, Deckelbaum RJ, Giddings SS, et al. Integrated cardiovascular health promotion in childhood. Circulation 1992;85:1638–1650.
8. Strong WB, Kelder SH. Pediatric preventive cardiology. In: Manson JE, Ridker PM, Gaziano JM, Hennekens GH, eds. Prevention of Myocardial Infarcation. New York: Oxford University Press, 1996;433–459.
9. Roig E, Castaner A, Simmons B, Patel R, Ford E, Cooper R. In-hospital mortality rates from acute myocardial infarction by race in US hospitals: findings from the National Hospital Discharge Survey. Circulation 1987;76:280–288.
10. Manuck SB. Cardiovascular reactivity in cardiovascular disease: "Once more unto the breach." Int J Behav Med 1994;1:4–31.
11. Matthews KA, Weiss SM, Detre T, et al. Handbook of Stress, Reactivity, and Cardiovascular Disease. New York: Wiley, 1986.
12. Murphy JK. Psychophysiological responses to stress in children and adolescents. In: La Greca PM, Siegal LJ, Wallander JL, Walker CE, eds. Advances in Pediatric Psychology: Stress and Coping in Child Health. New York: Guilford, 1992;44–71.
13. Sallis JF, Dimsdale JE, Caine C. Blood pressure reactivity in children. J Psychosom Res 1988;32:1–12.
14. Schneiderman N, Weiss SM, Kaufman PG. Handbook of Research Methods in Cardiovascular Behavioral Medicine. New York: Plenum, 1989.
15. Turner JR. Cardiovascular Reactivity and Stress: Patterns of Physiological Response. New York: Plenum, 1994.
16. Manuck SB, Kasprowicz AL, Muldoon MF. Behaviorally evoked cardiovascular reactivity and hypertension: conceptual issues and potential associations. Ann Behav Med 1990;12:17–29.
17. Kamarck TW, Lovallo WR. Cardiovascular reactivity to psychological challenge: conceptual and measurement considerations. Psychosom Med 2003;65:9–21.
18. Barnett PH, Hines Jr. EA, Schirger A, Gage RP. Blood pressure and vascular reactivity to the cold pressor test: restudy of 207 subjects 27 years later. JAMA 1963;183:845–848.
19. McGrath JJ, O'Brien WH. Pediatric impedance cardiography: temporal stability and intertask consistency. Psychophysiology 2001;38:479–484.
20. Taras HL, Sallis JF. Blood pressure reactivity in young children: comparing three stressors. J Dev Behav Pediatr 1992;13:41–45.
21. Giordani B, Manuck S, Farmer J. Stability of behaviorally-induced heart rate changes in children after one week. Child Dev 1981;52:533–537.
22. Mahoney LT, Schieken RM, Clarke WR, Lauer RM. Left ventricular mass and exercise responses predict future blood pressure: the Muscatine Study. Hypertension 1988;12:206–213.
23. Matthews K, Rakaczky C, Stoney C, Manuck S. Are cardiovascular responses to behavioral stressors a stable individual difference variable in childhood? Psychophysiology 1987;24:464–473.
24. Matthews KA, Woodall KA, Stoney CM. Changes in and stability of cardiovascular responses to behavioral stress: results from a four-year longitudinal study of children. Child Dev 1990;61:1134–1144.
25. Murphy JK, Alpert BS, Walker SS, Willey ES. Consistency of ethnic differences in children's pressor reactivity 1987 to 1992. Hypertension 1994;23:152–155.
26. Murphy JK, Alpert BS, Walker SS. Ethnicity, pressor reactivity, and children's blood pressure: five years of observation. Hypertension 1992;20:327–332.
27. Murphy JK, Alpert BS, Willey ES, Somes GW. Cardiovascular reactivity to psychological stress in healthy children. Psychophysiology 1988;25:144–152.
28. Murphy JK, Stoney CM, Alpert BS, Walker SS. Gender and ethnicity in children's cardiovascular reactivity: 7 years of study. Health Psychol 1995;14:48–55.
29. Treiber FA, Raunikar RA, Davis H, Fernandez T, Levy M, Strong WB. One year stability and prediction of cardiovascular functioning at rest and during laboratory stressors in youth with family histories of hypertension. Int J Behav Med 1994;1:335–353.
30. Sherwood A, Turner JR. Hemodynamic responses during psychological stress: implications for studying disease processes. Int J Behav Med 1995;2:193–218.
31. Kamarck TW, Jennings JR, Debski TT, et al. Reliable measures of behaviorally-evoked cardiovascular reactivity from a PC-based test battery: results from student and community samples. Psychophysiology 1992;29:17–28.
32. Kamarck TW, Jennings JR, Stewart CJ, Eddy MJ. Reliable responses to a cardiovascular reactivity protocol: a replication study in a biracial female sample. Psychophysiology 1993;30:627–634.
33. Manuck SB, Kamarck TW, Kasprowicz AS, Waldstein SR. Stability and patterning of behaviorally evoked cardiovascular reactivity. In: Blascovich J, Katkin ES, eds. Cardiovascular Reactivity to Psychological Stress and Disease. Washington, DC: APA, 1993;111–134.

34. Strong WB, Miller MD, Striplin M, Salehbhai M. Blood pressure response to isometric and dynamic exercise in healthy black children. Am J Dis Child 1978;132:587–591.
35. Verhaaren HA, Shieken RM, Mosteller M, Hewitt JK, Eaves LJ, Nance WE. Bivariate genetic analysis of left ventricular mass and weight in pubertal twins (The Medical College of Virginia Twin Study). Am J Cardiol 1991;68:661–668.
36. Parker FC, Croft JB, Cresanta JL, et al. The association between cardiovascular response tasks and future blood pressure levels in children: Bogalusa Heart Study. Circulation 1987;113:1174–1179.
37. Musante L, Raunikar RA, Treiber F, et al. Consistency of children's hemodynamic responses to laboratory stressors. Intl J Psychophysiol 1994;17:65–71.
38. Turner JR, Sherwood A, Light KC. Intertask consistency of hemodyamic responses to laboratory stressors in a biracial sample of men and women. Intl J Psychophysiol 1994;17:159–164.
39. Coates TJ, Parker FC, Kolodner K. Stress and heart disease: does blood pressure reactivity offer a link? In: Coates TJ, Peterson AC, eds. Promoting Adolescent Health. New York, Academic: 1982;305–321.
40. Ewart CK, Kolodner KB. Predicting ambulatory blood pressure during school: effectiveness of social and nonsocial reactivity tasks in black and white adolescents. Psychophysiology 1993;30:30–38.
41. Langewitz W, Ruddel H, Schachinger H, Schmieder R. Standardized stress testing in the cardiovascular laboratory: has it any bearing on ambulatory blood pressure values? J Hypertens 1989;7:S41–S48.
42. Matthews KA, Manuck SB, Saab PG. Cardiovascular responses of adolescents during a naturally occurring stressor and their behavioral and psychophysiological predictors. Psychophysiology 1986;23:198–209.
43. Treiber FA, Murphy JK, Davis H, Raunikar A, Pflieger K, Strong WB. Pressor reactivity, ethnicity, and 24-hour ambulatory monitoring in children from hypertensive families. Behav Med 1994;20:133–142.
44. Del Rosario JD, Treiber FA, Harshfield GA, Davis HC, Strong WB. Predictors of future ambulatory blood pressure in youth. J Pediatr 1998;132:693–698.
45. Fuster V, Badimon L, Badimon JJ, Chesebro JH. The pathogenesis of coronary artery disease and the acute coronary syndromes. N Engl J Med 1992;326:310–318.
46. Ross R. The pathogenesis of atherosclerosis: a perspective for the 1990s. Nature 1993;362:801–809.
47. Stary HS. Evolution and progression of atherosclerotic lesions in coronary arteries of children and young adults. Arteriosclerosis 1989;9:19–32.
48. Devereux RB, Alderman MH. Role of preclinical cardiovascular disease in the evolution from risk factor exposure to development of morbid events. Circulation 1993;88:1444–1455.
49. Devereux R, de Simone G, Koren M, Roman M, Laragh J. Left ventricular mass as a predictor of development of hypertension. Am J Hypertens 1991;4:603–607.
50. Devereux RB, Koren MJ, de Simone G, Roman MJ, Laragh JH. Left ventricular mass as a measure of preclinical hypertensive disease. Am J Hypertens 1992;5:175–181.
51. The sixth report of the Joint National Committee on Prevention, Detection, Evaluation, and Treatment of High Blood Pressure. Arch Intern Med 1997;157:2413–2445.
52. Hypertension Detection and Follow-up Program Cooperative Group: five-year findings of the Hypertension Detection and Follow-up Program: mortality by race-sex and blood pressure level—a further analysis. J Community Health 1984;9:314–327.
53. Burt VL, Whelton P, Roccella EJ, et al. Prevalence of hypertension in the US adult population: results from the Third National Health and Nutrition Examination Survey, 1988–1991. Hypertension 1995;25:305–313.
54. Update on the 1987 task force report on high blood pressure in children and adolescents: a working group report from the National High Blood Pressure Education Program National High Blood Pressure Education Program Working Group on Hypertension Control in Children and Adolescents. Pediatrics 1996;98:649–658.
55. Bao W, Threefoot SA, Srinivasan SR, Berenson GS. Essential hypertension predicted by tracking of elevated blood pressure from childhood to adulthood: The Bogalusa Heart Study. Am J Hypertens 1995;8:657–665.
56. Folkow B. "Structural Factor" in primary and secondary hypertension. Hypertension 1990;16:89–101.
57. Obrist PA. Cardiovascular Psychophysiology: A Perspective. New York: Plenum, 1981.
58. Levy D, Garrison RJ, Savage DD, Kannel WB, Castelli WP. Prognostic implications of echocardiographically determined left ventricular mass in the Framingham Heart Study. N Engl J Med 1990;322:1561–1566.
59. Levy D. Clinical significance of left ventricular hypertrophy: insights from the Framingham Study. J Cardiovasc Pharmacol 1991;17:1–6.
60. Kannel WB, Doyle JT, McNamara PM, Quickenton P, Gordon T. Precursors of sudden coronary death: factors related to the incidence of sudden death. Circulation 1975;51:606–613.
61. Mensah GA, Liao Y, Cooper RS. Left ventricular hypertrophy as a risk factor in patients with or without coronary artery disease. Cardiovasc Risk Fact 1995;5:67–74.

62. Bikkina M, Levy D, Evans JC, Larson MG, Benjamin EJ, Wolf PA, Castelli WP. Left ventricular mass and risk of stroke in an elderly cohort: The Framingham Heart Study. JAMA 1994;272:33–36.
63. Koren MJ, Devereux RB, Casale PN, Savage DD, Laragh JH. Relation of left ventricular mass and geometry to morbidity and mortality in uncomplicated essential hypertension. Ann Intern Med 1991;114:345–352.
64. Frohlich ED, Apstein C, Chobanian AV, et al. The heart in hypertension. N Engl J Med 1992;327:998–1008.
65. Levy DD, Garrison RJ, Savage DD, Kannel WB, Castelli WP. Left ventricular mass and incidence of coronary heart disease in an elderly cohort: The Framingham Study. Ann Intern Med 1989;110:101–107.
66. Liao Y, Cooper RS, McGee DL, Mensah GA, Ghali JK. The relative effects of left ventricular hypertrophy, coronary artery disease, and ventricular dysfunction on survival among black adults. JAMA1995;273: 1592–1597.
67. Wood DL, Sheps SG, Elveback LR, Schirger A. Cold pressor test as a predictor of hypertension. Hypertension 1984;6:301–306.
68. Hines EA. The hereditary factor in essential hypertension. Ann Intern Med 1937;11:593–601.
69. Hines EA. Reaction of the blood pressure of 400 school children to a standard stimulus. JAMA1937;108: 1249–1250.
70. Malpass D, Treiber FA, Turner JR, et al. Relationships between children's cardiovascular stress responses and resting cardiovascular functioning one-year later. Intl J Psychophysiol 1997;25:139–144.
71. Treiber FA, Turner JR, Davis H, Strong WB. Prediction of resting cardiovascular functioning in youth with family histories of essential hypertension: a 5-year follow-up. Int J Behav Med 1997;4:279–292.
72. Matthews KA, Woodall KL, Allen MT. Cardiovascular reactivity to stress predicts future blood pressure status. Hypertension 1993;22:479–485.
73. Newman JD, McGarvey ST, Steele MS. Longitudinal association of cardiovascular reactivity and blood pressure in Samoan adolescents. Psychosom Med 1999;61:243–249.
74. Treiber FA, Turner JR, Davis H, Thompson W, Levy M, Strong WB. Young children's cardiovascular stress responses predict resting cardiovascular functioning 2 1/2 years later. J Cardiovasc Risk 1996;3:95–100.
75. Treiber FA, Musante L, Kapuku G, Davis C, Litaker M, Davis H. Cardiovascular (CV) responsivity and recovery to acute stress and future CV functioning in youth with family histories of CV disease: a 4-year longitudinal study. Intl J Psychophysiol 2001;41:65–74.
76. Murphy JK, Alpert BS, Walker SS, Willey ES. Children's cardiovascular reactivity: stability of racial differences and relation to subsequent blood pressure over a one-year period. Psychophysiology 1991;28:447–457.
77. Treiber F, Del Rosario J, Davis H, Gutin B, Strong WB. Cardiovascular stress responses predict cardiovascular functioning: a four-year follow-up, Children and Exercise XIX. London: Chapman-Hall, 1997;366–372.
78. Murdison KA, Treiber FA, Mensah G, Davis H, Thompson W, Strong WB. Prediction of left ventricular mass in youth with family histories of essential hypertension. Am J Med Sci 1998;315:118–123.
79. Papavassiliou DP, Treiber FA, Strong WB, Malpass MD, Davis H. Anthropometric, demographic and cardiovascular predictors of left ventricular mass in young children. Am J Cardiol 1996;78:323–326.
80. Kapuku G, Treiber FA, Davis HC, Harshfield GA, Cook BB, Mensah GA. Hemodynamic function at rest, during acute stress, and in the field: predictors of cardiac structure and function 2 years later in youth. Hypertension 1999;34:1026–1031.
81. Light KC, Girdler SS, Sherwood A, et al. High stress responsivity predicts later blood pressure only in combination with positive family history and high life stress. Hypertension 1999;33:1458–1464.
82. Light KC. Hypertension and the reactivity hypothesis: the next generation. Psychosom Med 2001; 63:744–746.
83. Henry JP, Grim CE. Psychosocial mechanisms of primary hypertension. J Hypertens 1990;8:783–793.
84. Sanders BJ, Lawler JE. The borderline hypertensive rat (BHR) as a model for environmentally-induced hypertension: a review and update. Neurosci Biobehav Rev 1992;16:207–217.
85. Friedman R, Iwai J. Genetic predisposition and stress-induced hypertension. Science 1976;193:161–162.
86. Harshfield GA, Grim CE. Stress hypertension: the "wrong" genes in the "wrong" environment. Acta Physiol Scand 1997;640:129–132.
87. Ely D, Caplea A, Dunphy G, Smith D. Physiological and neuroendocrine correlates of social position in normotensive and hypertensive rat colonies. Acta Physiol Scand 1997;640:92–95.
88. Mormede P. Genetic influences on the responses to psychosocial challenges in rats. Acta Physiol Scand 1997;640:65–68.
89. Harrap SB, Louis WJ, Doyle AE. Failure of psychosocial stress to induce chronic hypertension in the rat. J Hypertens 1984;2:653–662.

90. Snieder H, vanDoornen LJP, Boomsma DI. Development of genetic trends in blood pressure levels and blood pressure reactivity to stress. In: Turner JR, Cardon LR, Hewitt JK, eds. Behavior Genetic Approaches in Behavioral Medicine. New York: Plenum, 1995;105–130.
91. Turner JR, Hewitt JK. Twin studies of cardiovascular response to psychological challenge: a review and suggested future directions. Ann Behav Med 1992;14:12–20.
92. Barbeau P, Kulharya A, Harshfield G, Snieder H, Davis H, Treiber F. Association between angiotensin II type I receptor polymorphism and resting hemodynamics in black and white youth. Ethn Dis 2002;12:S1-68–S1-71.
93. Barnes VA, Treiber FA, Musante L, Turner JR, Davis H, Strong WB. Ethnicity and socioeconomic status: impact on cardiovascular activity at rest and during stress in youth with a family history of hypertension. Ethn Dis 2000;10:4–16.
94. Jackson RW, Treiber FA, Turner JR, Davis H, Strong WB. Effects of race, sex, and socioeconomic status upon cardiovascular stress responsivity and recovery in youth. Intl J Psychophysiol 1999;31:111–119.
95. Snieder H, Barbeau P, Harshfield GA, et al. β2-adrenergic receptor gene and blood pressure in Black and White youth. The Georgia Twin Study. Hypertension 2001;38:17–18. Abstract.
96. Treiber FA, Davis H, Wells L, Musante L, Turner JR. Genetic and environmental contributions to cardiovascular responsivity to stress in youth. Psychosom Med 2000;62:106.
97. Anderson NB, McNeilly M, Myers H. A biopsychosocial model of race differences in vascular reactivity. In: Blascovich J, Katkin ESE, eds. Cardiovascular Reactivity to Psychological Stress and Disease. Washington, DC: APA, 1993;83–108.
98. Schneiderman N, Skyler JS. Insulin metabolism, sympathetic nervous system regulation, and coronary heart disease prevention. In: Orth-Gomer K, Schneiderman N, eds. Behavioral Medicine Approaches to Cardiovascular Disease Prevention. Mahwah, New Jersey: Lawrence Erlbaum Associates, 1996;105–133.
99. Snieder H, Harshfield GA, Barbeau P, Pollock DM, Pollock JS, Treiber FA. Dissecting the genetic architecture of the cardiovascular and renal stress response. Biol Psychol 2002;61:73–95.
100. Peltonen L, McKusick VA. Genomics and medicine. Dissecting human disease in the postgenomic era. Science 2001;291:1224–1229.
101. Treiber FA, Barbeau P, Harshfield G, et al. Endothelin-1 gene Lys198Asn polymorphism and blood pressure reactivity. Hypertension 2003;42(4):494–499.
102. Tiret L, Poirier O, Hallet V, et al. The Lys198Asn polymorphism in the endothelin-1 gene is associated with blood pressure in overweight people. Hypertension 1999;33:1169–1174.
103. Asai T, Ohkubo T, Katsuya T, et al. Endothelin-1 gene variant associates with blood pressure in obese Japanese subjects: the Ohasama Study. Hypertension 2001;38:1321–1324.
104. Bartels M, Van den Berg M, Sluyter F, Boomsma DI, De Geus EJC. Heritability of cortisol levels; review and simultaneous analysis of twin studies. Psychoneuroendocrinology 2003;28(2):121–137.
105. Inglis GC, Ingram MC, Holloway CD, et al. Familial pattern of corticosteroids and their metabolism in adult human subjects—the Scottish Adult Twin Study. J Clin Endocrinol Metab 1999;84:4132–4137.
106. Snieder H, Boomsma DI, Van Doornen LJ, De Geus EJ. Heritability of respiratory sinus arrhythmia: dependency on task and respiration rate. Psychophysiol 1997;34:317–328.
107. Williams RB, Marchuk DA, Gadde KM, et al. Central nervous system serotonin function and cardiovascular responses to stress. Psychosom Med 2001;63:300–305.
108. Francis DD, Caldji C, Champagne F, Plotsky PM, Meaney MJ. The role of corticotropin-releasing factor—norepinephrine systems in mediating the effects of early experience on the development of behavioral and endocrine responses to stress. Biol Psychiatry 1999;46:1153–1166.
109. Resnicow K. School-based obesity prevention: population versus high-risk interventions. In: Williams CL, Kimm SYS, eds. Prevention and Treatment of Childhood Obesity, Annals of the New York Academy of Sciences: 1993;154–166.
110. Ewart CK, Harris WL, Iwata MM, Coates TJ, Bullock R, Simon B. Feasibility and effectiveness of school-based relaxation in lowering blood pressure. Health Psychol 1987;6:399–416.
111. Barnes VA, Treiber FA, Davis H. Impact of transcendental meditation on cardiovascular function at rest and during acute stress in adolescents with high normal blood pressure. J Psychosom Res 2001;51:597–605.

# 15 Familial Aggregation of Blood Pressure

*Harold Snieder, PhD*

*CONTENTS*



## INTRODUCTION

In the first half of the last century, evidence for the familial aggregation of (elevated) blood pressure (BP) levels was largely anecdotal and based on case reports of clinicians. That is, until a number of large family studies in the 1960s showed familial resemblance of BP with correlations around $r = 0.20$ among first-degree relatives *(1,2)*.

Relatively few observations were made in children in these early studies, which initiated a number of research projects in the 1970s investigating whether familial aggregation of BP could be detected in childhood. Zinner et al. *(3)*, for example, measured BP in 721 children between 2 and 14 yr of age from 190 families. Sibling correlations of $r = 0.34$ and $r = 0.32$ were found for systolic BP and diastolic BP, respectively. Correlations between mother and child were $r = 0.16$ (systolic BP) and $r = 0.17$ (diastolic BP). These results were largely confirmed in a follow-up of the same cohort 4 yr later *(4)*. Findings were extended to even younger ages by two further studies that showed significant BP aggregation between 1-mo-old infants and their siblings *(5)*, and significant parent-offspring correlations between mothers and their newborn infants *(6)*.

These studies showed that a familial tendency to high (or low) BP is established early in life, but a number of questions remained unanswered. For example, it was unclear whether shared genes or shared environment caused the BP aggregation within families. Special study designs, such as adoption or twin studies, are necessary to effectively discriminate genetic from shared environmental influences, because these sources of familial resemblance are confounded within nuclear families. Furthermore, estimates of the relative influence of genetic and environmental factors derived from cross-sectional twin or family studies, are merely "snapshots" of a specific time. These estimates do not give information on underlying genetic and environmental sources of continuity, nor do they inform us of developmental change in cardiovascular disease

From: *Clinical Hypertension and Vascular Disease: Pediatric Hypertension*
Edited by: R. J. Portman, J. M. Sorof, and J. R. Ingelfinger © Humana Press Inc., Totowa, NJ

or its intermediate traits, such as BP or lipids *(7,8)*. Genetic (or environmental) influences on BP may therefore be age dependent and take two different forms *(9)*. First, the magnitude of these influences on BP can differ with age. Second, different genes or environmental factors may affect BP at different ages. For example, BP genes may switch on or off during certain periods in life, i.e., age-dependent gene expression.

Therefore, in this chapter the available literature of twin and family studies will be reviewed to address two issues: the potential causes of familial aggregation of BP, and the age dependency of genetic or environmental sources of BP variation and covariation within and between families.

## CAUSES OF FAMILIAL AGGREGATION OF BLOOD PRESSURE

### *Rationale Behind the Classic Twin Study*

Two approaches that have frequently been used to study the contributions of genes and environment to variations in BP levels are family and twin studies. The first approach studies the resemblance in BP between parents and offspring or between siblings in nuclear families. The second approach examines the similarity in BP of monozygotic (MZ) and dizygotic (DZ) twin pairs. Resemblance between family members (including twins) can arise from a common environment shared by family members and from a (partially) shared genotype. These sources of familial resemblance are confounded within nuclear families, because there is no differential sharing of genotype among first-degree relatives. Both parent–offspring and sibling pairs share an average of 50% of their genetic material. Therefore, special study designs are necessary to discriminate genetic from shared environmental influences. One possibility is the adoption design *(10)*, which has somewhat limited applicability due to practical considerations. Far more popular are twin studies, which examine phenotypic (e.g., BP) similarity of MZ and DZ twin pairs. They offer a unique opportunity to distinguish between the influences of environment and heredity on resemblance between family members. In a twin design, the separation of genetic and environmental variance is possible because MZ twins share 100% of their genetic make-up, whereas DZ twins only share an average of 50% of their genes. If a trait is influenced by genetic factors, MZ twins should resemble each other to a greater extent than DZ twins. In the classic twin method, the difference between intra-class correlations for MZ twins and those for DZ twins is doubled to estimate heritability [$h^2 = 2(r_{MZ} - r_{DZ})$], which can be defined as the proportion of total phenotypic variance explained by genetic factors. Whenever the DZ correlation is larger than half of the MZ correlation, this may indicate that part of the resemblance between twins is caused by shared environmental factors *(11)*. The twin method assumes that both types of twins share their environment to the same extent, which is known as the equal environment assumption. Although there has been some criticism of the equal environment assumption (e.g., *12*), most studies specifically carried out to test it have proved it to be valid. Even if shared environment differentially affects MZ and DZ twins, it is unlikely that this has a substantial effect on the trait under study *(11,13,14)*. Furthermore, BP levels in twins are representative of those in the general population *(15,16)*.

Use of quantitative genetic modeling to estimate these genetic and environmental variance components is now standard in twin research. Details of model-fitting to twin data have been described elsewhere *(17,18)*. In short, the technique is based on the comparison of the variance-covariance matrices (or correlations) in MZ and DZ twin pairs, and allows separation of the observed phenotypic variance, which can be decomposed into several contributing factors.

Additive genetic variance (A) is the variance that results from the additive effects of alleles at each contributing locus. Dominance genetic variance (D) is the variance that results from the nonadditive effects of two alleles at the same locus summed over all loci that contribute to the variance of the trait. Shared (common) environmental variance (C) is the variance that results from environmental events shared by both members of a twin pair (e.g., rearing, school, neighborhood, diet). Specific (unique) environmental variance (E) is the variance that results from environmental effects that are not shared by members of a twin pair and also includes measurement error. Dividing each of these components by the total variance yields the different standardized components of variance, for example the heritability which (in the absence of D) is the ratio of additive genetic variance to total phenotypic variance (A/A+C+E).

### *Heritability or Family Environment*

Over the last 30 yr a large number of twin studies have been conducted investigating the relative influence of genetic and environmental factors on BP variation. Tables 1 and 2 summarize pediatric and adult studies, respectively. Only twin studies with a reasonably large sample size (>50 twin pairs total) were included. Although studies used different methods to estimate heritability, it is immediately obvious from these tables that the evidence for a sizeable contribution of genetic factors to BP is overwhelming, with most heritability estimates around 50–60%. The majority of these studies found no evidence for influence of shared family environment on BP. For adult twins no longer living in the same family household, this result might have been expected. However, for children it is more surprising that environmental factors shared within families, such as salt in the diet or physical exercise, apparently explain a negligible amount of variation in BP. Part of the explanation might be that even apparently environmental variables such as diet and exercise have a heritable component *(19–21)*. Another part of the story might be that many twin studies may lack the power to detect moderate size influences of common environment *(22,23)*. A few studies that either had large sample sizes *(24,25)* or used a more powerful multivariate approach *(26)*, did find a small contribution of shared environment of around 10–20%. The conclusion seems nevertheless warranted that, if not entirely, the familial aggregation of BP is still largely owing to genes, not environmental factors shared within the family.

### *Sex Effects on Blood Pressure Heritability*

Sex differences, in influences of genetic and environmental factors on the phenotype, can take several forms. Although autosomal genes are not expected to be different between males and females as a result of the random nature of chromosomal segregation during meiosis, it is possible that some genes (or environments) differ in impact between women and men. It may also be true that some genes contributing to BP in women are distinct from genes contributing to BP in men *(27)*. Sex differences in the magnitude of genetic and environmental effects can be tested by comparing parameter estimates between males and females. Of the studies that considered sex differences in heritabilities, estimates for males and females are listed separately in Tables 1 and 2. However, heritability estimates for males and females are remarkably similar. A number of studies even report the same heritabilities for the two sexes, indicating that estimates for males and females could be set equal as part of the model-fitting process used in these studies. Lower correlations in DZ opposite- sex pairs compared to same-sex DZ pairs indicate that genetic or shared environmental influences may differ in kind between males and females, but this has never been reported for BP.

**Table 1**
**Pediatric Twin Studies Estimating Heritability ($h^2$) in Systolic (SBP) and Diastolic BP (DBP), in Ascending Order According to Age**

| | | *Age* | | | | $h^2$ | |
|---|---|---|---|---|---|---|---|
| *Study* | *Pairs of twins* | *Mean (SD)* | *Range* | *Race* | *Sex* | *SBP* | *DBP* |
| Yu et al. *(43)*[a] | 274 MZ, 65 DZ | ? ( ? ) | 0.0–1.0 | Chinese | m & f | 0.29 – 0.55 | 0.27 – 0.45 |
| Levine et al. *(28)*[b] | 67 MZ, 99 DZ | ? ( ? ) | 0.5–1.0 | b & w | m & f | 0.66 | 0.48 |
| Havlik et al. *(57)* | 72 MZ, 40 DZ | | | black | m & f | 0.46 | 0.51 |
| | 43 MZ, 42 DZ | | | white | m & f | 0.11 | 0.71 |
| | 115 MZ, 82 DZ | 7.0 (?) | ? | all | m & f | 0.23 | 0.53 |
| Wang et al. *(58)* | 75 MZ, 35 DZ | ? ( ? ) | 7.0–12.0 | Chinese | m & f | 0.32 | 0.46 |
| Schieken et al. *(59)* | 71 MZM, 74 MZF | 11.1 (0.25) | ? | white | male | 0.66 | 0.64 |
| | 23 DZM, 31 DZF, 52 DOS | | | | female | 0.66 | 0.51 |
| McIlhany et al. *(29)* | 40 MZM, 47 MZF | 14.0 (6.5) | 5.0–50.0 | b & w | male | 0.41 | 0.56 |
| | 32 DZM, 36 DZF, 45 DOS | | | | female | 0.78 | 0.61 |
| Snieder et al. *(30)* | 75 MZM, 91 MZF | 14.9 (3.0) | 10.0–26.0 | white | male | 0.57 | 0.45 |
| | 33 DZM, 31 DZF, 78 DOS | | | | female | 0.57 | 0.45 |
| | 52 MZM, 58 MZF | 14.6 (3.2) | 10.0–26.0 | black | male | 0.57 | 0.48 |
| | 24 DZM, 39 DZF, 50 DOS | | | | female | 0.57 | 0.58 |
| Snieder et al. *(7)* | 35 MZM, 33 MZF | 16.8 (2.0) | 13.0–22.0 | white | male | 0.49 | 0.69 |
| | 31 DZM, 29 DZF, 28 DOS | | | | female | 0.66 | 0.50 |

Abbreviations: MZF = Monozygotic Females; MZM = Monozygotic Males; DZF = Dizygotic Females; DZM = Dizygotic Males; DOS = Dizygotic Opposite-Sex; b & w = black and white combined; m & f = males and females combined.

[a] Range of heritability estimates between 2 mo and 1 yr are given.

[b] Heritability estimates reported by Levine et al. *(28)* were doubled as outlined by Kramer *(69)*.

**Table 2**
**Adult Twin Studies Estimating Heritability ($h^2$) in Systolic (SBP) and Diastolic Blood Pressure (DBP), in Ascending Order According to Age**

| | | *Age* | | | | $h^2$ | |
|---|---|---|---|---|---|---|---|
| *Study* | *Pairs of twins* | *Mean (SD)* | *Range* | *Race* | *Sex* | *SBP* | *DBP* |
| Sims et al. *(60)* | 40 MZM, 45 DZM | 19.4 (3.0) | ? | white | male | 0.68 | 0.76 |
| Ditto *(61)* | 20 MZM, 20 MZF | 20.0 (5.0) | 12.0–44.0 | white | male | 0.63 | 0.58 |
| | 20 DZM, 20 DZF, 20 DOS | | | | female | 0.63 | 0.58 |
| McCaffery et al. *(62)* | 129 MZ, 66 DZ | 21.3 (2.8) | 18.0–30.0 | 94% white | m & f | 0.48 | 0.51 |
| Bielen et al. *(63)* | 32 MZM | 21.7 (3.7) | 18.0–31.0 | white | male | 0.69 | 0.32 |
| | 21 DZM | 23.8 (3.9) | | | | | |
| Fagard et al. *(34)* | 26 MZM | 23.8 (4.2) | 18.0–38.0 | white | male | 0.64 | 0.73 |
| | 27 DZM | 24.7 (4.8) | | | | | |
| Busjahn et al. *(64)* | 100 MZ, 66 DZ | 29.8 (12.0) | ? | white | m & f | 0.74 | 0.72 |
| Slattery et al. *(65)* | 77 MZM, 88 DZM | ? ( ? ) | 22.0–66.0 | white | male | 0.60 | 0.66 |
| Vinck et al. *(35)* | 150 MZ, 122 DZ | 34.9 ( ? ) | 18.0–76.0 | white | m & f | 0.62 | 0.57 |
| Williams et al. *(66)* | 14 MZM, 44 MZF | 36.4 ( ? ) | 17.0–65.0 | white | male | 0.60 | 0.52 |
| | 9 DZM, 31 DZF, 11 DOS | | | | female | 0.60 | 0.43 |
| Austin et al. *(67)* | 233 MZF, 170 DZF | 42.0 ( ? ) | ? | 90% white | female | 0.35 | 0.26 |
| Baird et al. *(42)*[a] | 30 MZM, 28 MZF | 43.7 (1.4) | 40.5–46.5 | white | male | 0.48 | 0.30 |
| | 35 DZM, 45 DZF, 60 DOS | | | | female | 0.48 | 0.76 |
| Snieder et al. *(7)* | 43 MZM, 47 MZF | 44.4 (6.7) | 34.0–63.0 | white | male | 0.40 | 0.42 |
| | 32 DZM, 39 DZF, 39 DOS | | | | female | 0.63 | 0.61 |
| Snieder et al. *(25)* | 213 MZF, 556 DZF | 45.4 (12.4) | 18.0–73.0 | white | female | 0.17 | 0.22 |
| Feinleib et al. *(68)* | 250 MZM, 264 DZM | ? ( ? ) | 42.0–56.0 | white | male | 0.60 | 0.61 |
| Hong et al. *(24)* | 41 MZM, 66 MZF | 63.0 (8.0) | >50.0 | white | male | 0.56 | 0.32 |
| | 69 DZM, 111 DZF | | | | female | 0.56 | 0.32 |

Abbreviations: MZF = Monozygotic Females; MZM = Monozygotic Males; DZF = Dizygotic Females; DZM = Dizygotic Males; DOS = Dizygotic Opposite-Sex; m & f = males and females combined.

[a]DBP heritabilities were not reported in the original paper.

## *Ethnic Effects on Blood Pressure Heritability*

Genetic and environmental differences among ethnic populations may result in different BP heritabilities. As shown in Tables 1 and 2, most twin studies were conducted in Caucasian populations and a few combined twins from different ethnic groups without reporting separate heritability estimates *(28,29)*. To resolve the question of whether the relative influence of genetic and environmental factors on BP in youth is different between black and white Americans, we recently conducted a classic twin study, including both ethnic groups living in the same area. In this, the first study to estimate and compare the relative influence of genetic and environmental factors on BP in a large sample of young black and white twins, heritability estimates of BP in black and white youth were not significantly different *(30)*. Concurrent with the few other twin studies of non-Caucasians as reported in Table 1, there seems to be no evidence of large differences in BP heritabilities between different ethnic groups. The fact that a similar amount of BP variation is explained by genetic factors within different ethnicities does not exclude the possibility, however, that the actual genes responsible for this heritability differ between ethnic groups.

## *Twin Studies of Ambulatory Blood Pressure*

Conventional BP measures have shown their value in predicting adverse outcomes, but provide only a snapshot of 24-h BP variability as seen in real life, and might overestimate real BP as a result of the white coat effect. The value of ambulatory BP measurements is illustrated by studies showing that ambulatory BP is a better predictor of target organ damage and cardiovascular morbidity and mortality than BP measured in the clinic *(31)*.

In order to circumvent disadvantages of conventional BP measures several twin studies have examined ambulatory BP, but the sample sizes of initial studies have been small. Degaute et al. *(32)* evaluated 24-h ambulatory BP in a hospital research setting with 28 MZ and 16 DZ pairs of young adult males. The small sample size and the presentation of 33 different measures make interpretation of results difficult, but overall evidence suggested heritability on some characteristics of the 24-h profiles for diastolic BP. Somes et al. *(33)* examined the heritability of ambulatory BP in 38 pairs of MZ twins, 17 pairs of same-sex DZ twins, and 11 pairs of opposite-sex DZ twins. Heritability estimates of $h^2 = 0.22$ and $h^2 = 0.34$ were observed for 24-h systolic BP and diastolic BP, respectively.

Fagard et al. *(34)* measured 24-h ambulatory BP in 26 MZ and 27 DZ male twin pairs aged 18–38 yr. Using model-fitting techniques, heritability ranged from $h^2 = 0.51$ to $h^2 = 0.73$ for 24-h, daytime, and nighttime systolic BP and diastolic BP. The remaining variances were typically accounted for by unique environment (range = 0.27–0.40). In a recent study of a large sample of 150 MZ and 122 DZ twin pairs, Vinck et al. *(35)* measured conventional and ambulatory BP. Heritabilities were similar (around 50%) for laboratory and ambulatory (daytime and nighttime) systolic BP and diastolic BP. This finding shows that BP heritability is relatively insensitive to mode of measurement and provides strong confirmation of the robustness of the heritable effect on BP.

## *Influence of Obesity on Familial Aggregation of Blood Pressure*

In subjects of all ages, weight is probably the most important correlate of BP. The familial aggregation of BP may therefore, to a certain extent, be owing to the familial aggregation of obesity. Schieken et al. *(36)* addressed this question in a pediatric population of 11-yr-old twins. They observed highly significant correlations between systolic BP and weight ($r = 0.40$) as well as body mass index (BMI) ($r = 0.29$) that could largely be explained by common genes rather than common environmental effects influencing both systolic BP and weight (or BMI). The percentage of total systolic BP variance caused by genetic effects common to systolic BP and weight was 11.2%; for BMI this figure was 8%. The study found no significant correlations between diastolic BP and body size.

Two further twin studies in adult males *(37)* and females *(38)* found evidence for a direct effect of BMI on BP, rather than an effect of common genes (pleiotropy) on BP. Both mechanisms, however, imply that part of the genetic variation in BP can be explained by genes for obesity *(38)*.

### *Influence of Birthweight on Familial Aggregation of Blood Pressure*

The association between low birthweight and increased BP, although modest, has been well established, as shown by a meta-analysis of 34 studies; BP reduces 1–2 mmHg for every kg increase in birthweight for children. The effect increases to about 5 mmHg/kg in elderly people *(39)*. The fetal programming hypothesis states that this association is due to intrauterine malnutrition (reflected by low birthweight), which increases the risk of a number of chronic diseases in later life, including hypertension. However, other factors, such as socioeconomic status and genetics, may also explain the inverse relationship between birthweight and BP. The influence of confounding parental characteristics can be controlled by studying intrapair differences in twins (i.e., relate intrapair differences in birthweight with intrapair differences in outcome variables). Furthermore, the influence of genetic makeup can be eliminated in MZ twins and reduced in DZ twins. Using this intrapair twin design, Poulter et al. *(40)* found that BP tended to be lower among those twins of each pair that were heavier at birth, suggesting that the inverse association between birthweight and adult BP is independent of parental confounding variables. These results also point to the importance of environmental fetal nutrition factors that are different within twin pairs, such as placental dysfunction, rather than factors that are the same, such as maternal nutrition. A recent study of 1311 pairs of adolescent twins found a decrease in systolic BP of 1.88 mmHg for every kg increase in birthweight in the overall sample, but a reduction of this effect was observed when intrapair analyses were used *(41)*. Thus, the association between birthweight and systolic BP attenuated when genetic factors were controlled for suggesting that genetic factors do contribute to this association.

In summary, the relationship between birthweight and BP is most likely due to a combination of environmental and genetic factors. The contribution of genes that influence birthweight to the familial aggregation of BP, however, is likely to be small *(42)*.

## AGE DEPENDENCY OF GENETIC EFFECTS ON BLOOD PRESSURE

BP level changes as a function of age, but this trend is not simply linear. The age-specific increases in systolic BP and diastolic BP suggest that different (genetic and environmental) mechanisms exert their influences on BP during different periods of life. Not only mean BP, but also its population variance has been found to increase between adolescence and adulthood *(7)*. Such an increase in BP variance with age may be due to inter-individual variation in the rise of BP over time, and can only be explained by an increase in one or more underlying variance components, either genetic or environmental. These changes in variance components may imply age-related changes in heritabilities.

## *Twin Studies*

In Table 1 (mean age <18 yr) and Table 2 (mean age >18 yr), studies are listed in ascending order according to the age of the twin sample. A systematic overview of all studies such as this one may reveal any age-dependent trends in heritability, because each study yields heritability estimates representative of its specific age range. However, clear age trends in BP heritability can be detected within neither the adult nor the pediatric age range. Two studies in very young twins *(28,43)* confirm the conclusions of previously mentioned family studies that found that familial aggregation is established very early in life. These twin studies suggest that this aggregation can be ascribed to genetic factors. The above-mentioned study of Vinck et al. *(35)* specifically investigated stability of heritable and environmental influences on both conventional and ambulatory BP in three age groups: 18–29, 30–39, and ≥40 yr. Their large sample of 150 MZ and 122 DZ twin pairs had considerable power, but found no significant differences in genetic and environmental influences between age groups.

Therefore, the conclusion that the relative influence of genetic factors on BP is stable across the life span appears to be warranted.

## *Family Studies*

### Parent–Offspring and Sibling Correlations

Another approach to investigating the age-dependency of genetic and environmental effects is to compare parent–offspring data with data from siblings or twins. If there is an age-dependent genetic or envionmental effect on the phenotype, one would expect the parent–offspring correlation to be lower than sibling or DZ twin correlations, since siblings and DZ twins are measured at about the same age. This expectation was confirmed in a review by Iselius, Morton, and Rao *(44)*. They pooled the results from a large number of studies and arrived at a mean correlation for 14,553 parent–offspring pairs of $r = 0.165$ for systolic BP and $r = 0.137$ for diastolic BP. Corresponding values for 11,839 sibling and DZ twin pairs were $r = 0.235$ (systolic BP) and $r = 0.201$ (diastolic BP).

If, on the other hand, parents and their offspring are measured at the same age, a rise in parent–offspring correlations toward levels similar to sibling correlations is to be expected. This expectation was supported by data from Havlik et al. *(45)*, who measured systolic BP and diastolic BP for 1141 parent pairs aged 48–51. Twenty to thirty years later, BP was measured for 2497 of their offspring. At the time of testing, the offspring's ages were close to the ages of their parents when they were measured. Parent–offspring correlations ranged between $r =$ 0.13 and 0.25 for systolic BP, and between $r = 0.17$ and 0.22 for diastolic BP. These ranges were quite similar to the sibling-pair correlations, which were between $r = 0.17$ and 0.23 (systolic BP), and between $r = 0.19$ and 0.24 (diastolic BP). An alternative explanation for the lower parent–offspring correlation, compared to the sibling or DZ twin correlation, could be the influence of genetic dominance *(24,46)*. However, an effect of dominance is rarely found for BP and the similarity between correlations for parents and offspring (who do not share dominance variation) and siblings (who share 0.25 of their dominance variation) in the Havlik et al. study *(45)* also suggests that dominance variation is not important.

Lower values for parent–offspring correlations are also the most likely explanation for the peculiar finding that heritability estimates derived from family studies (which usually measure pairs of subjects at different ages) are generally lower than those derived from twin studies. Heritability estimates from family studies range from $h^2 = 0.17$ to $h^2 = 0.45$ for systolic BP, and from $h^2 = 0.15$ to $h^2 = 0.52$ for diastolic BP *(44,46,47)*. Estimates from twin studies typically range from 0.40 to 0.70 for both systolic BP and diastolic BP (*see* Tables 1 and 2).

### Age-Dependent Gene Expression

Two types of age-dependent effects could offer an explanation for the finding that the parent–offspring correlation is lower than the sibling and DZ twin pair correlations. First, the influence of unique environmental factors may accumulate over a lifetime. This accumulation, however, would lead to lower heritabilities with age, which is not supported by the evidence presented in Tables 1 and 2. Second, different genes could influence BP in childhood and adulthood. This possibility is still compatible with the results of Tables 1 and 2, as heritability can remain stable across time although different genes are influential at different times. The latter possibility is supported by data from Tambs et al. *(48)*. In a Norwegian sample with 43,751 parent–offspring pairs, 19,140 pairs of siblings, and 169 pairs of twins, correlations between relatives decreased as age differences between these relatives increased. A model specifying age-specific genetic additive effects and unique environmental effects fitted the data well. This model also estimated the extent to which genetic effects were age-specific. As an example, the researchers calculated expected correlations for systolic BP and diastolic BP in relatives with an age difference of 40 yr. For systolic BP, 62% of the genetic variance at age 20 and at age 60, for example, is explained by genes that are common to both ages, and 38% of the variance is explained by age-specific genetic effects. The same values for diastolic BP were 67% and 33%, respectively. The model used by Tambs et al. *(48)* assumes invariant heritabilities for BP throughout life. This assumption proved to be valid for systolic BP, whereas for diastolic BP a very slight increase in heritability was detected. Snieder et al. used an extended twin-family design *(49)* which included, in addition to younger twins and their parents, a group of middle-aged twins who were the same age as the parents. This design provided further support for age-specific genetic effects on BP that differ between childhood and adulthood *(7)*. Models allowing for these effects showed a slightly better fit for both systolic BP and diastolic BP with genetic correlations across time equal to $r = 0.76$ for systolic BP and $r = 0.72$ for diastolic BP. The slightly lower values found by Tambs et al. *(48)* ($r = 0.62$ for systolic BP and $r = 0.67$ for diastolic BP) might be explained by an age difference (40 yr) between parents and offspring that was greater than the age difference in this study (30 yr).

### Longitudinal Studies

During adulthood, the developmental genetics of BP might be similar to that reported for obesity. Although overall heritability of BMI remains relatively constant from young adulthood on, there are additional genetic influences in middle age that behave independently of those that influence young adults *(50)*. This possibility is supported by Colletto et al. *(51)*, who analyzed systolic BP and diastolic BP for 254 MZ and 260 DZ male twin pairs assessed in middle age (mean age: 48 yr), and again 9 and 24 yr later. Using a time series analysis of genetic and environmental components of variation, they found that shared family environmental effects were absent, and that specific environmental influences were largely occasion-specific. In contrast, genetic influences were, in part, the same across adulthood (60% of genetic variation at the later ages was already detected in middle age) and, in part, age-specific (the remaining 40% of the genetic variation at later ages was unrelated to that expressed earlier). Despite these changing genetic influences, the estimated heritabilities remain relatively constant across ages at around 0.5.

This is the only published longitudinal twin study reporting on BP data that I am aware of, which is unfortunate because only in longitudinal studies of genetically informative subjects can the stability of genetic and environmental factors be rigorously tested. Furthermore, the above study does not cover the important transition from childhood to adulthood. However, all the available evidence supports the conclusion that partly different genes are expressed in different periods of life.

We have recently used another type of longitudinal study to investigate the influence of genetic susceptibility to essential HTN on the development of systolic BP and left ventricular (LV) mass from childhood to adulthood *(52)*. Family history of HTN (physician-verified essential HTN in one or both biological parents) was used as the measure of genetic susceptibility to HTN. Individual systolic BP and LV mass growth curves across age were created for a sample of approx 700 subjects (age range: 4.9–27.5 yr), in approximately equal proportions of black, white, male, and female youth, with annual assessments over a 10-yr period. Subjects with a positive family history of HTN not only had higher systolic BP and LV mass levels ($p < 0.001$) across all ages, they also showed stronger increases in systolic BP over time ($p < 0.05$) than subjects with a negative family history of HTN. In addition, the effect of a family history of HTN on LV mass was stronger in females than males ($p < 0.025$). The effect of family history of HTV on LV mass appeared to be mediated by obesity, because it was no longer significant after adjustment for BMI. Nevertheless, the conclusion seems warranted that genetic susceptibility to essential HTN affects systolic BP and LV mass trajectories from childhood to adulthood. The challenge for future research will be to identify the genes responsible for individual differences in HTN and LV hypertrophy susceptibility.

## SUMMARY AND CONCLUSIONS

This chapter has examined causes of familial aggregation of BP, and whether and how underlying genetic or environmental influences, or both, are stable or change across the life span. Different types of genetically informative studies were discussed to shed some light on these questions.

Familial aggregation of BP is largely owing to genes rather than familial environment, and heritability estimates are very similar across sex, ethnicity, and modes of measurement. Genes for obesity and possibly birthweight can explain part of the genetic variation in BP. In twin studies of BP level, no age trend in heritability could be detected. Findings in family studies that reveal lower parent–offspring correlations than those for siblings and DZ twins indicate, however, that age may influence genetic or environmental effects on BP level. There are two possible explanations: the influence of unique environmental factors could increase with age, or different genes could influence BP in different periods of life. The lack of an age trend in heritabilities of twin studies is inconsistent with the first explanation, because an increase of unique environmental variance in adulthood, without a commensurate increase in genetic variance, would lower the heritability estimate. On the other hand, the twin data are not inconsistent with the second hypothesis of genes switching on and off with age, because the overall influence of genes can remain stable, although different genes are responsible for the effect. A number of further studies, including a longitudinal study of middle-aged twins, offered additional support for the second hypothesis that partly different genes affect BP in different periods of life, such as childhood, middle age, and old age.

The study of the genetics of the mechanisms involved in BP regulation in children might bring us closer to the causal mechanisms. There is considerable tracking of BP levels from childhood to adulthood *(53)*, making BP at a young age an important predictor of adult levels *(54)*. Longitudinal studies that follow children into adulthood can be used to study the influence of candidate genes for BP on the developmental trajectory of BP. Identification of these genes conferring susceptibility to the development of essential HTN in the general population will provide new avenues for treatment and prevention of this debilitating disease *(55,56)*.

## ACKNOWLEDGMENT

HS was supported in part by National Heart Lung and Blood Institute Grants HL56622 and HL69999, and a grant from the British Heart Foundation (FS/99050).

## REFERENCES

1. Johnson BD, Epstein FH, Kjelsberg MO. Distributions and family studies of blood pressure and serum cholesterol levels in a total community—Tecumseh, Michigan. J Chronic Dis 1965;18:147–160.
2. Miall WE, Heneage P, Khosla T, Lovell HG, Moore F. Factors influencing the degree of resemblance in arterial pressure of close relatives. Clin Sci 1967;33:271–283.
3. Zinner SH, Levy PS, Kass EH. Familial aggregation of blood pressure in childhood. N Engl J Med 1971;284(8):401–404.
4. Zinner SH, Martin LF, Sacks F, Rosner B, Kass EH. A longitudinal study of blood pressure in childhood. Am J Epidemiol 1974;100(6):437–442.
5. Hennekens CH, Jesse MJ, Klein BE, Gourley JE, Blumenthal S. Aggregation of blood pressure in infants and their siblings. Am J Epidemiol 1976;103(5):457–463.
6. Lee YH, Rosner B, Gould JB, Lowe EW, Kass EH. Familial aggregation of blood pressures of newborn infants and their mother. Pediatrics 1976;58(5):722–729.
7. Snieder H, van Doornen LJP, Boomsma DI. Development of genetic trends in blood pressure levels and blood pressure reactivity to stress. In: Turner JR, Cardon LR, Hewitt JK, eds. Behavior Genetic Approaches in Behavioral Medicine. New York: Plenum, 1995;105–130.
8. Snieder H, Boomsma DI, van Doornen LJP. Dissecting the genetic architecture of lipids, lipoproteins and apolipoproteins. Lessons from twin studies. Arterioscler Thromb Vasc Biol 1999;19:2826–2834.
9. Snieder H. Path analysis of age-related disease traits. In: Spector TD, Snieder H, MacGregor AJ, eds. Advances in Twin and Sib-pair Analyses. London: Greenwich Medical Media, 2000;119–129.
10. Biron P, Mongeau JG, Bertrand D. Familial aggregation of blood pressure in 558 adopted children. Can Med Assoc J 1976;115(8):773–774.
11. Plomin R, DeFries JC, McClearn GE. Behavioral Genetics. A Primer. 2nd ed. New York: W.H. Freeman and Company, 1990.
12. Phillips DI. Twin studies in medical research: can they tell us whether diseases are genetically determined? Lancet 1993;341(8851):1008–1009.
13. Kendler KS, Neale MC, Kessler RC, Heath AC, Eaves LJ. A test of the equal-environment assumption in twin studies of psychiatric illness. Behav Genet 1993;23(1):21–27.
14. Kyvik KO. Generalisability and assumptions of twin studies. In: Spector TD, Snieder H, MacGregor AJ, eds. Advances in Twin and Sib-Pair Analysis. London: Greenwich Medical Media, 2000;67–77.
15. Andrew T, Hart D, Snieder H, de Lange M, Spector TD, MacGregor AJ. Are twins and singletons comparable? A study of disease-related and lifestyle characteristics in adult women. Twin Res 2001;4:464–477.
16. De Geus EJC, Posthuma D, Ijzerman RG, Boomsma DI. Comparing blood pressure of twins and their singleton siblings: being a twin does not affect adult blood pressue. Twin Res 2001;4:385–391.
17. Neale MC, Cardon LR. Methodologies for genetic studies of twins and families. Dordrecht, The Netherlands: Kluwer Academic, 1992.
18. Spector TD, Snieder H, MacGregor AJ. Advances in Twin and Sib-Pair Analysis. London: Greenwich Medical Media, 2000.
19. de Castro JM. Heritability of diurnal changes in food intake in free-living humans. Nutrition 2001;17:713–720.
20. Simonen SL, Perusse L, Rankinen T, Rice T, Rao DC, Bouchard C. Familial aggregation of physical activity levels in the Quebec Family Study. Med Sci Sports Exerc 2002;34:1137–1142.

21. De Geus EJ, Boomsma DI, Snieder H. Genetic correlation of exercise with heart rate and respiratory sinus arrhythmia. Med Sci Sports Exerc 2003;35(8):1287–1295.
22. Hopper JL. Why 'common' environmental effects' are so uncommon in the literature. In: Spector TD, Snieder H, MacGregor AJ, eds. Advances in Twin and Sib-pair Analysis. London: Greenwich Medical Media, 2000;151–165.
23. Middelberg RP, Spector TD, Swaminathan R, Snieder H. Genetic and environmental influences on lipids, lipoproteins, and apolipoproteins: effects of menopause. Arterioscler Thromb Vasc Biol 2002;22(7):1142–1147.
24. Hong Y, de Faire U, Heller DA, McClearn GE, Pedersen NL. Genetic and environmental influences on blood pressure in elderly twins. Hypertension 1994;24(6):663–670.
25. Snieder H, Hayward CS, Perks U, Kelly RP, Kelly PJ, Spector TD. Heritability of central systolic pressure augmentation A twin study. Hypertension 2000;35:574–579.
26. Boomsma DI, Snieder H, de Geus EJ, van Doornen LJ. Heritability of blood pressure increases during mental stress. Twin Res 1998;1(1):15–24.
27. Reynolds CA, Hewitt JK. Issues in the behavior genetic investigation of gender differences. In: Turner JR, Cardon LR, Hewitt JK, eds. Behavior Genetics Approaches in Behavioral Medicine. New York: Plenum, 1995;189–199.
28. Levine RS, Hennekens CH, Perry A, Cassady J, Gelband H, Jesse MJ. Genetic variance of blood pressure levels in infant twins Am J Epidemiol 1982;116(5):759–764.
29. McIlhany ML, Shaffer JW, Hines EA. The heritability of blood pressure: an investigation of 200 pairs of twins using the cold pressor test. Johns Hopkins Med J 1974;136(2):57–64.
30. Snieder H, Harshfield GA, Treiber FA. Heritability of blood pressure and hemodynamics in African- and European-American youth. Hypertension 2003;41(6):1196–1201.
31. Verdecchia P. Prognostic value of ambulatory blood pressure: current evidence and clinical implications. Hypertension 2000;35:844–851.
32. Degaute JP, Van Cauter E, van de Borne P, Linkowski P. Twenty-four-hour blood pressure and heart rate profiles in humans. A twin study. Hypertension 1994;23(2):244–253.
33. Somes GW, Harshfield GA, Alpert BS, Goble MM, Schieken RM. Genetic influences on ambulatory blood pressure patterns. The Medical College of Virginia Twin Study. Am J Hypertens 1995;8(5 Pt 1):474–478.
34. Fagard R, Brguljan J, Staessen J, Thijs L, Derom C, Thomis M, Vlietinck R. Heritability of conventional and ambulatory blood pressures. A study in twins. Hypertension 1995;26(pt 1):919–924.
35. Vinck WJ, Fagard RH, Loos R, Vlietinck R. The impact of genetic and environmental influences on blood pressure variance across age-groups. J Hypertens 2001;19(6):1007–1013.
36. Schieken RM, Mosteller M, Goble MM, et al. Multivariate genetic analysis of blood pressure and body size. The Medical College of Virginia Twin Study. Circulation 1992;86(6):1780–1788.
37. Vinck WJ, Vlietinck R, Fagard RH. The contribution of genes, environment and of body mass to blood pressure variance in young adult males. J Hum Hypertens 1999;13(3):191–197.
38. Allison DB, Heshka S, Neale MC, Tishler PV, Heymsfield SB. Genetic, environmental, and phenotypic links between Body Mass Index and blood pressure among women. Am J Med Genet 1995;55:335–341.
39. Law CM, Shiell AW. Is blood pressure inversely related to birth weight? The strength of evidence from a systematic review of the literature. J Hypertens 1996;14(8):935–941.
40. Poulter NR, Chang CL, MacGregor AJ, Snieder H, Spector TD. Association between birth weight and adult blood pressure in twins: historical cohort study. Br Med J 1999;319(7221):1330–1333.
41. Christensen K, Stovring H, McGue M. Do genetic factors contribute to the association between birth weight and blood pressure? J Epidemiol Community Health 2001;55(8):583–587.
42. Baird J, Osmond C, MacGregor A, Snieder H, Hales CN, Phillips DIW. Testing the fetal origins hypothesis in twins: the Birmingham twin study. Diabetologia 2001;44:33–39.
43. Yu MW, Chen CJ, Wang CJ, et al. Chronological changes in genetic variance and heritability of systolic and diastolic blood pressure among Chinese twin neonates. Acta Genet Med Gemellol 1990;39:99–108.
44. Iselius L, Morton NE, Rao DC. Family resemblance for blood pressure. Hum Hered 1983;33(5):277–286.
45. Havlik RJ, Garrison RJ, Feinleib M, Kannel WB, Castelli WP, McNamara PM. Blood pressure aggregation in families. Am J Epidemiol 1979;110(3):304–312.
46. Tambs K, Moum T, Holmen J, et al. Genetic and environmental effects on blood pressure in a Norwegian sample. Genet Epidemiol 1992;9(1):11–26.

47. Hunt SC, Hasstedt SJ, Kuida H, Stults BM, Hopkins PN, Williams RR. Genetic heritability and common environmental components of resting and stressed blood pressures, lipids, and body mass index in Utah pedigrees and twins. Am J Epidemiol 1989;129(3):625–638.
48. Tambs K, Eaves LJ, Moum T, et al. Age-specific genetic effects for blood pressure. Hypertension 1993;22(5): 789–795.
49. Snieder H, van Doornen LJ, Boomsma DI. The age dependency of gene expression for plasma lipids, lipoproteins, and apolipoproteins. Am J Hum Genet 1997;60(3):638–650.
50. Fabsitz RR, Carmelli D, Hewitt JK. Evidence for independent genetic influences on obesity in middle age. Int J Obes Relat Metab Disord 1992;16(9):657–666.
51. Colletto GM, Cardon LR, Fulker DW. A genetic and environmental time series analysis of blood pressure in male twins. Genet Epidemiol 1993;10(6):533–538.
52. Dekkers JC, Treiber FA, Kapuku G, Snieder H. Differential influence of family history of hypertension and premature myocardial infarction on systolic blood pressure and left ventricular mass trajectories in youth. Pediatrics 2003;111(6 Pt 1):1387–1393.
53. van Lenthe FJ, Kemper HCG, Twisk JWR. Tracking of blood pressure in children and youth. Am J Human Biol 1994;6:389–399.
54. Bao W, Threefoot SA, Srinivasan SR, Berenson GS. Essential hypertension predicted by tracking of elevated blood pressure from childhood to adulthood: The Bogalusa Heart Study. Am J Hypertens 1995;8:657–665.
55. Snieder H, Harshfield GA, Barbeau P, Pollock DM, Pollock JS, Treiber FA. Dissecting the genetic architecture of the cardiovascular and renal stress response. Biol Psychol 2002;61(1–2):73–95.
56. Baker EH, Duggal A, Dong Y, et al. Amiloride, a specific drug for hypertension in black people with T594M variant? Hypertension 2002;40:13–17.
57. Havlik RJ, Garrison RJ, Katz SH, Ellison RC, Feinleib M, Myrianthopoulos NC. Detection of genetic variance in blood pressure of seven-year-old twins. Am J Epidemiol 1978;109(5):512–516.
58. Wang Z, Ouyang Z, Wang D, Tang X. Heritability of blood pressure in 7-to 12-year-old Chinese twins, with special reference to body size effects. Genet Epidemiol 1990;7:447–452.
59. Schieken RM, Eaves LJ, Hewitt JK, et al. Univariate genetic analysis of blood pressure in children (The Medical College of Virginia Twin Study). Am J Cardiol 1989;64:1333–1337.
60. Sims J, Carroll D, Hewitt JK, Turner JR. A family study of developmental effects upon blood pressure variation. Acta Genet Med Gemellol 1987;36:467–473.
61. Ditto B. Familial influences on heart rate, blood pressure, and self-report anxiety responses to stress: results from 100 twin pairs. Psychophysiol 1993;30:635–645.
62. McCaffery JM, Pogue-Geile M, Debski T, Manuck SB. Genetic and environmental causes of covariation among blood pressure, body mass and serum lipids during young adulthood: a twin study. J Hypertens 1999;17: 1677–1685.
63. Bielen EC, Fagard R, Amery AK. Inheritance of blood pressure and haemodynamic phenotypes measured at rest and during supine dynamic excercise. J Hypertens 1991;9:655–663.
64. Busjahn A, Li GH, Faulhaber HD, et al. β-2 adrenergic receptor gene variations, blood pressure, and heart size in normal twins. Hypertension 2000;35:555–560.
65. Slattery ML, Bishop TD, French TK, Hunt SC, Meikle AW, Williams RR. Lifestyle and blood pressure levels in male twins in Utah. Genet Epidemiol 1988;5:277–287.
66. Williams PD, Puddey IB, Martin NG, Beilin LJ. Platelet cytosolic free calcium concentration, total plasma calcium concentration and blood pressure in human twins: a genetic analysis. Clin Sci (Lond) 1992;82(5):493–504.
67. Austin MA, King MC, Bawol RD, Hulley SB, Friedman GD. Risk factors for coronary heart disease in adult female twins. Genetic heritability and shared environmental influences. Am J Epidemiol 1987;125(2):308–318.
68. Feinleib M, Garrison RJ, Fabsitz R, et al. The NHLBI twin study of cardiovascular disease risk factors: methodology and summary of results. Am J Epidemiol 1977;106(4):284–295.
69. Kramer AA. Re: "Genetic variance of blood pressure levels in infants twins". Am J Epidemiol 1984;119(4):651–552.

# 16 Influence of Dietary Electrolytes on Childhood Blood Pressure

*Dawn K. Wilson,* PhD

*CONTENTS*



## INTRODUCTION

Although the prevalence of hypertension (HTN) is relatively low during childhood and adolescence *(1)*, blood pressure (BP) patterns have been shown to track from childhood to the third and fourth decades of life *(1–2)*. Therefore, BP early in life may be a risk factor for the later development of HTN in young adulthood. Prevention programs are needed to reduce these risks in youth. Modification of sodium and/or potassium intake have been shown to be effective approaches to BP reduction in adults *(3–5)*, but there is less evidence of the benefits of these approaches in children and adolescents *(6)*. Current recommendations for primary prevention of HTN, published by The National High Blood Pressure Education Program Coordinating Committee *(7)*, involve a population approach and an intensive strategy for targeting individuals who are at increased risk for developing HTN in early adulthood. The Committee outlines a number of approaches that have proven effective for prevention of HTN. Two of these approaches include reducing sodium intake and maintaining an adequate intake of potassium.

Identifying precursors or markers of HTN is important for prevention of essential HTN. One marker for the development of essential HTN includes cardiovascular reactivity (CVR) *(8)*. CVR has been proposed as either a marker or a mechanism in the development of essential HTN. As a marker, hyperreactivity is conceptualized as a consequence of pre-existing cardiovascular damage, or of heightened sympathetic tone that results in vasoconstriction and/or excessive cardiac output. As a mechanism, hyperreactive peaks are proposed to damage the intimal layer of arteries, resulting in arteriosclerosis and subsequent HTN. Although there is

From: *Clinical Hypertension and Vascular Disease: Pediatric Hypertension*
Edited by: R. J. Portman, J. M. Sorof, and J. R. Ingelfinger © Humana Press Inc., Totowa, NJ

controversy about the predictive value of CVR, prospective studies have shown that increased CVR to mental stress is predictive of later development of essential HTN *(9)*. Only a limited number of studies have been conducted examining the relationship between dietary electrolytes and CVR in youth, and the results of these studies have been inconsistent *(8)*.

Recent evidence has suggested that ambulatory BP profiles may be an important predictor or risk factor of future HTN in youth. Ambulatory BP (APB) is a methodology for identifying and evaluating factors associated with individual differences in BP responses in the natural environment. Previous research indicates that most people display lower BP values at nighttime during sleeping hours and higher pressures during waking hours *(10)*. In healthy individuals, average BP declines by 15% or more during sleeping hours, while for hypertensive patients the circadian rhythm is generally preserved. The 24-h BP profile, however, is shifted upwards to a higher magnitude throughout the 24-h period *(11)*. A number of studies suggest that a blunted nocturnal decline in BP may be associated with greater cardiovascular risk *(10)*. For example, ambulatory BP nondipping status (defined as <10% decrease in BP from awake to asleep) is a risk factor for the development of end-organ disease in essential HTN. Specifically, patients who are characterized as nondippers show a more frequent history of stroke and left ventricular hypertrophy (LVH) *(12–14)*. Studies from our laboratory indicate that even among healthy African-American adolescents there is a 30% prevalence rate of nondipping status *(15–16)*. These findings have led us to investigate the factors that may influence the ABP pattern in youth.

Previous research indicates that dietary factors such as sodium and potassium significantly affect BP in adults, especially in industrialized and western countries *(17)*. Although some controversy exists about the differential effects of electrolyte intake on BP in childhood, some studies indicate that the relationship between environmental and genetic factors influence BP responses in children *(18–19)*. Specifically, some investigators have demonstrated that children as young as 0–3 yr of age may be at higher risk for future cardiovascular complications *(20)* because of differences in sodium handling and genetic phenotypes. Other investigators *(7)* have demonstrated that positive changes in dietary sodium and potassium in the first two decades of life can reduce BP. While the strongest support has been demonstrated for the effects of sodium on BP, the evidence concerning the effects of potassium have been less clear in children *(21)*. The purpose of this review is to summarize the nutritional electrolyte-related determinants of BP parameters in children and adolescents. In particular, this review focuses on the role of dietary sodium and potassium in shaping casual BP, BP reactivity, and circadian BP patterns in youth.

## DIETARY SODIUM AND BLOOD PRESSURE IN YOUTH

Previous research suggests that casual BP is important in understanding the influence of genetic, environmental, and nutritional influences on the progression and development of HTN in children and young adults. In a review paper, Simons-Morton and Obarzanck *(21)* critically evaluated 25 observational studies examining the association between sodium intake and casual BP in children and adolescents. Eight of the papers used self-report measures of dietary intake and 17 papers used urinary sodium excretion. Approximately 67% (two-thirds) of the urinary sodium studies that controlled for other factors (e.g., age, body mass index [BMI], weight) in the analysis found a significant positive association with casual BP. One-third of the studies that had no control variables found a significant association with casual BP.

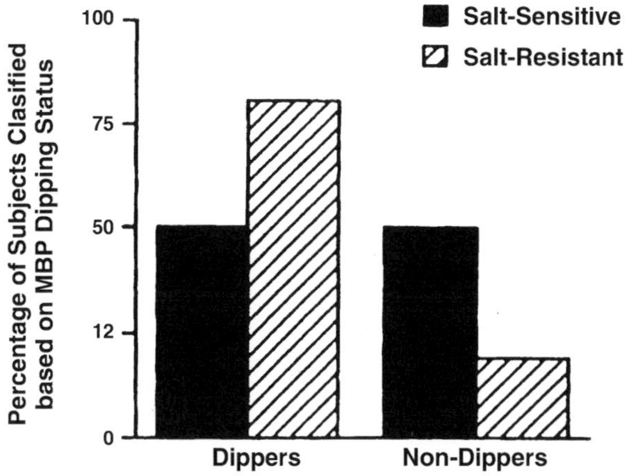


Fig. 1. Percentage of salt-sensitive versus salt-resistant normotensive African-American adolescents classified as dippers (>10 % decline in mean blood pressure from awake to asleep) or nondippers (<10 % decline in mean blood pressure from awake to asleep). Adapted with permission from ref. *26*.

Three of four of the studies which relied on self-report measures of dietary intake and that controlled for other variables found significant positive associations between dietary sodium and casual systolic BP, diastolic BP, or both. Taken together, the studies reviewed above provide fairly consistent support for the role of sodium intake on BP regulation in children and adolescents. Intervention studies that aim to reduce the intake of sodium may be beneficial.

Prior research shows that individuals who are at risk for cardiovascular complications such as African-Americans, hypertensive patients, and those with a positive family history of HTN are more likely to be salt-sensitive *(22,23)* (i.e. show increased BP in response to high sodium intake). Some of our recent work examined the prevalence of salt-sensitivity in normotensive African-American adolescents *(24)*. In this study, 22% of healthy normotensive African-American adolescents were characterized as salt-sensitive based on definitions established in the adult literature (25). Falkner et al. *(23)* have also shown that salt-sensitive adolescents with a positive family history of HTN had greater increases in BP with salt loading than did adolescents who were either salt-resistant or had a negative family history of HTN.

Several investigators have also examined the relationship between salt sensitivity and ambulatory BP profiles in children and adolescents. Wilson et al. examined the relationship between salt-sensitivity and ambulatory BP dipping status *(26)*. A significantly greater percentage of salt-sensitive adolescents were classified as nondippers according to mean BP (<10% decrease in BP from awake to asleep) as compared to salt-resistant individuals (Fig. 1). Harshfield et al. *(27)* also demonstrated that sodium intake is an important determinant of ambulatory BP profiles in African-American children and adolescents. These findings are consistent with de la Sierra et al. *(28)* who demonstrated higher awake BP values in normotensive salt-sensitive than in salt-resistant adults.

Rocchini et al. *(29)* conducted a series of studies examining BP sensitivity to sodium intake in obese adolescents. Obese adolescents showed greater decreases in casual BP after a shift from a high to low sodium intake compared to nonobese adolescents. This BP sensitivity to altering sodium intake was also positively correlated with plasma insulin concentration and with hyperinsulinemia *(29)*. Consequently, sodium retention may be a mechanism underlying the higher concentrations of plasma insulin in obese adolescents. In another study by Lurbe et

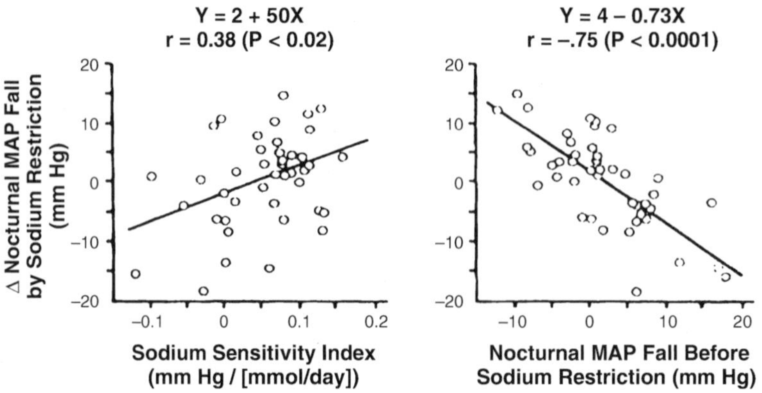


Fig. 2. Relationships of changes in nocturnal mean arterial pressure (MAP) fall induced by sodium restriction with the sodium-sensitivity index as well as with nocturnal MAP fall before sodium restriction. Adapted with permission from ref. *31*.

al. *(30),* 85 obese and 88 nonobese children (ages 3-19 yr) participated in 24-hr ambulatory BP monitoring and had their urinary sodium excretion rates determined. The interaction between sodium excretion and weight was negative, indicating a smaller rate of change in BP by sodium unit for obese than for nonobese participants. However, obese participants experienced higher ambulatory BP levels associated with the same levels of sodium excretion than nonobese participants. Taken together, these studies suggest that obesity may be associated with sodium regulation in that obese youth are more likely to be sensitive to alterations in sodium intake than nonobese children.

Salt-sensitivity is also associated with nondipping status in adults *(13–14)*. The role of sodium intake in nocturnal BP has been studied by several investigators. Uzu et al. *(31)* found that nondipper nocturnal BP in salt-sensitive patients was converted to a dipper pattern with sodium restriction (Fig. 2). Higashi et al. *(32)* also demonstrated that nocturnal decline in mean BP was significantly smaller in salt-sensitive subjects with hypertension when compared to salt-resistant subjects with hypertension during a sodium loading protocol.

The mechanism by which sodium sensitivity alters nighttime BP likely involves the sympathetic nervous system. Sympathetic nervous system arousal has been associated with differential handling of sodium following a behavioral challenge (video games) among individuals who are identified as retainers *(33)* (those who show little excretion of sodium load in urine). In a biracial sample of normotensive children, Harshfield et al. *(27)* demonstrated a stronger relationship between sodium handling and casual BP in African-American subjects. In Harshfield et al. *(27)*, African-American adolescents also showed a stronger association between 24-h urinary sodium excretion and casual BP, and BP during sleep independent of the urinary potassium excretion, than white adolescents. For casual BP and nighttime ambulatory BP, the slope was positive and significant for African-Americans, but no relationship was shown for white adolescents. The findings reported by Harshfield and colleagues *(27,33)*, and other investigators *(34)*, suggest an interactive role for the sympathetic nervous system in sodium retention which may, in part, explain blunted nocturnal decline in ambulatory BP profiles observed in salt-sensitive individuals.

## DIETARY POTASSIUM AND BLOOD PRESSURE IN YOUTH

In the review by Simons-Morton and Obarzanck *(21)*, 12 observational studies examined the association of potassium intake and casual BP in children and adolescents. Nine of the observational studies used urinary measures of potassium excretion, and 6 of these studies controlled for other factors such as weight. Two of these studies showed a significant inverse relationship between potassium intake and casual BP, while three studies showed no relationship. One study showed an unexpected positive association between potassium intake and casual BP. Two studies that relied on self-report estimates of intake showed a significant inverse relationship between potassium intake and systolic or diastolic BP, while two additional studies showed no relationship. Taken together, these studies only provide partial support for the beneficial effect of high potassium on casual BP levels in youth. However, as Wilson et al. *(16)* have noted, the effects of potassium may be most pronounced among salt-sensitive individuals, such as among African-Americans, or those with a positive family history of HTN. These factors were not specifically addressed in Simons-Morton and Obarzanck's *(21)* extensive review of the literature.

Research examining the effects of potassium intake on CVR has been scarce. In general, these studies have been correlational and have shown beneficial effects in only a subgroup of individuals. For example, Berenson and colleagues *(35)* reported that African-American boys in the highest BP strata, who showed significant increases in BP reactivity, had lower urinary potassium excretion than whites. Among adult populations, Morgan et al. *(36)* demonstrated in hypertensive patients that potassium supplementation (48 mmol/24 h) prevented the rise in BP produced by postural changes.

Very few reports have characterized the relationship between plasma potassium and ambulatory BP in adults. Goto et al. *(37)* showed a significant negative association between daytime plasma potassium concentration and 24-h systolic and diastolic BPs in patients with essential HTN. Plasma potassium was also inversely correlated with daytime and nighttime systolic and diastolic BP levels. Interpreting the relationship between a plasma electrolyte such as potassium and BP is difficult, however, because there are many factors known to influence plasma potassium values *(38,39)*. Although there are limitations of plasma potassium values, these results are consistent with prior epidemiological studies, which have shown a negative association between potassium intake, potassium excretion, and BP levels *(40)*.

## NUTRITION INTERVENTIONS AND BLOOD PRESSURE IN YOUTH

Several studies have examined the prevalence of consumption of high potassium/low sodium foods (e.g., fruit and vegetable intake) among adolescent populations. In a report by Falkner and Michel *(41)*, average sodium intakes of urban children and adolescents in Philadelphia well exceeded their nutritional needs (Fig. 3), determined by 24-h dietary recall assessments. Also noted in Fig. 3 is the high ratio of sodium to potassium in the diet, the reverse of the recommended ratio. These data are consistent with the Bogalusa Heart Study, a study that also assessed electrolyte intake among infants and children living in a rural biracial community *(43)*. Cullen et al. *(44)* had 5881 adolescents and young adults (aged 14–21 yr) complete a Survey on Youth Risk Behavior. Potassium intake related to fruit consumption declined for males and females during the high school years. Consistent with this finding, Neumark-Sztainer et al. *(45)* reported that among 30,000 adolescents who completed the Minnesota Health

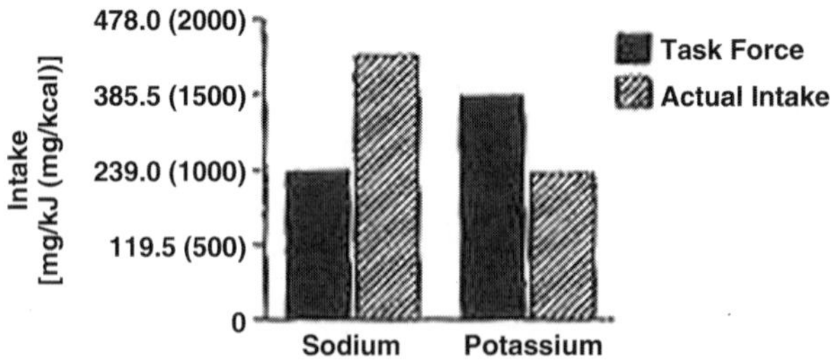


Fig. 3. Mean dietary intakes (actual intake) of sodium and potassium for urban adolescents aged 13–16 yr. These values are compared with the recommended dietary intake for adolescents *(42)*. Adapted with permission from ref. *41*.

Survey, and who had inadequate potassium intake, 28% had inadequate fruit intake and 36% had inadequate vegetable intake. Several investigators, including Berenson et al. *(27,46,47)* have also demonstrated that African-American children and adolescents show lower urinary potassium excretion rates than same-age whites. Thus, targeting adolescents and minority adolescents for dietary interventions that emphasize high potassium/low sodium food choices may be particularly needed at this age of development when emphasis on the importance of nutrition in youth seems to deteriorate.

Dietary electrolytes such as sodium, potassium, and the ratio of sodium/potassium are important in BP regulation. A number of studies have examined the influence of altering electrolyte intake on BP responses in children and adolescents. Miller et al. *(48)* examined the effect of sodium restriction for 12 wk (60 mEq/24h) on BP responses in white youth ages 3 to 30 yr. They found a decrease in diastolic BP after adjusting for age, sex, height, and weight; however, the magnitude of change was minimal (–2 mmHg). Other investigators have also not demonstrated significant decreases in casual BP in white children during sodium restriction ranging from 4 wk to 1 yr *(49,50)*.

Researchers have demonstrated that subgroups of children and adolescents show greater decreases in BP responses to changes in sodium restriction. For example, Rocchini et al. *(51)* demonstrated that obese adolescents had significantly greater decreases in mean BP than nonobese adolescents when they went from a high-salt diet to a low salt-diet. Other researchers have also demonstrated greater reductions in casual BP responses in African-American children compared to white children *(52)*.

In their review paper, Simons-Morton and Obarzanek *(21)* also identify 11 relevant intervention studies, 8 of which used a randomized controlled design, that examined the effects of reducing sodium intake on casual BP in children and adolescents. The studies ranged in size from 10 to 191 participants (children and/or adolescents). Duration of the interventions ranged from 3 wk to 3 yr, with half lasting 3–4 wk. Seven of 11 of the studies reported reduced systolic BP, diastolic BP, or both. However, only four of these studies reported statistically significant effects. Effects were stronger for girls and those with a BMI of less than 23. Two studies were identified that tested the effects of increasing potassium (one using supplementation and one using dietary change) on casual BP levels. Neither study, however, showed a significant effect from the intervention.

Several investigators have demonstrated longitudinal associations between potassium intake and casual BP responses in youth. Simons-Morton et al. *(53)* examined the associations between nutrients (including potassium) using 24-h recalls and casual systolic and diastolic BP in 662 youth who ranged in age from 8 to 11 yr. The participants were enrolled in the Dietary Intervention Study for Children (DISC), and had elevated low-density lipoprotein cholesterol. Assessments were done at baseline, 1 yr, and 3 yr. Longitudinal analyses revealed significant inverse associations between systolic BP and potassium, calcium, magnesium, protein, and fiber; and significant inverse associations between diastolic BP and potassium, calcium, magnesium, protein, carbohydrates, and fiber. Direct associations were also found between fat intake and both systolic and diastolic BP. Multivariate models showed calcium, fiber, and fat were the most important determinants of BP level in children with elevated low-density lipoprotein cholesterol.

Sinaiko et al. *(6)* tested the feasibility of a 3-yr potassium supplementation or sodium reduction in preventing the rise in BP among adolescents. Adolescents who were in the upper 15th percentile of BP distribution were randomly assigned to potassium chloride supplementation (1 mmol/kg potassium chloride/d), a low sodium diet (70 mmol sodium/d), or a placebo (normal diet plus placebo capsule). The results demonstrated that both the potassium supplementation and sodium restriction interventions were effective in reducing the rise in casual BP in girls, but not in boys. Consequently, the feasibility of long-term restriction of dietary sodium in boys may be limited.

Some evidence indicates that dietary electrolyte intake plays an influential role in circulatory responses to stress. Falkner and colleagues *(54)* have conducted a number of investigations into how altering dietary sodium affects CVR. One study evaluated 15 normotensive adolescent girls for 2 wk, at rest and during mental arithmetic exercises, and before and after adding 10 g of salt to their diet. The girls with a positive family history of essential HTN showed an increase in resting baseline and stress BP levels. The girls with a negative family history did not. These findings have been replicated in young adults *(55)*. However, for those with a positive family history of essential HTN, changes from baseline to stress were similar before and after salt-loading.

Sorof et al. *(56)* examined whether CVR was inversely related to the dietary intake of potassium in 39 children. At baseline, the 24-hr urinary potassium/creatinine ratio varied inversely with diastolic CVR in white children (who had a positive family history of HTN), however, CVR was not attenuated by potassium supplementation (1.5 mmol/kg/d of potassium citrate) compared to placebo. Urinary potassium/creatinine ratio was higher in white children than in African-American children and dietary potassium-modulated CVR in white children with a family history of HTN.

Consistent with this finding, Wilson et al. *(16)* demonstrated no significant change in BP reactivity in African-American adolescents who complied with a 3-wk high potassium diet. Wilson et al. *(16)* also demonstrated, in one of the first randomized control trials among adolescents, that increasing potassium was beneficial for reversing nondipping BP status and elevated nighttime BP in African-American adolescents. This study examined the effects of increasing dietary potassium on BP nondipping status in salt-sensitive and salt-resistant African-American adolescents. A sample of 58 normotensive (101/57 $\pm$ 9/4 mmHg) African-American adolescents (aged 13 to 16 yr) participated in a 5-d low sodium diet (50 mmol/24 h) followed by a 10-d high sodium diet (150 mmol/24 h NaCl supplement) to determine salt sensitivity status. Participants showed a significant increase in urinary sodium excretion (24 $\pm$ 19 to 224 $\pm$ 65 mmol/24 h) and were identified as salt-sensitive if their mean BP increase was $\geq$5 mm Hg from the low- to high- sodium diet. 16 salt-sensitive and 42 salt-resistant subjects were then randomly assigned to either a 3-wk high potassium diet (80 mmol/24 h) or usual diet control group. Urinary potassium excretion significantly increased in the treatment group (35 ± 7 to 57 ± 21 mmol/24 h). At baseline, a significantly greater percentage of salt-sensitive (44%) subjects were nondippers based on diastolic BP classifications ($p < 0.04$), compared to salt-resistant (7%) subjects.

After the dietary intervention, all of the salt-sensitive subjects in the high potassium group achieved a dipper BP status due to a drop in nocturnal diastolic BP (daytime 69 ± 5 vs 67 ± 5; nighttime 69 ± 5 vs 57 ± 6 mmHg). These results suggest that a positive relationship between dietary potassium intake and BP modulation can prevail, although daytime BP may be unchanged by a high potassium diet. Our data are the first to indicate that increasing dietary potassium reversed nondipping status in salt-sensitive subjects, while having no effect on daytime BP. These findings, in part, corroborate other investigations that have shown beneficial effects of increasing potassium on BP responses in salt-sensitive populations. For example, Fujita and Ando *(57)* demonstrated that salt-sensitive hypertensives who were given a potassium supplement (96 mmol/24h) while on a high sodium diet showed significantly greater decreases in MBP after 3 d when compared to nonsupplemented hypertensive patients. Svetkey et al. *(58)* demonstrated a significant drop in both systolic and diastolic BP after 8 wk of potassium supplementation (120 mmol/24h vs placebo) among mildly hypertensive patients. Siani et al. *(59)* reported similar findings among hypertensive patients who were given potassium supplements (48 mmol/24h) for 15 wk. In one of the most dramatic studies by Obel *(60)*, mildly hypertensive African-American men who received a potassium supplement (64 mmol/24h vs placebo) for 16 wk showed a drop in supine systolic BP from 175 ± 10 mmHg to 133 ± 10 mmHg and in supine diastolic BP from 100 ± 3 mmHg to 83 ± 4 mmHg, while no change was detected in the placebo group.

A number of reviews on the influence of potassium on BP responses have also shown positive inverse associations between high potassium intake and BP responses in primarily adult populations *(7,40,61)*. The mechanisms underlying BP nondipping status are unknown. One potential mechanism by which potassium may alter nighttime BP may involve potassium-related natriuresis *(62,63)*. Restricting potassium intake leads to sodium retention; potassium supplementation results in a natriuresis. Some investigators suggest that the effect of potassium on urinary sodium excretion, plasma volume, and mean arterial pressure could be evidence of a potassium-mediated vasodilator effect on BP *(40)*. If nondippers are characterized by elevated sympathetic nervous system activity and increased peripheral resistance during sleep, this potassium-mediated vasodilatory effect could explain the reversal of nondipping status in the Wilson et al. study *(16)*. Other studies that support this hypothesis show that intrabrachial arterial infusions of potassium chloride increase forearm blood flow and decrease forearm vascular resistance in healthy adults *(64,65)*. Potassium supplementation given in combination with a high sodium diet also suppresses the increase in catecholamine responses typically seen in response to salt-loading *(66)*. Previous studies have shown that total peripheral resistance and norepinephrine responses to stress are greater in offspring of hypertensives than in normotensives *(67)*. Several adult studies have also confirmed that sympathetic nervous system activation occurs in individuals with elevated nighttime BP. Kostic et al. *(68)* reported significantly higher BP values during sleeping hours for patients with severe HTN, and, in association with this, significantly higher daytime and nighttime cortisol and urinary catecholamine excretion. James and colleagues *(69)* found a positive association between nighttime BP and catecholamine excretion rates in normotensive working women. Taken together, these data support the hypothesis that the sympathetic nervous system may have a controlling influence on nondipping BP status.

## NUTRITION AND DIETARY COMPLIANCE IN YOUTH

Several lines of evidence suggest that targeting families may be important for promoting healthy dietary compliance in children and adolescents. Previous research has demonstrated moderate aggregation of dietary variables among adolescents and their parents *(70)*. Furthermore, because families share a genetic predisposition to health risk factors, family involvement may be important in motivating adolescents to improve their long-term eating habits. Parents and peers may serve as role models for adolescents by consuming foods that are healthy, and by reinforcing dietary knowledge and behaviors learned in schools *(71)*.

Social support from family members may be one way that parental involvement may influence compliance with dietary interventions. Parents may encourage adolescents to adopt healthy dietary behaviors, which in turn may decrease the risk for cardiovascular disease and chronic illness. Wilson and Ampey-Thornhill *(72)* examined the relationship between gender, dietary social support (emotional), and compliance to a low sodium diet. 184 healthy African-American adolescents participated in an intensive 5-d low sodium diet (50 mEq/2h) as part of a HTN prevention program. Girls who were compliant (urinary sodium excretion [UNaV] < 50 mEq/24h) reported higher levels of dietary support from family members than boys who were compliant (UNaV <50 mEq/24h). In contrast, boys who were compliant reported lower levels of dietary support from family members than boys who were not compliant.

In a study by Nader et al. *(73)*, White, African-American, and Mexican-American families were randomly assigned to a 3-mo low-sodium, low-fat diet program, or to a no-treatment group. The treatment group showed a greater increase in social support specific to diet than the no-treatment group. Taken together, these studies provide evidence that familial support may be important for increasing adolescents' compliance with healthy dietary programs that will ultimately decrease the risk of HTN and cardiovascular complications.

Another way that parents, teachers, and peers may influence adolescents' compliance with healthy eating habits is through role modeling. Cohen, Felix, and Brownell *(74)* randomly assigned adolescents to either peer-led or teacher-led promotions of a low-sodium, low fat dietary intervention. At the end of the intervention, both groups showed equal effectiveness in changing nutritional habits. The peer-led group, however, was more effective in reducing BP.

Previous research also suggests that the incorporation of behavioral skills training and developmentally appropriate dietary interventions may be most effective in promoting long-term changes in sodium and/or potassium change (e.g., increased fruit and vegetable intake). For example, in a study conducted by Gortmaker et al. *(75)* 1295 sixth- and seventh-grade students from public schools in Massachusetts participated in a school-based intervention over 2 yr to reduce the prevalence of obesity. The intervention was based on social cognitive theory (SCT) and behavioral choice theory. Treatment sessions were incorporated into the existing curricula, used classroom teachers, and included the students' increasing their fruit and vegetable intake. The results showed that the intervention schools that focused on increasing behavioral skills and choice were more effective for increasing fruit and vegetable consumption than control schools.

The Child and Adolescent Trial on Cardiovascular Health (CATCH) is one of the largest clinical trials *(76–78)* to examine the effects of an SCT approach to improving diet (e.g., lowering saturated fat, cholesterol, and sodium intake) in 96 elementary schools. Schools across four study sites were randomized to either an SCT treatment that focused on behavioral skills or a control condition. After 3 years, these intervention school children exhibited significant changes in improved knowledge, intentions, self-efficacy, dietary behavior, and perceived social reinforcement for healthy food choices.

Some studies have provided insight into the importance of targeting eating patterns for improving food choices related to high potassium/low sodium foods such as fruit and vegetable intake *(79)*. In 943 third to fifth graders, fruit juices accounted for 6.1% of the total food selections for boys and 6.6% for girls. Vegetables accounted for 15.7% of total selections for boys and 16.2% for girls. Fruit was more likely consumed for snacks than for meals, and vegetables were eaten at the same rate for snacks, at lunch, and at supper. Consequently, targeting an increase in fruits in all meals may be one effective approach to improving electrolyte intake in children. Further research is needed; specifically, more tests that systematically focus on the relevance of increasing fruit and vegetable intake throughout an entire day's eating episodes instead of sporadic episodes.

Several studies have demonstrated gender differences in compliance to sodium restriction and dietary potassium supplementation. Sinaiko et al. *(6)* reported urinary electrolyte excretion data over the course of a 3-yr intervention in fifth through eighth graders. Boys were less likely to comply with a sodium restriction of 70 mmol/d than girls. Subsequently, BP effects were only significant for girls. In a study by Wilson et al. *(80)*, boys were more likely than girls to comply with a 3-wk dietary intervention of increasing potassium to 80 mmol/d intake. These studies suggest that boys, in particular, may be more likely to comply with high potassium diets that emphasize adding foods to the diet compared to low sodium diets that focus on eliminating foods from the diet. Further research is needed to more fully explore the long-term effectiveness of dietary electrolyte interventions in boys vs girls.

## CONCLUSIONS AND IMPLICATIONS FOR FUTURE RESEARCH

In summary, the profile of elevated cardiovascular risk includes BP parameters such as high casual BP, elevated CVR, and nondipping ambulatory BP status. While much of the research to date has focused on adult populations, national efforts are moving in the direction of prevention at the childhood level.

Reducing sodium and increasing potassium intake have been shown to be effective approaches for reducing the risk and development of HTN, yet much work remains to be done among children and adolescent populations. This chapter provides the preliminary basis for promoting effective nutritional-electrolyte-focused interventions. However, other important factors must be considered, including those related to obesity and sedentary lifestyles. Minority populations, including African-Americans, are at particularly high risk for developing HTN in early adulthood, and efforts should focus on preventing HTN in these and underserved communities. Abnormal sympathetic nervous system activity may be most likely linked to elevated BP parameters reviewed in this chapter. The role of dietary intake on BP markers suggests that further attention should be paid to promoting positive dietary lifestyle skills in youth. Promoting healthy diets that target decreasing sodium and increasing potassium may help to decrease sympathetic nervous system activation. The precise physiological mechanisms that underlie the observations reported in this chapter should be another focus of future investigations.

## ACKNOWLEDGMENT

The projects described in this chapter were funded by a FIRST Award grant from NHLBI (HL#46736) and by a GCRC grant M01RR00065 at Virginia Commonwealth University. The author wishes to acknowledge Domenic A. Sica, MD, and Joel E. Williams, MPH for their input and assistance with the development of this manuscript.

## REFERENCES

1. Sinaiko AR, Gomez-Marin O, Prineas RJ. Prevalence of significant hypertension in junior high school-aged children. JPediatr 1989;114:664–669.
2. Lauer RM, Clarke WR. Childhood risk factors for high adult blood pressure: The Muscatine Study. Pediatrics 1989;84:633–644.
3. Carvalho JJ, Baruzzi FG, Howard PF, Poulter N, Alpers M, Stamler R. Blood pressure in four remote populations in the INTERSALT study. Hypertension 1989;14:238–246.
4. INTERSALT Cooperative Research Group. INTERSALT: an international study of electrolyte excretion and blood pressure. Results for 24-hour urinary sodium and potassium excretion. Br Med J 1988;297:319–328.
5. Whelton PK, He J, Cutler JA, et al. Effects of oral potassium on blood pressure: meta-analysis of randomized controlled clinical trials. JAMA 1997;277:1624–1632.
6. Sinaiko AR, Gomez-Marin O, Prineas R. Effect of low sodium diet or potassium supplementation on adolescent blood pressure. Hypertension 1993;21:989–994.
7. Whelton PK, He J, Appel LJ, et al. Primary prevention of hypertension: clinical and public health advisory from the National High Blood pressure Education Program. JAMA 2002;288:1882–1888.
8. Alpert BA, Wilson DK. Stress reactivity in childhood and adolescence. In: Turner JR, Sherwood A, Light K, eds. Individual Differences in Cardiovascular Response to Stress: Applications to Models of Cardiovascular Disease. New York: Plenum, 1992;187–201.
9. Borghi C, Costa FV, Boschi S, Mussi A, Ambrosioni E. Predictors of stable hypertension in young borderline subjects: a five-year follow-up study. J Cardiovasc Pharmacol 1986;8:S138–S141.
10. Sica DA, Wilson DK. Sodium, potassium, the sympathetic nervous system, and the renin-angiotensin system: impact on the circadian variability in blood pressure. In: White WB, ed. Cardiovascular Chronobiology and Variability in Clinical Practice. Totowa, NJ: Humana, 2001;171–189.
11. Verdecchia P, Schillaci G, Borgioni C, Porcellati C. Prognostic significance of the white-coat effect. Hypertension 1997;29:1218–1224.
12. Kobrin I, Oigman W, Kumar A, et al. Diurnal variation in blood pressure in elderly patients with essential hypertension. J Am Geriatrc Soc 1984;32:896–899.
13. Verdecchia P, Schillaci G, Guerrieri M, et al. Circadian blood pressure changes and left ventricular hypertrophy in essential hypertension. Circulation 1990;81:528–536.
14. Devereux RB, Pickering TG. Relationships between the level, pattern and variability of ambulatory blood pressure changes and left ventricular hypertrophy in essential hypertension. J Hypertens 1991;9(Suppl):S34–S38.
15. Wilson DK, Sica DA, Devens M, Nicholson S. The influence of potassium intake on Dipper and Non-Dipper blood pressure status in an African-American adolescent population. Blood Press Monit 1996;1:447–455.
16. Wilson DK, Sica DA, Miller SB. Effects of potassium on blood pressure in salt-sensitive and salt-resistant adolescents. Hypertension 1999;34:181–186.
17. Leong GM, Kainer G. Diet, salt, anthropological and hereditary factors in hypertension. Child Nephrol Urol 1992;12:96–105.
18. Kojima S, Inenaga T, Matsuoka H, et al. The association between salt sensitivity of blood pressure and some polymorphic factors. J Hypertens 1994;12:797–801.
19. Weinberger MH, et al. Association of haptoglobin with sodium sensitivity and resistence of blood pressure. Hypertension 1987;10:443–446.
20. Guerra A, Monteiro C, Breitenfeld L, et al. Genetic and environmental factors regulating blood pressure in childhood: prospective study from 0 to 3 years. J Hum Hypertens 1997;11:233–238.
21. Simons-Morton DG, Obarzanck E. Diet and blood pressure in children and adolescents. Pediatr Nephrol 1997;11:244–249.

22. Weinberger MH, Miller JZ, Luft FC, et al. Definitions and characteristics of sodium sensitivity and blood pressure resistance. Hypertension 1986;8:II127–II134.
23. Falkner B, Kushner H, Khalsa DK, et al. Sodium sensitivity, growth and family history of hypertension in young blacks. J Hypertens1986;4(Suppl):S381–S383.
24. Wilson DK, Bayer L, Krishnamoorthy JS, Ampey-Thornhill G, Nicholson S, Sica DA. The prevalence of salt-sensitivity in an African-American adolescent population. Ethn Dis 1999;9:350–358.
25. Sullivan JM, Ratts TE. Sodium sensitivity in human subjects: hemodynamic and hormonal correlates. Hypertension, 1988;11:717–723.
26. Wilson DK, Sica DA, Miller SB. Ambulatory blood pressure and nondipping status in salt-sensitive versus salt-resistant black adolescents. Am J Hypertens 1999;12:159–165.
27. Harshfield GA, Alpert BS, Pulliam DA, Willey ES, Somes GW, Stapleton FB. Sodium excretion and racial differences in ambulatory blood pressure patterns. Hypertension 1991;18:113–118.
28. de la Sierra A, del Mar Lluch M, Coca, et al. Assessment of salt-sensitivity in essential hypertension by 24-h ambulatory blood pressure monitoring. Am J Hypertens 1995;8:970–977.
29. Rocchini AP, Kolch V, Kveselis D, et al. Insulin and renal sodium retention in obese adolescents. Hypertension 1989;14:367–373.
30. Lurbe E, Alvarez V, Liao Y, et al. Obesity modifies the relationship between ambulatory blood pressure and natriuresis in children. Blood Press Monit 2000;5:275–280.
31. Uzu T, Ishikawa K, Fujita T, et al. Sodium restriction shifts circadian rhythm of blood pressure from nondipper to dipper in essential hypertension. Circulation 1997;96:1859–1862.
32. Higashi Y, Shima T, Ozono R, et al. Nocturnal decline in blood pressure is attenuated by NaCl loading in salt-sensitive patients with essential hypertension. Hypertension 1997;30(Pt 1):163–167.
33. Harshfield GA, Pulliam DA, Alpert BS. Pattern of sodium excretion during sympathetic nervous system arousal. Hypertension 1991;17:1156–1160.
34. Light KC, Koepke JP, Obrist PA, et al. Psychological stress induces sodium and fluid retention in men at high risk for hypertension. Science 1983;229:429–431.
35. Berenson GS, Voors AW, Webber LS, Dalferes ER Jr, Harsh DW. Racial differences of parameters associated with blood pressure levels in children–the Bogalusa Heart Study. Metabolism 1979;28:1218–1228.
36. Morgan T, Toew BH, Myers J. The role of potassium in control of blood pressure. Drugs 1984;28(Suppl I):I-188–I-195.
37. Goto A, Yamada K, Nagoshi H, et al. Relation of 24-h ambulatory blood pressure with plasma potassium in essential hypertension. J Hypertens 1997;10:337–340.
38. Solomon R,Weinberg MS, Dubey A. The diurnal rhythm of plasma potassium: relationship to diuretic therapy. J Cardiovasc Pharmacol 1991;17:854–859.
39. Struthers AD, Reid JL, Whitesmith R, et al. Effect of intravenous adrenaline on electrocardiogram, blood pressure and plasma potassium. Br Heart J 1983;49:90–93.
40. Linas SL. The role of potassium in the pathogenesis and treatment of hypertension. Kidney Int 1991;39:771–786.
41. Falkner B, Michel S. Blood pressure response to sodium in children and adolescents. Am J Clin Nutr 1997;65(Suppl):618–621.
42. Task Force on Blood Pressure Control in Children. Report of the Second Task Force on Blood Pressure Control in Children. Pediatrics 1987;79:1–25.
43. Frank GC, Webber LS, Nicklas TA, Berenson GS. Sodium, potassium, calcium, magnesium, and phosphorous intakes of infants and children: Bogalusa Heart Study. J Am Diet Assoc 1988;88:801–807.
44. Cullen KW, Koehly LM, Anderson C, et al. Gender differences in chronic disease risk behaviors through the transition out of high school. Am J Prev Med 1999;17:1–7.
45. Neumark-Sztainer D, Story M, Resnick MD, Blum RW. Lessons learned about adolescent nutrition from the Minnesota Adolescent Health Survey. J Am Diet Assoc 1998;98:1449–1456.
46. Berenson GS, Voors AW, Dalferes ER, Webber LS, Shuler SE. Creatinine clearance, electrolytes, and plasma renin activity related to the blood pressure of white and black children: the Bogalusa Heart Study. J Lab Clin Med 1979;93:535–548.
47. Pratt JH, Jones JJ, Miller JZ, Wagner MA, Fineberg NS. Racial differences in aldosterone excretion and plasma adolesterone concentrations in children. N Engl J Med 1989;321:1152–1157.
48. Miller JZ, Weinberger MH, Daugherty SA, Fineberg NS, Christian JC, Grim CE. Blood pressure response to dietary sodium restriction in healthy nomotensive children. Am J Clin Nutr 1988;47:113–119.

49. Gillum RF, Elmer PJ, Prineas RJ, Surbey D. Changing sodium intake in children: the Minneapolis children's blood pressure study. Hypertension 1981;3:698–703.
50. Watt GCM, Foy DJW, Hart JT, et al. Dietary sodium and arterial blood pressure: evidence against genetic susceptibility. Br Med J 1985; 291:1525–1528.
51. Rocchini AP, Key J, Bondie D, et al. The effect of weight loss on the sensitivity of blood pressure to sodium in obese adolescents. N Engl J Med 1989;321:580–585.
52. Wilson DK, Becker JA, Alpert BS. Prevalence of sodium sensitivity in black versus white adolescents. Circulation 1992;1(Suppl):13.
53. Simons-Morton DG, Hunsberger SA, Van Horn L, et al. Nutrient intake and blood pressure in the dietary intervention study in children. Hypertension 1997;29:930–936.
54. Falkner B, Onesti G, Angelakos ET. Effect of salt loading on the cardiovascular resonse to stress in adolescents. Hypertension 1981;3(II):195–199.
55. Falkner B, Kushner H. Effect of chronic sodium loading on cardiovascular response in young blacks and whites. Hypertension 1990;15:36–43.
56. Sorof JM, Forman A, Cole N, Jemerin JM, Morris RC. Potassium intake and cardiovascular reactivity in children with risk factors for essential hypertension. J Pediatr 1997;131:87–94.
57. Fujita T, Ando K. Hemodynamic and endocrine changes associated with potassium supplementation in sodium-loaded hypertensives. Hypertension 1984;6:184–192.
58. Svetkey LP, Yarger WE, Feussner JR, DeLong E, Klotman PE. Double-blind, placebo-controlled trial of potassium chloride in the treatment of mild hypertension. Hypertension 1987;9:444–450.
59. Siani A, Strazzulo P, Russo L, Guglielmi S, Ferrara LA, Mancini M. Controlled trial of long term oral potassium supplements in patients with mild hypertension. J Behav Med 1987;294:1453–1456.
60. Obel AO. Placebo-controlled trial of potassium supplements in black patients with essential hypertension. J Cardiovasc Pharmacol 1989;14:294–296.
61. Cappuccio FP, MacGregor GA. Does potassium supplementation lower blood pressure? A meta-analysis of published trials. J Hypertens 1991;9:465–473.
62. Krishna GG, Miller E, Kapoor S. Increased blood pressure during potassium depletion in normotensive man. N Engl J Med 1989;320:1177–1182.
63. Weinberger MH, Luft FC, Block R, et al. The blood pressure-raising effects of high dietary sodium intake: racial differences and the role of potassium. J Am Coll Nutr 1982;1:139–148.
64. Fujita T, Ito Y. Salt loads attenuate potassium-induced vasocilation of forearm vasculature in humans. Hypertension 1993;21:772–778.
65. Phillips RJW, Robinson BF. The dilator response to K+ is reduced in the forearm resistance vessels of men with primary hypertension. Clin Sci 1984;66:237–239.
66. Campese VM, Romoff MS, Levitan D, et al. Abnormal relationship between Na+ intake and sympathetic nervous activity in salt-sensitive patients with essential hypertension. Kidney Int 1982;21:371–378.
67. Stamler R, Stamler J, Riedlinger WF, Algera G, Roberts RH. Family (parental) history and prevalence of hypertension. Results of a nationwide screening program. JAMA 1979;241:43–46.
68. Kostic N, Secen S. Circadian rhythm of blood pressure and daily hormone variations. Med Pregl 1997;50: 37–40.
69. James GD, Schlussel YR, Pickering TG. The association between daily blood pressure and catecholamine variability in normotensive working women. Psychosom Med 1993;55:55–60.
70. Patterson TL, Rupp JW, Sallis JF, Atkins CJ, Nader PR. Aggregation of dietary calories, fats, and sodium in Mexican-American and Anglo families. Am J Prev Med 1988;14:75–82.
71. Perry CL, Luepker RV, Murray DM, Kurth C, Mullis R, Crockett S, Jacobs DR. Parental involvement with children's health promotion: The Minnesota Home Team. Am J Public Health 1988;78:1156–1160.
72. Wilson DK, Ampey-Thornhill G. Gender differences in social support and dietary compliance in African-American adolescents. Ann Behav Med 2001;23:59–67.
73. Nader PR, Sallis JF, Patterson TL, et al. A family approach to cardiovascular risk reduction: results from the San Diego Family Health Project. Health Educ Q 1989;16:229–244.
74. Cohen RY, Felix MRJ, Brownell KD. The role of parents and older peers in school-based cardiovascular prevention programs: implications for program development. Health Educ Q 1989;16:245–253.
75. Gortmaker SL, Cheung LW, Peterson KE, et al. Impact of school based interdisciplinary intervention on diet and physical activity among urban primary school children: eat well and keep moving. Arch Pediatr Adolesc Med 1999;153:975–983.

76. Stone EJ, Osganian SK, McKinlay SM, et al. Operational design and quality control in the CATCH Multicenter Trial. Prev Med 1996;25:384–399.
77. Edmundson E, Parcel GS, Feldman HA, et al. The effects of the child and adolescent trial for cardiovascular health upon psychosocial determinants of diet and physical activity behavior. Prev Med 1996;25:442–454.
78. Luepker RV, Perry CL, McKinlay SM, et al. Outcomes of a field trial to improve children's dietary patterns and physical activity: Child and Adolescent Trial for Cardiovascular Health (CATCH). JAMA 1996;257:768–776.
79. Simons-Morton BG, Baranowski T, Parcel GS, O'Hara NM, Matteson RC. Children's frequency of consumption of foods high in fat and sodium. Am J Prev Med 1990;6:218–227.
80. Wilson DK, Bayer L. The role of diet in hypertension prevention among African-American adolescents. Ann Beh Med 2002;24(Suppl):S198.

# 17 Ethnic Differences in Childhood Blood Pressure

*Gregory A. Harshfield,* PhD
*and Martha E. Wilson,* MA

*Contents*



## ETHNIC DIFFERENCES IN HYPTERTENSION

Essential hypertension (HTN) in the African-American community has reached epidemic proportions. According to the 2002 report of the American Heart Association *(1)*, the age-adjusted prevalence of HTN for African-Americans 20 yr and older was 36.7% for men and 36.6% for women. The high prevalence of HTN for African-Americans contributed to the increased morbidity and mortality among African-Americans compared to Caucasians including: (1) a 1.3 times greater rate of nonfatal stroke and a 1.8 times greater rate of fatal stroke; (2) a 1.5 times greater rate of heart disease and death; and (3) a 4.2 times greater rate of renal disease. Furthermore, African-American compared to Caucasian women have an 85% greater rate of hypertension-related ambulatory care visits. Perhaps the most telling statistic is that HTN contributes to 30% of all deaths for African-American males and 20% for all females.

## ETHNIC DIFFERENCES IN CASUAL OR RESTING BLOOD PRESSURE

Longitudinal studies clearly established that the development of HTN and blood pressure (BP)-related target organ damage begins in childhood. These studies are reviewed in other chapters in this book. However, it is not clear when ethnic differences in BP and HTN become apparent. Table 1 lists 47 studies, 2 meta-analyses, and 1 review that examined ethnic differences in BP of subjects from infancy to 18 yr of age. Of these, 26 reported higher BP for African-Americans, 8 reported higher BP for Caucasians, 2 reported higher BP for Hispanics, and 14 reported no differences between African-Americans and Caucasians.

From: *Clinical Hypertension and Vascular Disease: Pediatric Hypertension*
Edited by: R. J. Portman, J. M. Sorof, and J. R. Ingelfinger © Humana Press Inc., Totowa, NJ

### *African-American Blood Pressure Higher Than That of Caucasians, Asians, or Hispanics*

Many studies reported higher levels of casual or resting BP in African-American compared to Caucasian children and adolescents, as shown in Table 1. In 1993, Alpert and Fox *(2)* reviewed and performed a meta-analysis on 35 studies published in English. Of these, 6 (17%) did not report ethnic differences. The remaining 29 studies were divided into four groups based on the ages of the subjects: 0–12 yr ($n = 8$), 13–18 yr ($n = 17$), and 19–24 yr ($n = 3$), and studies spanning more than one range ($n = 3$). Data for two of these studies were longitudinal and presented in two age categories *(3,4)*, accounting for the 31 rather than 29 citations in the table in the article. Comparisons between African-Americans, Caucasians, and Asian subjects for both males and females were performed for both systolic and diastolic BP within each age grouping. The results were mixed, with the "plurality" of comparisons showing higher BP for African-Americans compared to either Caucasian or Asian males or females for either systolic BP or diastolic BP. Specifically, African-Americans had higher BP in 50% (19/38) of the comparisons for subjects 0–12 yr, in 66% (33/50) of the comparisons for subjects 13–18 yr, 80% (4/5) of the comparisons for 19–24 yr, and 100% (10/10) of the comparisons across the multiple age range.

Overall, these data suggest that ethnic differences may not become apparent until an older age. Consistent with this hypothesis are the results of a study by Manatunga, Jones, and Pratt *(5)* that examined ethnic differences in a prospective longitudinal assessment of BP in 164 African-American and 345 Caucasian children. Each child had his or her BP measured every 6 mo for 2 to 5.5 yr. The mean BP and the mean rate of increase in BP over time were compared between gender-specific African-American and Caucasian groups. For both boys and girls, the mean systolic BP was 2 mmHg higher in African-American compared to Caucasian children, and the mean diastolic BP was 1.5 mmHg higher for African-American compared to Caucasian children. More importantly, the rate of increase in BP over time was significantly greater in African-Americans than Caucasians. Age, weight, height, and body mass index (BMI) were highly correlated, with BP ranging between $r = 0.4$ and $r = 0.6$. When accounting for these variables, African-American children had consistently higher BP than Caucasian children, but the effect of ethnicity was only significant for systolic BP in girls. They concluded that the factors responsible for ethnic differences in HTN are apparent in childhood. Voors *(6)* reported on data from the Bogalusa Heart study. They measured BP, height, weight, maturation, triceps skinfold thickness, serum lipids, and hemoglobin as risk factors for coronary artery disease in 3524 children (93% of the eligible population) in Bogalusa, Louisiana. African-American children had significantly higher BP than Caucasian children. This difference, starting before age 10, was largest in the children in the upper 5% of the BP distribution. Body size, expressed by height and by weight/height$^3$ index, was a strong determinant of BP level. Other positive determinants were blood hemoglobin and external maturation.

A number of studies showed significant ethnic difference in African-American and Caucasian females. Daniels et al. *(7)* evaluated ethnic differences in BP in girls aged 9 to 10 yr in the National Heart, Lung, and Blood Institute Growth and Health Study (NGHS), and the extent to which these differences in BP are explained by sexual maturation and body size. The NGHS enrolled 539 African-American and 616 Caucasian girls aged 9 yr, and 674 African-American and 550 Caucasian girls aged 10 yr. The African-American girls had significantly higher systolic BP and diastolic BP compared to Caucasian girls (102/58 mmHg vs 100/56 mmHg). The stage of maturation was found to account for the difference in BP between African-

**Table 1**
**Studies Examining Ethnic Differences in Childhood BP[a]**

| *Author* | *AA* | *C* | *H* | *A* | *Boys* | *Girls* | *Total* | *Age* | *Effects* | *Comment* |
|---|---|---|---|---|---|---|---|---|---|---|
| Daniels *(8)* | 1213 | 1166 | | | | 2379 | 2379 | 9–14 | AA > C | longitudinal |
| Manatunga *(5)* | 164 | 345 | | | 266 | 243 | 509 | 9[b] | AA > C | longitudinal |
| Liebman *(9)* | 236 | 296 | | | | 532 | 532 | 12–16 | AA > C | longitudinal |
| Baron *(4)* | 2134 | 1794 | 414 | | 2039 | 2303 | 4339 | 13–18 | none | longitudinal |
| Schachter *(94)* | | | | | | | 232 | 0–2 | none | longitudinal |
| Schachter *(46)* | 75 | 135 | | | 106 | 104 | 209 | 0–5 | none | longitudinal |
| Schachter *(47)* | 122 | 195 | | | | | 318 | 0–6[c] | none | longitudinal |
| Donker *(48)* | 569 | 877 | | | 745 | 701 | 1446 | 0 to 1 | none | longitudinal |
| Levine *(49)* | 134 | 66 | | 4 | 109 | 95 | 204 | 0–6[c] | none | longitudinal |
| Dekkers *(43)* | 349 | 396 | | | 369 | 376 | 745 | 5–27 | AA > C | longitudinal |
| Hohn *(17)* | 1788 | 973 | 1365 | 451 | 2276 | 2301 | 4577 | 14.7[b] | A > AA,C | |
| Daniels *(7)* | 1213 | 1166 | | | | 2379 | 2379 | 9, 10 | AA>C | |
| Daniels *(50)* | 55 | 72 | | | 68 | 59 | 127 | 9–17 | AA > C | |
| Daniels *(51)* | 103 | 98 | | | 105 | 96 | 201 | 6–17 | AA > C | DBP |
| Rabinowitz | 2290 | 1059 | | | 1230 | 2119 | 3349 | 13–18 | AA > C | females |
| Gutgesell *(52)* | 657 | 769 | 1384 | | 1425 | 1385 | 2810 | 3–17 | AA > C, H | |
| Brandon *(53)* | 244 | 431 | | | 333 | 342 | 675 | 9, 12 | AA>C | |
| Burke *(13)* | | | | | | | 134 | 0–7 | C>AA | <1 yr |
| Berenson *(54)* | 1222 | 2072 | 401 | | 1857 | 1838 | 3695 | 5–17 | AA > C | |
| Kozinetz *(55)* | 142 | 361 | | | | 503 | 503 | 7–18 | AA > C | |
| Pratt *(56)* | 249 | 466 | | | 380 | 335 | 715 | 6–16 | AA > C | |
| Reed *(11)* | 1889 | 4430 | | | 3212 | 3107 | 6319 | 14–18 | AA > C | |
| Voors *(6)* | 1389 | 2335 | | | 1952 | 1772 | 3724 | 5–14 | AA > C | |
| Baranowski *(57)* | 54 | 57 | 52 | | | | 163 | 8–12 | H > AA,C | DBP |
| Burns *(12)* | 236 | 300 | | | 266 | 271 | 536 | 14–17 | C > AA | females |
| Webber *(58)* | 1605 | 2688 | | | 2234 | 2059 | 4293 | 8–17 | AA > C | |
| Fixler *(59)* | 4679 | 4500 | 1462 | | 10641 | 13, 14 | H,AA>C | C > AA < H | | SBP DBP |
| Garbus *(60)* | 3315 | 4183 | | | 3605 | 3893 | 7498 | 14–18 | AA > C | female SBP |
| Goldring *(61)* | 2050 | 4788 | | | 3494 | 3344 | 6838 | 14–18 | C > AA | |
| Harris *(3)* | 1620 | 4420 | 1464 | 336 | 3949 | 3891 | 7840 | 6–16 | AA > C,H,A | |
| Khaw *(14)* | 118 | 177 | | | 160 | 135 | 295 | 15, 16 | C > AA | Male SBP |
| Kilcoyne *(62)* | 2193 | 124 | 1220 | | 1515 | 2022 | 3537 | 14–16 | none | |
| Kotchen *(63)* | 590 | 207 | | | 365 | 432 | 797 | 17–20 | AA > C | SBP |
| Kotchen *(64)* | 787 | 1156 | | | 969 | 974 | 1943 | 14–18 | AA > C | SBP |
| Levin *(65)* | 446 | 480 | | | 468 | 458 | 926 | 3[c] | AA>C | SBP |
| Levinson *(66)* | 794 | 2380 | 302 | 313 | | | 3789 | 5–10 | AA,A > C,H | |
| Londe *(67)* | 1295 | 1186 | | | 1330 | 1151 | 2481 | 3–14 | C > AA | |
| Miller *(68)* | 748 | 12,468 | | | 6849 | 6367 | 13,216 | 15,16 | AA>C | DBP |
| Swartz *(69)* | 58 | 345 | 2 | 68 | 253 | 243 | 496 | 15–18 | C > AA,A | |
| Adrogue *(70)* | 3394 | 11,292 | | | | | 14,686 | 10–15 | none | |
| Cornoni-Huntley *(71)* | | | | | | | 2200 | 12–17 | none | |
| Morrison *(16)* | 178 | 504 | | | 353 | 329 | 682 | 6–19 | none | |
| Webber *(72)* | 1207 | 2072 | 401 | | 1855 | 1825 | 3680 | 5–17 | none | |
| Alpert *(73)* | 184 | 221 | | | | | 405 | 6–15 | none | |

(continued)

Table 1 (continued)

| *Author* | *AA* | *C* | *H* | *A* | *Boys* | *Girls* | *Total* | *Age* | *Effects* | *Comment* |
|---|---|---|---|---|---|---|---|---|---|---|
| Sinaiko *(74)* | 2701 | 7745 | | | | | 10,446 | 10–16 | none | |
| Park *(75)* | 952 | 2040 | 4315 | | | | 7207 | 5–17 | none | |
| Snieder *(76)* | 446 | 616 | | | 496 | 566 | 1062 | 10–26 | AA > C | twins |
| Alpert *(2)* | | | | | | | | | AA>C,H,A | meta-analysis |
| Rosner *(15)* | 17,466 | 29,730 | | | 24,048 | 23,148 | 47,196 | 5–17 | none | meta-analysis |
| Fixler *(77)* | 1874 | 11,513 | | | | | 13,387 | | C>AA | review |

Abbreviations: AA = African-American; C = Caucasian; H = Hispanic; A = Asian; SBP = systolic blood pressure; DBP = diastolic blood pressure.

[a]blank cells — data not provided in the study

[b]mean age,

[c]age in months

American girls and Caucasian girls in that the African-American girls were more mature than Caucasian girls. Daniels concluded that the effect of sexual maturation on BP appears to operate through height and body fat and that the effect of obesity may be more important for systolic BP than diastolic BP. Another study by Daniels and colleagues *(8)* assessed the longitudinal changes in BP in African-American and Caucasian adolescent girls and evaluated potential determinants of changes in BP, again including sexual maturation and body size. A total of 1213 African-American and 1166 Caucasian girls, ages 9 or 10 yr at study entry, were followed up through age 14 with annual measurements of height, weight, skinfold thickness, stage of sexual maturation, BP, and other cardiovascular risk factors. Average BPs in African-American girls were generally 1 to 2 mmHg higher than in Caucasian girls of similar age over the course of the study. Age, race, stage of sexual maturation, height, and BMI were all significant predictors of systolic BP and diastolic BP in longitudinal regression analyses. They observed that ethnic differences in BP were seen at all stages of maturation, which is consistent with the concept that additional factors other than sexual maturation are important in ethnic differences in BP in girls. BMI had a smaller impact on BP in African-American girls. However, BMI increased at a greater rate with age in African-American girls, which may have contributed to the ethnic differences in BP. Overall, in their study at higher BMIs there were no ethnic differences in BP. However, at lower BMIs African-American girls had higher BPs, which were not accounted for by maturation differences. Between ages 9 and 14 yr, BMI increased with age at a greater rate in African-American girls, which helped account for the maintenance of ethnic differences in BP between 9 and 14 yr, despite their findings of a lower increase in BP per unit increase in BMI in African-American girls compared to Caucasian girls.

Liebman et al. *(9)* assessed BP levels, anthropometric parameters, and dietary intakes in 1981 and 1983 in a population of African-American ($n$ = 236) and Caucasian ($n$ = 296) adolescent girls, aged 14 and 16 yr, in 1983. The 14-yr-old African-American girls exhibited significantly higher mean systolic BP and diastolic BP than Caucasians in both years. Body weight and Quetelet index were more strongly associated with BP than height and triceps skinfold thickness. Rabinowitz et al. *(10)* assessed differences in the prevalence of BP > or = 95th% (i.e., HTN on an initial screening of 3349 students by race, sex, and age). The overall prevalence of HTN in this urban adolescent population was 8.1%. Significant ethnic differences were present in females (African-Americans = 6.6% vs non-Hispanics = 2.9%, $p < 0.01$). Within the African-American females, HTN occurred more frequently among the girls attending predominantly African-American public schools (7.7%) compared to a more integrated parochial school (2.0%) $p < 0.001$. This difference could not be explained by weight, height, or the occurrence of obesity. However, the prevalence of obesity was higher in the adolescents with HTN and among females with HTN. Obesity was also present in a greater number of African-Americans than Caucasians. The observed BP differences within African-American females, by school, may reflect a family-environment effect on cardiovascular risk.

### *Caucasian Blood Pressure Higher Than That of African-Americans*

Other studies have found the BPs of Caucasian children were higher than African-American children. Reed *(11)* reported the results of an extensive high school BP screening program that found the BP levels of Caucasian youths equaled or exceed that of African-American youth. In their study, Caucasians had consistently higher systolic BP and diastolic BP. Burns et al. *(12)* assessed BP and anthropometric and demographic variables in 536 students, 14 to 17 yr of age, in integrated suburban and urban schools. They found suburban Caucasian females had higher systolic BP and diastolic BP ($p = 0.02$) than suburban African-American females. Burke *(13)* followed 440 children longitudinally from birth to 7 yr and found that Caucasian children had slightly higher levels of BP at 6 mo and 1 yr of age. Khaw and Marmot *(14)* conducted BP screenings on 357 students in London aged 15 to 16 yr. Caucasian males had significantly higher systolic BP than Black males, but diastolic BP was similar.

### *Studies Reporting No Ethnic Differences in Childhood Blood Pressure*

Many studies have not observed ethnic differences in BP. Rosner et al. *(15)* analyzed BPs from eight large epidemiologic studies published between 1978 and 1991 that included measurements of 47,196 children on 68,556 occasions for systolic BP and for 38,184 children on 52,053 occasions for diastolic BP. They conclude that "there are few substantive ethnic differences in either systolic BP or diastolic BP during childhood and adolescence. The differences that were observed were small, inconsistent, and often explained by differences in body size."

A longitudinal study by Baron and colleagues *(4)* did not observe ethnic differences in BPs between African-Americans, Caucasians, and Mexican-Americans prior to 20 yr of age. Morrison et al. *(16)* also found that in a bi-ethnic group of 682 schoolchildren, ages 6 through 19 yr, there were no significant African-American–Caucasian systolic BP or diastolic BP differences in children.

Hohn and colleagues' *(17)* study assessed racial differences in BP levels in youth of Asian, African-American, Hispanic, and non-Hispanic Caucasian descent. They obtained BP measurements from 4577 ninth grade students during the spring of the years 1985 to 1989 (39% African-American, 30% Hispanic, 21% Caucasian, 10% Asian; 50% female) with a mean age of 15 yr. They did not find differences between African-American and Caucasian youth; however, comparisons of the prevalence of elevated BP among ethnic groups within sexes were statistically significant only for Asian girls (systolic BP, 13.1%; diastolic BP, 14.0%) relative to other female subjects (systolic BP, 7.6%; diastolic BP, 8.8%). A similar trend for Asian boys was apparent only for diastolic BP (23% vs 18%).

Table 2
Studies Demonstrating Blunted Nocturnal Decline in BP in African-Americans

| |
|---|
| 35 normotensive African-American adults *(29)* |
| 60 normotensive African-American adults *(78)* |
| 27 normotensive African-American and 83 Caucasian females *(79)* |
| 22 normotensive African-American and 22 Caucasian adults *(31)* |
| 275 Hypertensive African-American and 246 Caucasian adults *(80)* |
| 31 normotensive African-American and 31 Caucasian adults *(81)* |
| 62 hypertensive African-American and 72 Caucasian adults *(82)* |
| 24 obese African-American and 55 Caucasian adults *(83)* |
| 46 hypertensive African-American and Caucasian adults *(32)* |
| 37 normotensive African-American and 62 Caucasian women *(84)* |
| 34 hypertensive African-American adults *(33)* |
| **107 African-American and 92 Caucasian youths *(30)*** |
| **32 African-American youths *(85)*** |
| **20 African-American and 20 Caucasian youths *(86)*** |
| **149 African-American and 151 Caucasian youths *(87)*** |
| **94 African-American and 92 Caucasian youths *(88)*** |
| **251 African-American and 244 Caucasian youths *(89)*** |
| 60 African-American and 60 Caucasian adults *(90)* |
| 29 African-American and 33 French Canadian adults *(91)* |
| African and Caucasian women *(92)* |

*Note:* pediatric studies in **bold**.

## ETHNIC DIFFERENCES IN AMBULATORY BLOOD PRESSURE PATTERNS

Automatic, noninvasive, ambulatory blood pressure monitoring (ABPM), which measures BP at preset intervals while the patient performs their normal activities, has been used to identify and treat HTN in adults for over 20 yr. There is a growing interest and acceptance of ABPM in pediatric patients *(18–22)*. Studies have consistently demonstrated that measures of BP derived from noninvasive ABPM have a relationship with indices of BP-related target organ damage that is approximately twice as strong as that found with casual BP. Furthermore, there is increasing evidence from prospective studies that ABPM is superior to casual BP as a predictor of cardiovascular morbidity and mortality (for reviews, *see 23–28*). The majority of these studies found that individuals who show a blunted nocturnal decline in BP, referred to as nondipping, are at the greatest risk because this pattern exposes these individuals to a greater cardiovascular load each day.

We *(29,30)* were the first to describe that African-American adults and adolescents are characterized by a blunted nocturnal decline in BP. Since our initial observation, a blunted nocturnal decline in BP has been described in 19 additional studies, as shown in Table 2. Of these, 6 were performed on pediatric subjects. Overall, these studies demonstrate that the nocturnal decline in BP for African-Americans is about 10% compared to the 15% normally seen in Caucasian subjects. These differences are reduced about a third in pediatric subjects. Comparative data for African-American and Caucasian youths by age, race, and height are presented in Table 3.

Several studies demonstrated the clinical significance of the blunted nocturnal decline in BP in African-Americans. Fumo et al. *(31)* were the first to observe that the blunted nocturnal

Table 3
The 10th, 50th, and 90th Percentiles for Daytime and Nighttime Systolic/Diastolic BP in Adolescents by Race, Sex, and Height

| | *Caucasian boys* | | | *African-American boys* | | | *Caucasian girls* | | | *African-American girls* | | |
|---|---|---|---|---|---|---|---|---|---|---|---|---|
| | *Percentile* | | | | | | | | | | | |
| *Height (cm)* | | | | | | | | | | | | |
| | *50th* | *90th* | *10th* | *50th* | *90th* | *10th* | *50th* | *90th* | *10th* | *50th* | *90th* | *10th* |
| *Daytime blood pressure (mmHg)* | | | | | | | | | | | | |
| 130–150 | 97/57 | 114/70 | 130/76 | 99/58 | 113/69 | 120/77 | 96/54 | 114/66 | 126/69 | 98/56 | 111/67 | 124/75 |
| 151–170 | 107/60 | 116/67 | 129/77 | 110/57 | 118/71 | 132/79 | 103/61 | 113/69 | 125/78 | 103/62 | 115/70 | 123/78 |
| 171–190 | 112/63 | 120/69 | 131/75 | 111/63 | 122/73 | 138/83 | 106/62 | 112/68 | 121/74 | 106/64 | 114/70 | 111/72 |
| *Nighttime blood pressure (mmHg)* | | | | | | | | | | | | |
| 130–150 | 95/52 | 103/60 | 126/69 | 101/53 | 108/64 | 114/68 | 98/54 | 91/54 | 104/62 | 120/73 | 91/54 | 104/62 |
| 151–170 | 95/49 | 105/58 | 125/70 | 97/50 | 110/62 | 127/73 | 94/50 | 98/53 | 106/62 | 120/70 | 98/53 | 106/62 |
| 171–190 | 101/50 | 108/57 | 120/64 | 101/50 | 110/62 | 131/73 | 94/51 | 90/49 | 105/62 | 109/70 | 90/49 | 105/62 |

Adapted from Harshfield and Trieber *(93)*.

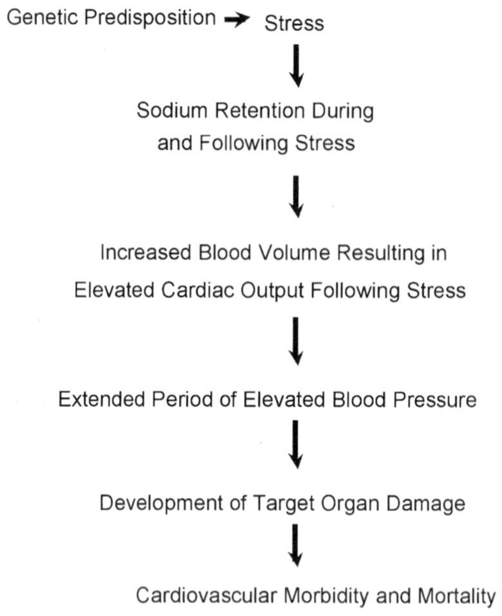


Fig. 1. Theoretical model to account for ethnic differences in the prevalence of hypertension and associated morbidity and mortality.

decline in BP in African-Americans was associated with target organ changes to the heart. This study is of particular interest because it compared African-Americans and Caucasians with South African blacks. The South Africans and Caucasians showed the same nocturnal decline in BP, which was greater than that of the African-Americans, who also had the greatest left ventricular (LV) mass.

Mayet et al. *(32)* took this work a step further. They examined an equal number of African-Americans and Caucasians on ambulatory BP patterns and LV mass. The African-Americans had a smaller nocturnal decline, which was inversely related to LVmass. These results have been replicated by Olutade et al. *(33)*. Finally, we demonstrated that the blunted nocturnal decline in African-American youth is associated with decreased renal function *(34)*.

## FACTORS RELATED TO ETHNIC DIFFERENCES IN AMBULATORY BLOOD PRESSURE PATTERNS

Relatively few studies examined the factors responsible for ethnic differences in ambulatory BP patterns. Our studies *(35–37)* identified three factors. Two of these factors, fitness *(35)* and body size *(36)*, are related, and both had a greater effect on nighttime BP African-Americans than in Caucasians. The third factor was sodium intake *(37)*. We observed that sodium intake, as determined by excretion, was related to daytime and nighttime BP in African-Americans, but not in Caucasians. These findings are consistent with the well-known differences in the influence of sodium intake on casual BP (for reviews, *see 38,39*).

We hypothesize that the interaction between salt and stress may account for the blunted nocturnal decline in BP in African-Americans, particularly obese African-Americans. Our theoretical model is presented in Fig. 1. We postulate that the physical and psychological demands of the day will lead to a sympathetic nervous system-induced increase in angiotensin

II (ANG II)-mediated sodium retention, similar to that observed in animal models of hypertension *(40)*. The sodium retention will increase blood volume and, therefore, will contribute to the increase in BP that is needed to meet the physical and psychological demands of waking hours. With sleep onset these demands are no longer present and the sympathetic nervous system becomes less active. Consequently, BP is reduced in most individuals. However, BP remains elevated at night in a large percentage of African-Americans because of the added contribution of the increase in blood volume to the increased BP, i.e., until pressure natriuresis occurs. We further hypothesize that obesity augments this pattern via adipose leptin-derived increases in catecholamines and adipose tissue-derived angiotensinogen.

We have preliminary data that support our hypothesis, which we refer to as "impaired stress-induced pressure natriuresis." Our initial study *(41)* demonstrated ethnic differences in stress-induced pressure natriuresis by showing that BP changes during a series of stressors was associated with slower natriuresis in African-American youth compared to Caucasian youth. Furthermore, this pattern was associated with cardiac remodeling in the Africans. In addition, we demonstrated that approx 30% of African-American youths show a delay in the return of BP to prestress levels following an extended stress period, which is mediated at least in part by ANG II *(42)*.

## SUMMARY AND CONCLUSION

In summary, the preponderance of studies indicate that African-American youths have higher casual and resting BP than other ethnic groups. Perhaps the bigger question posed by the longitudinal studies is not if differences exist, but when these differences become apparent. A recent longitudinal study by Dekkers et al. *(43)* was performed on 745 subjects over a 10-yr period. They observed that ethnic systolic BP differences in childhood females and early adolescent males tend to increase with age. Ethnic diastolic BP differences were apparent in childhood in both males and females, and remained relatively stable over time. The ethnic differences were not entirely explained by individual differences in socioeconomic status, growth, or adiposity. These results are consistent with studies conducted by Voors et al. *(6)* and Manatunga et al. *(5)*, discussed previously. It will be interesting to see if ethnic differences become apparent at an earlier age, concurrent with earlier onset of risk factors such as obesity and diabetes.

The data supporting ethnic differences in BP response to physical and psychological challenges are convincing. As reviewed in other chapters, there is convincing evidence that African-Americans' response to acute stress is an exaggerated increase in BP. Studies cited in this chapter extend these findings to differences in BP responses to the physical and psychological demands of the day. In this chapter, we provide a theoretical model to understand these ethnic differences, which is consistent with the pressure natriuresis theory of essential HTN *(44,45)*.

## REFERENCES

1. 2002 Heart and Stroke Statistical Update. American Heart Association, Dallas, TX.
2. Alpert BS, Fox ME. Racial aspects of blood pressure in children and adolescents. Pediatr Clin North Am 1993;40:13–22.
3. Harris RD, Phillips RL, Williams PM, Kuzma JW, Fraser GE. The child-adolescent blood pressure study: I. Distribution of blood pressure levels in Seventh-Day-Adventist (SDA) and non-SDA children. Am J Public Health 1981;71:1342–1349.
4. Baron AE, Freyer B, Fixler DE. Longitudinal blood pressures in blacks, whites, and Mexican Americans during adolescence and early adulthood. Am J Epidemiol 1986;123:809–817.

5. Manatunga AK, Jones JJ, Pratt JH. Longitudinal assessment of blood pressure in black and white children. Hypertension 1993;22:84–89.
6. Voors AW, Foster TA, Fredichs RR, Webber LS, Berenson GS. Studies of blood pressure in children, ages 5 to 14 years, in a total biracial community: The Bogalusa Heart Study. Circulation 1976;54:319–327.
7. Daniels SR, Obarzanek E, Barton BA, Kimm SYS, Similo SL, Morrison JA. Sexual maturation and racial differences in blood pressure in girls: The National Heart, Lung, and Blood Institute Growth and Health Study. J Pediatr 1996;129:208–213.
8. Daniels SR, McMahon RP, Obarzanek E, et al. Longitudinal correlates of change in blood pressure in adolescent girls. Hypertension 1998;31:97–103.
9. Liebman M, Chopin LF, Carter E, et al. Factors related to blood pressure in a biracial adolescent female population. Hypertension 1986;8:843–850.
10. Rabinowitz A, Kushner H, Falkner B. Racial differences in blood pressure among urban adolescents. J Adolesc Health 1993;14:314–318.
11. Reed WL. Racial differences in blood pressure levels of adolescents. Am J Public Health 1981;71:1165–1167.
12. Burns MD, Morrison JA, Khoury PR, Glueck CJ. Blood pressure studies in black and white inner-city and suburban adolescents. Prev Med 1980;9:41–50.
13. Burke GL, Arcilla RA, Culpepper WS, Weber LS, Chian Y, Berenson GS. Blood pressure and echocardiographic measures in children: the Bogalusa Heart study. Circulation 1987;75:106–114.
14. Khaw KT, Marmot MG. Blood pressure in 15- to 16-year-old adolescents of different ethnic groups in two London schools. Postgrad Med J 1983;59:630–631.
15. Rosner B, Prineas R, Daniels SR, Loggie J. Blood pressure differences between blacks and whites in relation to body size among US children and adolescents. Am J Epidemiol 2000;151:1007–1019.
16. Morrison JA, Khoury P, Kelly K, et al. Studies of blood pressure in schoolchildren (ages 6–19) and their parents in an integrated suburban school district. Am J Epidemiol 1980;111:156–165.
17. Hohn AR, Dwyer KM, Dwyer JH. Blood pressure in youth from four ethnic groups: the Pasadena Prevention Project. J Pediatr 1994;125:368–373.
18. Schieken RM. New perspectives in childhood blood pressure. Pediatrics 1995;10:87–91.
19. Alpert B, Daniels S. Twenty-four hour ambulatory blood pressure monitoring: now that technology has come of age–we need to catch up. J Peds 1997;130:167–169.
20. Harshfield GA, Hanevold CD. Ambulatory blood pressure monitoring in the evaluation of pediatric disorders. Pediatr Ann 1998;27:491–494.
21. Portman RJ, Yetman RJ. Clinical uses of ambulatory blood pressure monitoring. Ped Nephrol 1994;8:367–376.
22. Sorof JM, Portman RJ. Ambulatory blood pressure measurements. Curr Opin Pediatr 2001;13:133–137.
23. Consensus document on non-invasive ambulatory blood pressure monitoring. J Hypertens 1990;8:135–140.
24. Pickering TG, Alpert BS, deSwiet M, Harshfield GA, O'Brien E, Shennan AS. Ambulatory Blood Pressure. Redmond, Washington: SpaceLabs Medical, 1994.
25. White WB. How well does ambulatory blood pressure predict target-organ disease and clinical outcome in patients with hypertension? Blood Press Monit 1999;4:S17–S21.
26. Palatini P. Ambulatory blood pressure monitoring and borderline hypertension. Blood Press Monit 1999;4:233–240.
27. Pickering TG, Coats A, Mallion JM, Mancia G, Verdecchia P. Blood pressure monitoring. Task force V: White-coat hypertension. Blood Press Monit 1999;4:333–341.
28. Pickering TG. Ambulatory blood pressure monitoring. Curr Hypertens Rep 2000;2:558–564.
29. Harshfield GA, Hwang C, Edmunson J, Grim CE. Daily blood pressure patterns in blacks. CVD EPIDEM Newsletter 1987;41:137.
30. Harshfield GA, Alpert BS, Willey ES, Somes GW, Murphy JK, Dupaul LM. Race and gender influence ambulatory blood pressure patterns of adolescents. Hypertension 1989;14:598–603.
31. Fumo M, Teeger S, Lang R, Bednarz J, Sareli P, Murphy M. Diurnal blood pressure variation and cardiac mass in American blacks and whites and South African blacks. Am J Hypertens 1992;5:111–116.
32. Mayet J, Chapman N, Li CK, et al. Ethnic differences in the hypertensive heart and 24-hour blood pressure profile. Hypertension 1998;31:1190–1194.
33. Olutade BO, Gbadebo TD, Porter VD, Wilkening B, Hall WD. Racial differences in ambulatory blood pressure and echocardiographic left ventricular geometry. Am J Med Sci 1998;315:101–109.
34. Harshfield G, Pulliam D, Alpert B. Ambulatory blood pressure and renal function in healthy children and adolescents. Am J Hypertens 1994;7:282–285.

35. Harshfield GA, Dupaul LM, Alpert BS, et al. Aerobic fitness and the diurnal rhythm of blood pressure in adolescents. Hypertension 1990;15:810–814.
36. Harshfield GA, Barbeau P, Richey PA, Alpert BS. Racial differences in the influence of body size on ambulatory blood pressure in youths. Blood Press Monit 2000;5:59–63.
37. Harshfield GA, Alpert BS, Pulliam DA, Willey ES, Somes GW, Stapelton FB. Sodium excretion and racial differences in ambulatory blood pressure patterns. Hypertension 1991;18:813–818.
38. Weinberger MH, Miller JZ, Luft FC, Grim CE, Fineberg N. Definitions and characteristics of sodium sensitivity and blood pressure resistance. Hypertension 1986;8:II-127–II-134.
39. Campese VM. Salt sensitivity in hypertension: renal and cardiovascular implications. Hypertension 1994;23:531–550.
40. Harshfield GA, Grim CE. Stress hypertension: the "wrong" genes in the "wrong" environment. Acta Physiol Scand 1997;161:129–132.
41. Harshfield GA, Treiber FA, Davis H, Kapuku GK. Impaired stress-induced pressure natriuresis is related to left ventricle structure in blacks. Hypertension 2002;39:844–847.
42. Harshfield G, Wilson M, Hanevold C, et al. Impaired stress induced pressure-natriuresis increases cardiovascular load in African American youths. Am J Hypertens 2002;15(10 Pt 1):903–906.
43. Dekkers JC, Snieder H, Van Den Oord EJ, Treiber FA. Moderators of blood pressure development from childhood to adulthood: a 10-year longitudinal study. J Pediatr 2002;141(6):770–779.
44. Guyton AC. Renal function curve. A key to understanding the pathogenesis of hypertension. Hypertension 1987;10:1–6.
45. Hall JE, Guyton AC, Coleman TG, Woods LL, Mizelle HL. Renal excretory function and hypertension. In: Kaplan N, Brenner B, Laragh J, eds. The Kidney in Hypertension. New York: Raven, 1987;1–19.
46. Schachter J, Kuller LH, Perfetti C. Blood pressure during the first five years of life: relation to ethnic group (black or white) and to parental hypertension. Am J Epidemiol 1984;119:541–553.
47. Schachter J, Kuller LH, Perkins JM, Radin ME. Infant blood pressure and heart rate: relation to ethnic group (black or white), nutrition and electrolyte intake. Am J Epidemiol 1979;110:205–218.
48. Donker GA, Labarthe DR, Harrist RB, Selwyn BJ, Wattigney W, Berenson GS. Low birth weight and blood pressure at age 7–11 years in a biracial sample. Am J Epidemiol 1997;145:387–397.
49. Levine RS, Hennekens CH, Duncan RC, et al. Blood pressure in infant twins: birth to 6 months of age. Hypertension 1980;2:I29–I33.
50. Daniels SR, Morrison JA, Sprecher DL, Khoury P, Kimball TR. Association of body fat distribution and cardiovascular risk factors in children and adolescents. Circulation 1999;99:541–545.
51. Daniels SR, Kimball TR, Khoury P, Witt S, Morrison JA. Correlates of the hemodynamic determinants of blood pressure. Hypertension 1996;28:37–41.
52. Gutgesell M, Terrell G, Labarthe D. Pediatric blood pressure: ethnic comparison in a primary care center. Hypertension 1981;3:39–49.
53. Brandon LJ, Fillingim J. Body composition and blood pressure in children based on age, race, and sex. Am J Prev Med 1993;9:34–38.
54. Berenson GS, Wattigney WA, Webber LS. Epidemiology of hypertension from childhood to young adulthood in black, white, and Hispanic population samples. Public Health Rep 1996;111(Suppl 2):3–6.
55. Kozinetz CA. Sexual maturation and blood pressure levels of a biracial sample of girls. Am J Dis Child 1991;145:142–146.
56. Pratt JH, Jones JJ, Miller JZ, Wagner MA, Fineberg NS. Racial differences in aldosterone excretion and plasma aldosterone concentrations in children. N Engl J Med 1989;321:1152–1157.
57. Baranowski T, Tsong Y, Henske J, Dunn JK, Hooks P. Ethnic variation in blood pressure among preadolescent children. Pediatr Res 1988;23:270–274.
58. Webber LS, Berenson GS. Racial contrasts of blood pressure levels in two southern, rural communities. Prev Med 1985;14:140–151.
59. Fixler DE, Laird WP, Fitzgerald V, Stead S, Adams R. Hypertension screening in schools: results of the Dallas study. Pediatrics 1979;63:32–36.
60. Garbus SB, Young CJ, Hassinger G, Johnson W. Screening for hypertension in adolescents: the search for normal values. South Med J 1980;73:174–182.
61. Goldring D, Londe S, Sivakoff M, Hernandez A, Britton C, Choi S. Blood pressure in a high school population. I. Standards for blood pressure and the relation of age, sex, weight, height, and race to blood pressure in children 14 to 18 years of age. J Pediatr 1977;91:884–889.

62. Kilcoyne MM, Richter RW, Alsup PA. Adolescent hypertension. I. Detection and prevalence. Circulation 1974;50:758–764.
63. Kotchen JM, Kotchen TA, Schwertman NC, Kuller LH. Blood pressure distributions of urban adolescents. Am J Epidemiol 1974;99:315–324.
64. Kotchen JM, Kotchen TA. Geographic effect on racial blood pressure differences in adolescents. J Chronic Dis 1978;31:581–586.
65. Levin SE, Herman AA, Irwig LM. Systolic blood pressure differences in black, colored, and white infants. Am J Epidemiol 1987;125:221–230.
66. Levinson S, Liu K, Stamler J, et al. Ethnic differences in blood pressure and heart rate of Chicago school children. Am J Epidemiol 1985;122:366–377.
67. Londe S, Gollub SW, Goldring D. Blood pressure in black and in white children. J Pediatr 1977;90:93–95.
68. Miller RA, Shekelle RB. Blood pressure in tenth-grade students: results from the Chicago Heart Association Pediatric Heart Screening Project. Circulation 1976;54:993–1000.
69. Swartz H, Leitch CJ. Differences in mean adolescent blood pressure by age, sex ethnic origin, obesity and familial tendency. J Sch Health 1975;45:76–82.
70. Adrogue HE, Sinaiko AR. Prevalence of hypertension in junior high school-aged children: effect of new recommendations in the 1996 Updated Task Force Report. Am J Hypertens 2001;14:412–414.
71. Cornoni-Huntley J, Harlan WR, Leaverton PE. Blood pressure in adolescence. The United States Health Examination survey. Hypertension 1979;1:566–571.
72. Webber LS, Harsha DW, Phillips GT, Srinivasan SR, Simpson JW, Berenson GS. Cardiovascular risk factors in Hispanic, white, and black children: the Brooks County and Bogalusa Heart studies. Am J Epidemiol 1991;133:704–714.
73. Alpert BS, Dover EV, Booker DL, Martin AM, Strong WB. Blood pressure response to dynamic exercise in healthy children–black vs white. J Pediatr 1981;99:556–560.
74. Sinaiko AR, Gomez-Marin O, Prineas RJ. "Significant" diastolic hypertension in pre-high school black and white children. The children and adolescent blood pressure program. Am J Hypertens 1988;1:178–180.
75. Park MK, Menard SW, Yuan C. Comparison of blood pressure in children from three ethnic groups. Am J Cardiol 2001;87:1305–1308.
76. Snieder H, Harshfield GA, Treiber FA. Heritability of blood pressure and hemodynamics in African and European American Youth The Georgia Cardiovascular Twin Study. Hypertension 2003;41(6):1196–1201.
77. Fixler DE, Kautz JA, Dana K. Systolic blood pressure differences among pediatric epidemiological studies. Hypertension 1980;2:I3–I7.
78. Harshfield GA, Hwang C, Grim CE. Circadian variation of blood pressure in blacks: influence of age, gender and activity. J Human Hypertens 1990;4:43–47.
79. James GD. Race and perceived stress independently affect the diurnal variation of blood pressure in women. Am J Hypertens 1991;4:382–384.
80. Gretler DD, Fumo MT, Nelson KS, Murphy MB. Ethnic differences in circadian hemodynamic profile. Am J Hypertens 1994;7:7–14.
81. Osei K, Schuster DP. Effects of race and ethnicity on insulin sensitivity, blood pressure, and heart rate in three ethnic populations: comparative studies in African-Americans, African immigrants (Ghanaians), and white Americans using ambulatory blood pressure monitoring. Am J Hypertens 1996;9:1157–1164.
82. Hebert LA, Agarwal G, Ladson-Wofford SE, et al. Nocturnal blood pressure in treated hypertensive African Americans compared to treated hypertensive European Americans. J Am Soc Nephrol 1996;7:2130–2134.
83. Weir MR, Reisin E, Falkner B, Hutchinson HG, Sha L, Tuck ML. Nocturnal reduction of blood pressure and the antihypertensive response to a diuretic or angiotensin converting enzyme inhibitor in obese hypertensive patients. TROPHY Study Group. Am J Hypertens 1998;11:14–20.
84. Yamasaki F, Schwartz GE, Gerber LM, Warren K, Pickering TG. Impact of shift work and race/ethnicity on the diurnal rhythm of blood pressure and catecholamines. Hypertension 1998;32:417–423.
85. Belsha CW, Spencer HJ, Berry PL, Plummer JK, Wells TG. Diurnal blood pressure patterns in normotensive and hypertensive children and adolescents. J Hum Hypertens 1997;11:801–806.
86. Meininger JC, Liehr P, Mueller WH, Chan W, Chandler PS. Predictors of ambulatory blood pressure: identification of high-risk adolescents. ANS Adv Nurs Sci 1998;20:50–64.
87. Harshfield GA, Alpert BS, Pulliam DA, Somes GW, Wilson DK. Ambulatory blood pressure recordings in children and adolescents. Pediatrics 1994;94:180–184.

88. Harshfield GA, Treiber FA, Wilson ME, Kapuku GK, Davis HC. A longitudinal study of ethnic differences in ambulatory blood pressure patterns in youth. Am J Hypertens 2002;15:525–530.
89. Harshfield GA, Wilson ME, Treiber FA, Alpert BS. A comparison of ambulatory blood pressure patterns across populations. Blood Press Monit 2002;7(5):265–269.
90. Ituarte PH, Kamarck TW, Thompson HS, Bacanu S. Psychosocial mediators of racial differences in nighttime blood pressure dipping among normotensive adults. Health Psychol 1999;18:393–402.
91. Kotchen TA, Piering AW, Cowley AW, et al. Glomerular hyperfiltration in hypertensive African Americans. Hypertension 2000;35:822–826.
92. Sherwood A, Thurston R, Steffen P, Blumenthal JA, Waugh RA, Hinderliter AL. Blunted nighttime blood pressure dipping in postmenopausal women. Am J Hypertens 2001;14:749–754.
93. Harshfield GA, Treiber FA. Racial differences in ambulatory blood pressure monitoring-derived 24 h patterns of blood pressure in adolescents. Blood Press Monit 1999;4:107–110.
94. Schachter J, Kuller LH, Perfetti C. Blood pressure during the first two years of life. Am J Epidemiol 1982; 116(1):29–41.

# 18 Childhood Obesity and Blood Pressure Regulation

*Albert P. Rocchini,* MD

*CONTENTS*



## INTRODUCTION

Childhood obesity is the most common nutritional problem among children in developed countries. From the 1960s to 1990s, the prevalence of obesity in children grew from 5 to 11% *(1)*. In adults, obesity is recognized as an independent risk factor for the development of hypertension (HTN) and cardiovascular disease (CVD). In childhood, there are data to demonstrate a strong relationship between childhood obesity and HTN, type 2 diabetes mellitus, dyslipidemia, obstructive sleep apnea, left ventricular hypertrophy (LVH), and orthopedic problems. This chapter will cover: (1) The epidemiologic evidence that substantiates obesity as an independent risk factor for the development of HTN in adults and children; (2) An explanation of how obesity may cause HTN; (3) A brief summary of other cardiovascular (CV) abnormalities associated with obesity; and (4) A brief summary of how to manage the child with HTN and obesity.

## RELATIONSHIP BETWEEN OBESITY AND HIGH BLOOD PRESSURE

### *Epidemiological Studies Linking Obesity to Hypertension*

The association between obesity and HTN has been recognized since the early 1900s. Several large epidemiological studies documented the association between increasing body weight and an increase in blood pressure (BP) *(2–13)*. Symonds *(4)* analyzed 150,419 policy-

From: *Clinical Hypertension and Vascular Disease: Pediatric Hypertension*
Edited by: R. J. Portman, J. M. Sorof, and J. R. Ingelfinger © Humana Press Inc., Totowa, NJ

holders in the Mutual Life Insurance Corporation and documented that systolic and diastolic BP increased with both age and weight. The Framingham study *(5)* documented that the prevalence of HTN in obese individuals was twice that of those individuals who were of normal weight. This relationship held up in all age groups for women and for men. Stamler, in a study of 1 million North Americans *(3)*, found that the odds ratio of HTN was significantly increased in obese compared to nonobese individuals (comparing obese with nonobese subjects aged 20–39 yr the odds ratio for HTN was 2.42:1, and 1.54:1 in subjects aged 40–64 yr).

The association of obesity and HTN in children has also been well-documented. Rosner and co-workers *(14)* pooled data from eight large US epidemiological studies involving over 47,000 children. Regardless of race, gender, and age, the risk of elevated BP was significantly higher for children in the upper compared to the lower decile of body mass index (BMI). Freedman et al. *(15)* reported that overweight children were 4.5 to 2.4 times as likely to have elevated systolic and diastolic BP respectively. Similarly, Sorof et al. *(16)* reported a 3 times greater prevalence of HTN in obese compared to nonobese adolescents in a school-based HTN and obesity screening study. As we have indicated, a large number of population-based studies have documented a strong association between obesity and HTN in both sexes, in all age groups, and for virtually every geographical and ethnic group.

### *Relationship of Weight Gain to Blood Pressure Level*

There have been no studies in humans that have investigated the effect of weight gain on BP. However, it has been shown that weight gain is directly related to an increase in BP in dogs. Cash and Wood in 1938 *(17)* demonstrated that weight gain in dogs with renal vascular HTN was responsible for an additional increase in BP. Rocchini et al. *(18,19)* found that normal mongrel dogs fed a high fat diet gained weight and developed HTN. In these dogs, the HTN was associated with sodium retention, hyperinsulinemia, and activation of the sympathetic nervous system. Hall et al. *(20)* have also observed that weight gain in the dog is directly associated with an increase in arterial BP.

### *Effect of Weight Loss on Blood Pressure Level*

Weight loss is associated with a lowering of BP. Haynes *(21)* reviewed the literature dated to the mid 1980s on the relationship of weight loss to reductions in arterial pressure. He used strict criteria to examine only well-done studies and noted that there were only six studies available. Three of the six studies that met Haynes' criteria clearly demonstrated the effect of weight loss on lowering arterial pressure. Overall, many clinical trials that have been published since the late 1970s have clearly documented the BP-lowering effect of weight loss *(21–35)*. The Hypertension Prevention Trial *(23)* found that a mean weight loss of 5 kg was associated with as much as a 5/3 mmHg decrease in BP in individuals with borderline elevations in BP. However, one of the controversial aspects of these studies is whether the weight loss alone, independent of alterations in dietary sodium, was responsible for the observed reductions in BP. Dahl *(31)* concluded that the reduced salt intake inherent in hypocaloric diets, rather than weight loss, is responsible for the lowering of BP. Similarly, Fagerberg et al. *(25)* noted no decrease in BP in individuals after weight loss using a 1230 calorie, unrestricted sodium diet. However, in another group of individuals, similar caloric restriction combined with a low sodium diet resulted in a significant BP reduction.

Reisen et al. *(29)* reported that hypertensive individuals placed on diets designed to produce weight loss, but without sodium restriction, resulted in a substantial reduction in BP. Tuck et al. *(32)* reported that weight loss decreased BP in individuals who received either a 40-mmol/d sodium diet or a 120-mmol/d sodium diet. Maxwell et al. *(26)* reported that in obese subjects, weight loss resulted in the same BP reduction whether sodium intake was restricted to 40 mmol/d, or maintained at 240 mmol/d. Gillum and coworkers *(27)* found that weight loss without significantly altered sodium intake resulted in BP decreases. Rocchini et al. *(30)* demonstrated that prior to weight loss, the BP of a group of obese adolescents was very sensitive to dietary sodium intake; however, after weight loss, the obese adolescents lost their BP sensitivity to sodium.

A limitation with the use of studies documenting that weight loss is associated with a reduction in BP is that most studies do not address the long-term effect of weight change on BP in subjects who are again placed on unrestricted diets. Dornfield and coworkers *(34)* documented that long-term changes in BP correlate with changes in body weight. In obese subjects whose BP fell during a very low-calorie, protein-supplemented fast, when weight loss stopped and body weight was maintained for one month, BP did not increase. In compliant patients who regained less than 15 pounds 6 mo after discontinuation of the very low-calorie, protein-supplemented fast, BP increased minimally. Therefore, calorie restriction and weight loss are associated with a reduction in BP. In addition, it is clear that even modest weight loss (i.e., 10% of body weight) improves BP, and many individuals achieve normal BP levels without attaining their calculated ideal weight.

However, recent data suggest that long-term weight loss may not reduce the incidence of HTN. Sjostrom et al. *(36)* compared the incidence of HTN and diabetes in 346 patients undergoing gastric surgery with 346 obese control subjects who were matched on 18 variables. After 8 yr, the surgical group had maintained a 16% weight loss, whereas, the control subjects had a 1% weight gain. These investigators demonstrated that the weight reduction in the surgical group had a dramatic effect on the 8-yr incidence of diabetes, but had no effect on the 8-yr incidence of HTN. They *(37)* and others *(38)* previously documented that surgical weight loss positively affected BP at 2 and 4 yr of follow-up, but that this effect on BP is lost after 8 yr of follow-up. These authors have speculated "that remaining obesity in the surgically treated patients could have induced a reappearance of HTN during the course of the study independent of ongoing weight increase"; therefore, Sjostrom's study suggests that the relapse of BP after surgically induced weight loss is more related to aging and recent small weight increase than to either initial weight or initial weight losses *(39)*.

### *Effect of Body Fat Distribution on Blood Pressure*

Obesity is defined not just as an increase in body weight but rather as an increase in adipose tissue mass. Adipose tissue mass can be estimated by multiple techniques, such as skinfold thickness, BMI ([weight in kg]/[height in meters]$^2$), hydrostatic weighing, bioelectrical impedance, and water dilution methods. In most clinical studies, BMI is usually used as the index of adiposity. Obesity is generally defined as a BMI of greater than 30 kg/m$^2$. In 1956, Jean Vague *(40)* reported that the CV and metabolic consequences of obesity were greatest in individuals whose fat distribution pattern favored the upper body segments. Since that observation, several population-based studies have demonstrated that upper body obesity is a more important CV risk factor than BMI alone *(41–47)*. The Normative Aging Study *(41)* has demonstrated that there is a significant relationship between abdominal circumference and diastolic BP.

In fact, the risk of developing HTN was better predicted by upper body fat distribution than by either body weight or BMI. In both children and young adults, Shear et al. *(42)* reported that

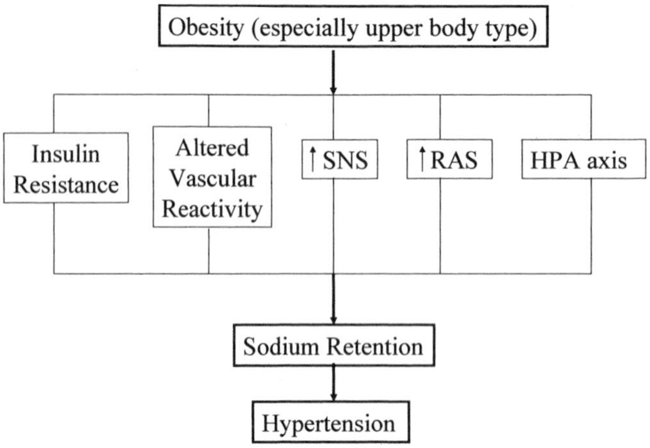


Fig. 1. A schematic representation for how obesity might result in HTN.

BP correlated strongly with upper body fat pattern, but not with measures of global obesity. Many investigators have demonstrated that the association of obesity to increased CV risk is primarily related to upper body adiposity *(48,49)*. There is limited information relating fat distribution to BP in the pediatric population.

## MECHANISM WHEREBY OBESITY MIGHT CAUSE HYPERTENSION

The exact pathophysiologic mechanism whereby obesity causes HTN is still unknown. Obesity HTN is complex and multifactorial. It appears to involve insulin resistance, activation of the sympathetic nervous system, activation of the renin-angiotensin system (RAS), abnormal renal sodium handling, possible leptin-resistance, altered vascular reactivity, and alterations in the hypothalamic–pituitary–adrenal axis (Fig. 1).

### *Enhanced Sodium Retention*

Most investigators believe that fluid retention is the final common pathway that links obesity to HTN. There are ample human and animal data linking obesity HTN to fluid retention. Rocchini et al. *(33)* demonstrated that when compared to nonobese adolescents, obese adolescents have a renal-function relation (plot of urinary sodium excretion as a function of arterial pressure) that has a shallower slope. The renal-function relationship is also normalized by weight loss (Fig. 2). The relationship between urinary sodium excretion and mean arterial pressure can be altered by intrinsic and extrinsic factors known to affect the ability of the kidney to excrete sodium (Table 1).

Insulin resistance and/or hyperinsulinemia can result in chronic sodium retention. Insulin can enhance renal sodium retention directly, through its effects on renal tubules *(50–52)*, and indirectly, through stimulation of the sympathetic nervous system and augmenting angiotensin II (ANG II)-mediated aldosterone secretion *(53,54)*. There are data to suggest that insulin resistance is directly related to sodium sensitivity in both obese and nonobese subjects. Rocchini et al. *(33)* demonstrated in obese adolescents that insulin resistance and sodium sensitivity of BP are directly related. They demonstrated that the BP of obese adolescents is more dependent on dietary sodium intake than that of nonobese adolescents, and that hyperinsulinemia and increased sympathetic nervous system activity appear to be responsible for the observed sodium

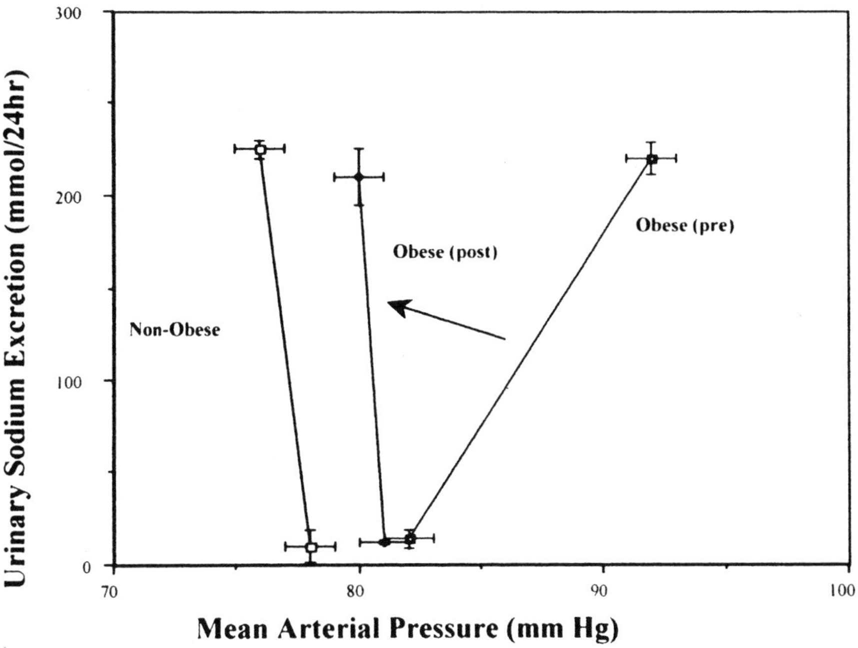


Fig. 2. Renal-function relations for 18 nonobese (open square), 60 obese adolescents before a weight loss program (closed square), and the 36 obese adolescents who lost weight during a 20-wk weight loss program (closed diamond). In comparison with the nonobese adolescents' renal-function relation, the obese adolescents' renal-function relation has a shallow slope ($p < 0.001$). In those who lost weight, the slope increased (arrow). This increase was owing to a decrease in the mean arterial pressure during the two weeks of the high salt diet. From Rocchini et al. *(33)*.

sensitivity and HTN. Finta et al. *(55)* showed that the endogenous hyperinsulinemia that occurs in obese subjects following a glucose meal can result in urinary sodium retention (Fig. 3). In that study, the investigators also demonstrated that the most sodium-sensitive obese adolescents had significantly higher fasting insulin concentrations, higher glucose-stimulated insulin levels, and greater urine sodium retention in response to the oral glucose load. Finally, there is a direct relationship between sodium sensitivity and insulin resistance in nonobese subjects with *(52)* or without *(56)* essential HTN.

There are also animal data that suggests that insulin resistance may be partly responsible for the sodium retention associated with obesity HTN. In a dog model of obesity-induced HTN, Rocchini et al. *(18,19)* demonstrated that during the first week of the high fat diet, the increase in sodium retention appeared to best relate to an increase in plasma norepinephrine activity whereas, during the latter weeks of the high fat diet, an increase in plasma insulin appeared to be the best predictor of sodium retention. Finally, Rocchini et al. demonstrated that HTN associated with weight gain in the dog occurs only if adequate salt is present in the diet *(56)*.

In non-insulin resistant subjects, both a concomitant decrease in proximal tubular sodium reabsorption, and an increase in glomerular filtration, oppose the direct effect of insulin to increase distal sodium retention. Hall and co-workers *(57)* demonstrated that obesity-induced HTN in the dog is associated with increased renal tubular sodium reabsorption, since marked sodium retention occurred despite large increases in glomerular filtration and renal plasma flow. Ter Maaten el al. *(58)* demonstrated that insulin-mediated glucose uptake was positively

Table 1
Factors That Produce Alterations in Renal-Function Curves

| | |
|---|---|
| 1. | Constriction of the renal arteries and arterioles |
| 2. | Changes in glomerular filtration coefficients |
| 3. | Changes in the rate of tubular reabsorption |
| 4. | Reduced renal mass |
| 5. | Changing levels of renin-angiotensin activation |
| 6. | Changing levels of aldosterone |
| 7. | Changing levels of vasopressin |
| 8. | Changing levels of insulin |
| 9. | Changing levels of sympathetic nervous system activation |
| 10. | Changing levels of atrial natriuretic hormone |

correlated with changes in glomerular filtration, but not with changes in either proximal tubular sodium reabsorption or overall fractional sodium excretion. They speculated that insulin could only cause abnormal sodium retention if an additional antinatriuretic stimulus is present, such as through stimulation of the sympathetic activity, or augmenting ANG II-mediated aldosterone production.

Another mechanism that may link insulin and insulin resistance to salt-sensitive HTN is that of alterations in insulin receptor structure or function. Rocchini et al. characterized the change in insulin-mediated glucose uptake that occurs with feeding dogs a high fat diet *(59)* (Fig. 4). After 1 wk of the high fat diet there was a significant increase in the amount of insulin that was required to produce a half maximal response in glucose uptake (insulin $ED_{50}$ dose), and little change in the maximal glucose uptake response.

However, by 3 wk of the high fat diet there was a further increase in the insulin $ED_{50}$ dose and a significant reduction in the maximal insulin induced glucose uptake. Laasko et al. *(60)* reported, in obese humans, similar changes in the insulin-mediated glucose uptake/dose response relationship. Kolterman et al. *(61)* has suggested that insulin resistance in obesity is owing to target-tissue defects (i.e., reduced sensitivity to insulin; reduced responsiveness to insulin; or a combined defect). Reduced sensitivity to insulin is believed to result from a prereceptor or receptor defect. In this type of resistance, high concentrations of insulin overcome the defect and evoke a maximum insulin stimulation of the tissue. Alternatively, reduced responsiveness to insulin is associated with a reduced maximum insulin stimulation of the tissue, and is believed to result from a defect that is distal to the insulin-receptor complex. Since weight gain is associated with both a reduced maximum insulin-stimulated glucose uptake and a shift of the dose response curve to the right (i.e., a significantly reduced insulin $ED_{50}$ dose), using Kolterman's terminology, weight gain in the dog results in both a reduced sensitivity and responsiveness to insulin. Therefore, insulin resistance appears to be important in producing the salt-sensitive HTN observed in obese humans and dogs. Sechi *(62)* reported that dietary salt content can alter insulin receptor function in the SHR rat and the fructose fed rat. An increase in dietary salt content decreases insulin receptor number and mRNA levels only in the kidney of WKY, but not SHR. Similarly, Sechi reported that when control Sprague-Dawley rats are fed a high salt diet, renal insulin receptor number and mRNA levels decrease. However, when fructose is added to the high salt diet, renal insulin receptor number and mRNA levels did not decrease. Therefore, Sechi has speculated that in both SHR and fructose fed rats, the sensitivity

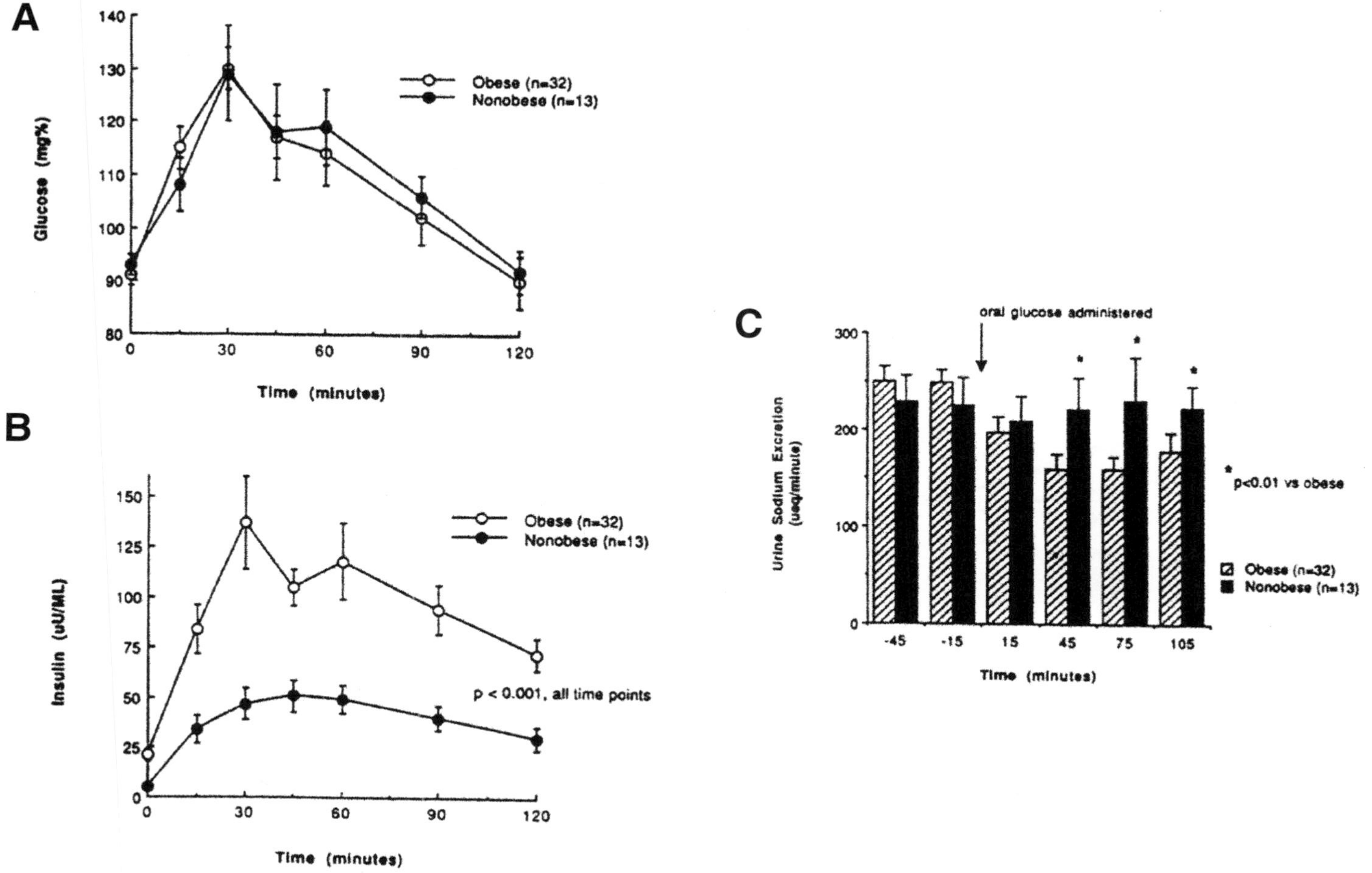


Fig. 3. (A) Serum glucose levels following an oral glucose tolerance test in 32 obese and 13 nonobese adolescents. There was no significant difference between the two groups. (B) Serum insulin levels following an oral glucose tolerance test in the same group of obese and nonobese subjects. The obese subjects experienced a significant larger increase in insulin concentration compared with the nonobese subjects ($p < 0.001$). (C) Change in urinary sodium excretion during water diuresis in this same group of subjects. In the nonobese subjects (black), there is no change in urine sodium excretion following the oral glucose tolerance test. However, there is a significant decrease in urine sodium excretion after the oral glucose tolerance test in the obese subjects ($p < 0.01$). Adapted from Finta et al. *(55)*.

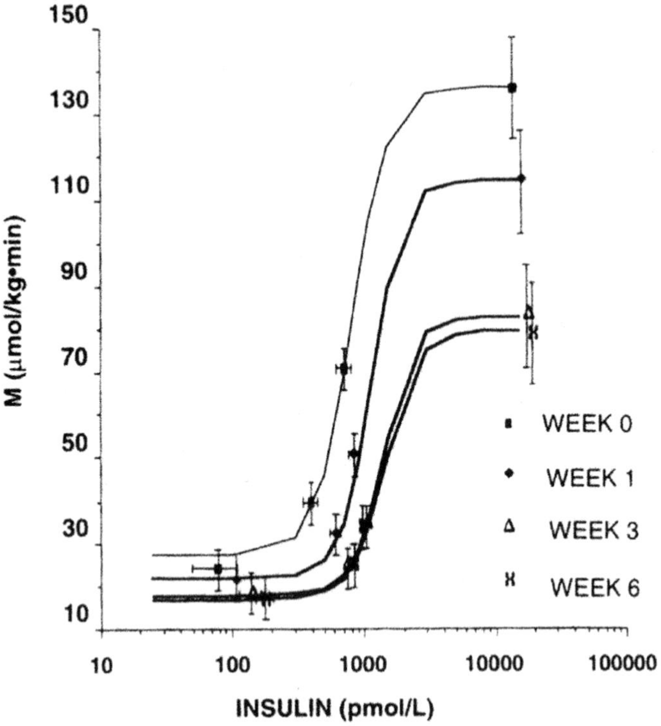


Fig. 4. Rates of whole body glucose uptake (M) determined during euglycemic clamp studies over a wide range of steady-state insulin concentrations serially in four dogs fed a high-fat diet. Weight gain resulted in a shift to right and a decrease in maximal rate of M ($p < 0.001$). From Rocchini et al. *(59)*.

to insulin of the kidney is unresponsive to manipulations of dietary sodium. He believes that this abnormality may contribute to sodium retention and HTN.

Finally, there are structural changes in the kidneys of obese individuals that can cause fluid retention. The kidneys from obese animals and humans are tightly encapsulated with fat tissue. Some of the fat penetrates the renal hilum into the sinuses surrounding the renal medulla *(63)*. The interstitial fluid hydrostatic pressure is elevated to 19 mmHg in obese dogs compared with only 9–10 mmHg in lean dogs. The elevated interstitial pressure reduces medullary blood flow and causes tubular compression, thereby slowing tubular flow rate and increasing fraction tubular reabsorption.

Therefore, obesity, either from hormonal changes or because of physical changes in the kidney, causes fluid retention.

### *Insulin Resistance*

For years it has been recognized that HTN is common in obese and diabetic individuals. Glucose intolerance independent of obesity is also associated with HTN *(64)*. In children, several studies have demonstrated a positive association between fasting insulin level and resting BP *(65–69)*. Analysis of data from the San Antonio Heart Study has demonstrated an impressive pattern of overlap among HTN, diabetes, and obesity. It has been estimated that by the fifth decade of life, 85% of diabetic individuals are hypertensive and obese, 80% of obese subjects have abnormal glucose tolerance and are hypertensive, and 67% of hypertensive subjects are both diabetic and obese *(8,70)*. The relationship between insulin resistance and BP has been observed in most populations *(71–74)*. Many investigators have suggested that insulin resistance may be the metabolic link that connects obesity to HTN.

Factors known to improve insulin resistance are also associated with reductions in BP. It has been documented that weight loss is associated with a decrease in BP, as well as an improvement in insulin sensitivity *(75,76)*. The decline in BP associated with exercise training programs seems to be limited to individuals who are initially hyperinsulinemic and have the greatest fall in plasma insulin level as a result of the training program *(76,77)*.

In addition to human data linking insulin and BP, there are also animal data that suggests that insulin is an important regulator of BP *(18,19,78–85)*.

Finally, there is evidence to suggest that in individuals of normal weight, hyperinsulinemia and insulin resistance precede the development of HTN. Young black males with borderline high BP have been reported to have higher insulin levels and more insulin resistance than normotensive black men *(71,72)*. According to the Tecumseh Study *(86)*, individuals with borderline HTN have higher plasma insulin levels and greater weight than normotensive individuals. Normotensive children with a family history of HTN have higher insulin levels and more insulin resistance than children with no family history of HTN *(87)*.

However, in contrast to these and other reports *(8,71–76,88–92)* linking hyperinsulinemia to HTN, there have been other studies that have been unable to establish a relationship between hyperinsulinemia and high BP. There is at least one study in obese hypertensive individuals *(93)* which did not find a correlation between hyperinsulinemia and HTN. In normal dogs, a chronic infusion of insulin, with or without an infusion of norepinephrine, failed to increase BP *(25,94)*. In addition, even in those reports that have documented a relationship between insulin and BP, there is significant overlap in insulin resistance between those individuals who are hypertensive and those who are normotensive. No correlation has been found between BP and plasma insulin or insulin sensitivity in Pima Indians *(95)* or obese Mexican-American women *(48)*. Drawing from all of these studies, it is clear that not all hypertensive subjects are insulin resistant, and that not all insulin resistant subjects are hypertensive.

Based on available data in the literature, it appears that selective insulin resistance, and not only hyperinsulinemia, is more likely the metabolic link that is responsible for the observed epidemiological relationship between obesity and HTN. The term selective insulin resistance implies that, although an individual or animal may have an impaired ability of insulin to cause whole body glucose uptake, some of the other physiological actions of insulin may be preserved. With respect to HTN, one of the potentially important actions of insulin is the ability to induce renal sodium retention. Obese adolescents have selective insulin resistance in that they are resistant with respect to insulin's ability to stimulate glucose uptake, yet are still sensitive to the renal sodium-retaining effects of insulin *(50)* (Fig. 5). In nonobese patients with essential HTN, insulin resistance has been demonstrated to involve glucose metabolism, but not lipid or potassium metabolism, and is limited to the nonoxidative pathways of intracellular glucose disposal *(51,88)*.

Consequently, there is evidence to indicate that in obese hypertensive subjects, insulin resistance is *selective* (mostly involving glucose metabolism), *tissue specific* (predominantly effecting skeletal muscle), and *pathway specific* ( insofar as only glycogen synthesis is usually affected). Therefore, in any individual or animal, the degree to which insulin resistance is tissue- and/or pathway-specific may determine whether or not HTN will develop.

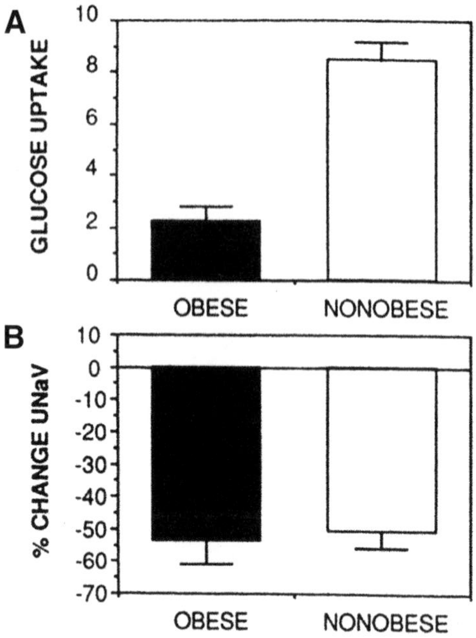


Fig. 5. (A) depicts the change in glucose uptake (M) (mg/kg/min) during euglycemic hyperinsulinemia in seven obese and five nonobese subjects. Compared to the nonobese individuals, a 40 μU/m$^2$/min infusion of insulin resulted in a significant depression in whole body glucose uptake in the obese subjects ($p < 0.001$). The plasma insulin response to the insulin infusion was not significantly different between obese and nonobese subjects. (B) depicts the percent change in urinary sodium excretion (% change UNaV) that occurred in the same 7 obese and 5 nonobese subjects during water diuresis and euglycemic hyperinsulinemia. Insulin infusion resulted in a significant (approx 50%) decrease in urinary sodium excretion in both the obese and nonobese subjects. There was no significant difference in the response of urinary sodium excretion to hyperinsulinemia observed between the two groups. Adapted from Rocchini et al. *(50)*.

In addition to sodium retention, selective insulin resistance may modulate the development of HTN through changes in vascular structure and function, alterations in cation flux, activation of the renin angiotensin aldosterone system, and activation of the sympathetic nervous system.

### *Alterations in Vascular Structure and Function*

Another way that obesity can cause HTN is through alterations in vascular structure and function. Cellular metabolism of cations and other molecules may be altered in obesity and lead to changes in vascular responsiveness. Vascular abnormalities are also known to exist in obese individuals. In normal, nonobese volunteers, insulin induces peripheral arterial vasodilation *(96)*. In obese adolescents, Rocchini et al. *(97)* demonstrated that ischemic exercise results in a decreased maximal forearm blood flow and an increased minimum vascular resistance. These investigators demonstrated that the abnormal vascular responses to ischemic exercise directly correlate with fasting insulin and whole body glucose uptake, and that the vascular and metabolic abnormalities improve with weight loss. Ultrasound of the carotid artery has demonstrated increased intimal-medial thickness in diabetic children *(98,99)*. Decreased vascular compliance has also been reported in obese children. Tounian et al. *(100)* demonstrated lower arterial compliance, lower distensibility, and lower endothelium-dependent and independent function in severely obese children compared to control children.

Steinberg et al. *(101)* demonstrated that insulin enhances the release of endothelium-derived nitric oxide (NO). Baron et al. *(102)* demonstrated that insulin-resistant individuals exhibit blunted insulin-mediated vasodilation and impaired endothelium-dependent vasodilation. Others have also demonstrated that salt-sensitive and insulin-resistant hypertensive patients manifest impaired endothelium-dependent relaxation mediated by NO *(103,104)*.

The development of vascular changes may possibly be associated with insulin resistance; in addition, data also suggest that abnormalities in skeletal muscle vascular regulation may be a cause. In both dogs *(97)* and man *(96)*, euglycemic hyperinsulinemia has been documented to result in vasodilation, not vasoconstriction. Even though the exact mechanism by which insulin induces vasodilation in non-insulin resistant individuals is unknown, some investigators believe that this vasodilator response is in part a result of stimulation of endothelial-dependent relaxing factor *(105,106)*. Type II, but not type I, diabetic subjects respond abnormally to acetylcholine, which induces vasodilation by stimulation of endothelial-dependent relaxing factor *(107)*.

Insulin-mediated glucose uptake is determined both by insulin's ability to stimulate glucose extraction at the tissue and cell levels and by the rate of glucose and insulin delivery (blood flow). Therefore, the relative contributions of tissue and blood flow actions of insulin will determine the overall rate of glucose uptake (i.e., degree of insulin resistance). In obese individuals with insulin resistance, an attenuated limb vasodilator response to hyperinsulinemia has been reported *(108,109)*. Insulin's lack of ability to produce vasodilation has led Baron *(110)* to speculate that abnormalities of skeletal muscle vascular regulation may be a cause, and not a result, of insulin resistance. This hypothesis is also supported by the fact that antihypertensive drugs that are vasodilators ( i.e., captopril, calcium channel blockers, and prazosin) tend to improve insulin resistance; whereas other antihypertensive drugs—such as diuretics or β-blockers—do not *(111–113)*.

### *Alterations in Ion Transport*

The fourth method by which obesity could cause HTN is through alterations in cation transport. Insulin has been shown to have an effect on sodium and calcium transport, although controversy still exists regarding the molecular mechanism of this effect. A direct effect of insulin on sodium/hydrogen exchange has been demonstrated in vitro *(114)*. Insulin has been reported to both increase and decrease Na-K-ATPase activity *(115)*. Insulin has been linked to both Na-Li countertransport and Na-K cotransport *(115)*. In a study of leukocyte sodium content and sodium pump activity in overweight and lean hypertensive subjects, it was observed that overweight hypertensive subjects accumulated intracellular sodium, most likely through abnormalities of sodium pump activity *(116)*. Consequently, alteration in intracellular sodium concentration could lead to an increased intracellular calcium, an increase in vascular smooth muscle tone, and HTN. Insulin alone has also been demonstrated to elevate cytosolic-free calcium levels in adipocytes of normal subjects *(117)*. In addition, weight loss in obese individuals is reported to be accompanied by a significant decrease in platelet-free calcium levels *(118)*.

Insulin-mediated glucose transport is dependent upon an intracellular calcium concentration of between 40 and 375 nm/L *(119)*. Therefore, increased intracellular calcium concentration may lead to insulin resistance, increased vascular resistance and HTN *(76)*. In hypertensive type II diabetics, a decrease in calcium adenosine-triphosphate activity is associated with increased intracellular calcium concentration *(120)*. Insulin has also been shown to stimulate plasma membrane calcium adenosine-triphosphate activity *(107)* and sodium-potassium adenosine-triphosphate activity *(115)*. Insulin resistance may blunt these pump functions and could lead to chronic increases in intracellular calcium, increased peripheral vascular resistance and HTN. Finally, reduced intracellular levels of magnesium are also associated with increased vascular resistance and insulin resistance *(121)*. With the use of magnetic resonance imaging to evaluate the aorta of normal and hypertensive subjects, Resnick et al. *(122)* found that increased abdominal visceral fat, decreased intracellular magnesium, and advanced age were closely associated with reduced aortic distensibility vessels. Therefore, in obesity alterations in either intracellular calcium and/or magnesium could result in the development of both HTN and insulin resistance.

### *Stimulation of the Renin-Angiotensin-Aldosterone System*

A fifth way by which obesity could cause HTN is through alterations in the renin-angiotensin-aldosterone system (RAAS). The RAAS is an important determinant of efferent glomerular arteriolar tone, and tubular sodium reabsorption. Its activity is modulated by dietary salt ingestion and BP. Therefore, alterations in the RAAS could be expected to alter pressure-natriuresis. Enhanced activity of the RAAS has been reported in obese humans and dogs *(32,54,123–128)*. Tuck et al. *(32)* demonstrated in obese hypertensives that plasma renin activity decreases with weight loss, and that the decrease in plasma renin activity was statistically correlated with the weight loss associated decrease in mean arterial pressure. Granger and co-workers *(128)* reported that plasma renin activity is 170% higher in obese dogs than in control dogs. However, Hall et al. *(57)* demonstrated that weight-related changes in BP can occur in dogs independent of changes in ANG II.

Obesity is also associated with abnormalities in the angiotensin-aldosterone system. Tuck and associates *(32)* demonstrated in obese adults that weight loss lowered both plasma renin activity and aldosterone concentration. Hiramatsu et al. *(124)* documented in obese hypertensives that, with increasing body weight, there is a progressive increase in the ratio of plasma aldosterone to plasma renin activity. Scavo et al. *(125,126)* reported that although obese adults have a normal plasma renin activity, they have an increased plasma aldosterone concentration and an increased aldosterone secretion rate. Sparks and co-workers *(127)* reported that, in obese patients, during the early stages of fasting there is a dissociation between plasma renin activity and aldosterone. Rocchini et al. *(123)* measured supine and 2-h upright plasma renin activity and aldosterone in 10 nonobese and 30 obese adolescents before and after a 20-wk weight loss program. The obese adolescents had significantly higher supine and 2-h upright aldosterone concentrations. Although plasma renin activity was not significantly different between the two groups of adolescents, they observed that a given increment in plasma renin activity produced a greater increment in aldosterone in the obese adolescents. Compared with an obese control group, weight loss resulted in a significant decrease in plasma aldosterone. After weight loss there was also a significant decrease in the slope of the posture-induced relation between plasma renin activity and aldosterone. In addition, after weight loss there was a significant correlation between the change in plasma aldosterone and the change in mean BP. The authors speculated that increased plasma aldosterone concentration in some obese subjects is caused by increased adrenal sensitivity to ANG II.

Insulin has been shown to influence the renin-angiotensin aldosterone system in both normal subjects *(53,129)* and in patients with diabetes *(130)*. Since hyperinsulinemia is a characteristic feature of obesity, Rocchini et al. *(54)* hypothesized that increased aldosterone levels observed in obese individuals are caused by hyperinsulinemia and insulin's ability to augment ANG II-mediated aldosterone production. Rocchini et al. *(84)* measured the increase in plasma aldosterone after intravenous ANG II (5, 10, and 20 ng/kg/min for 15 min each) before and after euglycemic hyperinsulinemia in seven chronically instrumented dogs. Euglycemic hyperinsulinemia resulted in a significantly greater ($p < 0.01$) change in the ANG II-stimulated increments of plasma aldosterone than that observed when ANG II was administered alone. However, there was no dose dependence of insulin's effect on ANG II-stimulated aldosterone. Weight gain significantly increased ANG II-stimulated aldosterone; however, with hyperinsulinemia, the response was not significantly different than that observed in the dogs prior to weight gain. The authors speculated that possible mechanisms by which insulin could increase ANG II-stimulated aldosterone production include: increased intracellular potassium, reduced plasma free fatty acids and a direct action of insulin to induce increased adrenal steroidogenesis.

Hollenberg and Williams *(131,132)* have described a group of subjects with essential HTN that they have called nonmodulators. These normal renin subjects appear to have a defect in their sodium-modulated tissue responsiveness to ANG II. Ferri et al. *(133)* have shown that nonmodulating hypertensives are insulin resistant. Similarly, Trevisan et al. *(134)* have demonstrated that insulin-dependent diabetes mellitus (IDDM) patients have both an enhanced renal response to ANG II and insulin resistance.

### *Increased Activation of the Sympathetic Nervous System*

The sixth way in which obesity could cause HTN is through stimulation of the sympathetic nervous system. For over 20 yr it has been recognized that diet affects the sympathetic nervous system. Fasting suppresses sympathetic nervous system activity, whereas overfeeding with either a high carbohydrate or high fat diet simulates the sympathetic nervous system *(135–138)*. Insulin is believed to be the signal that networks dietary intake and nutritional status to sympathetic activity. Glucose and insulin-sensitive neurons in the ventromedial portion of the hypothalamus have been demonstrated to alter the activity of inhibitory pathways between the hypothalamus and brainstem *(139)*. It is believed that the physiological role of the link between dietary intake and sympathetic nervous system activity is to regulate energy expenditure in the hope of maintaining weight homeostasis. Landsberg *(140)* has suggested that in obese individuals the sympathetic nervous system is chronically activated in an attempt to prevent further weight gain, and that HTN is a byproduct of the overactive sympathetic nervous system. They and their associates, as have others, clearly documented that euglycemic hyperinsulinemia in normal and obese humans and animals causes activation of the sympathetic nervous system, documented by increases in heart rate (HR), BP, and plasma norepinephrine *(30,54,140–143)*. More recently, it has been shown that hyperinsulinemia in normal humans is associated not only with an increase in circulating catecholamines, but also with an increase in sympathetic nerve activity *(96)*. The Bogalusa Heart Study reported that in a biracial group of children resting HR was positively correlated with BP and subscapular skinfold thickness *(144)*. These investigators also demonstrated that a hyperdynamic CV state was associated with obesity *(145)*. Obese children are also reported to have increased HR variability and BP variability compared to nonobese children *(146)*. Although many studies in obese individuals have demonstrated increased sympathetic nervous system activity, this has not been a universal finding *(147)*. Part of the controversy regarding the role of the sympathetic nervous system in obesity relates to relying on plasma levels of catecholamines as the index of sympathetic activity. Data from the Normative Aging Study *(41)* strongly suggest that obesity is associated with increased sympathetic nervous system activity. This study demonstrated that sympathetic activity, assessed by measuring 24-h urinary norepinephrine excretion, is directly related to abdominal girth, waist-to-hip ratio, and BMI. Other studies, using the appearance rate of norepinephrine in the circulation *(148)* and the effects of somatostatin-induced suppression of insulin on plasma norepinephrine levels *(149)*, provide additional corroboration for an increase in sympathetic activity linked to obesity and driven by insulin. Sondergaard et al. *(150)* demonstrated that measurements of resting and 24 h sympathoadrenal activity may differ in obese individuals. They demonstrated that sympathic activity at rest, evaluated by forearm venous plasma norepinephrine levels, was increased in obese subjects. However, thrombocyte norepinephrine and epinephrine levels, which likely reflect 24-h plasma catecholamine concentrates, were reduced in obese subjects with body fat above 40%. They speculate that the reduced thrombocyte catecholamine levels are most likely due to a reduced physical activity in these subjects.

Finally, there are ethnic differences in sympathetic tone. Weyer et al. *(151)* examined the relation among HR, BP, percentage of body fat, fasting insulin, and muscle sympathetic nerve activity in male normotensive whites and Pima Indians. These investigators demonstrated that in both ethnic groups, HR and BP positively related to percent body fat and muscle sympathetic nerve activity, and both were independent determinants of HR and BP. However, muscle sympathetic nerve activity was positively related to body fat percentage and fasting insulin concentration in white subjects, but not in Pima Indian subjects. This study emphasizes that the roles of hyperinsulinemia and increased sympathetic nervous system activity as a mediator of the relationship between obesity and HTN can differ among ethnic groups. Weyer's study may explain why the Pima Indians have a low prevalence of HTN in this population, despite their high incidence of obesity and insulin resistance.

Abnormalities in the sympathetic nervous system may also play a role in the actual pathogenesis of some forms of obesity. The recent identification and cloning of the β3-adrenergic receptor have spurred great interest in the potential of this receptor in the regulation of energy expenditure and, ultimately, in the development of obesity. The β3-adrenergic receptor is predominantly expressed in omental fat tissue and in the gall bladder, at low levels in ileum and colon, and absent in muscle, heart, liver, lung, kidney, thyroid, and lymphocytes *(152)*. Mutations in the β3-adrenergic receptor gene have been detected in Pima Indians and Mexican Americans, two populations with a high incidence of obesity and diabetes *(153)*. Finally, preliminary studies in obese humans have demonstrated that the administration of an agent with high specificity for the β3-adrenergic receptor results in increased energy expenditure that is accompanied by a marked improvement in insulin sensitivity and glucose tolerance *(154)*.

### *Natriuretic Peptides*

Natriuretic peptides are important regulators of volume and pressure. There are at least three natriuretic peptides that have been identified: atrial natriuretic peptide, brain natriuretic peptide, and C-type peptide. Few studies have examined the role of natriuretic peptides in obesity. Licata and co-workers *(155)* demonstrated that, following a sodium load, obese subjects have delayed urinary sodium excretion and a blunted rise in atrial natriuretic peptide levels. Maoz and co-workers *(156)* demonstrated that weight loss was associated with a significant diuresis and natriuresis, together with an early increase in plasma atrial natriuretic peptide levels. Finally, Dessi-Fulgheri et al. *(157)* reported that, after caloric restriction in obese hypertensive subjects, atrial natriuretic peptide infusion caused a more pronounced diuresis, natriuresis, fall in BP, and an elevation in plasma cGMP levels than was observed in these subjects prior to caloric restriction. These authors suggested that relative overt expression of inactive receptor Npr-C in adipose tissue might trap and clear more atrial natriuretic peptide from the circulation, thereby reducing its biologic effects on the kidney.

### *Leptin*

Leptin is a 167 amino acid hormone that is secreted exclusively by adipocytes. By binding to the leptin receptor in the hypothalamus, and by activating multiple neuropeptide pathways, leptin decreases appetite and increases energy expenditure, thereby decreasing adipose tissue mass and body weight. Serum leptin level is low in lean individuals and is elevated in most obese subjects *(158)*. Since there is a strong relationship between serum leptin levels and body fat mass, some authors have concluded that obesity may be associated with leptin-resistance *(159)*.

Leptin has been shown to have significant CV effects. Leptin-treated animals have a higher metabolic rate and core temperature. This may be owing to the fact that leptin increases sympathetic outflow and norepinephrine turnover in adipose tissue *(160)*. Despite the increase in sympathetic outflow associated with leptin administration, no BP elevation has been reported with the acute infusion of leptin *(161)*. However, the chronic administration of leptin is associated with an increase in BP, HR, and renal vascular resistance, despite a decrease in food intake *(162)*. Transgenic mice that overexpress leptin are also hypertensive. In these mice, the elevated BP can be prevented by an α-receptor blocker *(163)*. Leptin has also been found to increase insulin sensitivity and inhibit glucose-mediated insulin secretion *(164)*.

### *Hypothalamic Origins of Obesity Hypertension*

The similarities between Cushing's syndrome and the metabolic abnormalities associated with obesity HTN has led Bjorntorp to speculate that hypercortisolemia is involved in the pathogenesis of obesity HTN *(165)*. Cortisol secretion has been measured repeatedly in obesity, but there have been conflicting results. There is evidence of increased secretion and turnover, resulting in normal, or even lower than normal, circulating concentration *(166)*. Measuring salivary cortisol, investigators have been able to demonstrate that normally regulated cortisol secretion is associated with "healthy" anthropometric, metabolic, and hemodynamic variables. However, upon perceived stress, cortisol secretion is increased and followed by insulin resistance, abdominal obesity, elevated BP, and hyperlipidemia *(167,168)*. In a small portion of the population a defective, "burned-out" cortisol secretion occurs. This "burn-out" is also associated with decreased sex steroid and growth hormone secretions, and is strongly associated with visceral adiposity, insulin resistance, and HTN. Rosmond and Bjorntorp *(169)* have demonstrated that diminished dexamethasone suppression is directly associated with obesity and elevation of leptin levels. These authors suggest that a poor control of the hypothalamic pituitary axis may be associated with obesity and inefficient leptin signals. Zahrezewska et al. *(170)* demonstrated in rats that glucocorticoids diminish leptin signals.

Bjorntorp and Rosmond *(165)* speculate that the two ways that elevated activity of the hypothalamic–pituitary–adrenal (HPA) axis could occur are an elevated stimulation and/or a diminished feedback control. Elevated stimulation of the HPA axis can occur because of psychosocial and socioeconomic handicaps such as living alone, divorce, poor education, low social class, unemployed family members, and problems at school, or even excessive food intake *(171)*. With respect to causes of diminished feedback control of the HPA axis, Bjorntorp and others *(172–174)* demonstrated that a restriction fragment length polymorphism of the glucocorticoid receptor gene is associated with poorly controlled HPA axis function, as well as abdominal obesity, insulin resistance, and HTN. Therefore, Bjorntorp has suggested that many of the CV and physiologic consequences found in obese individuals could be the result of "a discretely elevated cortisol secretion, discoverable during reactions to perceived stress in everyday life" *(175)*.

### *Summary*

In summary, there are conclusive data to suggest that obesity, especially upperbody fat distribution, is an independent risk factor for the development of HTN. Caloric restriction and weight loss are associated with a reduction in BP. In addition, it is clear that even modest weight loss (i.e., 10% of body weight) improves BP, and many individuals achieve normal BP levels without attaining their calculated ideal weight. Although there is controversy over the role that insulin resistance and hyperinsulinemia play in the pathogenesis of obesity HTN, there are ample data suggesting that selective insulin resistance and HTN are related. Other hormonal systems (leptin, renin-angiotensin-aldosterone, sympathetic nervous system, and HPA axis) have also been identified as having a relationship with obesity, HTN, and insulin resistance. Further studies will be necessary, not only to clarify the origin of defects in insulin action that are responsible for the development of insulin resistance, but also to more precisely define the exact role that insulin resistance and the regulatory abnormalities in these other hormone systems play in BP homeostasis.

## OBESITY AS A CARDIOVASCULAR RISK FACTOR

The Framingham Heart Study *(5)* identified obesity and HTN as independent risk factors in the development of CVD. Obese normotensive and hypertensive men have a higher rate of coronary heart disease (CHD) *(47)*. Manson et al. *(176)* have also reported that, in women, the relative risk of fatal and nonfatal CHD increased from the lowest to the highest quartiles of obesity. Childhood obesity is associated with the development of early coronary artery pathology. The autopsies of 210 children aged 5–15 yr who had suffered violent death were evaluated by Kortelainen *(177)*. Ponderal index was a significant predictor of heart weight and the presence of coronary artery intimal fatty streaks. In the Bogalusa Heart Study, Berenson et al. demonstrated that children and young adults who died of trauma showed an association between BMI, systolic and diastolic BP, and the presence of fatty streaks and fibrous plaques in the aorta and coronary arteries *(15,68)*.

Long-standing obesity is associated with preclinical and clinical left ventricular (LV) dilatation *(178)* and impaired systolic function *(179,180)*, with heart failure frequently the ultimate cause of death in markedly overweight individuals *(181)*.

A physiologic change that may contribute to the association of obesity with LV dilatation is sodium retention and a concomitant increase in blood volume and cardiac output (CO). Many investigators *(182)* have reported that obesity is associated with an increased blood volume and CO. However, the increment in CO associated with obesity cannot be explained by an increase in adipose tissue perfusion alone; some have suggested that blood flow to the nonadipose mass must also be increased in obese subjects *(183,184)*. Consequently, obesity is characterized by a relative volume expansion in the presence of restricted vascular capacity. The increase in volume in the presence of restricted vascular capacity may lead to LV dilatation, increased LV wall stress, and compensatory LVH *(178,183,185)*. HTN increases afterload and, as a consequence, the left ventricle adapts with an increase in wall thickness. The combination of obesity and HTN, therefore, creates a double burden on the heart, ultimately leading to the development of impaired ventricular function *(179–181,186,187)*.

MacMahon et al. *(178)* reported that 50% of individuals who are more than 50% overweight have LVH. In children, adiposity is also one of the determinants of left ventricular mass. Urbina et al. reported that the major factor influencing LV mass in childhood was linear growth, defined by height and measures of ponderosity *(188)*. Daniels et al. reported that in children, lean body mass was the strongest determinant of LV mass, but that fat mass and systolic BP were also important predictors *(189,190)*. Similar to BP, weight loss can result in LVH regression *(178,185,191)*.

Unlike the universal finding of LVH in obese individuals, not all studies have demonstrated an impairment in LV function. Schmeider and Messerli *(192)* reported that obese hypertensive individuals have normal global LV systolic function, measured by LV fractional shortening and the velocity of circumferential fiber shorting. However, since both of these indices of LV systolic function are dependent on ventricular preload and afterload, the results of Schmeider's study do not show that LV contractility is normal. In fact, Blake and co-workers *(185)* demonstrated that despite a normal LV ejection fraction (LVEF) at rest, obese individuals have an impaired LVEF in response to dynamic exercise. Guilermo et al. *(186)* reported that the end-systolic wall stress to end-systolic volume index, a load independent index of LV function, is also abnormal in even mild or moderately obese individuals. These investigators also documented a significant inverse relationship between the index of end-systolic wall stress to end-systolic volume and BMI, diastolic diameter and LV mass index.

Abnormalities in left ventricular filling have also been reported to occur in obese individuals, i.e., decreased peak filling rate, duration of peak filling, and left atrial emptying index *(191)*, an increased isovolumic relaxation time, and an abnormal mitral valve Doppler filling pattern *(187)*. Harada et al. *(193)* demonstrated that BMI predicts LV diastolic filling rate in asymptomatic obese children. Kanoupakis et al. *(194)* demonstrated that weight loss improves diastolic function.

LVH, depressed myocardial contractility, and diastolic dysfunction can predispose individuals to excessive ventricular ectopy. Messerli et al. *(195)* reported that the prevalence of premature ventricular contractions was 30 times higher in obese individuals with eccentric LVH than in lean individuals.

Finally, similar to HTN, insulin resistance may be related to both the cardiac hypertrophy and abnormal cardiac function that is observed in many obese individuals. Nakajima et al. *(196)* reported a direct relationship between intraabdominal fat accumulation and the cardiac abnormalities associated with obesity. Since increased upperbody and intraabdominal fat accumulation relate to the presence of insulin resistance, although without significant overall obesity, these investigators speculated that the cardiac dysfunction observed in obese individuals may be related to insulin resistance.

In summary, obesity is recognized as an independent risk factor in the development of CVD. Obesity in both children and adults is associated with the development of cardiac dysfunction.

Table 2
Cardiovascular Consequences of Obesity

1. Premature development of coronary atherosclerosis
2. Left ventricular hypertrophy
3. Left ventricular dilation
4. Left ventricular diastolic dysfunction
5. Left ventricular systolic dysfunction
6. Congestive heart failure

Obese individuals have an increased risk for developing LV dilatation, impaired systolic and diastolic dysfunction, and the development of LVH (Table 2).

## MANAGEMENT OF THE OBESE CHILD WITH HYPERTENSION

Weight loss is the cornerstone of hypertensive management in the obese individual. Weight loss in both adolescents and adults improves all of the CV abnormalities associated with obesity, including: HTN, dyslipidemia, and sodium retention; structural abnormalities in resistant vessels; and LVH and dysfunction. The method by which weight loss is accomplished is important. Although weight loss, in general, results in a drop in resting systolic/diastolic BP and HR, when the weight loss is incorporated with physical conditioning the greatest decrease in resting systolic BP, peak exercise diastolic pressure, and HR can be achieved *(30)*. Similarly, a weight loss program that incorporates exercise along with caloric restriction produces the most favorable effects on insulin resistance *(30,77)*, dyslipidemia *(77,197)*, and vascular reactivity *(30,97)*. Endurance training in obese and nonobese individuals improves insulin resistance, in part by increasing muscle oxidative capacity and capillary density *(198,199)*, Most investigators believe that the additive effect of exercise to weight loss is related to the fact that exercise improves insulin resistance, independent of weight loss.

Although weight loss and exercise are the cornerstones of BP management in obese hypertensive individuals, most obese individuals are either unable or unwilling to lose weight or are unable to keep from regaining lost weight. Therefore, pharmacological therapy is frequently required in the hypertensive obese individual. This therapy is divided into treatment of obesity and/or treatment of HTN. The role of drug therapy in the treatment of childhood obesity is controversial. Many of the obesity drugs that have been tried in adults have resulted in complication, such as fenfluramine/dexfenfluramine *(200)*. There have been few well-controlled studies to show that the available obesity drugs are well tolerated and effective for use in obese children. One medication that is currently showing promise for treatment of obesity in adolescents is sibutramine, a reuptake inhibitor of serotonin and norepinephrine. However, sibutramine is also associated with an increase in BP in some patients and therefore may not be ideal for the very hypertensive child. Orlistat is a gastrointestinal lipase inhibitor that may hold promise for the effective pharmacological treatment of childhood obesity.

When choosing an antihypertensive agent for the obese child, it is important to remember that, depending on the antihypertensive agents used, insulin resistance has been reported to improve, worsen, or remain unchanged. In general, thiazide diuretics *(92,111,201)* and β-blockers *(92,111)* are known to impair insulin sensitivity and glucose tolerance, calcium blockers do not seem to adversely affect carbohydrate metabolism *(202–204)*, indapamide and potassium-sparing diuretics do not influence glucose homeostasis *(205)*, and, finally, angiotensin-converting enzyme (ACE) inhibitors *(111)* and α1-blockers *(112,206)* may improve glucose metabolism and insulin resistance. Recently, Rocchini et al. *(207)* demonstrated that clonidine, a centrally acting sympathetic agent, not only improved the HTN associated with obesity, but also improved the insulin resistance. Guigliano et al. *(208)* demonstrated that transdermal clonidine was effective in reducing BP and improving insulin resistance in hypertensive individuals with non-insulin-dependent diabetes mellitus. Based on these two preliminary studies, it would appear that clonidine or other similar drugs have a favorable profile for obese individuals with HTN.

In addition to their unfavorable effect on insulin resistance, thiazide diuretics impair pancreatic insulin secretion *(209,210)* and increase low-density lipoprotein and total cholesterol *(111,211)*. β-Blockers are associated with a two- to threefold incidence of inducing diabetes mellitus *(212)* and are associated with a significant lowering of high-density lipoprotein (HDL) cholesterol *(213,214)*. However, despite the different pharmacologic profiles of the antihypertensive drugs, there are no clear recommendations for obese hypertensive individuals.

There are increasing data that confirm that ACE inhibitors have specific benefits for individuals with diabetes, atherosclerosis, LV dysfunction, and renal insufficiency *(215)*.

Finally, there are two other classes of agents, biguandines (metformin) and thiazolidinediones (pioglitazone, rosiglitazone, and troglitazone), that also appear to reverse insulin resistance, HTN, and dyslipidemia *(216,217)*. However, troglitazone has recently been associated with significant liver toxicity *(218)*. It is too early to know the role that these or similar agents will play in the treatment of childhood obesity HTN.

Although weight loss is the cornerstone of hypertensive management in the obese individual, many individuals will also require pharmacologic therapy. When choosing an antihypertensive medication it is important to individualize the agent to the patient. Some agents, such as thiazide diuretics and β-blockers, can impair glucose tolerance and adversely alter plasma lipid levels. On the other hand, ACE inhibitors and centrally-acting sympathetic agents improve the HTN and insulin resistance associated with obesity. Finally, ACE inhibitors are also effective in reducing the development of congestive heart failure, and in reducing CV mortality.

## FUTURE PERSPECTIVES

The prevalence and severity of obesity is increasing in children and adolescents. Based on this increased incidence of childhood obesity, we are currently facing an epidemic of childhood type II diabetes and HTN. In the past, most pediatricians were taught that HTN in children is a rare condition associated with renal disease. In reality, secondary HTN in children has become far less common relative to primary (essential) HTN. In a large pediatric HTN practice, the typical hypertensive child is an otherwise healthy adolescent, but afflicted with obesity and some combination of CV risk factors associated with obesity. Obesity in childhood is a chronic medical condition and requires long-term treatment. It is hoped that with new discoveries such as leptin more effective forms of treatment of childhood obesity will be developed.

## ACKNOWLEDGMENT

This work was supported in part by grants 1RO1 HL 52205, HL-18575, 2RO1-HL-35743, 2P60 AM 20572, and 2P01HL18575-24 from the National Institutes of Health.

## REFERENCES

1. Ogden CL, Troiano RP, Briefel RR, Kuczmarski RJ, Flegal KM, Johnson CL. Prevalence of overweight among preschool children in the United States, 1971 through 1994. Pediatrics 1997;99:E1.
2. Dublin LI. Report of the Joint Committee on Mortality of the Association of Life Insurance Medical Directors. The Actuarial Society of America, 1925.
3. Stamler R, Stamler J, Riedlinger WF, Algera G, Roberts R. Weight and blood pressure. Findings in hypertension screening of 1 million Americans. J Am Med Assoc 1978;240:1607–1609.
4. Symonds B. Blood pressure of healthy men and women. J Am Med Assoc 1923;8:232.
5. Hubert HB, Feinleib M, McNamara PM, Castelli WP. Obesity as an independent risk factor for cardiovascular disease: a 26-year follow-up of participants in the Framingham Heart Study. Circulation 1983;67:968–977.
6. McMahon SW, Blacket RB, McDonald GJ, Hall W. Obesity, alcohol consumption and blood pressure in Australian men and women: National Heart Foundation of Australia Risk Factor Prevalence Study. J Hypertens 1984;2:85–91.
7. Bloom E, Swayne R, Yano K, MacLean C. Does obesity protect hypertensives against cardiovascular disease? J Am Med Assoc 1986;256:2972–2975.
8. Ferannini E, Haffner SM, Stern MP. Essential hypertension: an insulin-resistance state. J Cardiovasc Pharmacol 1990;15(Suppl 5):S18–S25.
9. Manolio TA, Savage PJ, Burke GL, et al. Association of fasting insulin with blood pressure and lipids in young adults. The CARDIA Study. Atherosclerosis 1990;10:430–436.
10. Larimore JW. A study of blood pressure in relation to type of bodily habitus. Arch Int Med 1923;31:567.
11. Levy RL, Troud WD, White PD. Transient hypertension: its significance in terms of later development of sustained hypertension and cardiovascular-renal diseases. JAMA 1944;126:82.
12. Hypertension Detection and Follow-Up Program Cooperative Group. Race, education and prevalence of hypertension. Am J Epidemol 1977;106:351–361.
13. Kannel WB, Brand N, Skinner JJ Jr, Dawber TR, McNamara PM. The relation of adiposity to blood pressure and development of hypertension. The Framingham study. Ann Intern Med 1967;67:48–59.
14. Rosner B, Prineas R, Daniels SR, Loggie J. Blood pressure differences between blacks and whites in relation to body size among US children and adolescents. Am J Epidemiol 2000;151:1007–1019.
15. Freedman DS, Dietz WH, Srinivasan SR, Berenson GS. The relation of overweight to cardiovascular risk factors among children and adolescents: the Bogalusa Heart Study. Pediatrics 199;103:1175–1182.
16. Sorof JM, Poffenbarger T, Franco K, Bernard L, Portman RJ. Isolated systolic hypertension. Obesity, and hyperkinetic hemodynamic states in children. J Pediatr 2002;140:660–666.
17. Cash JR, Wood JR. Observations upon the blood pressure of dogs following changes in body weight. South Med J 1938;31:270–282.
18. Rocchini AP, Moorehead C, Wentz E, Deremer S. Obesity-induced hypertension in the dog. Hypertension 1987;9(Suppl III):III64–III68.
19. Rocchini AP, Moorehead CP, DeRemer S, Bondie D. Pathogenesis of weight-related changes in blood pressure in dogs. Hypertension 1989;13:922–928.
20. Hall JE, Brands MW, Dixon WN, Smith MJ Jr. Obesity-induced hypertension. Renal function and systemic hemodynamics. Hypertension 1993;22:292–299.
21. Haynes R. Is weight loss an effective treatment for hypertension. Can J Physiol Pharmacol 1985;64:825–830.
22. Langford H, Davis B, Blaufox D, et al. Effect of drug and diet treatment of mild hypertension on diastolic blood pressure. Hypertension 1991;17:210–217.
23. Hypertension Prevention Treatment Group. The Hypertension Trial: three-year effects of dietary changes on blood pressure. Arch Intern Med 1990;150:153–162.
24. Davis BR, Blaufox D, Oberman A, et al. Reduction in long-term antihypertensive medication requirements: effects of weight reduction by dietary intervention in overweight persons with mild hypertension. Arch Intern Med 1993;153:1773–1782.
25. Fagerberg B, Andersson O, Isaksson B, Bjorntorp P. Blood pressure control during weight reduction in obese hypertensive men: separate effects of sodium and energy restriction. Br Med J 1984;288:11–14.
26. Maxwell M, Kushiro T, Dornfeld L, Tuck ML, Waks AU. BP changes in obese hypertensive subjects during rapid weight loss. Comparison of restricted v unchanged salt intake. Arch Intern Med 1984;144:1581–1584.
27. Gillum RF, Prineas RJ, Jeffrey RW, et al. Nonpharmacological therapy of hypertension: the independent effects of weight reduction and sodium restriction in overweight borderline hypertensive patients. Am Heart J 1983;105:128–133.

28. Reisin E. Weight reduction in the management of hypertension: epidemiologic and mechanistic evidence. Can J Physiol Pharmacol 1985;64:818–824.
29. Reisin E, Abel R, Modan M, et al. Effect of weight loss without salt restriction on the reduction of blood pressure in overweight hypertensive patients. N Engl J Med 1978;298:1–6.
30. Rocchini AP, Katch V, Anderson J, et al. Blood pressure and obese adolescents: effect of weight loss. Pediatrics 1988;82;116–123.
31. Dahl LK, Silver L, Christie RW. The role of salt in the fall of blood pressure accompanying reduction in obesity. N Engl J Med 1958;258:1186–1192.
32. Tuck MI, Sowers J, Dornfield L, Kledzik G, Maxwell M. The effect of weight reduction on blood pressure plasma renin activity and plasma aldosterone level in obese patients. N Engl J Med 1981;304:930–933.
33. Rocchini AP, Key J, Bondie D, et al. The effect of weight loss on the sensitivity of blood pressure to sodium in obese adolescents. N Engl J Med 1989;321:580–585.
34. Dornfield TP, Maxwell MH, Waks AU, Schroth P, Tuck ML. Obesity and hypertension: long-term effects of weight reduction on blood pressure. Int J Obes 1985;9:381–389.
35. Reisen E, Frohlich ED. Effects of weight reduction on arterial pressure. J Chronic Dis 1982;33:887–891.
36. Sjöström CD, Peltonen M, Wedel H, Sjöström L. Differential long-term effects of intentional weight loss on diabetes and hypertension. Hypertension 2000;36:20–25.
37. Sjöström CD, Lissner L, Wedel H, Sjöström L. Reduction in incidence of diabetes, hypertension, and lipid disturbances after intentional weight loss induced by bariatric surgery: the SOS Intervention Study. Obes Res 1999;7:477–484.
38. Carson JL Ruddy ME, Duff AE, Holems NJ, Cody RP, Brolin RE. The effect of gastric bypass surgery on hypertension in morbidly obese patients. Arch Intern Med 1994;154:193–200.
39. Sjöström CD, Peltonen M, Sjöström L. Blood pressure and pulse pressure during long-term weight loss in the obese: The Swedish Obese Subjects (SOS) Intervention Study. Obesity Research 2001;9:188–195.
40. Vague J. The degree of masculine differentiation of obesities: a factor determining predisposition to diabetes, atherosclerosis, gout, and uric calculous disease. Am J Clin Nutr 1956;4:20–34.
41. Landsberg L. Obesity and hypertension: experimental data. J Hypertens 1992;10:S195–S201.
42. Shear CL, Freedman DS, Burke GL, Harsha DW, Berenson GS. Body fat patterning and blood pressure in children and young adults: The Bogalusa Heart Study. Hypertension 1987;9:236–244.
43. Van Itallie TB. Health implications of overweight and obesity in the United States. Ann Intern Med 1985;103:983–988.
44. Kalkhoff R, Hartz A, Rupley D, Kissebah AH, Kelber S. Relationship of body fat distribution to blood pressure, carbohydrate tolerance, and plasma lipids in healthy obese women. J Lab Clin Med 1983;102:621–627.
45. Kissebah A, Vydelingum N, Murray R, et al. Relation of body fat distribution to metabolic complications of obesity. J Clin Endocrinol Metab 1982;54:254–260.
46. Peiris A, Sothmann M, Hoffmann R, et al. Adiposity, fat distribution, and cardiovascular risk. Ann Intern Med 1989;110:867–872.
47. Donahue RP, Abbot RD, Bloom E, Reed DM, Yano K. Central obesity and coronary heart disease in men. Lancet 1987;1:882–884.
48. Lapidus L, Bengtsson C, Lissner L. Distribution of adipose tissue in relation to cardiovascular and total mortality as observed during 20 years in a prospective population study of women in Gothenburg, Sweden. Diabetes Res Clin Pract 1990;10(Suppl 1):S185–S189.
49. Bjorntorp P. Portal adipose tissue as a generator of risk factors for cardiovascular disease and diabetes. Atheriosclerosis 1990;289:333–345.
50. Rocchini AP, Katch V, Kveselis D, et al. Insulin and renal sodium retention in obese adolescents. Hypertension 1989;14:367–374.
51. DeFronzo RA, Cooke CR, Andres R, Fabona GR, Davis PJ. The effect of insulin on renal handling of sodium, potassium, calcium and phosphate in man. J Clin Invest 1975;55:845–855.
52. Baum M. Insulin stimulates volume absorption in the proximal convoluted tubule. J Clin Invest 1987;79:1104–1109.
53. Vierhapper H, Waldhausl W, Nowontny P. The effect of insulin on the rise in blood pressure and plasma aldosterone after angiotensin II in normal man. Clin Sci 1983;64:383–386.
54. Rocchini AP, Moorehead C, DeRemer S, Goodfriend TL, Ball DL. Hyperinsulinemia and the aldosterone and pressor responses to angiotensin II. Hypertension 1990;15:861–866.
55. Finta KM, Rocchini AP, Moorehead C, Key J, Katch V. Sodium retention in response to an oral glucose tolerance test in obese and nonobese adolescents. Pediatrics 1992;90:442–446.

56. Rocchini AP. Insulin resistance, obesity, and hypertension. J Nutr 1995;125(6 Suppl):1718S–1724S.
57. Hall JE, Granger JP, Hester RL, Montani JP. Mechanisms of sodium balance in hypertension: role of pressure natriuresis. J Hypertens 1986;4(Suppl 4):S57–S65.
58. Ter Maaten JC, Bakker SJ, Serne EH, ter Wee PM, Donker AJ, Gans RO. Insulin's acute effects on glomerular filtration rate correlate with insulin sensitivity whereas insulin's acute effects on proximal tubular sodium reabsorption correlate with salt sensitivity in normal subjects. Nephrol Dial Transplant 1999;14:2357–2363.
59. Rocchini A, Marker P, Cervenka T. Time course of insulin resistance associated with weight gain in the dog: relationship to the development of hypertension. Am J Physiol 1996;272:E147–E154.
60. Laakso M, Edelman SV, Brechtel G, Baron AD. Impaired insulin-mediated skeletal muscle blood flow in patients with NIDDM. Diabetes 1992;41:1076–1083.
61. Kolterman O, Insel J, Saekow M, Olefsky J. Mechanisms of insulin resistance in human obesity: evidence for receptor and post-receptor defects. J Clin Invest 1980;65:1272–1284.
62. Sechi LA. Mechanisms of insulin resistance in rat models of hypertension and their relationships with salt sensitivity. J Hypertens 1999;17:1229–1237.
63. Hall JE, Brands MW, Henegar JR, Shek EW. Abnormal kidney function as a cause and a consequence of obesity hypertension. Clin Exp Pharmacol Physiol 1998;25:58–64.
64. Modan M, Halkin H, Almog S, et al. Hyperinsulinemia: a link between hypertension, obesity and glucose intolerance. J Clin Invest 1985;75:809–817.
65. Voors AW, Radhakrishnamurthy B, Srinivasan SR, Webber LS, Berenson GS. Plasma glucose level related to blood pressure in 272 children, ages 7–15 years, sampled from a total biracial population. Am J Epidemiol 1981;113:347–356.
66. Kanai H, Matsuzawa Y, Tokunaga K, et al. Hypertenison in obese children: fasting serum insulin levels are closely correlated with blood pressure. Int J Obes 1990;14:1047–1056.
67. Saito I, Nishino M, Kawabe H, et al. Leisure time physical activity and insulin resistance in young obese students with hypertension. Am J Hypertens 1992;5(12 Pt 1):915–918.
68. Chen W, Srinivasan SR, Elkasabany A, Berenson GS. Cardiovascular risk factors clustering features of insulin resistance syndrome (Syndrome X) in a biracial (black-white) population of children, adolescents, and young adults: the Bogalusa Heart Study. Am J Epidemiol 1999;150:667–674.
69. Young-Hyman D, Schlundt DG, Herman L, De Luca F, Counts D. Evaluation of the insulin resistance syndrome in a 5- to 10-year-old overweight/obese African-American children. Diabetes Care 2001;24:1359–1364.
70. Haffner SM, Ferrannini E, Hazuda HP, Stern MP. Clustering of cardiovascular risk factors in confirmed prehypertensive individuals: The San Antonio heart study. Diabetes 1992;41:715–722.
71. Falkner B. Differences in blacks and whites with essential hypertension: biochemistry and endocrine. Hypertension 1990;15:681–686.
72. Falkner B, Hulman S, Tannenbaum J, Kushner H. Insulin resistance and blood pressure in young black males. Hypertension 1988;12:352–358.
73. Shen DC, Shieh SM, Fuh MM, Wu DA, Chen YD, Reaven GM. Resistance to insulin-stimulated-glucose uptake in patients with hypertension. J Clin Endocrinol Metab 1988;66:580–583.
74. Darwin CH, Alpizar M, Buchanan TA, et al. Insulin resistance does not correlate with hypertension in Mexican American women. In: 75th Annual Meeting Abstracts, Endocrine Society, Bethesda, MD: 1993;233.
75. Pollare T, Lithell H, Berne C. Insulin resistance is a characteristic feature of primary hypertension independent of obesity. Metabolism 1990;39:167–174.
76. Rocchini AP, Katch V, Schork A, Kelch RP. Insulin's role in blood pressure regulation during weight loss in obese adolescents. Hypertension 1987;10:267–273.
77. Krotkorwski M, Mandroukas K, Sjostrom L, Sullivan L, Wetterquist H, Bjorntorp P. Effect of long-term physical training on body fat, metabolism and blood pressure in obesity. Metabolism 1979;28:650–658.
78. Zavaroni I, Sander S, Scott S, Reaven GM. Effect of fructose feeding of insulin secretion and insulin action in the rat. Metabolism 1980;29:970–973.
79. Hwang IS, Ho H, Hoffman BB, Reaven GM. Fructose-induced insulin and hypertension in rats. Hypertension 1987;10:512–516.
80. Reaven GM, Ho H, Hoffman BB. Attenuation of fructose-induces hypertension in rats by exercise drainage. Hypertension 1988;12:129–132.
81. Reaven GM, Ho H, Hoffamn BB. Somatostatin inhibition of fructose-induced hypertension. Hypertension 1989;14:117–120.

82. Kurtz TW, Morris RC, Pershadsingh HA. The Zucker fatty rat as a genetic model of obesity and hypertension. Hypertension 1989;13(6 pt 2):896–901.
83. Mondon CE, Reaven GM. Evidence of abnormalities of insulin-stimulated glucose uptake in adipocytes isolates from spontaneously hypertensive rats with spontaneous hypertension. Metabolism 1988;37: 303–305.
84. Reaven GM, Chang H, Hoffman BB, Azhar S. Resistance to insulin-stimulated glucose uptake in adipocytes isolates from spontaneously hypertensive rats. Diabetes 1989;38:1155–1160.
85. Finch D, Davis G, Bower J, Kirchner K. Effect of insulin on renal sodium handling in hypertensive rats. Hypertension 1990;15:514–518.
86. Julius S, Jamerson K, Mejia A, Krause L, Schork N, Jones K. The association of borderline hypertension with target organ changes and higher coronary risk. Tecumseh Blood Pressure Study. JAMA 1990;264:354–358.
87. Ferrari P, Weidmann P, Shaw S, et al. Altered insulin sensitivity, hyperinsulinemia, and dyslipidemia in individuals with a hypertensive parent. Am J Med 1991;91:589–596.
88. Ferrannini E, Buzzigoli G, Bonadonna R, et al. Insulin resistance in essential hypertension. N Engl J Med 1987;317:350–357.
89. Welborn TA, Breckneridge A, Rubinstein HT, Dollery CT, Russel-Fraser T. Serum insulin in essential hypertension and in peripheral vascular disease. Lancet 1966;II:1336–1337.
90. Lucas CP, Estigarribia JA, Daraga LL, Reaven GM. Insulin and blood pressure in obesity. Hypertension 1985;7:702–706.
91. Sowers JR. Insulin resistance, hyperinsulinemia, dyslipidemia, hypertension, and accelerated atherosclerosis. J Clin Pharmacol 1992;32:529–535.
92. Swislocki ALM, Hoffman BB, Reaven GM. Insulin resistance, glucose intolerance, and hyperinsulinemia in patients with hypertension. Am J Hypertens 1989;2:419–423.
93. Grugni G, Ardizzi A, Dubini A, Guzzaloni G, Sartorio A, Morabito F. No correlation between insulin levels and high blood pressure in obese subjects. Horm Metab Res 1990;22(2):124–125.
94. Hall JE, Brands MW, Kivlighn SD, Mizelle HL, Hidebrandt DA, Gaillard CA. Chronic hyperinsulinemia and blood pressure: interaction with catecholamines? Hypertension 1990;15:519–527.
95. Berchtold P, Jorgens V, Finke C, Berger M. Epidemiology and hypertension. Int J Obes 1981;5(Suppl 1):1–7.
96. Anderson EA, Hoffman RP, Balon TW, Sinkey CA, Mark AL. Hyperinsulinemia produces both sympathetic neural activation and vasodilation in normal humans. J Clin Invest 1991;87:2246–2252.
97. Rocchini AP, Moorehead C, Katch V, Key J, Finta KM. Forearm resistance vessel abnormalities and insulin resistance in obese adolescents. Hypertension 1992;19:615–620.
98. Peppa-Patrikiou M, Scordili M, Antoniou A, Giannaki M, Dracopoulou M, Dacou-Voutetakis C. Carotid atherosclerosis in adolescents and young adults with IDDM. Relation to urinary endothelin, albumin, free cortisol, and other factors. Diabetes Care 1998;21:1004–1007.
99. Javisalo MJ, Putto-Laurila A, Jartti L, et al. Carotid artery intimal-media thickness in children with Type 1 diabetes. Diabetes 2002;51:493–498.
100. Tounian P, Aggoun Y, Dubern B, et al. Presence of increased stiffness of the common carotid artery and endothelial dysfunction in severely obese children: a prospective study. Lancet 2001;358:1400–1404.
101. Steinberg HO, Brechtel G, Johnson A. Insulin mediated skeletal muscle vasodilation is nitric oxide dependent. A novel action of insulin to increase nitric oxide release. J Clin Invest 1994;94:1172–1179.
102. Baron AD, Steinberg HO, Chaker H. Insulin mediated skeletal muscle vasodilation contributed to both insulin sensitivity and responsiveness in lean humans. J Clin Invest 1995;96:786–792.
103. Miyoshi A, Suzuki H, Fujiwara M. Impairment of endothelial function in salt-sensitive hypertension in humans. Am J Hypertens 1997;10:1083–1090.
104. Facchini FS, DoNascimento C, Reaven GM, Yip JW, Ni XP, Humphreys MH . Blood pressure, sodium intake, insulin resistance, and urinary nitrate excretion. Hypertension 1999;33:1008–1012.
105. Wu HY, Jeng YY, Yue CJ, Chyu KY, Hsueh WA, Chan TM. Endothelial-dependent vascular effects of insulin and insulin-like growth factor-I in the rat perfused mesenteric artery and aortic rings. Diabetes 1994;43(8): 1027–1032.
106. Yagi S, Takata S, Kiyokawa H, et al. Effects of insulin on vasoconstrictive responses to norepinephrine and angiotensin II in rabbit femoral artery and vein. Diabetes 1988;37:1064–1067.
107. Zemel MB, Sowers JR, Shehin S, Walsh MF, Levy J. Impaired calcium metabolism associated with hypertension in Zucker obese rats. Metabolism 1990;39:704–708.

108. Natali A, Buzzigoli G, Taddei S, et al. Effects of insulin on hemodynamics and metabolism in human forearm. Diabetes 1990:39:490–500.
109. Laakso M, Edelman SV, Brechtel G, Baron AD. Decreased effect of insulin to stimulate skeletal muscle blood flow in obese man. J Clin Invest 1990;85:1844–1952.
110. Baron AD, Laasko M, Brechtel G, Edelman SV. Mechanism of insulin resistance in insulin-dependent diabetes mellitus: a major role for reduced skeletal muscle blood flow. J Clin Endocrinol Metab 1991;73:637–643.
111. Pollare T, Lithell H, Berne C. A comparison of the effects of hydrochlorothiazide and captopril on glucose and lipid metabolism in patients with hypertension. N Engl J Med 1989;321:868–873.
112. Swislocki AL, Hoffman BB, Sheu WH, Chen YD, Reaven GM. Effect of prazosin treatment on carbohydrate and lipoprotein metabolism in patients with hypertension. Am J Med 1989;86:14–18.
113. Pollare T, Lithell H, Morlin C, Prantare H, Hvarfner A, Ljunghall S. Metabolic effects of diltiazem and atenolol: results from a randomized, double-blind study with parallel groups. J Hypertens 1989;7:551–559.
114. Lagadie-Grossman D, Chesnais JM, Fewray D. Intracellular pH regulation in papillary muscle cells from streptozotocin diabetic rats: an ion-sensitive microelectrode study. Pflugers Arch 1988;412:613–617.
115. Tedde R, Sechi LA, Marigliano A, Scano L, Pala A. In vitro action of insulin on erythrocyte sodium transport mechanisms: its possible role in the pathogenesis of arterial hypertension. Clin Exp Hypertens 1988;10:545–559.
116. Ng LL, Harker M, Abel ED. Leucocyte sodium content and sodium pump activity in overweight and lean hypertensives. Clin Endocrinol (Oxf) 1989;30(2):191–200.
117. Draznin B, Kao M, Sussman KE. Insulin and glyburide increase in cytosolic free calcium concentration in isolated rat adipocytes. Diabetes 1987;36:174–178.
118. Jacobs DD, Sowers JR, Hmeidan A, Niyogi T, Simpson L, Standley PR. Effects of weight reduction on cellular cation metabolism and vascular resistance. Hypertension 1993;21:308–314.
119. Dranzin B, Sussman K, Kao M, Lewis D, Sherman N. The existence of an optimal range of cystolic free calcium for insulin-stimulated glucose transport in rat adipocytes. J Biol Chem 1987;262:14,385–14,388.
120. Schaefer W, Priessen J, Mannhold R, Gries AF. $CA^{2+}$-$MG^{2+}$-ATPase activity of human red blood cells in healthy and diabetic volunteers. Klin Wochenschr 1987;65:17–21.
121. Resnick LM, Gupta RK, Gruenspan H, Laragh JH. Intracellular free magnesium in hyprtension: relation to peripheral insulin resistance. J Hypertens 1988;6:S199–S201.
122. Resnick LM, Militianu D, Cummings AJ, Pipe JG, Evelhoch JL, Soulen RL. Direct magnetic resonance determination of aortic distensibility in essential hypertension, relation to age, abdominal visceral fat, and in situ intracellular free magnesium. Hypertension 1997;30:654–659.
123. Rocchini AP, Katch VL, Grekin R, Moorehead C, Anderson J. Role for aldosterone in blood pressure regulation of obese adolescents. Am J Cardiol 1986;57:613–618.
124. Hiramatsu K, Yamada T, Ichikawak T, Izumiyama T, Nagata H. Changes in endocrine activity to obesity in patients with essential hypertension. J Am Geriatr Soc 1981;29:25–30.
125. Scavo D, Borgia C, Iacobelli A. Aspetti di funzione corticosurrenalica nell'obesita'. Nota VI. Il comportamento della secrezione di aldosterone e della escrezione dei suoi metabolite nel corso di alcune prove dinamiche. Folia Endocrinol 1968;21:591–602.
126. Scavo D, Iacobelli A, Borgia C. Aspetti fi funzione corticosurrenalica nell'obesita'. Nota V. La secrezonia giornlieia di aldosterone. Folia Endocrinol 1968;21:577–590.
127. Spark RF, Arky RA, Boulter RP, Saudek CD, Obrian JT. Renin, aldosterone and glucagon in the natriureses of fasting. N Engl J Med 1975;292:1335–1340.
128. Granger JP, West D, Scott J. Abnormal pressure natriuresis in the dog model of obesity-induced hypertension. Hypertension 1994;23(Suppl I):I8–I11.
129. Trovati M, Massucco P, Anfossi G, et al. Insulin influences the renin-angiotensin-aldosterone system in humans. Metabolism 1989;38:501–503.
130. Farfel Z, Iania A, Eliahou HE. Presence of insulin-renin-aldosterone-potassium interrelationship in normal subjects, disrupted in chronic hemodialysis patients. Clin Endrocrinol Metab 1978;47:9–17.
131. Shoback DM, Williams GH, Moore TJ, Dluhy RG, Podolsky S, Hollenberg NK. Defect in the sodium-modulated tissue responsiveness to angiotensin II in essential hypertension. J Clin Metab 1983;57:764–770.
132. Hollenberg NK, Moore TJ, Shoback D, Redgrave J, Rabinowe S, Williams GH. Abnormal renal sodium handling in essential hypertension: relation to failure of renal and adrenal modulation of responses to angiotensin II. Am J Med 1986;81:412–418.
133. Ferri C, Bellini C, Desideri G, et al. Relationship between insulin resistance and nonmodulating hypertension: linkage of metabolic abnormalities and cardiovascular risk. Diabetes 1999;48:1623–1630.

134. Trevisan R, Bruttomesso D, Vedovato M, et al. Enhanced responsiveness of blood pressure to sodium intake and to angiotensin II is associated with insulin resistance in IDDM patients with microalbuminuria. Diabetes 1998;47:1347–1353.
135. Young JB, Landsberg L. Suppression of sympathetic nervous system during fasting. Science 1977;196:1473–1475.
136. Young JB, Landsberg L. Stimulation of the sympathetic nervous system during sucrose feeding. Nature 1977;269:615–617.
137. Landsberg L, Young JB. Fasting, feeding and regulation of the sympathetic nervous system. N Engl J Med 1978;298:1295–1301.
138. Young JB, Saville ME, Rothwell NJ, Stock MJ, Landsberg L. Effect of diet and cold exposure on norepinephrine turnover in brown adipose tissue in the rat. J Clin Invest 1982;69:1061–1071.
139. Landsberg L, Young JB. Insulin-mediated glucose metabolism in the relationship between dietary intake and sympathetic nervous system activity. Int J Obes 1985;9:63–68.
140. Landsberg L, Krieger DR. Obesity, metabolism and the sympathetic nervous system. Am J Hypertens 1989;2:125s–132s.
141. Young JB, Kaufman LN, Saville ME, Landsberg L. Increased sympathetic nervous system activity in rats fed a low protein diet: evidence against a role for dietary tyrosine. Am J Physiol 1985;248(5 Pt 2):R627–R637.
142. Rowe JW, Young BY, Minaker KL, Stevens AL, Pallatta J, Landsberg L. Effect of insulin and glucose infusions on sympathetic nervous system activity in normal human man. Diabetes 1981;30:219–225.
143. O'Hare JA, Minaker K, Young JB, Rowe JW, Pallotta JA, Landsberg L. Insulin increases plasma norepinephrine (NE) and lowers plasma potassium equally in lean and obese men (abstract). Clin Res 1985;33:441a.
144. Voors AW, Webber LS, Berenson GS. Resting heart rate and pressure-rate product of children in a total biracial community: the Bogalusa Heart Study. Am J Epidemiol 1982;116:276–286.
145. Jiang X, Srinivasan SR, Urbina E, Berenson GS. Hyperdynamic circulation and cardiovascular risk in children and adolescents: the Bogalusa Heart Study. Circulation 1995;91:1101–1106.
146. Riva P, Martini G, Rabbia F, Milan A, Paglieri C, Chiandussi L, Veglio F. Obesity and autonomic function in adolescents. Clin Exp Hypertens 2001;23:57–67.
147. Young JB, Macdonald IA. Sympathoadrenal activity in human obesity: heterogeneity of findings since 1980. Int J Obes 1992;16:959–967.
148. Elahi D, Sclater A, Waksmonski C, et al. Insulin resistance, sympathetic activity and cardiovascular function in obesity (abstract). Clin Res 1991;39:355a.
149. Elahi D, Krieger DR, Young JB, Landsberg L. Effects of somatostatin infusion on plasma or norepinephrine (NE) and cardiovascular function in men (abstract). Clin Res 1991;39:385a.
150. Sondergaard SB, Verdich C, Astrup A, Bratholm P, Christensen NJ. Obese male subjects show increased resting forearm venous plasma noradrenaline concentration but decreased 24-hour sympathetic activity as evaluated by thrombocyte noradrenaline measurements. Int J Obes Relat Metab Disord 1999;23:810–815.
151. Weyer C, Pratley RE, Snitker S, Spraul M, Ravussin E, Tataranni A. Ethnic differences in insulinemia and sympathetic tone as links between obesity and blood pressure. Hypertension 2000;36:531–542.
152. Krief S, Lonnquest F, Raimbault S. Tissue distribution of B3-adrenergic receptor RNA in man. J Clin Invest 1993;91:344–349.
153. Walston J, Silver K, Bogardus C, et al. Time of onset of non-insulin-dependent diabetes mellitus and genetic variation in the beta 3-adrenergic-receptor gene. N Eng J Med 1995;333(6):343–347.
154. Wheeldon NM, McDevitt DG, McFarlane LC, Lipworth BJ. Beta-adrenoceptor subtypes mediating the metabolic effects of BRL 35135 in man. Clinical Science 1994;86:331–337.
155. Licata G, Volpe M, Scanglione R, Rubattu S. Salt-regulating hormones in your normotensive obese subjects: effect of saline load. Hypertension 1994;3(Suppl I):120–124.
156. Maoz E, Shamiss A, Peleg E, Salzberg M, Rosenthal T. The role of atrial natriuretic peptide in the natriuresis of fasting. J Hypertens 1992:10:1041–1044.
157. Dessi-Fulgheri P, Sarzani R, Tamburrini P, et al. Plasma atrial natriuretic peptide and natriuretic peptide receptor gene expression in adipose tissue of normotensive and hypertensive obese patients. J Hypertens 1997;15:1695–1699.
158. Golden P, MacCagnan TJ, Pardridge WM. Human blood brain barrier leptin receptor binding and endocytosis in isolated human brain microvessels. J Clin Invest 1997;99:14–18.
159. Considine RV, Sinha MK, Heiman ML, Kriauciunas A, Stephens TW. Serum immunoreactive leptin concentrations in normal-weight and obese humans. N Engl J Med 1996;334:292–295.

160. Collins S, Kuhn CM, Petro AE, Swick AG, Chrunyk BA, Surwit RS. Role of leptin in fat regulation. Nature 1996;380:667.
161. Haynes WG, Morgan DA, Walsh SA, Mark AL, Sivitz WI. Receptor mediated regional sympathetic nerve activation by leptin. J Clin Invest 1997;100:270–278.
162. Shek EW, Brands MW, Hall JE. Chronic leptin infusion increases arterial pressure. Hypertension 1998;31: 409–414.
163. Ogawa Y, Masuzaki H, Aizawa M, et al. Blood pressure elevation in transgenic mice over-expressing leptin, the obe gene product. J Hypertens (abstract) 1989;16:S7.
164. Haynes WG, Morgan DA, Walsh SA, Sivitz W, Mark AL. Cardiovascular consequences of obesity: role of leptin. Clin Exp Pharmacol Physiol 1998;2565–2569.
165. Bjorntorp P, Rosmond R. Neuroendocrine abnormalities in visceral obesity. Int J Obes Relat Metab Disord 2000;24(Suppl 2):S80–S85.
166. Strain GW, Zumoff B, Strain JL. Cortisol production in obesity. Metabolism 1980;29:980–985.
167. Rosmond R, Dallman MF, Bjorntorp P. Stress-related cortisol secretion in men: relationships with abdominal obesity and endocrine, metabolic and hemodynamic abnormalities. J Clin Endocrinol Metab 1998;83: 1853–1859.
168. Kvist H, Chowdhury B, Grangard U, Tylen U, Sjostrom L. Total and visceral adipose tissue volumes derived from measurements with computed tomography in adult men and women. Predicative equations. Am J Clin Nutr 1988;48:1351–1361.
169. Rosmond R, Bjorntorp P. The interactions between hypothalamic-pituitary-adrenal axis activity, testosterone, insulin-like growth factor I and abdominal obesity with metabolism and blood pressure in man. Int J Obes Relat Metab Disord 1998;22:1184–1196.
170. Zahrezewska KE, Cusin J, Sainbury A, Pohner F, Jeanrenaud FR, Jeanrenaud B. Glucocorticoids are counterregulatory hormones to leptin. Towards an understanding of leptin resistance. Diabetes 1997;46:717–719.
171. Rosmond R, Holm G, Bjorntorp P. Food-induced cortisol secretion relation to anthropometric, metabolic and hemodynamic variables in men. Int J Obes Relat Metab Disord 2000;24:95–105.
172. Rosmond R, Chagnon YC, Holm G, et al. A glucocorticoid receptor gene marker is associated with abdominal obesity, leptin, and dysregulation of the hypothalamic-pituitary-adrenal axis. Obesity Research 2000; 8:211–218.
173. Weaver J, Hitman GA, Kopelaman PG. An association between a Bc/I restriction fragment length polymorphism of the glucocorticoid receptor gene locus and hyperinsulinemia in obese women. J Mol Endocrinol 1992;9:295–300.
174. Buemann B, Vohl MC, Chagnon M, et al. Abdominal visceral fat is associated with a Bc/I restriction fragment length polymorphism at the glucocorticoid receptor gene locus. Obes Res 1997;5:186–189.
175. Bjorntorp P, Rosmond R. Hypothalamic origin of the metabolic syndrome X. Ann N Y Acad Sci 1999;892;308–311.
176. Manson JE, Colditz GA, Stampfer MJ, et al. A prospective study of obesity and risk of coronary heart disease in women. N Engl J Med 1990;322:882–889.
177. Kotelainen ML. Adiposity, cardiac size and precursors of coronary atherosclerosis in 5 to 15 year old children: a retrospective study of 210 violent deaths. Int J Obesity 1997;21:691–697.
178. MacMahon SW, Wicken DEL, MacDonald GJ. Effect of weight loss on left ventricular mass, a randomized controlled trail in young overweight hypertensive patients. N Engl J Med 1985;314:334–339.
179. Alpert MA, Singh A, Terry BE, Kelly DL, Villarreal D, Mukerji V. Effect of exercise on left ventricular systolic function and reserve in morbid obesity. Am J Cardiol 1989;63:1478–1482.
180. De Divittis O, Fazio S, Petitto M, Maddalena G, Contaldo F, Mancini M. Obesity and cardiac function. Circulation 1981;64:477–482.
181. Alexander JK, Pettigrove JR. Obesity and congestive heart failure. Geriatrics 1967;22:101–108.
182. Raison HJ, Achimastos A, Bouthier J, London G, Safar M. Intravascular volume, extracellular fluid volume, and total body water in obese and non-obese hypertensive patients. Am J Cardiol 1983;51:165–170.
183. Reisin E, Frohlich ED, Messerli FH, et al. Cardiovascular changes after weight reduction in obesity hypertension. Ann Int Med 1983;98:315–319.
184. Lesser GT, Deutsch S. Measurement of adipose tissue blood flow and perfusion in man by uptake of 85-Kr. J Appl Physiol 1967;23:621–631.

185. Blake J, Devereux RB, Borer JS, Szulc M, Pappas TW, Laragh JH. Relation of obesity, high sodium intake, and eccentric left ventricular hypertrophy to left ventricular exercise dysfunction in essential hypertension. Am J Med 1990;88:477–485.
186. Guillerno E, Garavaglia E, Messerli FH, Nunez BD, Schmieder RE, Grossman E. Myocardial contractility and left ventricular function in obese patients with essential hypertension. Am J Cardiol 1988;62:594–597.
187. Stoddard MF, Tseuda K, Thomas M, Dillon S, Kupersmith J. The influence of obesity on left ventricular filing and systolic function. Am Heart J 1992;124:694–699.
188. Urbina EM, Gidding SS, Bao W, Pickoff AS, Berdusis K, Berenson GS. Effect of body size, ponderosity, and blood pressure on left ventricular growth in children and young adults in the Bogalusa Heart Study. Circulation 1995;91:2400–2406.
189. Daniels SR, Kimball TR, Morrison JA, Khoury P, Witt S, Meyer RA. Effect of lean body mass, fat mass, blood pressure, and sexual maturation on left ventricular mass in children and adolescents. Statistical, biological, and clinical significance. Circulation 1995;92:3249–3254.
190. Daniels SR, Loggie JM, Khoury P, Kimball TR. Left ventricular geometry and severe left ventricular hypertrophy in children and adolescents with essential hypertension. Circulation 1998;97:1907–1911.
191. Grossman E, Orren S, Messerli FH. Left ventricular filling in the systemic hypertension of obesity. Am J Cardiol 1991;60:57–60.
192. Schmeider RE, Messerli FH. Does obesity influence early target organ damage in hypertensive patients? Circulation 1993;87:1482–1488.
193. Harada L, Orino T, Takada G. Body mass index can predict left ventricular diastolic filling in asymptomatic obese children. Pediar Cardiol 2001;22:273–278.
194. Kanoupalis E, Michaloudis D, Fraidakis O, Parthenakis F, Vardas P, Melissas J. Left ventricular function and cardiopulmonary performance following surgical treatment of morbid obesity. Obes Surg 2001;11:552–558.
195. Messerli FH, Nunez BD, Ventura HO, Snyder DW. Overweight and sudden death: increased ventricular ectopy in cardiopathy in obesity. Arch Intern Med 1987;147:1725–1728.
196. Nakajima T, Fugiola S, Tokunaga K, Matsuzawa Y, Tami S. Correlation of intraabdominal fat accumulation and left ventricular performance in obesity. Am J Cardiol 1989;64:369–373.
197. Becque MD, Katch VL, Rocchini AP, Marks CR, Moorehead C. Coronary risk incidence of obese adolescents: reductions of exercise plus diet intervention. Pediatrics 1988;81:605–612.
198. Anderson P, Henriksson J. Capillary supply of the quadriceps femoris muscle of man: adaptive response to exercise. J Physiol 1977;270:677–690.
199. Chi MMY, Hintz CS, Henriksson J. Chronic stimulation of mammalian muscle: enzyme changes in individual fibers. Am J Physiol 1986;251:c633–c642.
200. Ryan DH, Bray GA, Helmcke F, et al. Serial echocardiographic and clinical evaluation of valvular regurgitation before, during, and after treatment with fenfluramine or dexfenfluramine and mazindol or phentermine. Obes Res 1999;7:313–322.
201. Beardwood DM, Alden JS, Graham CA, Beardwood JT Jr, Marble A. Evidence for a peripheral action of chlorothiazide in normal man. Metabolism 1965;14:561–567.
202. Gill JS, Al-Hussary N, Anderson DC. Effect of nifedipine on glucose tolerance, serum insulin, and serum fructosamine in diabetic patients. Clin Ther 1987;9:304–310.
203. Klauser R, Prager R, Gaube S, et al. Metabolic effects on isradipine versus hydrochlorothiazide in diabetes mellitus. Hypertension 1991;17:15–21.
204. Pollare T, Lithell H, Morlin C, Prantare H, Hvarfner A, Ljunghall S. Metabolic effects of diltiazem and atenolol: results from a randomized, double blind study with parallel groups. J Hypertens 1989;7:551–559.
205. Grunfeld CM, Chappell DA. Prevention of glucose intolerance of thiazide diuretics by maintenance of body potassium. Diabetes 1983;32:106–111.
206. Pollare T, Lithell H, Selinus I, Berne C. Application of prazosin is associated with an increase of insulin sensitivity in obese patients with hypertension. Diabetologia 1988;31:415–420.
207. Rocchini AP, Mao HZ, Babu K, Marker P, Rocchini AJ. Clonidine prevents insulin resistance and hypertension in obese dogs. Hypertension 1999;33(part II):548–553.
208. Giugliano D, Acampora R, Marfella R, et al. Hemodynamic and metabolic effects of transdermal clonidine in patients with hypertension and non-insulin dependent diabetes mellitus. Am J Hypertens 1998;11:184–189.
209. Fajans SS, Floyd JC Jr, Knopf RF, Rull J, Guntsche EM, Conn JW. Benthiadiazine suppression of insulin release from normal and abnormal islet cell tissue of a man. J Clin Invest 1966;45:481–492.

210. Amery A, Birkenhager W, Brixko P, et al. Glucose intolerance during diuretic therapy in elderly hypertensive patients. A second report from the European Working Party on high blood pressure in the elderly (EWPHE). Postgrad Med J 1986;62:919–924.
211. Morgan TO. Metabolic effects of various antihypertensive agents. J Cardiovascular Pharmacol 1990;15 (Suppl 5):s39–s45.
212. Bergtsson C, Blohme G, Lapidus L, et al. Do antihypertensive drugs precipitate diabetes? Br Med J (Clin Res Ed) 1984;289:1495–1497.
213. Greenberg G, Brennan PJ, Miall WE. Effects of diuretic and β-blocker therapy in the MRC trial. Am J Med 1984;76:45–51.
214. Gemma G, Montanari G, Suppa G, et al. Plasma lipid and lipoprotein changes in hypertensive patients treated with propranolol and prazosin. J Cardiovasc Pharmacol 1982;4(Suppl 2):S233–S237.
215. Ferdinand KC. Update in pharmacologic treatment of hypertension. Cardiol Clin 2001;19(2):279–294.
216. Kobayashi M, Iwanishi M, Egawa K, Shigeta Y. Pioglitazone increases insulin sensitivity by activation insulin receptor kinase. Diabetes 1992;41:476–483.
217. King AB. A comparison in a clinical setting of the efficacy and side effects of three thiazolidinediones. Diabetes Care 2000;23:557–558.
218. Wagenaar LJ, Kuck EM, Hoekstra JB. Troglitazone. Is it all over? Neth J Med1999;55(1):4–12.

# 19 Social Environments, Agonistic Stress, and Elevated Blood Pressure in Urban Youth

*Craig K. Ewart,* PhD

***Contents***



## INTRODUCTION

The social environment strongly affects cardiovascular (CV) health during childhood and adolescence *(1,2)*. An extensive scientific literature suggests that family living conditions and social and economic resources influence children's access to health care, their quality of care, and the development of behavior patterns (e.g., smoking, poor nutrition and weight control, sedentary lifestyle, emotional stress) that increase risk of hypertension (HTN) and cardiovascular disease (CVD). Among the known behavioral risk factors, environmentally induced emotional stress responses are perhaps the most provocative and least well understood contributors to CVD *(2)*. Recent research with urban adolescents provides promising insights into psychological mechanisms linking neighborhood environments with chronic stress and elevated blood pressure (BP). New evidence suggests that exposure to neighborhood poverty, disorder, and violence may undermine youths' social competence and encourage forms of interpersonal behavior that, although responsive to environmental demands, may impair emotion regulation capabilities, undermine social ties, and contribute to persistent CV stress and related illness.

From: *Clinical Hypertension and Vascular Disease: Pediatric Hypertension*
Edited by: R. J. Portman, J. M. Sorof, and J. R. Ingelfinger © Humana Press Inc., Totowa, NJ

## RELATIONSHIPS BETWEEN SOCIOECONOMIC STATUS AND HEALTH

Socioeconomic status (SES) is defined in terms of personal resources and prestige *(3)*. Resources are typically indexed by measures of income, wealth, and educational attainment; prestige (or social status) refers to a person's access to goods, services, and knowledge, and is usually measured by occupation and education. SES can be measured at the level of the individual, household, neighborhood, or wider community. Although individual-level indices are often used, neighborhood-level indices predict health outcomes beyond this *(1)*.

Epidemiologic research in the US and other industrial nations indicates that SES is associated with a wide range of health outcomes *(4)*. This is partly explained by differences in access to health care, nutrition, and other resources. Yet the association is not limited to groups living in poverty. Differences in health outcomes show a monotonic relationship to SES; even at the highest levels of income, better health is associated with greater affluence. Emotional stress and related disorders have been proposed as a possible explanation *(5)*.

It is important to note that some SES indices, such as income and occupation, may be affected by *reverse causation*—that is, emotional problems or illness may cause a decline in SES. Although researchers usually assume that social conditions affect health outcomes, the possibility that health problems cause people to "drift downward" in socioeconomic standing must be considered *(1)*.

## SOCIOECONOMIC STATUS AND CHILDREN'S CARDIOVASCULAR HEALTH

A recent review of the literature on SES and health in childhood finds strong support for a childhood SES effect; as in adulthood, decreases in SES are associated monotonically with increases in children's health problems *(2)*. This relationship exists across all causes of child mortality, as well as across a variety of acute illnesses (e.g., pneumonia, influenza, injury) and chronic health conditions (e.g., asthma, vision and hearing disorders, blood lead levels). With decreasing SES, children are less likely to see a physician, and more likely to be treated in emergency departments and hospitalized, associations that again display a monotonic effect. As SES drops, rates of cigarette smoking, exposure to tobacco smoke, and sedentary lifestyles increase.

Patterns of relationships between SES and health outcomes may change over the course of development, a fact that tends to be obscured in cross-sectional studies. The relationship between SES and smoking is strongest in adolescence, for example, suggesting an "adolescent-emergent" pattern. BP presents a somewhat complicated picture, with the association between BP and SES appearing strong throughout childhood until approximately age 13 yr. During the teenage years, the relationship is not significant. Existing data do not clearly demonstrate whether BP of lower SES children improves in adolescence, or if BP of higher SES children worsens during this period. An inverse relationship between SES and BP is apparent in adulthood, and childhood BP predicts adult BP 20–30 yr later. This pattern might be explained by a common adolescent culture that homogenizes youth during the high school years, temporarily obscuring the effects of SES *(6)*. Physical inactivity has been found to be related to SES only in adolescence (among youth aged 12 yr and older), suggesting preliminary support for an adolescent-emergent model.

In addition to SES, it is important to consider the role of race in shaping health outcomes. In the US, African-American and Hispanic families have lower average incomes than Caucasian families. Although minority groups have made economic gains in recent decades, the gains have been small relative to Caucasians; these economic differences are associated with substantial health care gaps *(7)*. Despite these differences, studies comparing the health effects of SES and race have found that SES is significantly related to child health, even after controlling for race. Moreover, similar monotonic associations between SES and blood pressure are found in both African American and Caucasian children *(8)*. Therefore, although race is an important factor in children's health, SES is not merely a proxy for race. Both SES and race contribute to illness risk in childhood, and each must be considered.

## HOW DOES SOCIOECONOMIC STATUS AFFECT CARDIOVASCULAR HEALTH IN YOUTH?

Recent reviews have proposed a variety of mechanisms by which SES might influence CV health during childhood and adolescence *(1,2,9)*. Low-SES women are more likely to smoke during pregnancy, and smoking is associated with lower infant birthweight and slower growth in childhood *(10)*. Health information is often less available as SES declines. People in very poor neighborhoods also have less contact with others, smaller social networks, and less social support *(11)*. Lower levels of social support curtail opportunities for help with behavioral lifestyle modification; moreover, reduced supportive contacts are associated with cardiovascular, neuroendocrine, and immune changes that increase CVD risk *(12)*. Aspects of impoverished neighborhood environments can affect health also. Residents of lower SES neighborhoods report more stressful life events, and have higher blood lead levels *(13)*. In neighborhoods characterized by disorder and decay, neighbors are less able to monitor and protect children, or to curb behaviors that threaten safety and health *(14)*. Lower SES families also have fewer health care options, make fewer physician visits, and are less compliant with medical recommendations *(13)*. Crowded living conditions have been associated with higher resting BP in boys *(15)*.

## SOCIOECONOMIC STATUS, EMOTIONAL STRESS, AND BLOOD PRESSURE

Much has been learned in recent years about behavioral and biological mechanisms through which cigarette smoking, consumption of dietary fats and sodium, and levels of physical exercise may adversely affect CV health. Far less is known about how environmentally induced emotional stress increases risk. Growing evidence suggests that negative emotions can damage the CV system. Emotional processes related to hostility, anger, and depression have been shown to generate physiologic changes linked to increased CV morbidity and mortality, including dysregulation of the hypothalamic–pituitary–adrenocortical axis, hyperactivity of the sympathetic adrenal-medullary (SAM) system, reduced heart rate (HR) variability, increased platelet reactivity, heightened inflammatory processes, and stress-induced ischemia *(16–18)*. The *metabolic syndrome*, a clustering of disorders involving insulin resistance, hyperglycemia, dislipidemia, visceral obesity, and hypertension *(19,20)*, confers substantial risk of CVD and non-insulin-dependent diabetes *(21,22)*. A number of studies have linked individual components of metabolic syndrome separately to hostility *(23)*; including positive relationships between hostility and CVD risk factors such as fasting insulin and glucose *(24,25)*, waist-to-hip ratio (WHR) *(24,26)*, body mass index (BMI) *(27,28)*, hypertension *(29,31)*, and cholesterol *(28,32–34)*. A recent meta-analysis of 45 studies found that hostility was an independent risk factor for coronary heart disease (CHD), with a weighted mean of $r = .18$ *(17)*, an effect size equal to or greater in magnitude than those reported for CHD risk factors such as elevated serum cholesterol, elevated BP, and cigarette smoking *(35)*.

The possible links between SES, emotional stress, and risk factors such as elevated BP thus deserve greater attention. Gallo and Matthews reviewed evidence for relationships between SES, health outcomes, "maladaptive emotions" (ones that are inappropriate, frequent, intense), and "emotional disorders" (syndromes comprising a cluster of symptoms, behaviors, and affective processes) *(1)*. Their review focused on depression, hopelessness, anxiety, and hostility–anger. They found that evidence for a relationship between SES and negative emotions was especially strong in the case of depressive, hopeless, anxious, and hostile symptoms, with some evidence for a link between SES and depressive and anxiety disorders. Low SES is associated with higher levels of hostility, which has been linked to CHD incidence, mortality, and severity in adults *(17)* and increased left ventricular (LV) mass and heightened cardiovascular reactivity (CVR) in African-American children *(36)*. Low SES is also associated with higher levels of hopelessness and depression in adults. In children and adolescents, lower SES is associated with hostile attribution bias, a tendency to attribute another person's ambiguous actions to hostile intent *(37)*. This bias has been shown to mediate the relationship between low SES and CVR in youth *(38)*. Hostility and depression gradually increase during childhood, suggesting that they may exert the greatest influence on health outcomes during adolescence.

The evidence for an association between negative emotions and health was reviewed also. Research into relationships between maladaptive emotions and emotional disorders suggests that a variety of negative emotions predict health outcomes; the evidence is most compelling for the effects of depression, hopelessness, and hostility on CV morbidity and mortality, and for anxiety on risk of sudden cardiac death. Evidence for an association between hostility and all-cause mortality is especially strong. It should be noted that these associations were observed in initially healthy populations as well as in individuals with diagnosed CVD. Moreover, a number of the studies reviewed suggested a dose–response relationship between emotional symptoms and health risks. The weight of the evidence indicates that SES is consistently related to negative emotions, and that health outcomes worsen as symptoms of negative emotion increase *(1)*.

Negative emotions appear to affect health through several interrelated behavioral and physiological pathways. These include direct effects of emotional arousal on physiologic processes (e.g., cardiovascular, immune, and metabolic function), as well as indirect effects through health-damaging behaviors. Depressed people are more likely to smoke and less likely to exercise *(39)*. High levels of hostility and anxiety in youth increase the probability that young people will engage in health-damaging behaviors later in life *(2)*. But this research has also shown that such health practices do not entirely account for the association between negative emotions and disease *(1)*. The evidence argues for multicomponent longitudinal models that, in addition to positing a direct causal role for emotion, allow for the possibility of bidirectional relationships in which emotions can cause and be caused by disease, and also consider that the psychosocial aspects of low SES environments do not affect health exclusively through emotional paths *(1,2)*. Low-SES environments also directly affect behavioral and biological mechanisms that influence health *(40)*.

## HOW MIGHT LOW SOCIOECONOMIC STATUS IMPAIR EMOTION REGULATION?

If SES affects health by influencing emotion regulation, how might this process work? To address this question, it is necessary to clarify what is meant by "emotion," a term that has been applied to a wide array of affective phenomena, ranging from mild feelings of contentment or unease to intense and complex episodes of rage, joy, or grief. Many investigators emphasize the episodic and multifaceted nature of emotions *(41,42)*. Emotion episodes are triggered by external or internal events of major importance to the individual, and consist of coordinated changes in physiologic arousal, motor behavior (expression), and subjective feeling, as well as in the cognitive processes involved in evaluating the triggering events and in regulating ongoing emotions *(43)*. An emotion episode lasts for a limited period and gradually fades away.

The multifaceted nature of emotion has given rise to disagreements about definition, conceptualization, and measurement. Different theories of emotion often appear to disagree because they address different parts of the emotion process—for example, "appraisal" models tend to focus on the cognitive triggers at the "front end" of the episode, whereas neural circuitry models tend to focus on the final adaptive response pattern, or "back end," of the process *(43)*. Other disagreements reflect failures to distinguish between "emotions" and "moods." Emotions are relatively brief episodes of synchronized responses to events judged to be of major significance; examples include fear, anger, sadness, shame, joy, and pride. Moods are diffuse affective states characterized primarily by changes in subjective feeling. Moods tend to be of lower intensity than emotions, of longer duration, and often have no apparent cause, as when one feels irritable, gloomy, listless, cheerful, or euphoric *(43)*. Moods and emotions may be interconnected—for example, moods may bias cognitive appraisal processes that trigger emotion episodes.

## REGULATING STRESSFUL EMOTIONS

Single episodes of emotion, while capable of raising BP or altering immune responses temporarily, are too brief to cause the lasting physiologic changes associated with a chronic disease like HTN. Instead, the effects of emotion are probably cumulative. Pathogenetic changes occur only after a persistent failure to regulate emotions has caused negative arousal to become frequent and prolonged. Important clues to unraveling the mystery of stress-related illness may lie in understanding the processes by which emotions are regulated, and in identifying factors that impair regulation and prolong stress exposure.

Emotions can be regulated by altering the antecedent conditions that elicit affect at the front-end phase of an emotion episode, or by modifying the physiologic and behavioral responses that follow at the back end *(44)*. One may try to control anxiety, for example, by avoiding threatening situations or trying to alter them by diverting one's attention to less threatening aspects of the situation, or by construing the situation differently, thereby changing its meaning. An important class of antecedent regulation mechanisms targets cognitive attribution processes, as when one copes with a bout of nerves by attributing a racing pulse to "excitement" rather than to debilitating fear. When antecedent control fails, regulation of emotion may be achieved through back-end response-focused maneuvers that target the behavioral manifestations of affect. Anxiety, for example, may be moderated by inducing competing physiologic responses through progressive muscle relaxation.

Stressful emotions often have no external trigger, but arise from internal stimuli involving distressing trains of thought. Research on the sociocognitive origins of emotional stress suggests that chronic stress results less from the frequency of emotionally unpleasant events than from a perceived inability to effect emotion regulation through behavioral, cognitive, and affective control *(45)*. Studies of anxiety and depression reveal that interventions to increase self-perceived ability (self-efficacy) to control thoughts, through mechanisms of attention or construing, are effective in reducing anxiety and the frequency of intrusive negative thoughts. Raising self-efficacy to modulate stressful responses through relaxation lowers stress *(45)*.

This research suggests that sustained emotional stress may result from a self-perceived inability to regulate negative emotions.

## AGONISTIC STRIVING IMPAIRS EMOTION REGULATION CAPABILITIES

The ability to regulate stressful emotions is part of the more general construct of social–economic competence (SEC), defined broadly as the ability to select and pursue desired, attainable goals by controlling one's actions and emotions, and by understanding, relating to, and influencing others *(46)*. Recent studies of "emotional adaptiveness" and "emotional intelligence" in children and adults suggest that SEC affects developmental outcomes throughout the life span *(47)*. SEC in youth has been found to influence peer relationships and school success, for example *(48,49)*.

A Social Competence Model (SCM) of emotion regulation, chronic stress exposure, and CVD risk in youth has been developed from the research of "Project Heart," a series of community-based studies conducted in public high schools in Baltimore, supported by the National Heart, Lung, and Blood Institute (NHLBI). This research tested the hypothesis that impaired emotion regulation related to interpersonal conflict and persistent environmental stress induces chronic emotional arousal and elevates CV risk factors (e.g., BP, lipid profiles) in urban youth. In the first Project Heart study (PH1; 1987–1991), a preliminary version of the SCM *(50)* of stress exposure was developed along with a behavioral assessment procedure, the Social Competence Interview (SCI), to measure hypothesized dimensions of social–emotional competence *(46,51)*. Initial studies with the SCI showed that adolescents' CVR to the interview procedure, assessed by measuring changes in BP and HR, were greater in youths whose stress narratives disclosed recurring interpersonal conflict *(52)*. Moreover, higher levels of emotional lability and frequent anger were associated with elevated ambulatory BP in African-American and Caucasian boys *(53)*. Subsequent research (PH2; 1992–1995) revealed that, in girls, heightened CVR during the SCI was associated with "sociotropic" stress (emotional distress over being disliked or rejected by peers) *(54,55)*.

Research building on this work identified distinct patterns of social–emotional and interpersonal skill deficits that are associated with recurring stress. SCI data from stress interviews with more than 700 adolescents revealed three major groups of youth. One group experiences recurring emotional arousal related to other-directed goals (e.g., attempts to defend oneself from attack or to win sympathy, support, or affection), whereas a second group of youth report stress related to self-directed goals (i.e., attempts to achieve a valued performance standard, experience, or personal quality). Goals of the first type represent what we have called "agonistic striving," defined as struggle that pits one's personal needs, desires, or tendencies against those of others. Goals of the second type represent what we have labeled "transcendence striving," defined as a struggle to rise above or to move beyond one's present state or condition. Agonistic striving is associated with increased interpersonal conflict and stress.

Although the SCM highlights the agonistic and transcendent stress patterns, the SCI data from PH1 and PH2 also revealed a third group of youths who reported problems with other people, but who were reserved and emotionally unexpressive during the SCI, and gave little sign of an active agonistic struggle to influence those who caused them stress. We have labeled this third group "avoidant."

A further study in the Project Heart series (PH3; 1995–2000) compared social skills, CVR (to stress interview), and ambulatory BP in groups of youths who exhibited the agonistic, transcendent, and avoidant stress patterns, in a high school sample that included 212 African-

American (66% of sample) and Caucasian participants. Stress narratives obtained with the SCI were coded by trained observers to yield indices of social–emotional competence *(56)*.

Results disclosed that youths with the agonistic coping profile believed themselves less capable of solving recurrent problems than did peers who displayed the transcendent profile. Ratings provided independently by the trained observers supported these misgivings; the proposed problem-solving strategies of youths in the agonistic group were judged comparatively unrealistic and ineffective. Moreover, the possibility that youths exhibiting the agonistic profile might be treated more negatively by others was supported by the observers' ratings of hostile social impact. Youths in the agonistic group were rated as appearing more aggressive, guarded, or "oppositional" during the interview, suggesting that those with the agonistic pattern may provoke negative responses from others, and may therefore experience a stressful social environment.

Significant group differences were also evident in CV responses recorded during the SCI. Youths with the agonistic profile exhibited larger increases in total peripheral resistance (TPR) when discussing their problems than did youths with the transcendent profile, possibly reflecting increased vasoconstriction associated with greater interpersonal distress *(57)*.

Implications for long-term CV health were suggested by the 24-h ambulatory BP levels, which are known to be more strongly associated with indices of CV dysfunction and to have greater prognostic value than casual readings taken in a clinic setting *(58,59)*. Group comparisons disclosed that, as predicted, the agonistic group exhibited higher mean elevations of BP, suggesting greater CVD risk, than did youths in the other groups. The mean diastolic BP of adolescents in the agonistic group was significantly higher than the diastolic BP of peers in the lower-risk transcendent group when readings were averaged over all waking hours, and was higher than the diastolic BP of both the transcendent and avoidant groups in social situations when the adolescent interacted with others (this difference remained significant even after possible artifacts of body posture and movement were excluded). The fact that ambulatory *diastolic* pressure discriminated between the groups is consistent with the interpretation that CV responses of agonistic youths during the SCI reflect increased systemic vasoconstriction.

## HOW DOES LOWER SOCIOECONOMIC STATUS FOSTER AGONISTIC BEHAVIOR?

The Project Heart studies suggest that, in adolescents, agonistic striving is associated with diminished social–emotional competence, heightened CVR to interpersonal stress, and elevated ambulatory BP. The data obtained in Project Heart using the SCI are consistent with data from adult samples that link interview-based measures of hostility to CHD *(17)*. Is there evidence that associations between SES and increased CVD risk might be explained, in part, by heightened agonistic striving? Research on connections between neighborhood disorder, exposure to violence, and child health problems suggest that this might be the case. This research suggests that lower SES environments may induce defensive states of interpersonal vigilance that intensify and prolong emotions of anxiety and anger, undermine social ties, and thereby impair ability to regulate emotional stress.

Data showing that residents of low-income neighborhoods encounter more difficulties and daily hassles support this hypothesis; increased hardship reduces the "reserve capacity" for coping *(1)*. Investigators of the effects of neighborhood environments on health have proposed that community SES may affect health through three complementary but distinct pathways *(14)*. These pathways include institutional resources (e.g., quantity or quality of educational and employment opportunities), social relationships and ties (e.g., family and network characteristics), and community norms and collective efficacy (e.g., organizations, peer groups, physical threats). All are compatible with the view that living in an impoverished neighborhood may increase agonistic striving.

### *Inadequate Institutional Resources*

People who live in lower SES neighborhoods have fewer employment opportunities. Those who are able to find work report lower job status, less control over the work process, and higher levels of job stress than do residents of more affluent communities. The former also tend to be at the lower end of social status hierarchies in the workplace *(60,61)*. Adults who thus experience more negative interpersonal interactions at work may develop an agonistic orientation and convey this to neighborhood youth.

### *Impaired Social Relationships and Ties*

The difficulty of coping from day to day may exhaust parents' energy and induce negative moods (fatigue, irritability) that foster hostile attribution biases *(9)*. Residents of lower SES communities are more prone to marital conflict, which can model agonistic behavior to children *(62)*. Increased hardship also reduces parents' coping alternatives, and this may curtail opportunities for children to observe effective emotion regulation skills and strategies, or to see the value of perseverance in pursuit of long-range goals (transcendent focus) *(45)*.

Finally, lower SES parents have been found to display less parental warmth and to use harsher discipline than parents in higher SES communities *(63,64)*. The former tend to exercise "authoritarian" control, use more restrictive parenting practices, and are more verbally aggressive toward their children *(65,66)*. Although these practices may protect children from many immediate dangers (e.g., by ensuring that children comply promptly with parental restrictions in threatening circumstances), harsh parenting may model an agonistic outlook and interpersonal style.

### *Peer Group Norms and Activities*

Children in lower SES neighborhoods are more often exposed to violence in the community, and are more likely to be influenced by aggressive peers than are children who live in higher SES neighborhoods *(67)*. The threat of violence can foster involvement in peer group activities (e.g., gangs) that induce chronic interpersonal vigilance and aggressiveness associated with the agonistic profile.

## HOW DOES AGONISTIC STRIVING FOSTER PERSISTENT STRESS?

The SCM proposes that environmentally induced agonistic striving impairs emotion regulation and undermines social relationships, conserving and amplifying the emotional impact of daily hassles. More specifically, the model suggests that an agonistic interpersonal focus impedes emotion regulation by disrupting behavioral, cognitive, and response-based control processes. Research on social cognition identifies a number of mechanisms through which interpersonal conflicts and struggles may impair emotion regulation capabilities and induce chronic health-damaging arousal.

### *Interpersonal Control*

It is more difficult to control another person's actions than to control one's own behavior. During a challenging interpersonal encounter, coping is interdependent; each person's action elicits a response from the other that, in turn, shapes further responses *(68)*. When trying to influence another person, it is necessary to monitor and evaluate the other's behavior as well as one's own. Moreover, efforts to influence or control others often evoke negative counter responses that, in turn, generate new threats that must be controlled. The need to attend simultaneously to self and other can tax cognitive information processing resources and reduce one's ability to monitor and modulate emotional responses *(69)*.

Some interpersonal threats can be difficult to discern or alter. An example is "stereotype threat," in which a member of a stereotyped social group expects to be judged by a negative (e.g., racist) group stereotype *(70)*. In such circumstances, it may be difficult to know if those with whom one is interacting subscribe to the stereotype, or to know how to disprove it. Stereotype threat has been shown to induce negative affect and to impair performance on cognitive tasks *(71–73)*. One recent experiment compared the BP responses of African Americans and whites while they performed a cognitive task under threat or no-threat conditions *(74)*. The African Americans in the stereotype threat condition exhibited impaired task performance and increased BP relative both to the whites and to the African Americans who were not exposed to stereotype threat.

## *Cognitive Control*

Interpersonal challenges may impair the cognitive processing of social information, thus inducing and prolonging stressful arousal. The SCM identifies a set of social cognitive mechanisms that impair emotional control under these circumstances.

### Heightened Interpersonal Vigilance

During a challenging encounter, one must simultaneously formulate a response, monitor the other person's reaction, and prepare an appropriate counter-response, in a continuous sequence of moves and counter moves. This induces active coping, which has been associated with increased cardiac output *(75)*, and which fosters a mental state of alert vigilance known to elicit heightened systemic vasoconstriction *(76,77)*. This state of vigilance does not necessarily cease after the encounter has ended, however. The experience may trigger recollection of similar past events and contemplation of possible future scenarios *(78)*. Such thinking may help one identify possible threats and envision ways to cope. Yet it may also lead one to imagine the many unpleasant things that others might say or do, and give rise to trains of disturbing rumination that prolong and intensify emotional arousal and elevate blood pressure long after the initial exchange has ended *(79,80)*.

### Biased Information Processing

Interpersonal challenges often call for an immediate response, and proper timing can be critical. Yet preparing oneself to recognize threats and respond quickly may negatively bias the processing of social information. Readiness to detect imminent danger is enhanced by a low threshold for judging threat. Yet a lower threshold for alarm reduces perceptual specificity. Avoiding the danger of unnoticed threats (false negatives) raises the likelihood that one will misconstrue a neutral or even friendly act as hostile (false positive). The result is a perception of the interpersonal world as dangerous, leading to more frequent episodes of negative emotion. A lowered threshold for threat detection contributes to the "hostile attribution bias" of highly aggressive children who tend to misconstrue ambiguous acts of unfamiliar peers as hostile *(37)*. Such bias is associated with increased negative affect and CVR to challenges even in children who are not highly aggressive *(38)*.

### Attribution Errors

Hostile attribution bias also may contribute to the "fundamental attribution error," or tendency to ascribe another's hostile actions to enduring personal traits rather than situational circumstances *(81)*. This error involves a two-step process: first, the perceiver evaluates another's behavior negatively; then, the perceiver considers possible situational explanations *(82)*. When a perceiver is emotionally aroused (e.g., feeling threatened), the process can be cut short. The perceiver makes the initial judgment that the other's behavior is hostile but fails subsequently to consider possible situational explanations (e.g., the annoying individual may be having a bad day). The perceiver mistakenly concludes that the other person isfundamentally and perpetually hostile, and that future encounters with this individual will therefore be equally unpleasant, when this may not necessarily be the case.

### Error-Prone Cognitive Heuristics

Negative ruminations about interpersonal threats involve mentally replaying stressful encounters or envisioning possible future scenarios. Such rumination may be productive when it discloses more effective ways to handle similar challenges in the future. Yet, if an effective coping response fails to emerge, rumination may have the unfortunate consequence of heightening the mental vividness and cognitive availability of possible dangers. Heightened cognitive availability has been shown to increase the likelihood that imagined events will actually occur *(83)*. Rumination about past encounters may also involve "counterfactual thinking" (e.g., "If only I had said . . . ") *(84)*. Again, counterfactual thinking may reveal better ways to handle future challenges, but can also heighten awareness of past failures and reduce one's confidence and ability to cope.

### Negative Priming Effects

Ruminations about interpersonal threats may increase a sense of personal danger by giving rise to negative "priming." This occurs when a cognitive predisposition to detect possible threats increases the likelihood that a perceiver will notice something unpleasant about another person *(85)*. If the first thing the perceiver notices is negative, albeit minor, this initial negative perception is likely to bias subsequent perceptions in an unfavorable direction by preventing the perceiver from noticing the person's more positive qualities. This is especially likely when the perceiver is tired or emotionally stressed *(86)*. Afterward, the mere act of thinking about the person may bring the negative perceptions to mind and thereby convince the perceiver that the hostile impressions are accurate *(87)*.

### Negative Stereotyping

Negative rumination may contribute to group stereotyping. When angry at or frightened by someone, a perceiver is more likely to infer that all persons who resemble that individual, even in trivial ways, may share that person's negative qualities or hostile intentions *(88)*. Such stereotyping can magnify the apparent threat by multiplying the number of people who thereafter may be perceived as dangerous. The perception that one is personally threatened at all times by large social groups or classes, rather than by certain individuals under specific circumstances, may contribute to a sense of isolation, powerlessness, victimization, and lowered self-esteem. Under such threats, efforts to rebuild self-esteem can take the form of disparaging social out-groups and favoring one's own in-group *(89)*. All too often, an unfriendly interpersonal world is the cost of repaired self esteem, and may lead to behavior that elicits hostility from others in a "self-fulfilling prophecy" *(90)*.

### *Response Control*

Exerting influence in a difficult social encounter may require one to engage in "impression management" by concealing negative emotional reactions or striving to present a socially appropriate facade *(91)*. It is often helpful to suppress affective responses that could undermine a desired image. Emotional suppression, while tactically useful, can impose physiologic costs. Concealment of anxiety and revulsion aroused by films of injuries has been shown to raise BP levels during stress exposure, reduce positive affect, and cause one to be perceived more negatively by others *(92)*. These difficulties magnify perceived dangers and undermine confident regulation of distressing affect. Lowered self-efficacy for coping contributes to negative emotions and intrusive thoughts that maintain arousal when threats are not present *(45)*.

## CONCLUSIONS AND IMPLICATIONS

The SCM posits that low-SES neighborhoods expose children and adolescents to an array of environmental stressors that may foster agonistic stress involving heightened vigilance, interpersonal conflict, impaired emotion regulation, and the disruption of social ties. Agonistic stress fosters patterns of thought and behavior that, while responsive to immediate environmental demands, unfortunately conserve and amplify negative emotional responses that contribute to persistent physiologic stress. In youths susceptible to chronic diseases such as essential HTN, persistent emotional stress owing to impaired emotion regulation and disrupted social ties may accelerate disease progression *(50,93)*.

The SCM specifies social cognitive mechanisms through which these processes may operate, and thereby advances understanding of pediatric illness and suggests directions for preventive interventions. One of our early studies of stress in urban youth was a clinical trial of progressive muscle relaxation to lower BP in black and white high school students at increased HTN risk *(94)*. At the end of the 3-mo study, adolescent participants in the experimental condition enjoyed practicing relaxation exercises in school, mastered the technique, and achieved lower BPs relative to the controls in laboratory assessments.. But practice of relaxation was difficult to maintain over time; at a later follow-up the BPs of experimental and control groups did not differ. Subsequent SCM analysis suggests that a broader approach, targeting cognitive front-end antecedent emotional triggers as well as back-end relaxation responses, may be needed. The SCM highlights the importance of altering social perception processes, enhancing interpersonal skills, and addressing the personal goals and strivings that guide youths' social interactions and shape their emotional responses. We are currently researching youths' day-to-day interpersonal encounters and the cognitive, affective, and CV responses that these experiences evoke. This research utilizes experience sampling using electronic diaries and is designed to help youth identify sources of personal stress and modulate emotions by improving interpersonal skills and building supportive social ties.

Finally, preventive measures aimed at children and adolescents require supportive interventions targeting communities and institutions. Experimental and quasi-experimental studies of neighborhood environments have randomly selected families to receive assistance in relocating to better public housing, or to receive vouchers to rent homes in more advantaged neighborhoods *(95)*. Children who moved to less-impoverished neighborhoods were found to enjoy better health and school achievement relative to peers who remained where they were *(96)*. Multilevel approaches to building key social and emotion-regulation skills within supportive neighborhood, school, and other institutional contexts promise the most success in promoting youths' CV health *(97,98)*.

## ACKNOWLEDGMENT

Preparation of this manuscript was supported in part by a grant from the Center for Health and Behavior, Syracuse University, and by grant R01-HL52080 from the National Heart, Lung, and Blood Institute, Bethesda, Maryland.

## REFERENCES

1. Gallo LC, Matthews KA. Understanding the association between socioeconomic status and physical health: do negative emotions play a role? Psychol Bull 2003;129:10–51.
2. Chen E, Matthews KA, Boyce WT. Socioeconomic differences in children's health: how and why do these relationships change with age? Psychol Bull 2002;128:295–329.
3. Lynch J, Kaplan G. Socioeconomic position. In: Berkman LF, Kawachi I, eds. Social Epidemiology. New York: Oxford University Press, 2000;13–35.
4. Adler NE, Marmot M, McEwen BS, Stewart J, eds. Socioeconomic Status and Health in Industrialized Nations. Ann N Y Acad Sci No. 896. New York: New York Academy of Sciences, 1999.
5. Kaplan G, Keil JE. Socioeconomic factors and cardiovascular disease: a review of the literature. Circulation 1993;88:1973–1998.
6. West P. Health inequalities in the early years: is there equalisation in youth? Soc Sci Med. 1997;44:833–858.
7. Williams DR, Yu Y, Jackson JS, Anderson NB. Racial differences in physical and mental health: socioeconomic status, stress, and discrimination. J Health Psychol 1997;2:335–351.
8. Walter HJ, Hofman A. Socioeconomic status, ethnic origin, and risk factors for coronary heart disease in children. Am Heart J. 1987;113:812–818.
9. Repetti RL, Taylor SE, Seeman T. Risky families: family social environments and the mental and physical health of offspring. Psychol Bull 2002;128:330–336.
10. Gazmararian JA, Adams MM, Pamuk ER. Associations between measures of socioeconomic status and maternal health behavior. Am J Prev Med 1996;12:108–115.
11. Bosma H, Van de Mheen HD, Mackenbach JP. Social class in childhood and general health in adulthood: questionnaire study of contribution of psychological attributes. Br Med J 1999;318:18–22.
12. Uchino BN, Cacioppo JT, Kiecolt-Glaser JK. The relationship between social support and physiological processes: a review with emphasis on underlying mechanisms and implications for health. Psychol Bull 1996;119:488–531.
13. Pamuk ER, Makuc D, Heck K, Reuben C, Lochner K. Socioeconomic status and health chartbook: Health, United States, 1998. Hyattsville, MD: National Center for Health Statistics, 1998.
14. Leventhal T, Brooks-Gunn J. The neighborhoods they live in: the effects of neighborhood residence on child and adolescent outcomes. Psychol Bull 2000;126:309–337.
15. Evans GW, Lepore SJ, Shejwal BR, Palsane MN. Chronic residential crowding and children's well-being: an ecological perspective. Child Dev 1998;69:1514–1523.
16. Krantz DS, McCeney MK. Effects of psychological and social factors on organic disease: a critical assessment of research on coronary heart disease. Annu Rev Psychol 2002;53:341–369.
17. Miller TQ, Smith TW, Turner CW, Guijarro ML, Hallet AJ. Meta-analytic review of research on hostility and physical health. Psychol Bull 1996;119:322–348.
18. Van Kanel R, Mills PJ, Fainman C, Dimsdale JE. Effects of psychological stess and psychiatric disorders on blood coagulation and fibrinolysis: a biobehavioral pathway to coronary artery disease. Psychosom Med 2001;63:531–544.
19. Kissebah AH, Krakower GR. Regional adiposity and morbidity. Physiol Rev 1994;74:761–811.
20. Timar O, Sestier F, Levy E. Metabolic syndrome X: a review. Can J Cardiol 2000;16:779–789.
21. Bjorntorp P. "Portal" adipose tissue as a generator of risk factors for cardiovascular disease and diabetes. Arteriosclerosis 1990;10:493–496.
22. Lebovitz HE. Insulin resistance: definition and consequences. Exp Clin Endocrinol Diabetes 2001;109: S135–S148.
23. Niaura R, Todaro JF, Stroud L, Spiro III A, Ward KD, Weiss S. Hostility, the metabolic syndrome, and incident coronary heart disease. Health Psychol 2002;21:588–593.
24. Niaura R, Banks SM, Warad KD, Stoney CM, Spiro III A, Aldwin CM. Hostility and the metabolic syndrome in older males: the Normative Aging Study. Psychosom Med 2000;62:7–16.

25. Vitaliano PP, Scanlan JM, Krenz C, Fujimoto W. Insulin and glucose: relationships with hassles, anger, and hostility in nondiabetic older adults. Psychosom Med 1996;58:489–499.
26. Scherwitz LW, Perkins LL, Chesney MA, Hughes GH, Sidney S, Manolio TA. Hostility and health behaviors in young adults: the CARDIA Study (Coronary Artery Risk Development in Young Adults Study). Am J Epidemiol 1992;136:136–145.
27. Houston BK, Vavak CR. Cynical hostility: developmental factors, psychosocial correlates, and health behaviors. Health Psychol 1991;10:9–17.
28. Siegler IC, Peterson BL, Barefoot JC, Williams RB. Hostility during late adolescence predicts coronary risk factors at mid-life. Am J Epidemiol 1992;136:146–154.
29. Barefoot JC, Dahlstrom WG, Williams RB. Hostility, CHD incidence, and total mortality: a 25-year follow-up study of 255 physicians. Psychosom Med 1983;51:46–57.
30. Barefoot JC, Dodge KA, Peterson BL, Dahlstrom WG, Williams RB, Jr. The Cook-Medley Hostility Scale: item content and ability to predict survival. Psychosom Med 1989;51:46–57.
31. Irvine J, Garner DM, Craig HM, Logan AG. Prevalence of Type A behavior in untreated hypertensive individuals. Hypertension 1991;18:72–78.
32. Dujovne VF, Houston BK. Hostility-related variables and plasma lipid levels. J Behav Med 1991;14:553–563.
33. Lundberg U, Hedman M, Melin B, Frankenhauser M. Type A behavior in healthy males and females as related to physiological activity and blood lipids. Psychosom Med 1989;49:112–122.
34. Weidner G, Sexton G, McLellarn R, Conner SL, Matarazzo JD. The role of Type A behavior in an elevation of plasma lipids in adult women and men. Psychosom Med 1987;49:136–145.
35. Review Panel on Coronary-Prone Behavior and Coronary Heart Disease. Coronary-prone behavior and coronary heart disease: a critical review. Circulation 1978;65:1199–1215.
36. Gump BS, Matthews KA, Raikkonen K. Modeling relationships among socioeconomic status, hostility, cardiovascular reactivity, and left ventricular mass in African American and white children. Health Psychol 1999;18:140–150.
37. Crick NR, Dodge KA. A review and reformulation of social information-processing mechanisms in children's social adjustment. Psychol Bull 1994;115:74–101.
38. Chen E, Matthews KA. Cognitive appraisal biases: an approach to understanding the relation between socioeconomic status and cardiovascular reactivity in children. Ann Behav Med 2001;23(2):101–111.
39. Horowitz MJ, Berfari R, Hulley S, et al. Life events, risk factors, and coronary disease. Psychosomatics 1979;20:586–592.
40. Taylor SE, Repetti RL, Seeman T. What is an unhealthy environment and how does it get under the skin? Annu Rev Psychol 1997;48:411–447.
41. Ekman P. An argument for basic emotions. Cognition Emotion 1992;6:169–200.
42. Scherer KR. Neuroscience projections to current debates in emotion psychology. Cognition Emotion 1993;7:1–41.
43. Scherer KR. Psychological models of emotion. In: Borod JC, ed. The Neuropsychology of Emotion. New York: Oxford University Press, 2000;137–162.
44. Gross JJ. Antecedent- and response-focused emotion regulation: divergent consequences for experience, expression, and physiology. J Pers Soc Psychol 1998;74:224–237.
45. Bandura A. Self-Efficacy: The Exercise of Control. New York: W.H. Freeman, 1997.
46. Ewart CK, Jorgensen RS, Suchday S, Chen E, Matthews KA. Measuring stress resilience and coping in vulnerable youth: the Social Competence Interview. Psychol Assess 2002;14(3):339–352.
47. Wallander JL. Social-emotional competence and physical health. Center for the Advancement of Health, Washington, DC: 2000.
48. Abe JA, Izard CE. A longitudinal study of emotion expression and personality relations in early development. J PersSoc Psychol 1999;77:566–577.
49. Izard CE, Fine SE, Schultz D, Mostow AJ, Ackerman BP, Youngstrom EA. Emotion knowledge as a predictor of social behavior and academic competence in children at risk. Psychol Sci 2001;12:18–23.
50. Ewart CK. Familial transmission of essential hypertension: genes, environments, and chronic anger. Ann Behav Med 1991;13:40–47.
51. Ewart CK, Kolodner KB. Social competence interview for assessing physiological reactivity in adolescents. Psychosom Med 1991;53:289–304.
52. Ewart CK. Nonshared environments and heart disease risk: concepts and data for a model of coronary-prone behavior. In: Hetherington E, Reiss D, Plomin R, eds. The Separate Social Worlds of Siblings. Hillsdale, NJ: Erlbaum, 1994:175–203.

53. Ewart CK, Kolodner KB. Negative affect, gender, and expressive style predict ambulatory blood pressure in adolescents. J Pers Soc Psychol 1994;66:596–605.
54. Ewart CK, Jorgensen RS, Kolodner KB. Sociotropic cognition moderates blood pressure response to interpersonal stress in high-risk adolescent girls. Int J Psychophysiol 1998;28:131–142.
55. Sauro MD, Jorgensen RS, Larson CA, Frankowski JJ, Ewart CK, White J. Sociotropic cognition moderates stress-induced cardiovascular responsiveness in college women. J Behav Med 2001;24:423–439.
56. Ewart CK, Jorgensen RS. Agonistic interpersonal striving: social-cognitive mechanism of cardiovascular risk in youth? Health Psychol 2004;23:75–85.
57. Herrald MM, Tomaka J. Patterns of emotion-specific appraisal, coping, and cardiovascular reactivity during an ongoing emotional episode. J Pers Soc Psychol 2002;83(2):434–450.
58. Perloff D, Sokolow M, Cowan R. The prognostic value of ambulatory blood pressure. J Am Med Assoc 1983;249:2792–2798.
59. White WB, Schulman P, McCabe EJ, Dey M. Average daily blood pressure, not office blood pressure, determines cardiac function in patients with hypertension. J Am Med Assoc 1989;261:873–877.
60. Marmot M, Theorell T. Social class and cardiovascular disease: the contribution of work. Int J Health Serv 1988;18:659–674.
61. Stansfeld SA, Head J, Marmot M. Explaining social class differences in depression and well-being. Soc Psychiatry Psychiatr Epidemiol 1998;33:1–9.
62. Tseng JM, Mare RD. Labor market and socioeconomic effects on marital stability. Soc Sci Res 1995;24:329–351.
63. Klebanov PK, Brooks-Gunn J, Duncan GJ. Does neighborhood and family poverty affect mothers' parenting, mental health, and social support? J Marriage Fam 1994;56:441–445.
64. Simons RI, Johnson C, Beaman JJ, Conger RD, Whitbeck LB. Parents and peer group as mediators of the effect of community structure on adolescent behavior. Am J Community Psychol 1996;24:145–171.
65. McLoyd VC. The impact of economic hardship on Black families and development. Child Dev1990;61:311–346.
66. Earls F, McGuire J, Shay S. Evaluating a community intervention to reduce the risk of child abuse: methodological strategies in conducting neighborhood surveys. Child Abuse Negl 1994;18:473–485.
67. Sampson RJ. Collective regulation of adolescent misbehavior: validation results from eight Chicago neighborhoods. J Adolesc Res 1997;12:227–244.
68. Kelley HH, Berscheid E, Christensen A, et al. Analyzing close relationships. In: Kelley HH, Berscheid E, Christensen A, et al., eds. Close Relationships. New York: W.H. Freeman, 1983:20–67.
69. Wilson BJ, Gottman JM. Attention—The shuttle between emotion and cognition: risk, resiliency, and physiological bases. In: Hetherington EM, Blechman EA, eds. Stress, Coping, and Resiliency in Children and Families. Mahwah, NJ: Lawrence Erlbaum, 1996; 189–228.
70. Steele C. A threat in the air: how stereotypes shape intellectual identity and performance. Am Psychol 1997;52: 613–629.
71. Steele C, Aronson J. Contending with a stereotype: African-American intellectual test performance and stereotype threat. J Pers Soc Psychol 1995;69:797–811.
72. Spencer SJ, Steele C, Quinn D. Stereotype threat and women's math performance. J Exp Soc Psychol 1999; 35:4–28.
73. Frederickson BL, Roberts TA, Noll SM, Quinn DM, Twenge JM. The swimsuit becomes you: sex differences in self-objectification, restrained eating, and math performance. J Pers Soc Psychol 1998;75:269–284.
74. Blascovich J, Spencer SJ, Quinn D, Steele C. African Americans and high blood pressure: the role of stereotype threat. Psychol Sci 2001;12(3):225–229.
75. Obrist PA. Cardiovascular psychophysiology: a perspective. New York: Plenum, 1981.
76. Schneiderman N, McCabe PM. Psychophysiologic strategies in laboratory research. In: Schneiderman N, Weiss SM, Kaufmann PG, eds. Handbook of Research Methods in Cardiovascular Behavioral Medicine. New York: Plenum, 1989; 349–364.
77. Smith TW, Ruiz JM, Uchino BN. Vigilance, active coping, and cardiovascular reactivity during social interaction in young men. Health Psychol 2000;19(4):382–392.
78. Rusting CL, Nolen-Hoeksema S. Regulating responses to anger: effects of rumination and distraction on angry mood. J Pers Soc Psychol 1998;74:790–803.
79. Ewart CK, Jorgensen RS, Schroder KE, Suchday S, Sherwood A. Vigilance to a persisting personal threat: unmasking cardiovascular consequences in adolescents with the Social Competence Interview. Psychophysiology 2004, in press.

80. Brosschot JF, Thayer JF. Anger inhibition, cardiovascular recovery, and vagal function: a model of the link between hostility and cardiovascular disease. Ann Behav Med 1998;20(4):326–332.
81. Ross L. The intuitive psychologist and his shortcomings: distortions in the attribution process. In: Berkowitz L, ed. Advances in Experimental Social Psychology. Vol 10. New York: Academic, 1977;174–221.
82. Gilbert DT, Malone PS. The correspondence bias. Psychol Bull 1995;117:21–38.
83. MacLeod C, Campbell L. Memory accessibility and probability judgments: an experimental evaluation of the availability heuristic. J Pers Soc Psychol 1992;63:890–902.
84. Roese NJ. Counterfactual thinking. Psychol Bull 1997;121:133–148.
85. Bargh JA, Chen M, Burrows L. Automaticity of social behavior: direct effects of trait construct and stereotype activation on action. J Pers Soc Psychol 1996;71:230–244.
86. Webster DM, Richter L, Kruglanski AW. On leaping to conclusions when feeling tired: mental fatigue effects on impressional primacy. J Exp Soc Psychol 1996;32:181–195.
87. Tesser A. Self-generated attitude change. In: Berkowitz L, ed. Advances in Experimental Social Psychology. Vol 11. New York: Academic, 1978;288–338.
88. Ryan CS, Judd CM, Park B. Effects of racial stereotypes on judgments of individuals: the moderating role of perceived group variability. J Exp Soc Psychol 1996;32:71–103.
89. Turner JC. Rediscovering the Social Group: A Self-categorization Theory. Oxford: Basil Blackwell, 1987.
90. Copeland JT. Prophecies of power: motivational implications of social power for behavioral confirmation. J Pers Soc Psychol 1994;67:264–277.
91. Baumeister RF. A self-presentational view of social phenomena. Psychol Bull 1982;91:3–26.
92. Gross JJ. Emotion regulation in adulthood: timing is everything. Curr Dir Psychol Sci 2001;10(6):214–219.
93. Ewart CK, Harris WL, Zeger S, Russell GA. Diminished pulse pressure under mental stress characterizes normtensive adolescents with parental high blood pressure. Psychosom Med 1986;48:489–501.
94. Ewart CK, Harris WL, Iwata M, Bullock R, Coates TJ, Simons B. Feasibility and effectiveness of school-based relaxation to lower blood pressure. Health Psychol 1987;6:399–416.
95. Leventhal T, Brooks-Gunn J. Children and youth in neighborhood contexts. Curr Dir Psychol Sci 2003;12: 27–31.
96. Katz LF, Kling JR, Liebman JB. Moving to opportunity in Boston: early results of a randomized mobility experiment. Q J Econ 2001;116:607–654.
97. Ewart CK. Social action theory for a public health psychology. Am Psychol 1991;46:931–946.
98. Ewart CK. How integrative theory building can improve health promotion and disease prevention. In: Frank RG, Wallander J, Baum A, eds. Models and Perspectives in Health Psychology. Washington, DC: American Psychological Association, 2004, in press.

# 20 Neonatal Hypertension

*Joseph T. Flynn,* MD, MS

***Contents***



## INTRODUCTION

Hypertension (HTN) as a clinical problem in newborn infants was first recognized in the 1970s *(1)*. However, advances in the management for premature infants have led to an increased awareness of neonatal HTN, not only in the neonatal intensive care unit (NICU), but also in the neonatal follow-up clinic. This chapter will focus on the differential diagnosis of HTN in the neonate, the optimal diagnostic evaluation, and both acute and chronic antihypertensive therapy.

## INCIDENCE/EPIDEMIOLOGY

It is difficult to ascertain the actual incidence of HTN in neonates because no generally accepted definition of HTN exists for this age group *(2,3)*. In a recent study of preterm infants admitted to six NICUs in New England, 28% of infants with birthweights <1500 g had at least one blood pressure (BP) reading that was considered "hypertensive" *(2)*. Clearly, few of these infants had sustained HTN. At the other extreme, HTN is considered so unusual in otherwise healthy term infants that routine BP determination is not advocated for this group *(4)*.

Despite these issues, most authors agree that the actual incidence of HTN in neonates is quite low, ranging from 0.2 to 3% in most reports *(1,5–8)*. The incidence may be somewhat higher in premature and otherwise high-risk newborns. In a review of over 3000 infants admitted to a Chicago NICU, the overall incidence of HTN was found to be 0.81% *(8)*. Hypertension was

From: *Clinical Hypertension and Vascular Disease: Pediatric Hypertension*
Edited by: R. J. Portman, J. M. Sorof, and J. R. Ingelfinger © Humana Press Inc., Totowa, NJ

considerably more common (approx 9%) in infants with bronchopulmonary dysplasia, patent ductus arteriosus, intraventricular hemorrhage, and in those who had in-dwelling umbilical arterial catheters.

It is important to note that HTN may also be detected well after discharge from the NICU. In a retrospective review of over 650 infants seen in follow-up after discharge from a teaching hospital NICU, Friedman found an incidence of HTN (defined as a systolic BP of greater than 113 mmHg on three consecutive visits over 6 wk) of 2.6% *(9)*. HTN in this study was detected at a mean age of approx 2 mo postterm when corrected for prematurity. Although the differences were not significant, infants in this study who developed HTN tended to have lower initial Apgar scores and longer NICU stays compared to infants who remained normotensive, indicating a trend toward a greater likelihood of developing HTN in sicker babies, a finding similar to that of Singh *(8)*. Even with the increasing survival rates of premature infants, however, HTN remains a relatively infrequent clinical problem that is primarily confined to the NICU or neonatal follow-up clinic.

## DIFFERENTIAL DIAGNOSIS

As in older infants and children, the causes of HTN in neonates are numerous (Table 1), the two largest categories being renovascular and other renal parenchymal diseases *(1,5–10)*. More specifically, umbilical artery catheter-associated thromboembolism, affecting the aorta and/or the renal arteries, probably accounts for the majority of cases of HTN seen in the typical NICU. A clear association between the use of umbilical artery catheters and the development of arterial thrombi was first demonstrated in the early 1970s by Neal and colleagues *(11)*. They performed aortography at the time of umbilical artery removal in 19 infants, demonstrating thrombus formation in 18 of the 19 infants, as well as several instances of clot fragmentation and embolization. Thrombosis was also seen at autopsy in 7 of 12 additional infants who had died, for an overall incidence of 25 out of 31 infants, or approx 81% of infants studied.

Following the Neal et al. report, the association between umbilical arterial catheter-associated thrombi and the development of neonatal HTN was confirmed by several other investigators *(12–17)*. HTN was demonstrated in infants who had undergone umbilical artery catheterization even when thrombi could not be demonstrated in the renal arteries. Reported rates of thrombus formation have generally been much lower than noted in the Neal et al. study, however, typically about 25% *(12,18,19)*. Although there have been several studies that examined duration of line placement and line position ("low" vs "high") as factors involved in thrombus formation, data have been inconclusive *(18–20)*. Consequently, the assumption has been made that the cause of HTN in such cases is related to thrombus formation at the time of line placement, probably related to disruption of the vascular endothelium of the umbilical artery. Such thrombi may then embolize to the kidneys, causing areas of infarction and increased renin release. A similar phenomenon has been reported in infants who have undergone catheter-based dilatation of the ductus arteriosus *(21)*.

The Cochrane Group has recently attempted to resolve the controversy regarding umbilical artery catheter placement *(22)*. They analyzed 11 randomized clinical trials and one study using alternate assignments to compare the incidence of morbidity and mortality for high vs low catheter tip placement. The placement of a catheter tip was defined as high when located in the descending aorta above the diaphragm, and as low when in the descending aorta above the bifurcation but below the renal arteries. The reviewers concluded that high catheter position causes fewer clinically obvious ischemic complications and possibly decreases the frequency

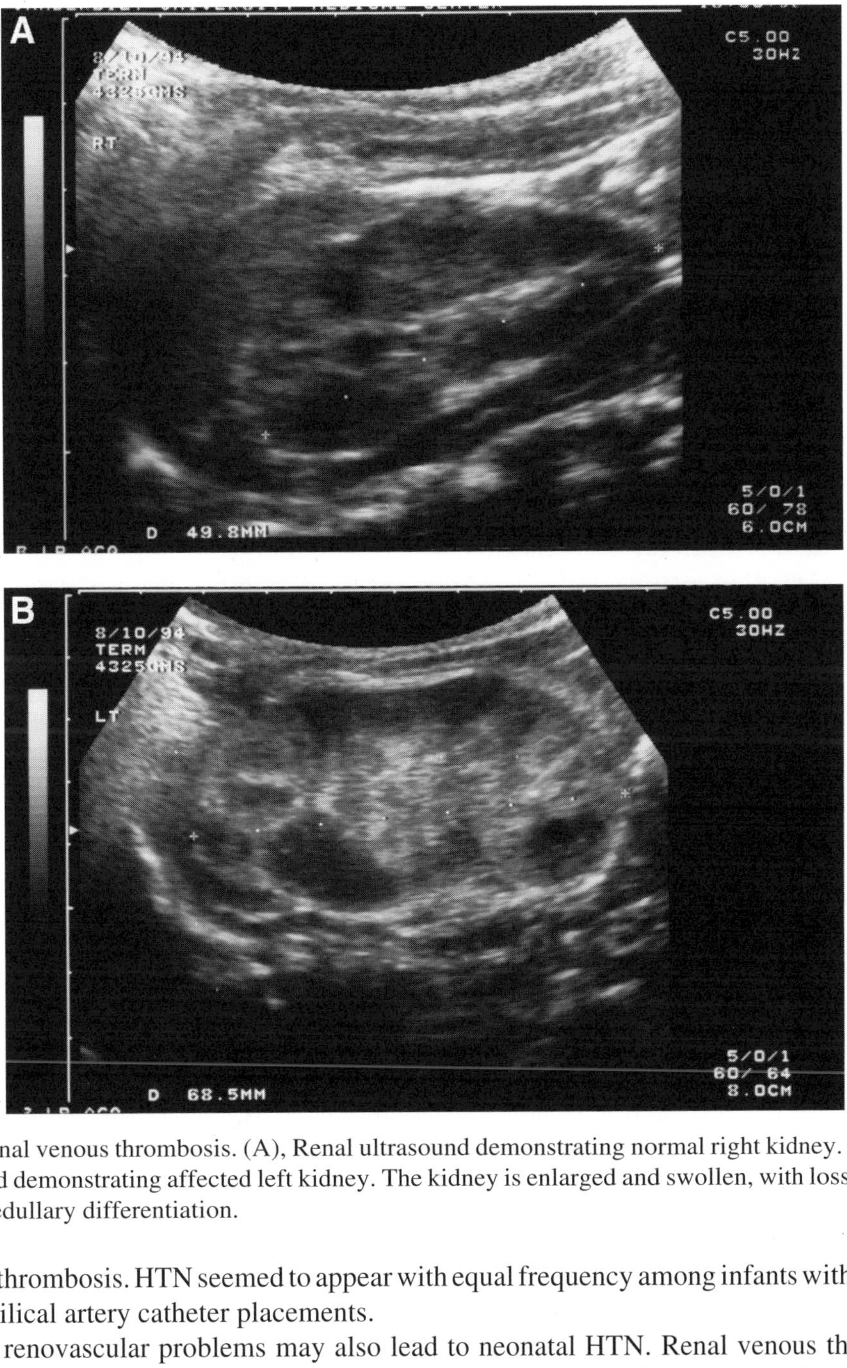


Fig. 1. Renal venous thrombosis. (A), Renal ultrasound demonstrating normal right kidney. (B), Renal ultrasound demonstrating affected left kidney. The kidney is enlarged and swollen, with loss of normal corticomedullary differentiation.

of aortic thrombosis. HTN seemed to appear with equal frequency among infants with high and low umbilical artery catheter placements.

Other renovascular problems may also lead to neonatal HTN. Renal venous thrombosis (Fig. 1) classically presents with the triad of HTN, gross hematuria, and an abdominal mass. HTN associated with renal venous thrombosis may be quite severe and may persist beyond the neonatal period *(23,24)*. Fibromuscular dysplasia leading to renal arterial stenosis is another important cause of renovascular HTN in the neonate. Arteriography often demonstrates normal main renal arteries, but clinically significant branch vessel disease that can cause severe HTN *(25)*. In addition, renal arterial stenosis may also be accompanied by mid-aortic coarctation and cerebral vascular stenoses *(25)*. Other vascular abnormalities may lead to HTN in the neonate as well, including idiopathic arterial calcification *(26,27)* and renal artery stenosis secondary to congenital rubella infection *(28)*. Congenital aortic aneurysm is a rare condition producing renovascular HTN that may be fatal because of intractable congestive heart failure *(29)*. Finally, mechanical compression of one or both renal arteries by tumors, hydronephrotic kidneys, or other abdominal masses may also lead to HTN.

Congenital intrinsic renal parenchymal abnormalities constitute the next large group of infants with HTN. It is well known that both autosomal dominant polycystic kidney disease (ADPKD) and autosomal recessive polycystic kidney disease (ADPKD) may present in the newborn period with severe nephromegaly and HTN *(30,31)*. The majority of infants with ARPKD will be discovered to be hypertensive during the first year of life *(30)*; the most severely affected are at risk for development of congestive heart failure because of severe, malignant HTN. Although much less common than in PKD, HTN has also been reported in infants with unilateral multicystic dysplastic kidneys *(6,32–34)*. This is somewhat paradoxical because these kidneys are usually thought to be nonfunctioning. In fact, the case has been made that HTN in such patients is the result of another coexisting urologic abnormality, such as renal parenchymal scarring in the contralateral functioning kidney *(35)*.

Renal obstruction may be accompanied by HTN, even in the absence of renal arterial compression, as seen in infants with congenital ureteropelvic-junction obstruction *(6,8,9)*. Such HTN may sometimes persist following surgical correction of the obstruction *(36)*. Hypertension has also been described in babies with congenital primary megaureter *(37)*. Ureteral obstruction by other intraabdominal masses may also be accompanied by HTN. The mechanism of HTN in such instances is unclear, although the renin-angiotensin system has been implicated *(38,39)*. Finally, unilateral renal hypoplasia may also present with HTN *(40)*, although this is uncommon.

Hypertension caused by acquired renal parenchymal disease is less common than that caused by congenital renal abnormalities. However, severe acute tubular necrosis (ATN), interstitial nephritis, or cortical necrosis may be accompanied by significant HTN *(6,8)*, usually on the basis of volume overload or hyperreninemia.

Hemolytic uremic syndrome, which has been described in both term and preterm infants *(41)*, is usually also accompanied by HTN. Such HTN may be extremely difficult to control, requiring treatment with multiple antihypertensive agents *(41)*.

HTN as a consequence of bronchopulmonary dysplasia (BPD) was first described in the mid-1980s by Abman and colleagues *(42)*. In a study of 65 infants discharged from a NICU, the instance of HTN in infants with BPD was 43% compared to 4.5% in infants without BPD. The investigators were unable to identify a clear cause of the observed HTN, but postulated that hypoxemia might be involved. Over half of the infants with BPD who developed HTN did not display elevated BP until after discharge from the NICU, highlighting the need for measurement of BP in NICU "graduates," whether or not they have lung disease *(9)*.

Abman's findings have been reproduced by other investigators, most recently in 1998 by Alagappan *(43)*, who found that HTN was twice as common in very low birthweight infants with BPD compared to all very low birthweight infants. Since all of the hypertensive infants required supplemental oxygen and aminophylline, development of HTN appeared to be correlated with the severity of pulmonary disease. Anderson and colleagues have demonstrated that the more severe the bronchopulmonary dysplasia (BPD), the higher the likelihood of the development of increased BP *(44)*. Severe BPD was defined as a greater need for diuretics

(91% of the hypertensive group vs 55% of the normotensive group, $p < 0.05$) and bronchodilators (91% of the hypertensive group vs 37% of the normotensive group, $p < 0.001$).

These observations reinforce the impression that infants with severe BPD are clearly at increased risk and need close monitoring for the development of HTN. This is especially true in infants who require ongoing treatment with theophylline preparations and/or corticosteroids.

HTN may also be seen in disorders of several other organ systems. Coarctation of the thoracic aorta is easily detected in the newborn period and has been reported in numerous case series of neonatal HTN *(5,6,8–10)*. HTN may persist after surgical repair of the coarctation. Repair early in infancy seems to lead to an improved long-term outcome compared to delayed repair *(45)*. Endocrine disorders, particularly congenital adrenal hyperplasia, hyperaldosteronism, and hyperthyroidism constitute easily recognizable clinical entities that have been reported to cause HTN in neonates *(46–49)*. Similarly, pseudohypoaldosteronism type II (Gordon's Syndrome) should be suspected in the hypertensive infant with hyperkalemia and metabolic acidosis.

Iatrogenic causes of HTN comprise another important category. Medications such as dexamethasone and aminophylline, commonly administered to infants for treatment of pulmonary disease, have clearly been shown to elevate BP *(50–52)*. The risks of dexamethasone were recently highlighted by the Neonatal Research Network *(52)* in a study of 220 very low birthweight infants (birthweight 501–1000 g) randomized to receive either dexamethasone or placebo because of the need for mechanical ventilation; the incidence of systolic BP >90 mmHg was significantly higher in the dexamethasone group ($p = 0.01$ compared to placebo), as was the likelihood of being treated for HTN ($p = 0.04$).

In addition, high doses of adrenergic agents, prolonged use of pancuronium, or administration of phenylephrine ophthalmic drops *(53)* may raise BP in the newborn. HTN associated with these medications typically resolves when the offending agent is discontinued or its dose reduced. Infants receiving prolonged parenteral nutrition (TPN), may develop HTN from salt and water overload, or from hypercalcemia, either caused directly by excessive calcium intake, or indirectly by vitamin A or D intoxication.

Substances ingested during pregnancy may also lead to clinically significant problems with HTN in the neonate. In particular, maternal cocaine use may have a number of undesirable effects on the developing kidney that may lead to HTN *(54)*. HTN has also been reported to occur in infants of drug-addicted mothers withdrawing from heroin.

Tumors, including neuroblastoma, Wilms tumor, and mesoblastic nephroma may all present in the neonatal period and may produce HTN, either because of compression of the renal vessels or ureters, or because of production of vasoactive substances such as renin or catecholamines *(9,55–58)*. Neurologic problems such as seizures, intracranial HTN, and pain constitute fairly common causes of episodic HTN. In the typical modern NICU, postoperative pain must not be overlooked as a cause of HTN. Provision of adequate analgesia may constitute the only required "antihypertensive medication" in such infants.

There are numerous other miscellaneous causes of HTN in neonates, the most common of which are listed in Table 1. Of these, HTN associated with extracorporeal membrane oxygenation (ECMO) deserves comment. Elevated BP may be seen in up to 50% of infants requiring ECMO *(59,60)*, and may result in serious complications, including intracranial hemorrhage *(61)* and increased mortality *(60)*. Despite extensive investigation, the exact pathogenesis of ECMO-associated HTN remains poorly understood. Fluid overload, altered handling of sodium and water, and derangements in atrial baroceptor function have all been proposed as potential

Table 1
Causes of Neonatal HTN

| | |
|---|---|
| *Renovascular* | *Medications/Intoxications* |
| Thromboembolism | Infant |
| Renal artery stenosis | Dexamethasone |
| Mid-aortic coarctation | Adrenergic agents |
| Renal venous thrombosis | Vitamin D intoxication |
| Compression of renal artery | Theophylline |
| Abdominal aortic aneurysm | Caffeine |
| Idiopathic arterial calcification | Pancuronium |
| Congenital rubella syndrome | Phenylephrine |
| *Renal parenchymal disease* | Maternal |
| Congenital | Cocaine |
| Polycystic kidney disease | Heroin |
| Multicystic-dysplastic kidney disease | *Neoplasia* |
| Tuberous sclerosis | Wilms tumor |
| Ureteropelvic junction obstruction | Mesoblastic nephroma |
| Unilateral renal hypoplasia | Neuroblastoma |
| Primary megaureter | Pheochromocytoma |
| Congenital nephrotic syndrome | *Neurologic* |
| Acquired | Pain |
| Acute tubular necrosis | Intracranial HTN |
| Cortical necrosis | Seizures |
| Interstitial nephritis | Familial dysautonomia |
| Hemolytic-Uremic Syndrome | Subdural hematoma |
| Obstruction (stones, tumors) | *Miscellaneous* |
| *Pulmonary* | Total parenteral nutrition (TPN) |
| Bronchopulmonary dysplasia | Closure of abdominal wall defect |
| Pneumothorax | Adrenal hemorrhage |
| *Cardiac* | Hypercalcemia |
| Thoracic aortic coarctation | Traction |
| *Endocrine* | ECMO |
| Congenital adrenal hyperplasia | Birth asphyxia |
| Hyperaldosteronism | Essential HTN ? |
| Hyperthyroidism | HTN |
| Pseudohypoaldosteronism type II (Gordon's Syndrome) | |

causative factors *(59,61)*. Given the widespread and increasing use of ECMO in both neonates and older children, further investigation of this problem is clearly needed.

## DEFINITION OF HYPERTENSION

Defining what is considered a normal BP in newborn infants is a complex task. Just as BP in older children has been demonstrated to increase with increasing age and body size, studies in both term and preterm infants have demonstrated that BP in neonates increases with both gestational and postconceptional age, as well as with birthweight *(62–68)*. Extremely useful

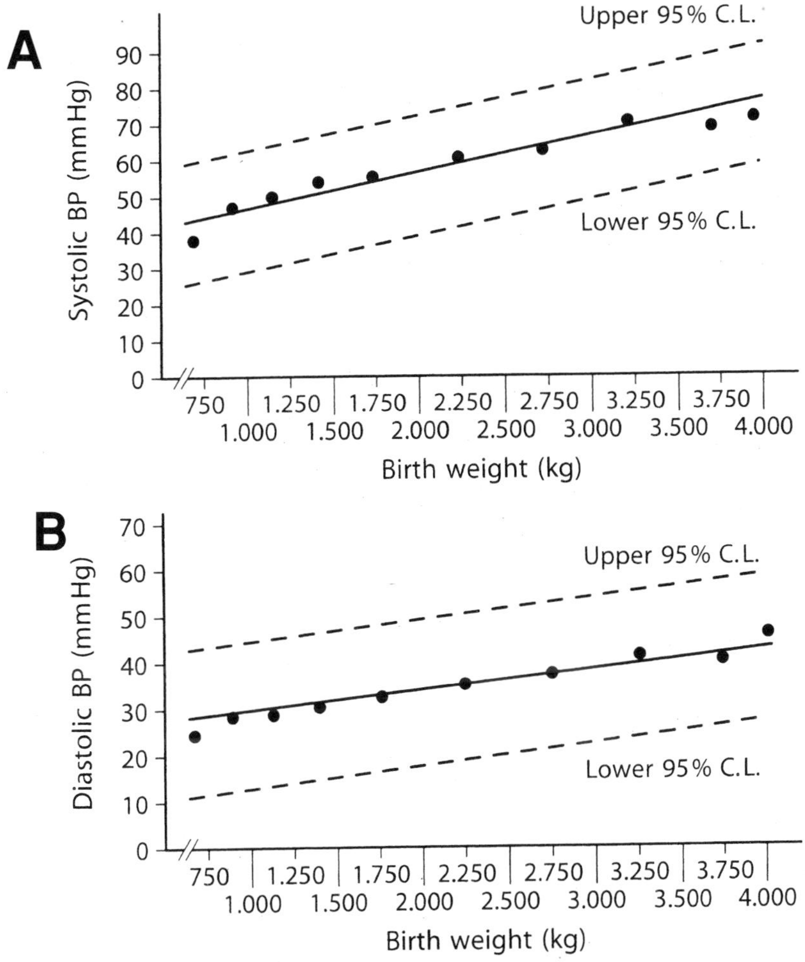


Fig. 2. Linear regression of mean systolic (A) and diastolic (B) BPs by birthweight on d 1 of life, with 95% confidence limits (upper and lower dashed lines). Reproduced from Zubrow et al. *(66)* with permission from Nature Publishing Group.

data in this regard have been published by Zubrow and associates *(66)*, who prospectively obtained serial BP measurements from 695 infants admitted to several NICUs in a large metropolitan area over a period of 3 mo. They then defined the mean BPs and upper and lower 95% confidence limits for the infants studied. Their data clearly demonstrated that BP increases with increasing gestational age, birthweight and postconceptional age (Figs. 2–4). Using these data, we would consider an infant's BP to be elevated if it was consistently above the upper 95% confidence interval for infants of similar gestational or postconceptional age.

For older infants found to be hypertensive following discharge from the NICU, the percentile curves published in the Second Task Force report (Fig. 5) appear to be the most useful. Based on serial BP measurements obtained from nearly 13,000 infants, these curves allow BP to be characterized as normal or elevated, not only by age and gender, but also by size, albeit to a somewhat limited extent. HTN in this age group would be defined as sustained BP elevation above the 95th percentile for infants of similar age, size, and gender.

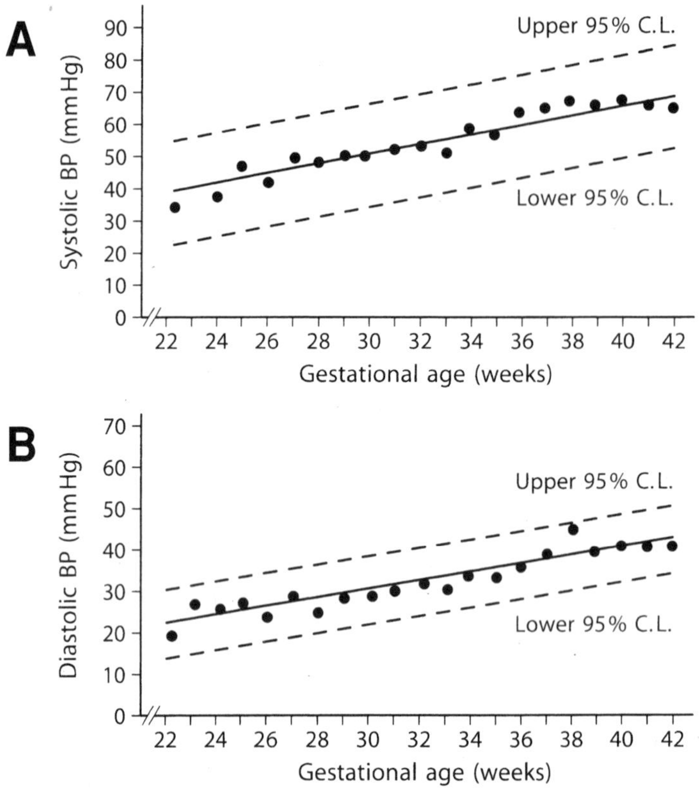


Fig. 3. Linear regression of mean systolic (A) and diastolic (B) BPs by gestational age on d 1 of life, with 95% confidence limits (upper and lower dashed lines). Reproduced from Zubrow et al.*(66)* with permission from Nature Publishing Group.

## BLOOD PRESSURE MEASUREMENT

As in older children, it is crucial that BP is measured accurately so that hypertensive infants will be correctly identified. Fortunately, in most acutely ill neonates, BP is usually monitored directly via an indwelling arterial catheter in the radial or umbilical artery. This method provides the most accurate BP readings and is clearly preferable to other methods *(70)*. In addition to accurately measuring BPs, these catheters are also crucial in the careful management of HTN, particularly in infants with severe BP elevation. This will be discussed in more detail later in the chapter.

Automated, oscillometric devices are the most common alternative method of BP measurement in most NICUs. Although accurate, readings obtained by these devices may differ significantly from intra-arterial readings. When comparing BPs obtained from 31 newborns with these two techniques, Low *(71)* reported that the average oscillometric pressures were lower than the intra-arterial pressures, a significant finding. The systolic was lower by 1 mmHg, the mean by 5.3 mmHg, and the diastolic by 4.6 mmHg. These differences may need to be considered when determining whether an infant's BP is normal or elevated.

Despite the fact that BP readings obtained by oscillometric devices may differ slightly from intra-arterial BP measurements, they are easy to use and provide the ability to follow BP trends over time. They are especially useful for infants who require BP monitoring after discharge

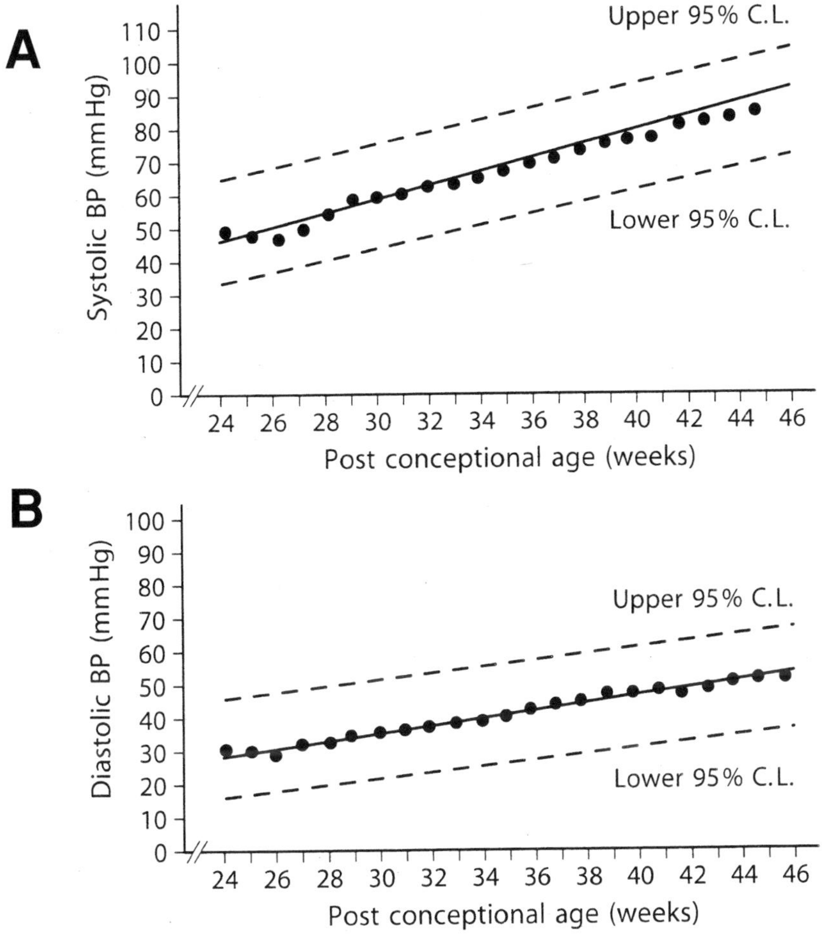


Fig. 4. Linear regression of mean systolic (A) and diastolic (B) BPs by postconceptional age in weeks, with 95% confidence limits (upper and lower dashed lines). Reproduced from Zubrow et al. *(66)* with permission from Nature Publishing Group.

from the NICU *(72)*. When using these devices, however, attention should be paid to using a arm *(69)*. Since BPs obtained in the leg may be higher than those obtained in the arm *(73–75)*, the use of other extremities for routine BP determination may complicate the evaluation of HTN. Nursing staff should document the extremity used for BP determinations and, if possible, try to use the same extremity for subsequent determinations. Finally, the infant's state of activity may also affect the accuracy of BP readings. Increased activity, including oral feeding, increases BP *(75)*. It may therefore be important to obtain BP readings while infants are sleeping in order to obtain the most accurate readings.

These issues were recently highlighted in a study of BP in low birthweight term and preterm infants by Nwanko et al. *(76)*. It was demonstrated that BP was significantly lower in the prone than in the supine position, and that the first reading was significantly higher than the third. Nwanko et al. concluded that a standardized protocol is necessary to correctly identify HTN. They recommended checking BPs 1.5 h after the last feeding or intervention, applying an appropriately sized cuff (covering at least two-third the length of the limb segment and 75%

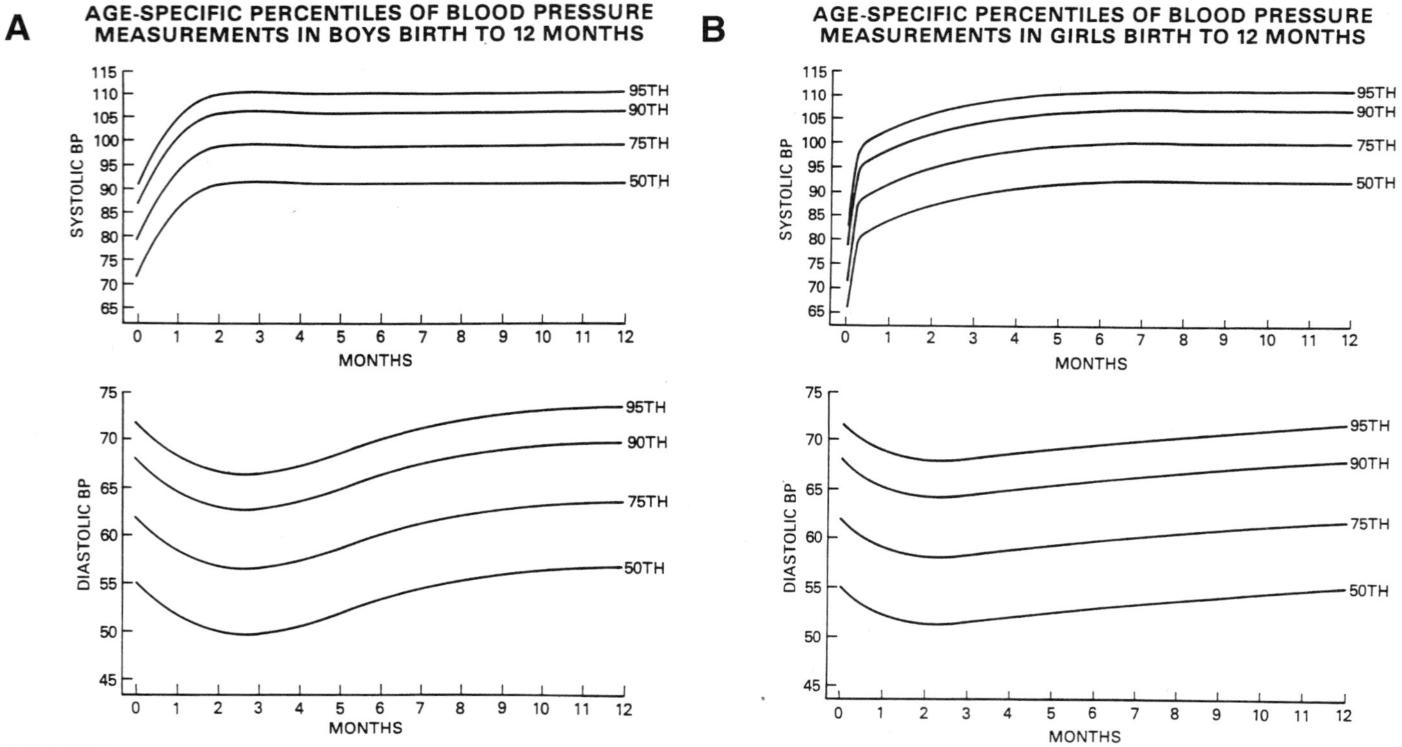


A

| 90TH PERCENTILE | 0 | 1 | 2 | 3 | 4 | 5 | 6 | 7 | 8 | 9 | 10 | 11 | 12 |
|---|---|---|---|---|---|---|---|---|---|---|---|---|---|
| SYSTOLIC BP | 87 | 101 | 106 | 106 | 106 | 105 | 105 | 105 | 105 | 105 | 105 | 105 | 105 |
| DIASTOLIC BP | 68 | 65 | 63 | 63 | 63 | 65 | 66 | 67 | 68 | 68 | 69 | 69 | 69 |
| HEIGHT CM | 51 | 59 | 63 | 66 | 68 | 70 | 72 | 73 | 74 | 76 | 77 | 78 | 80 |
| WEIGHT KG | 4 | 4 | 5 | 5 | 6 | 7 | 8 | 9 | 9 | 10 | 10 | 11 | 11 |

B

| 90TH PERCENTILE | 0 | 1 | 2 | 3 | 4 | 5 | 6 | 7 | 8 | 9 | 10 | 11 | 12 |
|---|---|---|---|---|---|---|---|---|---|---|---|---|---|
| SYSTOLIC BP | 76 | 98 | 101 | 104 | 105 | 106 | 106 | 106 | 106 | 106 | 106 | 105 | 105 |
| DIASTOLIC BP | 68 | 65 | 64 | 64 | 65 | 65 | 66 | 66 | 66 | 67 | 67 | 67 | 67 |
| HEIGHT CM | 54 | 55 | 56 | 58 | 61 | 63 | 66 | 68 | 70 | 72 | 74 | 75 | 77 |
| WEIGHT KG | 4 | 4 | 4 | 5 | 5 | 6 | 7 | 8 | 9 | 9 | 10 | 10 | 11 |

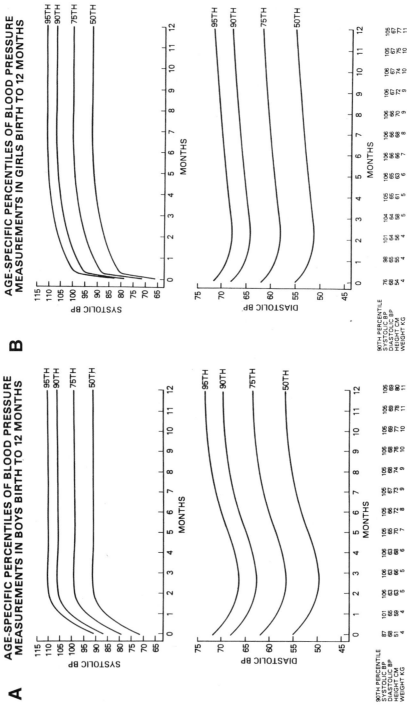

Fig. 5. Age-specific percentiles for blood pressure in boys (A) and girls (B) from birth to 12 mo of age. Reproduced with permission from ref. *69*.

Table 2
Diagnostic Testing in Neonatal HTN

| *Generally useful* | *Useful in selected infants* |
|---|---|
| Urinalysis (+/– culture) | Thyroid studies |
| CBC and platelet count | Urine VMA/HVA |
| Electrolytes | Aldosterone |
| BUN, creatinine | Cortisol |
| Calcium | Echocardiogram |
| Plasma renin | Abdominal/pelvic ultrasound |
| Chest x-ray | VCUG |
| Renal ultrasound with Doppler | Aortography |
| | Renal angiography |
| | Nuclear scan (DTPA/Mag-3) |

of the limb circumference), waiting an additional 15 min for the infant to be quiet and calm, and then obtaining three successive readings at 2-min intervals. Using proper technique, it should be possible to correctly identify infants with HTN requiring further evaluation.

## DIAGNOSTIC EVALUATION

Diagnosing the etiology of HTN is a straightforward task in most hypertensive neonates. A relatively focused history should be obtained, with attention to determining whether there were any pertinent prenatal exposures, as well as to the particulars of the infant's nursery course and any concurrent conditions. The procedures that the infant has undergone (e.g., umbilical catheter placement) should be reviewed, and the current medication list should be scrutinized.

The physical examination, likewise, should be focused on obtaining pertinent information to assist in narrowing the differential diagnosis. BP readings should be obtained in all four extremities in order to rule out coarctation of the thoracic aorta. The general appearance of the infant should be assessed, with particular attention paid to the presence of dysmorphic features that may indicate an obvious diagnosis such as congenital adrenal hyperplasia. Careful cardiac and abdominal examination should be performed. The presence of a flank mass, or of an epigastric bruit, may point the clinician towards diagnosis of either ureteropelvic junction obstruction or renal artery stenosis, respectively.

In most instances, few laboratory data are needed in the evaluation of neonatal HTN; the correct diagnosis is usually suggested by the history and physical examination. It is important to assess renal function, as well as to examine a specimen of the urine in order to ascertain the presence of renal parenchymal disease. Chest x-rays may be useful as an adjunctive test in infants with congestive heart failure, or in those with a murmur on physical examination. Other diagnostic studies, such as cortisol, aldosterone, or thyroxine levels, should be obtained when there is a history suggesting endocrine HTN (Table 2).

Determination of plasma renin activity is frequently recommended in the assessment of neonates with HTN *(6)*, although there are few data on what constitutes normal values for infants, particularly premature infants. The available data indicate that renin values are typically high in infancy, at least in term newborns *(77,78)*. Although renal artery stenosis and thromboembolic phenomenon are typically considered high renin forms of HTN, a peripheral renin level may not be elevated in such infants despite the presence of significant underlying pathology. Conversely, plasma renin may be falsely elevated by medications that are commonly used in the NICU, such as aminophylline *(79)*. Despite these difficulties, assessment of plasma renin activity may be helpful in the evaluation of some infants, especially when elevated, and is therefore usually included as part of the initial laboratory evaluation.

Ultrasound imaging of the genitourinary tract is a relatively inexpensive, noninvasive, and quick study that should be obtained in all hypertensive infants. As demonstrated in Fig. 1, an accurate renal ultrasound can help uncover potentially correctable causes of HTN such as renal venous thrombosis *(23)*, may detect aortic and/or renal arterial thrombi *(12,17)*, and can identify anatomic renal abnormalities or other congenital renal diseases. For these reasons, ultrasound has largely replaced intravenous pyelography, which has little if any use in the routine assessment of neonatal HTN.

For infants with extremely severe BP elevation, angiography may be necessary. A formal angiogram utilizing the traditional femoral venous approach offers the most accurate method of diagnosing renal arterial stenosis, particularly given the high incidence of intrarenal branch vessel disease in children with fibromuscular dysplasia *(25)*. In extremely small infants, or where appropriate facilities are not available, it may be acceptable to defer angiography, managing the HTN medically until the infant is large enough for an angiogram to be performed safely.

Although nuclear scanning has been shown in some studies to demonstrate abnormalities of renal perfusion caused by thromboembolic phenomenon *(1,7,8,16,21)*, in our practice it has had little role in the assessment of infants with HTN, primarily because of the difficulties in obtaining accurate, interpretable results in this age group. Other studies, including echocardiograms and voiding cystourethrograms, should be obtained as indicated.

## TREATMENT

With a few exceptions (for example, congestive heart failure) generally accepted indications for treatment of hypertensive neonates have not been established. It is therefore up to the individual clinician to decide which infants should receive antihypertensive medications. Although long-term follow-up data of untreated hypertensive infants are not available, it is reasonable to assume that, as in older children, long-standing HTN in the neonate may cause left ventricular hypertrophy or other target organ damage. Therefore, consideration should be given to treatment of any infant with sustained HTN (as defined above).

Although today's clinician has available an ever-expanding list of agents that can be used for treatment of neonatal HTN (Tables 3 and 4), practically none of these medications has been systematically studied in neonates, and there are no antihypertensive medications with Food and Drug Administration (FDA)-approved indications for use in hypertensive infants. It is unfortunate that infants remain "therapeutic orphans" *(80)* despite the increased number of cardiovascular agents that have been studied in children under the auspices of the 1997 FDA Modernization Act *(81)*. Physicians who care for hypertensive neonates must therefore rely on data from case series and older clinical trials, as well as on expert opinion, for guidance in selecting the appropriate agent for a particular neonate.

Prior to initiating antihypertensive drug therapy, however, the infant's clinical status should be assessed and any easily correctable iatrogenic causes of HTN addressed. These may include infusions of inotropic agents or administration of other medications known to elevate BP,

Table 3
Intravenous Agents for Acute HTN and Hypertensive Emergencies/Urgencies

| *Drug* | *Class* | *Dose* | *Route* | *Comments* |
|---|---|---|---|---|
| *Diazoxide* | Vasodilator (arteriolar) | 2–5 mg/kg/dose | RAPID bolus injection | Slow injection ineffective; duration unpredictable. |
| *Enalaprilat* | ACE Inhibitor | 15 ± 5 μg/kg/dose Repeat Q 8–24 h | Injection over 5–10 min | USE WITH CAUTION. May cause prolonged hypotension and acute renal insufficiency. |
| *Esmolol* | β-blocker | Drip: 100–300 μg/kg/min | IV infusion | Very short-acting—constant infusion necessary. |
| *Hydralazine* | Vasodilator (arteriolar) | Bolus: 0.15–0.6 mg/kg/dose Drip: 0.75–5.0 μg/kg/min | IV bolus or infusion | Tachycardia frequent side-effect; must administer Q4h when given IV bolus |
| *Labetalol* | α- and β-blocker | Bolus: 0.20–1.0 mg/kg/dose Drip: 0.25–3.0 mg/kg/h | IV bolus or infusion | Heart failure, BPD relative contraindications |
| *Nicardipine* | $Ca^{++}$ channel blocker | Drip: 1–4 μg/kg/min | IV infusion | May cause reflex tachycardia |
| Sodium *Nitroprusside* | Vasodilator (arteriolar & venous) | Drip: 0.5–10 μg/kg/min | IV infusion | Thiocyanate toxicity can occur with prolonged (>72 h) use or in renal failure. |

volume overload, or pain. Following this, an antihypertensive agent should be chosen that is not only appropriate for the specific clinical situation, but also directed to the pathophysiology of the infant's HTN whenever possible.

For the majority of acutely ill infants, particularly those with severe HTN, the most appropriate approach is continuous intravenous infusions. There are numerous advantages to intravenous infusions, most importantly the ability to quickly increase or decrease the rate of infusion to achieve the desired level of BP control. Infusions may also allow the infant's BP to be kept within a relatively narrow range. This approach stands in stark contrast to the wide fluctuations in BP frequently seen when intermittently administered intravenous agents are used. As in patients of any age with malignant HTN, care should be taken to avoid too rapid a reduction in BP *(82,83)* in order to avoid cerebral ischemia and hemorrhage, a problem that premature infants in particular are already at increased risk for because of the immaturity of their periventricular circulation. Here again, continuous infusions of intravenous antihypertensives offer a distinct advantage over intermittently administered agents.

Although comprised of single-center, retrospective studies, a growing body of literature suggests that the intravenous calcium channel antagonist nicardipine is appropriate for use as a first-line agent in severely hypertensive infants *(84–86)*. This drug offers the advantage of quick onset action, which allows the patient's BP to be easily titrated to and maintained at the desired level *(87)*. It may also be continued for prolonged periods of time without an apparent decrease in antihypertensive efficacy *(86)*. Other drugs that have been successfully used in neonates include esmolol *(88)*, labetalol, and nitroprusside *(82)*. Whichever agent is used, BP should be monitored continuously via an indwelling arterial catheter, or by frequently repeated

Table 4
Oral Agents Useful for Hypertension in Infants

| *Drug* | *Class* | *Dose* | *Interval* | *Comments* |
|---|---|---|---|---|
| *Amlodipine* | $Ca^{++}$ channel blocker | 0.05–0.17 mg/kg/dose Max 0.34 mg/k/d | QD–BID | Less likely to cause sudden hypotension than isradipine |
| *Captopril* | ACE Inhibitor | <3m: 0.01–0.5 mg/kg/dose Max 2 mg/kg/d >3m: 0.15–0.3 mg/kg/dose Max 6 mg/kg/d | TID | Avoid in preterm infants? First dose may cause rapid drop in BP; monitor serum creatinine and $K^+$ |
| *Chlorothiazide* | Thiazide diuretic | 5–15 mg/kg/dose | BID | Monitor electrolytes |
| *Clonidine* | Central α agonist | 0.05–0.1 mg/dose | BID–TID | Side effects include dry mouth and sedation; rebound hypertention with abrupt discontinuation |
| *Enalapril* | ACE Inhibitor | 0.08–0.58 mg/kg/d | QD–BID | Avoid in preterm infants? Monitor serum creatinine and $K^+$ |
| *Hydralazine* | Vasodilator (arteriolar) | 0.25–1.0 mg/kg/dose Max 7.5 mg/kg/d | TID–QID | Suspension stable up to 1 wk; tachycardia and fluid retention common side-effects; lupus-like syndrome may develop in slow acetylators |
| *Hydrochlorothiazide* | Thiazide diuretic | 1–3 mg/kg/dose | QD | Monitor electrolytes |
| *Isradipine* | $Ca^{++}$ channel blocker | 0.05–0.15 mg/kg/dose Max 0.8 mg/kg/d | QID | Suspension may be compounded; useful for both acute and chronic HTN |
| *Labetalol* | α and β blocker | 0.5–1.0 mg/kg/dose Max 10 mg/kg/d | BID–TID | Monitor heart rate; avoid in infants with BPD |
| *Minoxidil* | Vasodilator (arteriolar) | 0.1–0.2 mg/kg/dose | BID–TID | Most potent oral vasodilator; excellent for refractory HTN |
| *Propranolol* | β-blocker | 0.5–1.0 mg/kg/dose Max 8–10 mg/kg/d | TID | Maximal dose depends on heart rate; avoid in infants with BPD |
| *Spironolactone* | Aldosterone antagonist | 0.5–1.5 mg/kg/dose | BID | Potassium sparing; monitor electrolytes. Takes several days to see maximum effectiveness. |

(Q 10–15 min) cuff readings so that the dose can be titrated to achieve the desired degree of BP control.

For some infants, intermittently administered intravenous agents have a role in therapy. Hydralazine and labetalol in particular may be useful in infants with mild-to-moderate HTN who aren't yet candidates for oral therapy because of gastrointestinal dysfunction. Enalaprilat, the intravenous angiotensin-converting enzyme (ACE) inhibitor, has also been reported to be useful in the treatment of neonatal renovascular HTN *(89,90)*. However, in our experience, this agent should be used with great caution. Even doses at the lower end of published ranges may lead to significant, prolonged hypotension and oliguric acute renal failure. Furthermore, the potential effects on renal maturation in preterm infants give additional rationale for avoiding this agent in the NICU.

Oral antihypertensive agents (Table 4) are best reserved for infants with less severe HTN or infants whose acute HTN has been controlled with intravenous infusions and are ready to be transitioned to chronic therapy. Captopril, in particular, is a useful agent for many causes of neonatal HTN *(91)* and is commonly used in many NICUs, despite the concerns of some pediatric nephrologists about the effects of ACE inhibitors on renal maturation in premature infants. Care must be taken to avoid giving a dose that is too high to premature infants, as they may have an exaggerated fall in BP following captopril administration *(91,92)*. Adverse neurologic effects have been described in infants following captopril-related hypotension *(92)*, highlighting the need for close BP monitoring after administration of this agent.

If captopril is chosen as the initial agent, and if the infant's BP is not controlled by captopril alone, the addition of a diuretic will frequently result in the desired degree of BP control. Beta-blockers may need to be avoided in chronic therapy of neonatal HTN, particularly in infants with chronic lung disease. In such infants, diuretics may have a beneficial effect, not only in controlling BP, but also in improving pulmonary function *(93)*.

When a vasodilator is indicated, isradipine may be superior to the older agents hydralazine and minoxidil, since it can be compounded into a stable suspension *(95)* that can be dosed with accuracy, even in tiny infants *(94)*. We no longer use nifedipine at our center because of the difficulty in administering small doses, and because of the rapid, profound, and short-lived BP reduction typically produced by this agent *(87,96)*. The calcium channel blocker amlodipine may also be useful for long-term management of neonatal HTN. Like isradipine, it may be compounded into a stable suspension and can therefore be dosed accurately, even in small infants *(87)*.

Surgery is indicated for treatment of neonatal HTN in a limited set of circumstances *(97)*. In particular, HTN caused by ureteral obstruction or aortic coarctation *(45)* is best approached surgically. For infants with renal arterial stenosis, it may be necessary to manage the infant medically until it has grown sufficiently to undergo definitive repair of the vascular abnormalities *(98)*. Outcome of such surgical procedures can become quite good if performed at centers with a large experience *(99)*. Infants with HTN secondary to Wilms tumor or neuroblastoma will require surgical tumor removal *(55,56,97)*, possibly following chemotherapy. Although controversial, a case has also been made by some authors for removal of multicystic-dysplastic kidneys because of the risk of development of HTN *(32–35)*. Infants with malignant HTN secondary to polycystic kidney disease may require bilateral nephrectomy. Fortunately, such severely affected infants are rare.

## LONG-TERM OUTCOME

Few studies examining the long-term outcome of neonatal HTN have been published. Fortunately, data are available for the largest category of hypertensive infants, namely those with HTN related to an umbilical arterial catheter *(100,101)*. In such babies, HTN will usually resolve over time. In our experience, these infants may require increases in their antihypertensive medications in the first several months following discharge from the nursery as they undergo rapid growth. Following this, it is usually possible to "wean" their antihypertensives by making no further dose increases as the infant continues to grow. Home BP monitoring by the parents is a crucially important component of this process. It should be standard practice to arrange for home BP equipment, either a Doppler or oscillometric device, for all infants discharged from the NICU on antihypertensive medications. Ultimately, antihypertensive medications should be able to be discontinued in most of these infants.

Some forms of neonatal HTN may persist beyond infancy. In particular, PKD and other forms of renal parenchymal disease may continue to cause HTN throughout childhood *(30,31,102)*. Infants with renal venous thrombosis may also remain hypertensive *(24)*, and some of these children will ultimately benefit from removal of the affected kidney *(23,24)*. Persistent or late HTN may also be seen in children who have undergone repair of renal artery stenosis *(99)* or thoracic aortic coarctation *(45)*. Reappearance of HTN in these situations should prompt a search for re-stenosis by the appropriate imaging studies.

True long-term outcome studies of infants with neonatal HTN are sorely needed at this point. Since many of these infants are delivered prior to the completion of nephron development, it is possible that they may not develop the full complement of glomeruli normally seen in term infants. Reduced nephron mass has been hypothesized to be a risk factor for the development of HTN in adulthood *(103)*. Thus, it may be possible that hypertensive neonates (and, possibly, normotensive premature neonates) are at increased risk compared to term infants for the development of HTN in late adolescence or early adulthood. Since we are now entering the era in which the first significantly premature NICU "graduates" are reaching their second and third decades of life, it is possible that appropriate studies will be conducted to address this question.

## CONCLUSIONS

BP in neonates depends on a variety of factors, including gestational age, postconceptional age, and birthweight. HTN can be seen in a variety of situations in the modern NICU, and is especially common in infants who have undergone umbilical arterial catheterization. A careful diagnostic evaluation should lead to determination of the underlying cause of HTN in most infants. Treatment decisions should be tailored to the severity of the HTN, and may include intravenous and/or oral therapy. Most infants will resolve their HTN over time, although a small number may have persistent BP elevation throughout childhood. Further study is needed to better define the long-term outcome of hypertensive neonates.

## REFERENCES


1. Adelman RD. Neonatal hypertension. Ped Clin North Am 1978;25:99–110.
2. Al-Aweel I, Pursley DM, Rubin LP, Shah B, Weisberger S, Richardson DK. Variations in prevalence of hypotension, hypertension and vasopressor use in NICUs. J Perinatol 2001;12:272–278.
3. Watkinson M. Hypertension in the newborn baby. Arch Dis Child Fetal Neonatal Ed 2002;86:F78–F81.
4. American Academy of Pediatrics Committee on Fetus and Newborn. Routine evaluation of blood pressure, hematocrit and glucose in newborns. Pediatrics 1993;92:474–476.
5. Inglefinger JR. Hypertension in the first year of life. In: Inglefinger JR. Pediatric Hypertension. Philadelphia: W.B. Saunders, 1982;229–240.
6. Buchi KF, Siegler RL. Hypertension in the first month of life. J Hypertens 1986;4:525–528.
7. Skalina MEL, Kliegman RM, Fanaroff AA. Epidemiology and management of severe symptomatic neonatal hypertension. Am J Perinatol 1986;3:235–239.
8. Singh HP, Hurley RM, Myers TF. Neonatal hypertension: incidence and risk factors. Am J Hypertens 1992;5:51–55.
9. Friedman AL, Hustead VA. Hypertension in babies following discharge from a neonatal intensive care unit. Pediatr Nephrol 1987;1:30–34.

10. Arar MY, Hogg RJ, Arant BS, Seikaly MG. Etiology of sustained hypertension in children in the southwestern United States. Pediatr Nephrol 1994;8:186–189.
11. Neal WA, Reynolds JW, Jarvis CW, Williams HJ. Umbilical artery catheterization: demonstration of arterial thrombosis by aortography. Pediatrics 1972;50:6–13.
12. Seibert JJ, Taylor BJ, Williamson SL, Williams BJ, Szabo JS, Corbitt SL. Sonographic detection of neonatal umbilical-artery thrombosis: clinical correlation. Am J Roentgenol 1987;148:965–968.
13. Ford KT, Teplick SK, Clark RE. Renal artery embolism causing neonatal hypertension. Radiology 1974;113:169–170.
14. Bauer SB, Feldman SM, Gellis SS, Retik AB. Neonatal hypertension: a complication of umbilical-artery catheterization. N Engl J Med 1975;293:1032–1033.
15. Plumer LB, Kaplan GW, Mendoza SA. Hypertension in infants—a complication of umbilical arterial catheterization. J Pediatr 1976;89:802–805.
16. Merten DF, Vogel JM, Adelman RD, Goetzman, BW, Bogren HG. Renovascular hypertension as a complication of umbilical arterial catheterization. Radiology 1978;126:751–757.
17. Brooks WG, Weibley RE. Emergency department presentation of severe hypertension secondary to complications of umbilical artery catheterization. Pediatr Emerg Care 1987;3:104–106.
18. Goetzman BW, Stadalnik RC, Bogren HG, Balnkenship WJ, Ikeda RM, Thayer J. Thrombotic complications of umbilical artery catheters: a clinical and radiographic study. Pediatrics 1975;56:374–379.
19. Wesström G, Finnström O, Stenport G. Umbilical artery catheterization in newborns. I. Thrombosis in relation to catheter type and position. Acta Paediatr Scand 1979;68:575–581.
20. Stork EK, Carlo WA, Kliegman RM, Fanaroff AA. Neonatal hypertension appears unrelated to aortic catheter position (Abstract). Pediatr Res 1984;18:321A.
21. Durante D, Jones D, Spitzer R. Neonatal arterial embolism syndrome. J Pediatr 1976;89:978–981.
22. Barrington KJ. Umbilical artery catheters in the newborn: effects of position of the catheter tip (Cochrane Review). In: The Cochrane Library, Issue 4. Oxford: Update Software, 2001.
23. Evans DJ, Silverman M, Bowley NB. Congenital hypertension due to unilateral renal vein thrombosis. Arch Dis Child 1981;56:306–308.
24. Mocan H, Beattie TJ, Murphy AV. Renal venous thrombosis in infancy: long-term follow-up. Pediatr Nephrol 1991;5:45–49.
25. Deal JE, Snell MF, Barratt TM, Dillon MJ. Renovascular disease in childhood. J Pediatr 1992;121:378–384.
26. Milner LS, Heitner R, Thomson PD, et al. Hypertension as the major problem of idiopathic arterial calcification of infancy. J Pediatr 1984;105:934–938.
27. Ciana G, Colonna F, Forleo V, Brizzi F, Benettoni A, de Vonderweid U. Idiopathic arterial calcification of infancy: effectiveness of prostaglandin infusion for treatment of secondary hypertension refractory to conventional therapy: case report. Pediatr Cardiol 1997;18:67–71.
28. Dorman DC, Reye RDK, Reid RR. Renal-artery stenosis in the rubella syndrome. Lancet 1966;1:790–792.
29. Kim ES, Caitai JM, Tu J, Nowygrod R, Stolar CJ. Congenital abdominal aortic aneurysm causing renovascular hypertension, cardiomyopathy and death in a 19-day-old neonate. J Pediatr Surg 2001;36:1445–1449.
30. Zerres K, Rudnik-Schöneborn S, Deget F, et al. Autosomal recessive polycystic kidney disease in 115 children: clinical presentation, course and influence of gender. Acta Paediatr 1996;85:437–435.
31. Fick GM, Johnson AM, Strain JD, et al. Characteristics of very early onset autosomal dominant polycystic kidney disease. J Am Soc Nephrol 1993;3:1863–1870.
32. Susskind MR, Kim KS, King LR. Hypertension and multicystic kidney. Urology 1989;34:362–366.
33. Angermeier KW, Kay R, Levin H. Hypertension as a complication of multicystic dysplastic kidney. Urology 1992;39:55–58.
34. Webb NJA, Lewis MA, Bruce J, et al. Unilateral multicystic dysplastic kidney: the case for nephrectomy. Arch Dis Child 1997;76:31–34.
35. Husmann DA. Renal dysplasia: the risks and consequences of leaving dysplastic tissue in situ. Urology 1998;52:533–536.
36. Gilboa N, Urizar RE. Severe hypertension in newborn after pyeloplasty of hydronephrotic kidney. Urology 1983;22:179–182.
37. Oliveira EA, Diniz JS, Rabelo EA, et al. Primary megaureter detected by prenatal ultrasonography: conservative management and prolonged follow-up. Int Urol Nephrol 2000;32:13–18.
38. Cadnapaphornchai P, Aisenbrey G, McDonald KM, Burke TJ, Schrier RW. Prostaglandin-mediated hyperemia and renin-mediated hypertension during acute ureteral obstruction. Prostaglandins 1978;16:965–971.

39. Riehle RA Jr, Vaughan ED Jr. Renin participation in HTN associated with unilateral hydronephrosis. J Urol 1981;126:243–246.
40. Tokunaka S, Osanai H, Hashimoto H, Takamura T, Yachiku S, Mori Y. Severe hypertension in infant with unilateral hypoplastic kidney. Urology 1987;29:618–620.
41. Wilson BJ, Flynn JT. Familial, atypical hemolytic uremic syndrome in a premature infant. Pediatr Nephrol 1998;12:782–784.
42. Abman SH, Warady BA, Lum GM, Koops BL. Systemic hypertension in infants with bronchopulmonary dysplasia. J Pediatr 1984;104:929–931.
43. Alagappan A, Malloy MH. Systemic hypertension in very low-birth weight infants with bronchopulmonary dysplasia: incidence and risk factors. Am J Perinatol 1998;15:3–8.
44. Anderson AH, Warady BA, Daily DK, Johnson JA, Thomas MK. Systemic hypertension in infants with severe bronchopulmonary dysplasia: associated clinical factors. Am J Perinatol 1993;10:190–193.
45. Beekman RH. Coarctation of the aorta. In: Emmanouilides GC, Riemenschneider TA, Allen HD, Gutgesell HP, eds. Moss and Adams' Heart Disease in Infants, Children and Adolescents: Including the Fetus and Young Adult, 5th ed. Baltimore: Williams and Wilkins, 1995;1111–1133.
46. Mimouni M, Kaufman H, Roitman A, Moraq C, Sadan N. Hypertension in a neonate with 11 beta-hydroxylase deficiency. Eur J Pediatr 1985;143:231–233.
47. White PC. Inherited forms of mineralocorticoid hypertension. Hypertens 1996;28:927–936.
48. Pozzan GB, Armanini D, Cecchetto G, et al. Hypertensive cardiomegaly caused by an aldosterone-secreting adenoma in a newborn. J Endocrinol Invest 1997;20:86–89.
49. Schonwetter BS, Libber SM, Jones D Jr, Park KJ, Plotnick LP. Hypertension in neonatal hyperthyroidism. Am J Dis Child 1983;137:954–955.
50. Greenough A, Emery EF, Gamsu HR. Dexamethasone and hypertension in preterm infants. Eur J Pediatr 1992;151:134–135.
51. Smets K, Vanhaesebrouck P. Dexamethasone associated systemic hypertension in low birth weight babies with chronic lung disease. Eur J Pediatr 1996;155:573–575.
52. Stark AR, Carlo WA, Tyson JE, et al. Adverse effects of early dexamethasone treatment in extremely-low-birth-weight infants. N Engl J Med 2001;344:95–101.
53. Greher M, Hartmann T, Winkler M, Zimpfer M, Crabnor CM. Hypertension and pulmonary edema associated with subconjunctival phenylephrine in a 2-month old child during cataract extraction. Anesthesiology 1998;88:1394–1396.
54. Horn PT. Persistent hypertension after prenatal cocaine exposure. J Pediatr 1992;121:288–291.
55. Weinblatt ME, Heisel MA, Siegel SE. Hypertension in children with neurogenic tumors. Pediatrics 1983;71: 947–951.
56. Malone PS, Duffy PG, Ransley PG, Risdon RA, Cook T, Taylor M. Congenital mesoblastic nephroma, renin production, and hypertension. J Pediatr Surg 1989;24:599–600.
57. Steinmetz JC. Neonatal hypertension and cardiomegaly associated with a congenital neuroblastoma. Pediatr Pathol 1989;9:577–582.
58. Haberkern CM, Coles PG, Morray JP, Kennard SC, Sawin RS. Intraoperative hypertension during surgical excision of neuroblastoma: case report and review of 20 years' experience. Anesth Analg 1992;75:854–858.
59. Boedy RF, Goldberg AK, Howell CG Jr, Hulse E, Edwards EG, Kanto WP. Incidence of hypertension in infants on extracorporeal membrane oxygenation. J Pediatr Surg 1990;25:258–261.
60. Becker JA, Short BL, Martin GR. Cardiovascular complications adversely affect survival during extracorporeal membrane oxygenation. Crit Care Med 1998;26:1582–1586.
61. Sell LL, Cullen ML, Lerner GR, Whittlesey GC, Shanley CJ, Klein MD. Hypertension during extracorporeal membrane oxygenation: cause, effect and management. Surgery 1987;102:724–730.
62. de Swiet M, Fayers P, Shinebourne EA. Systolic blood pressure in a population of infants in the first year of life: the Brompton study. Pediatrics 1980;65:1028–1035.
63. Versmold HT, Kitterman JA, Phibbs RH, Gregory GA, Tooley WH. Aortic blood pressure during the first 12 hours of life in infants with birth weight 610 to 4220 grams. Pediatrics 1981;67:607–613.
64. Tan KL. Blood pressure in very low birth weight infants in the first 70 days of life. J Pediatr 1988;112: 266–270.
65. McGarvey ST, Zinner SH. Blood pressure in infancy. Semin Nephrol 1989;9:260–266.
66. Zubrow AB, Hulman S, Kushner H, Falkner B. Determinants of blood pressure in infants admitted to neonatal intensive care units: a prospective multicenter study. J Perinatol 1995;15:470–479.

67. Hegyi T, Anwar M, Carbone MT, et al. Blood pressure ranges in premature infants: II. The first week of life. Pediatrics 1996;97:336–342.
68. Georgieff MK, Mills MM, Gomez-Marin O, Sinaiko AR. Rate of change of blood pressure in premature and full term infants from birth to 4 months. Pediatr Nephrol 1996;10:152–155.
69. Report of the Second Task Force on Blood Pressure Control in Children—1987. Task Force on Blood Pressure Control in Children. National Heart, Lung, and Blood Institute, Bethesda, Maryland. Pediatrics 1987;79:1–25.
70. Elliot SJ, Hansen TN. Neonatal hypertension. In: Long WA, ed. Fetal and Neonatal Cardiology. Philadelphia: W.B. Saunders, 1990;492–498.
71. Low JA, Panagiotopoulos C, Smith JT, Tang W, Derrick EJ. Validity of newborn oscillometric blood pressure. Clin Invest Med 1995;18:163–167.
72. Park MK, Menard SM. Normative oscillometric blood pressure values in the first 5 years of life in an office setting. Am J Dis Child 1989;143:860–864.
73. DeSwiet M, Peto J, Shinebourne EA. Difference between upper and lower limb blood pressure in neonates using Doppler technique. Arch Dis Child 1974;49:734–735.
74. Crapanzano MS, Strong WB, Newman IR, Hixon RL, Casal D, Linder CW. Calf blood pressure: clinical implications and correlations with arm blood pressure in infants and young children. Pediatrics 1996;97: 220–224.
75. Park MK, Lee D. Normative arm and calf blood pressure values in the newborn. Pediatrics 1989;83:240–243.
76. Nwanko MU, Lorenz JM, Gardiner JC. A standard protocol for blood pressure measurement in the newborn. Pediatrics 1997;99:E10.
77. Tannenbaum J, Hulman S, Falkner B. Relationship between plasma renin concentration and atrial natriuretic peptide in the human newborn. Am J Perinatol 1990;7:174–177.
78. Krüger C, Rauh M, Dörr HG. Immunoreactive renin concentration in healthy children from birth to adolescence. Clinica Chim Acta 1998;274:15–27.
79. Cannon ME, Twu BM, Yang CS, Hsu CH. The effect of theophylline and cyclic adenosine 3', 5'-monophosphate on renin release by afferent arterioles. J Hypertens 1989;7:569–576.
80. Shirkey H. Therapeutic orphans. Pediatrics 1968;72:119–120.
81. Flynn JT. Successes and shortcomings of the Food and Drug Modernization Act. Am J Hypertens 2003;16(10):889–891.
82. Deal JE, Barratt TM, Dillon MJ. Management of hypertensive emergencies. Arch Dis Child 1992;67:1089–1092.
83. Adelman RD, Coppo R, Dillon MJ. The emergency management of severe hypertension. Pediatr Nephrol 2000;14:422–427.
84. Gouyon JB, Geneste B, Semama DS, Francoise M, Germain JF. Intravenous nicardipine in hypertensive preterm infants. Arch Dis Child 1997;76:F126–F127.
85. Milou C, Debuche-Benouachkou V, Semama DS, Germain JF, Gouyon JB. Intravenous nicardipine as a first-line antihypertensive drug in neonates. Intensive Care Med 2000;26:956–958.
86. Flynn, JT, Mottes TA, Brophy PB, Kershaw DB, Smoyer WE, Bunchman TE. Intravenous nicardipine for treatment of severe hypertension in children. J Pediatr 2001;139:38–43.
87. Flynn JT, Pasko DA. Calcium channel blockers: pharmacology and place in therapy of pediatric hypertension. Pediatr Nephrol 2000;15:302–316.
88. Wiest DB, Garner SS, Uber WE, Sade RM. Esmolol for the management of pediatric hypertension after cardiac operations. J Thorac Cardiovas Surg 1998;115:890–897.
89. Wells TG, Bunchman TE, Kearns GL. Treatment of neonatal hypertension with enalaprilat. J Pediatr 1990;117:664–667.
90. Mason T, Polak MJ, Pyles L, Mullett M, Swanke C. Treatment of neonatal renovascular hypertension with intravenous enalapril. Am J Perinatol 1992;9:254–257.
91. Sinaiko AR, Kashtan CE, Mirkin BL. Antihypertensive drug therapy with captopril in children and adolescents. Clin Exp Hypertens 1986;A8:829–839.
92. Perlman JM, Volpe JJ. Neurologic complications of captopril treatment of neonatal hypertension. Pediatrics 1989;83:47–52.
93. Englehardt B, Elliott S, Hazinski TA. Short- and long-term effects of furosemide on lung function in infants with bronchopulmonary dysplasia. J Pediatr 1986;109:1034–1039.
93. Flynn JT, Warnick SJ. Isradipine treatment of hypertension in children: a single-center experience. Pediatr Nephrol 2002;17(9):748–753.

94. MacDonald JL, Johnson CE, Jacobson P. Stability of isradipine in an extemporaneously compounded oral liquid. Am J Hosp Pharm 1994;51:2409–2411.
95. Blaszak RT, Savage JA, Ellis, EN. The use of short-acting nifedipine in pediatric patients with hypertension. J Pediatr 2001;139:34–37.
96. Leonard MB, Kasner SE, Feldman HI, Schulman SL. Adverse neurologic events associated with rebound hypertension after using short-acting nifedipine in childhood hypertension. Pediatr Emerg Care 2001;17: 435–437.
97. Hendren WH, Kim SH, Herrin JT, Crawford JD. Surgically correctable hypertension of renal origin in childhood. Am J Surg 1982;143:432–442.
98. Bendel-Stenzel M, Najarian JS, Sinaiko AR. Renal artery stenosis: long-term medical management before surgery. Pediatr Nephrol 1995;10:147–151.
99. Stanley JC, Zelenock GB, Messina LM, Wakefield TW. Pediatric renovascular hypertension: a thirty-year experience of operative treatment. J Vasc Surg 1995;21:212–227.
100. Adelman RD. Long-term follow-up of neonatal renovascular hypertension. Pediatr Nephrol 1987;1:35–41.
101. Caplan MS, Cohn RA, Langman CB, Conway JA, Ahkolnik A, Brouillette RT. Favorable outcome of neonatal aortic thrombosis and renovascular hypertension. J Pediatr 1989;115:291–295.
102. Roy S, Dillon MJ, Trompeter RS, Barratt TM. Autosomal recessive polycystic kidney disease: long-term outcome of neonatal survivors. Pediatr Nephrol 1997;11:302–306.
103. Mackenzie HS, Lawler EV, Brenner BM. Congenital olionephropathy. The fetal flaw in essential hypertension? Kidney Int 1996;55:S30–S34.

# 21 Hypertension in Chronic Kidney Disease

*Franz Schaefer, MD, PhD and Otto Mehls, MD*

*CONTENTS*



## PREVALENCE OF RENAL HYPERTENSION IN CHILDHOOD

Persistent arterial hypertension (HTN) is observed in approx 0.1% of children. In contrast to adults, secondary forms of HTN are more frequent than essential HTN, which accounted for only 20% of cases in a meta-analysis of 1575 children and adolescents compiled from nine published studies *(1)*. Essential HTN is diagnosed almost exclusively in adolescent patients, whereas secondary causes prevail in prepubertal children.

Although the spectrum of secondary HTN in childhood comprises a wide range of renal, cardiovascular, endocrine, neurological and iatrogenic diseases, renoparenchymal disorders are responsible for 75%, and renovascular disease for another 10% of cases *(1)*. Hypertensive renoparenchymal disease is most commonly caused by acute or chronic glomerulonephritis (28%), pyelonephritic scars with or without reflux (23%), obstructive uropathies (10%), hemolytic-uremic syndrome (5%), and polycystic kidney disease (4%). In these disorders, the prevalence of HTN varies directly with the prevalence of concomitant chronic renal failure (CRF).

In a recent survey of 508 children with moderate chronic renal failure (CRF) (mean glomerular filtration rate [GFR] 47 mL/min/1.73 m$^2$), mean standardized systolic and diastolic blood pressure (BP) were 0.6 and 1.1 standard deviation (SD) above the means for age, respectively (Fig. 1) *(2)*. The survey also indicated that 35% of patients received antihypertensive medication. Additionally, 11% of untreated patients had (diastolic) BPs above the 95th percentile, indicating an HTN prevalence of 46% in early CRF in children. 30% of the patients receiving antihypertensive treatment had elevated BP. The prevalence of (diastolic) HTN was 88% in patients with acquired glomerulopathies, 38% in children with hypo/dysplastic kidney disorders and 57% in other congenital or hereditary renal diseases. Notably, the degree of HTN

From: *Clinical Hypertension and Vascular Disease: Pediatric Hypertension*
Edited by: R. J. Portman, J. M. Sorof, and J. R. Ingelfinger © Humana Press Inc., Totowa, NJ

(expressed as standard deviation score) was not correlated with the GFR, indicating that the mechanisms underlying HTN in CRF are operative early in the course of disease.

## UNDERLYING DISEASES

### *Renovascular Disease*

Renovascular HTN is defined as HTN resulting from lesions that impair blood flow to a portion, or all, of one or both kidneys *(3,4)*. Renovascular HTN accounts for about 10% of pediatric patients (20% of infants) presenting with persistent HTN. Renal artery stenosis caused by fibromuscular dysplasia is the most frequent underlying disorder (70%), affecting the main renal artery and/or, more commonly, intrarenal vessels *(5)*. Fibromuscular dysplasia most often occurs in a familial pattern *(6)*; the genetics are consistent with an autosomal dominant inheritance with variable (and often no) clinical effect. Neurofibromatosis Type 1 (NF-1, von Recklinghausen disease) constitutes a major subgroup among children with fibromuscular dysplasia, accounting for at least 15% of all pediatric cases of renal artery stenosis *(3,7)*. Another frequent genetic cause of renal artery stenosis is Williams Beuren syndrome *(8)*. In these and other hereditary syndromes, renal artery stenosis is usually combined with anomalies of extrarenal arteries. When renal artery disease is seen in combination with aortic coarctation, it is known as the mid-aortic syndrome *(9)*. Apart from vascular malformation complexes, mid-aortic syndrome is most often caused by Takayasu disease, an unspecific aorto-arteritis of autoimmune origin common in non-white populations *(10)*. Renovascular HTN may also be caused by other systemic vasculitic disorders, such as periarteritis nodosa or scleroderma.

### *Renoparenchymal Disesase*

HTN is extremely common in various forms of glomerulonephritis. Whereas acute, e.g., poststreptococcal, glomerulonephritis usually induces a reversible rise in BP, chronic glomerular disease, typically manifesting as steroid-resistant nephrotic syndrome, is commonly associated with persistent HTN. The most frequent underlying histopathological entities associated with HTN, even in the absence of renal failure, are focal-segmental glomerulosclerosis, membranoproliferative glomerulonephritis, and crescentic glomerulonephritis. Persistent HTN is also common in patients who recovered from hemolytic uremic syndrome. A high prevalence of secondary HTN is observed in glomerulonephritis secondary to systemic vasculitis, such as lupus erythematosus.

Renoparenchymal HTN is not limited to glomerular disease, but is also observed in tubulointerstitial disorders that lead to renal scarring. Recurrent pyelonephritis, reflux nephropathy, obstructive uropathies, and polycystic kidney disease all result in tubulointerstitial fibrosis and tubular atrophy. By mechanisms not entirely understood, scarring processes induce local renin and angiotensin synthesis, along with synthesis of other vasoactive substances, although peripheral renin activity is frequently normal.

### *Chronic Renal Failure*

HTN is an inevitable consequence of CRF. While HTN is most severe in patients approaching end-stage renal disease, BP increases with even mild impairment of renal function. CRF-related HTN is characterized by increased peripheral vascular resistance, whereas cardiac output (CO) may be normal or increased. An expanded extracellular fluid volume is usually present only in advanced predialytic or end-stage renal disease (ESRD). The degree of HTN is affected by the underlying disease. At any given level of GFR, children with acquired glomerulopathies or polycystic kidney disease tend to have higher BP than patients with renal hypoplasia and/or uropathies.

## PATHOGENESIS OF HYPERTENSION IN CHRONIC RENAL FAILURE

### *Sodium and Water Retention*

In a seminal study, Coleman and Guyton *(11)* showed that infusion of normal saline in anephric dogs led to HTN characterized by an initial increase in plasma volume and CO, followed by an increased peripheral vascular resistance *(11)*. Extracellular fluid expansion is most consistently found in hypertensive ESRD patients. Strict enforcement of dry weight by reduced salt intake, slow, long hemodialysis (8 h twice weekly) or additional ultrafiltration sessions, have been shown to normalize BP in adults, without the need for antihypertensive agents in the majority of hemodialysis patients *(12,13)*. Plasma volume is elevated and correlated with BP in renal disease, but not in essential HTN. However, the correlation between interdialytic weight gain and BP is poor, suggesting that additional, fluid-independent mechanisms must affect BP in ESRD *(14–19)*. The correlation of BP and interdialytic weight gain seems to be higher in hypertensive than in normotensive patients *(16)*, suggesting individual differences in vascular autoregulation. At a certain level of extracellular fluid expansion, HTN may become manifest only in those patients who fail to suppress vasoconstrictor systems.

Early in the course of CRF, the prevalence of HTN is high, although plasma and extracellular fluid volumes tend to be normal *(20)* (Fig. 1). This is particularly remarkable in patients with renal hypo/dysplasia, who tend to lose considerable amounts of sodium and water. In addition, as nephron loss progresses in mild and moderate CRF, the remaining nephrons have an increased responsiveness to natriuretic factors *(21)*. Diuretics are effective in decreasing BP in early CRF. This fact alone is insufficient to prove a role for salt and water retention in the pathogenesis of HTN, since loop diuretics interfere with the vascular actions of angiotensin II (ANG II), independent of their saluretic effect *(22,23)*. The most compelling evidence for volume-independent mechanisms of HTN in CRF comes from hypertensive hemodialysis patients undergoing bilateral nephrectomy. The removal of the native kidneys markedly reduced BP and total peripheral vascular resistance, suggesting that an excessive vasopressor function of the scarred kidneys plays a major role in the pathophysiology of HTN in ESRD. Of interest, previously hypertensive patients, but not previously normotensive patients, responded to salt and water loading with an increase of BP. Therefore, in ESRD, vascular tone must be affected by kidney-related, as well as kidney-unrelated mechanisms.

### *Renin-Angiotensin-Aldosterone System*

Although plasma renin activity is typically in the normal range in hypertensive CRF patients, the lack of renin suppression, despite HTN and expansion of the intracellular fluid space, has been interpreted as a state of relative hyperreninemia *(22,24)*. In keeping with this notion, the infusion of normal saline fails to suppress plasma renin activity in hemodialysis patients *(25)*. In recent years, the traditional view of the renin-angiotensin system, as an endocrine system mediating systemic vasoconstriction and fluid retention, has been complemented by the understanding that angiotensin is synthesized locally and regulates growth and differentiation of many tissues, including the kidneys. The local effects of ANG II in the diseased kidney are

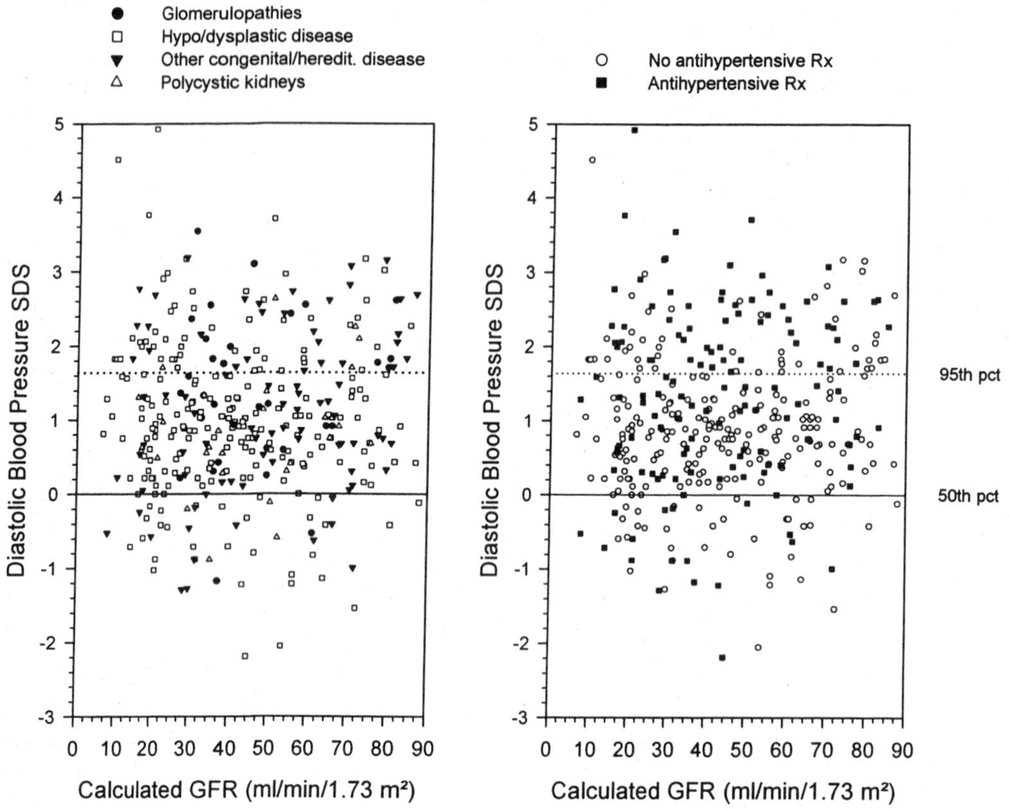


Fig. 1. BP in 508 children with chronic kidney disease. Distribution of diastolic BP SDs is depicted according to underlying disease (left panel) and by prevalent antihypertensive medication (right panel). Data were obtained as part of a trial screening procedure in 33 pediatric nephrology units throughout Europe (ESCAPE Study group). Diastolic BP values were converted to SDs using the European pediatric reference values for casual BP from De Man et al. *(105)*.

affected by multiple mechanisms, independent of plasma renin activity. Apart from its hemo- and glomerulodynamic actions, locally formed ANG II stimulates glomerular hypertrophy and tubulointerstitial scar formation, directly and via regulation of endothelin-1 (ET-1), tissue growth factor (TGF)-β, and multiple other growth factors, as well as chemokines. Of importance with respect to the pathogenesis of renal HTN, intrarenal ANG II upregulates afferent neuronal activity originating from the kidney, resulting in sympathetic overstimulation in chronic renal disease.

### *Increased Sympathetic Tone*

Recent clinical and experimental evidence suggests that sympathetic overactivity triggered by afferent signals from the diseased kidneys may play a key role in the pathogenesis of HTN in CRF. In rats undergoing 5/6-nephrectomy, afferent sensory neural pathways in the remnant kidneys are activated and transmit impulses to the hypothalamic vasomotor control center, resulting in a rise in BP that is sustained by noradrenergic mechanisms *(26)*. The clinical relevance of this mechanism has been demonstrated impressively by microneurographic studies in patients with CRF. Sympathetic nerve activity is markedly increased in predialysis *(27)*, as well as hemodialysis patients *(28)*. This increased activity persists after renal transplanta-

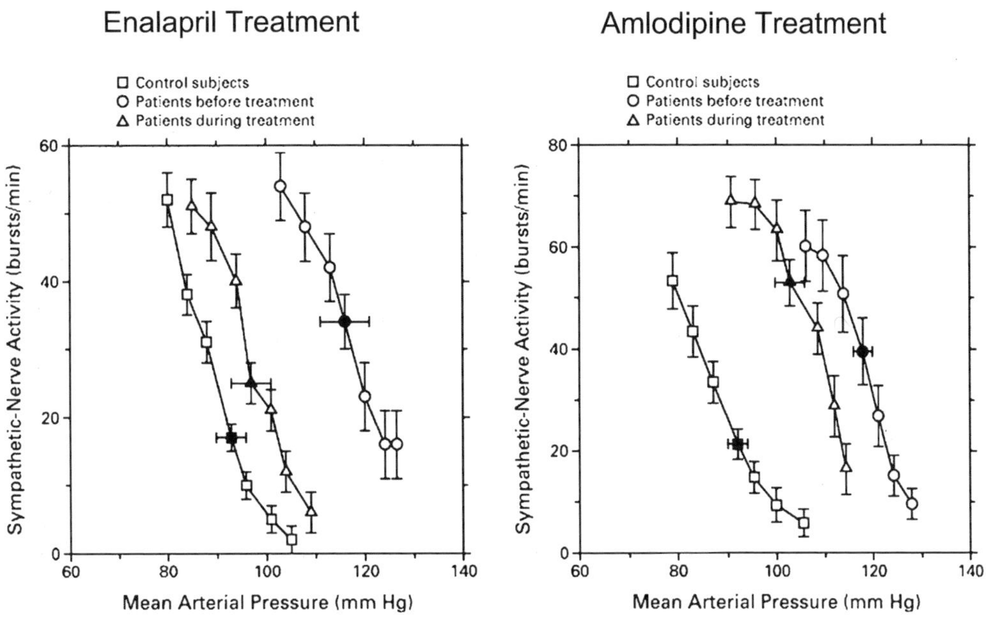


Fig. 2. Baroreflex response of sympathetic nerve activity to changes in mean arterial pressure in patients with CRF before and after 4 wk of treatment with enalapril ($n = 14$, left panel) or amlodipine ($n = 10$, right panel) and in control subjects. Both drugs lowered baseline BP to the same degree. Enalapril, which lowered resting sympathetic-nerve activity and heart rate, shifted baroreflex curves downward and nearly normalized sympathetic nerve activity. By contrast, amlodipine increased resting muscle sympathetic-nerve activity and the baroreflex response curve was shifted upward, implying that sympathetic activity remained elevated over a range of BP levels. Adapted with permission from *27*.

tion, provided the native kidneys are in place. After bilateral nephrectomy, sympathetic nerve activity normalizes, with a concomitant reduction of BP *(28)*. Treatment with angiotensin-converting enzyme (ACE) inhibitors, but not with calcium channel blockers, normalizes sympathetic activity, suggesting that the tone induced by intrarenal ANG II strongly influences afferent neural signaling *(27)* (Fig. 2).

### *Endothelial Factors*

The vascular endothelium exerts important endocrine and paracrine functions, including active control of vascular tone. The key vasodilator factor secreted by the endothelium is nitric oxide (NO), the absence of which causes severe HTN *(29)*. In uremia, endothelium-dependent (but not endothelium-independent) vasodilatation is impaired *(30)*. This endothelial dysfunction has been ascribed to deficient NO synthesis. The stable NO metabolites nitrite and nitrate are decreased in patients receiving chronic peritoneal and hemodialysis *(31,32)*. Uremic plasma suppresses NO synthase (NOS) activity in cultured endothelial cells, suggesting the presence of a circulating NOS inhibitor. Indeed, asymmetric dimethylarginine (ADMA), a potent NOS inhibitor, accumulates in CRF *(33)*, with 6- to 10-fold elevated concentrations in hemodialysis patients *(31,34)*. While NOS suppression by accumulating ADMA would provide a ready explanation for volume-independent HTN in ESRD, some doubt concerning the role of NO has been raised by the poor correlation between ADMA concentrations and BP *(35)*, as well as the normal NO production rate observed by direct assessment of exhaled NO in hemodialysis patients *(36)*. Moreover, the specificity of ADMA accumulation in uremia has been ques-

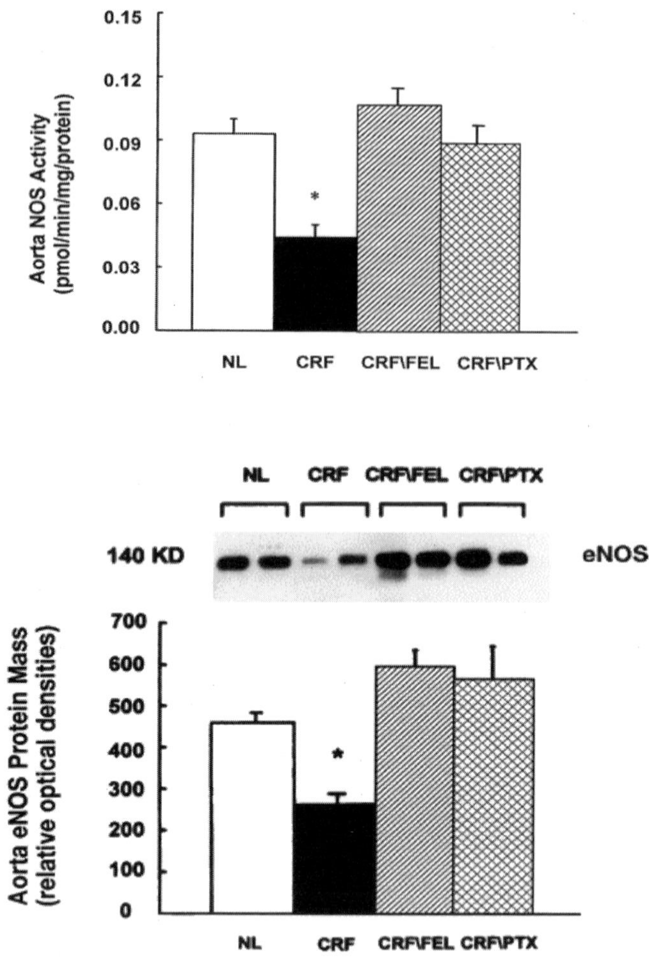


Fig. 3. Reduced NOS activity (upper panel) and eNOS protein expression in thoracic aorta of 5/6 nephrectomized uremic rats: NOS protein abundance and activity are restored both by calcium channel blockade (FEL=felodipine treatment) and parathyroidectomy (PTX). Adapted with permission from *37*.

tioned, since ADMA is also elevated in patients with atherosclerotic disease and normal kidney function *(34)*.

Animal studies have suggested reduced eNOS protein expression in CRF, with a causative role of hyperparathyroidism (Fig. 3) *(37)*.

ET-1, a peptide secreted mainly by vascular endothelial cells, is the most potent vasoconstrictor currently known. In addition, ET-1 affects salt and water homeostasis via interaction with the renin-angiotensin-aldosterone system, vasopressin and atrial natriuretic peptide, and stimulates the sympathetic nervous system *(38)*. ET-1 overexpression renders mice susceptible to salt-induced HTN and renal damage *(39)*. In patients with ESRD, as well as in the rat remnant kidney model of CRF, ET-1 plasma levels increase directly with BP *(40)*. Therefore, circulating and, possibly, renal ET-1 may contribute to HTN in CRF. Notably, ACE inhibitors reduce ET-1 expression and attenuate ET-1-induced HTN by inhibiting the catabolism of vasodilatory kinins *(41,42)*.

### *Calcium and Parathyroid Hormone*

Secondary hyperparathyroidism starts early in the course of CRF. Parathyroid hormone (PTH) has multiple effects on the cardiovascular system. Acute infusion of PTH lowers BP in a dose-dependent fashion via its well established vasodilatory effect *(43)*. In contrast, a high correlation between BP and serum PTH levels is observed in patients with chronic secondary hyperparathyroidism *(44)*.

This relationship has been explained by the increase in intracellular calcium levels caused by chronically elevated PTH, which may render vascular smooth muscle cells more susceptible to vasoconstrictors. For example, calcium infusions increase BP more effectively in parathyroid intact uremic rats than in parathyroidectomized animals *(45)*. Similarly, patients with early CRF exhibit an excessive pressor response to norepinephrine infusion, and calcium channel blocker administration normalizes this response, as well as that of free cytosolic calcium levels *(46)*.

The enhancement of pressor responses by PTH, and dysregulation of cytosolic calcium, may be mediated in part via suppression of eNOS expression. In the remnant kidney rat model of CRF, reduced aortic eNOS protein abundance was observed; it can be reversed by parathyroidectomy, and by calcium channel blockade *(37)* (Fig. 3). Apart from PTH, cytosolic calcium is regulated by (Na,K)-ATPase. The activity of this transmembrane carrier protein is reduced in CRF by accumulated, circulating, digitalis-like substances, which may contribute to the proposed cytosolic, calcium-mediated hyperresponsiveness of vascular smooth muscle cells to endogenous vasoconstrictors.

### *Intrauterine Programming*

Recent epidemiological and experimental evidence has suggested that environmental influences in intrauterine life may predispose individuals to HTN, dyslipidemia, and cardiovascular disease (CVD) in later life. Barker et al. first proposed that intrauterine malnutrition, indicated by relatively low birth weight, is associated with type II diabetes mellitus, HTN, dyslipidemia, and CVD in adult life *(47)*. Furthermore, intrauterine malnutrition appears to be associated with reduced nephrogenesis. Adequate maternal protein intake appears critical for normal fetal nephron endowment. Similarly, exposure to excess glucocorticoids leads to a decrease in nephron number by 30 to 40% in rodents and sheep *(48)*, associated with marked HTN in postadolescent life.

Disproportionately small kidney size, suggesting reduced nephron mass, has been reported as evident on ultrasound in children with intrauterine growth retardation, even antenatally *(49)*. A reduction of nephron numbers by 13% was found in humans born with a weight of less than 2.5 kg *(50)*. A possible link between reduced nephron endowment and the development of HTN has recently been suggested by an autopsy study. In the study, ten subjects with essential HTN were compared to matched nonhypertensive controls. The essential HTN subjects disclosed a reduction in total kidney nephron number by almost 50%, which was compensated by a two-fold increase in glomerular size *(51)*. Of note in this context, we unexpectedly found a 38% prevalence of HTN in children with severe renal hypoplasia, despite the common presence of polyuria and salt wasting in this population *(2)*. These observations are consistent with Brenner's concept, which implies that a congenital reduction of nephron endowment predisposes individuals to HTN as a consequence of long-term glomerular hyperfiltration and glomerulosclerosis *(52)*. On the other hand, glomerulosclerosis was very mild in the hypertensive oligonephronic humans, and absent in the sheep model *(48,51)*. Also, only unilateral nephrectomy during the period of active nephrogenesis is associated with the later development of HTN in rats and sheep *(53,54)*. Children with unilateral renal agenesis have higher 24-h BP than children losing one kidney shortly after birth *(55)*. Additional mechanisms of prenatal BP imprinting have been suggested, such as persistent upregulation of renal angiotensinogen and angiotensin receptors and increased sodium channel expression *(56,57)*, which may operate independently of nephron endowment. Consequently, HTN and reduced renal mass may not be causally related, but may both be secondary to the condition of intrauterine malnutrition. This is supported by the observation that selective supplementation of low-protein diets with additional nitrogen sources in pregnant rats normalized nephron number, regardless of the supplement composition. Only glycine supplementation, however, could reverse the hypertensinogenic effect of an antenatal low-protein diet *(58)*. Finally, it is possible that abnormalities in genes controlling nephron development could also affect the predisposition for HTN *(59)*.

## EFFECT OF HYPERTENSION ON PROGRESSION OF CHRONIC RENAL FAILURE

### *Association of Hypertension With Progressive Renal Failure*

A large body of evidence from clinical trials and epidemiological studies indicates that HTN is an important risk factor for progressive renal disease. In the Multiple Risk Factor Intervention Trial (MRET), more than 330,000 men were followed over a 16-yr period. The initial BP quantitatively predicted the risk of ESRD, with a twofold increase in risk even among the men with BPs in the high normal range *(60)*. In diabetic nephropathy, an almost linear relationship between mean arterial BP and the annual decrease in glomerular filtration rate has been observed *(61)*.

Apart from BP, the presence of proteinuria is associated with an accelerated progression of renal failure in people with diabetic *(62)* and nondiabetic nephropathies *(63)*. A large, prospective trial in children with CRF designed to evaluate the renoprotective effect of a low protein diet, failed to slow down progression by restricted protein intake. However, the trial identified HTN and proteinuria as two major independent predictors of progressive CRF in children *(64)*. The distinction between fast and slow progressors was greatest when low cut-off levels for BP (i.e., 120 mmHg systolic) and proteinuria (50 mg/m$^2$/d) were chosen (Fig. 4).

Although these observational studies cannot rule out the possibility that proteinuria and HTN are markers of more active renal disease rather than active factors in the progression of CRF, a large body of experimental and clinical research has provided evidence for a definitive role of BP and proteinuria in the pathogenesis of progressive CRF.

### *Pathogenic Mechanisms of Chronic Renal Failure Progression*

The current views of the mechanisms leading to progressive renal failure are summarized in Fig. 5. In healthy kidneys, the glomerular tufts are protected from the effects of systemic BP variations by judicious adaptation of the afferent arteriolar tone, leading to a stable filtration pressure over a wide range of systemic BP. This autoregulation is thought to be defective in CRF *(65)*, resulting in disinhibited transmission of systemic BP to the glomeruli. HTN and preexisting renal damage converge at the level of glomerular transcapillary pressure. According to the Brenner hypothesis, any critical reduction of functional renal mass leads to hyperfiltration and intraglomerular HTN in the remaining nephrons *(52)*. The increased filtra-

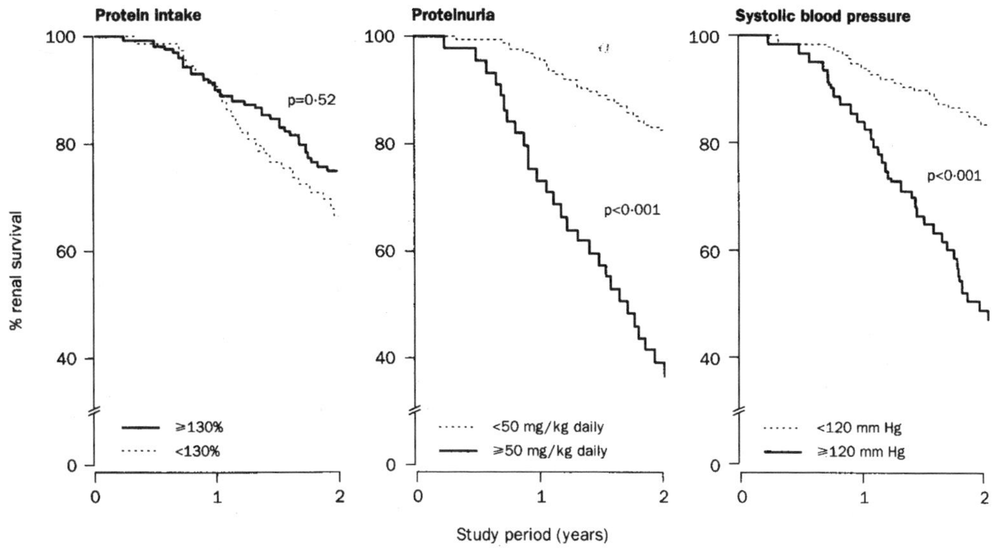


Fig. 4. Lacking effect of restricted protein intake on renal survival (defined as less than 10 mL/min/1.73 $m^2$ GFR loss during 2 yr of observation) in 200 children with CRF (left panel). Secondary analysis revealed markedly lower renal survival rates in children with proteinuria >50 mg/kg/d (middle panel) and systolic BP greater than 120 mmHg (right panel). Adapted with permission from ref. *64*.

tion pressure causes, or aggravates, preexisting proteinuria. The exposure of tubular and mesangial structures to macromolecular proteins elicits a marked and persistent tissue response. This is characterized by the release of vasoactive peptides and growth factors such as ANG II, ET-1, and others *(66)*, which further increase intraglomerular HTN by preferentially constricting the efferent arterioles and/or by inducing glomerular hypertrophy.

Independent of its glomerular hemodynamic effects, ANG II interferes with tubulointerstitial tissue homeostasis. ANG II stimulates the synthesis and release of TGF-β which, via its downstream mediator connective tissue growth factor (CTGF), stimulates collagen and matrix protein synthesis. In addition, angiotensin and aldosterone induce the local release of inhibitors of tissue proteases, such as TIMP-1, TIMP-2 and PAI-1. Increased production and diminished degradation of matrix proteins results in excessive deposition of fibrous filaments. Moreover, proteinuria and enhanced ANG II formation stimulate the synthesis and release of several pro-inflammatory cytokines and chemokines, such as RANTES and MCP-1, and of the transcription factor NFκB *(67,68)*. These mediators enhance macrophage infiltration, matrix deposition, interstitial fibrosis, and tubular cell apoptosis.

In addition to the stimulation of vasoactive factors and cytokines, proteinuria induces complement activation on the luminal surface of tubular epithelial cells. Recent studies in rats unable to form C5b-9 membrane attack complexes demonstrated that complement induction is required for the development of tubulointerstitial damage in nonimmunological proteinuric disease models, as well as for progression of CRF in the remnant kidney model *(69,70)*. Proteinuria may cause tubular complement activation via multiple mechanisms, one of which is the apotransferrin component of filtered transferrin *(71)*. Moreover, iron dissociating from accumulating internalized transferrin causes oxidative damage in tubular cells *(72)*.

Recently, another possible mechanism of progressive renal damage has been identified in animal models of hypertensive glomerulopathy *(73)*. Once glomerulosclerosis is established,

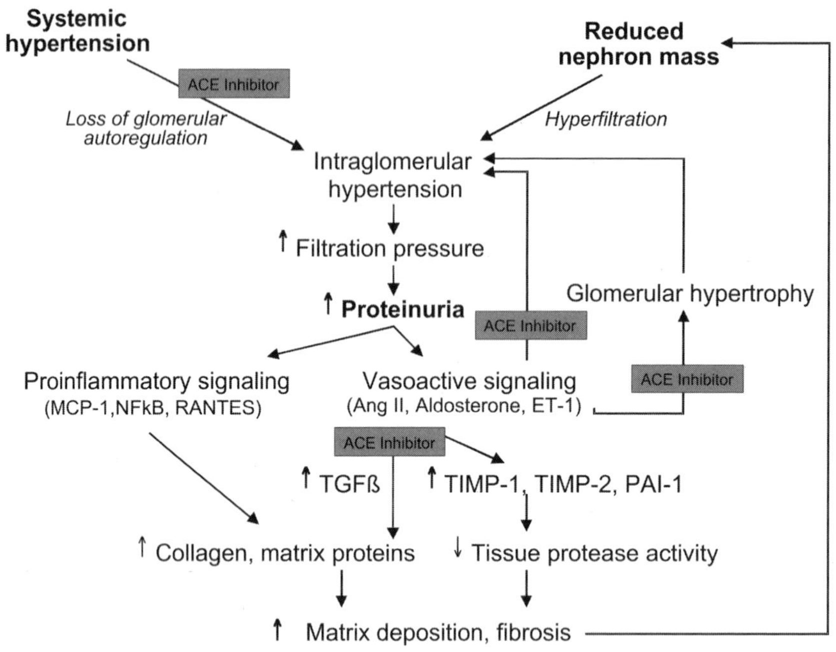


**Fig. 5.** Mechanisms of disease progression in CRF, and sites of action of ACE inhibitors.

synechial glomerular capillaries may continue to produce ultrafiltrate, which is misdirected into the paraglomerular and peritubular space, resulting in local inflammation, a fibrotic tissue response and atrophy of the nephron.

### *Renoprotective Effect of Antihypertensive Treatment in Chronic Renal Failure*

Several interventional trials have provided evidence that lowering BP in hypertensive patients at risk for progressive renal disease preserves kidney function (Table 1) *(63,74–84)*. In view of the multiple mechanisms by which ANG II stimulates glomerulosclerosis and tubulointerstitial fibrosis, together with promising results from animal research, it was hoped that renin-angiotensin system (RAS) antagonists might confer specific renoprotection beyond their antihypertensive properties. Therefore, most trials assessing renoprotection by intensified BP control have used ACE inhibitors in comparison to other antihypertensive agents. To date, most comparative trials suggested a superior renoprotective efficacy of RAS antagonists. The renoprotective potential of $AT_1$ receptor blockers was first demonstrated 10 yr ago in patients with diabetic nephropathy *(77,83,84)* and subsequently confirmed in various nondiabetic renal diseases *(63,74–76,78,80–82)*. A recent meta-analysis of 11 randomized controlled trials in patients with nondiabetic nephropathies showed that ACE inhibition decreased the risk of doubling serum creatinine or developing ESRD by 36% *(85)*. In line with hypotheses based on pathophysiology, the renoprotection afforded by ACE inhibitors appeared, in part, independent of their antihypertensive, and even their antiproteinuric, action. Even after adjusting for BP and proteinuria, the risk for progressive renal failure was reduced by 30%.

In recent years, the advent of angiotensin type I receptor blockers (ARBs) has added an additional therapeutic option. ACE inhibitors and ARBS have slightly different modes of action. ACE inhibitors nonselectively antagonize angiotensin type I and type II receptor-mediated events, and enhance the action of vasodilatory kinins by interfering with their deg-

Table 1
Clinical Trials Demonstrating Renoprotective Effect of Antihypertensive Treatment in Adult Patients

| *Source* | *Patient population* | *Renal outcome* | *ACEI/ARB comparison vs. other AHT* | *ACEI/ARB superior* |
|---|---|---|---|---|
| Parving et al. *(79)* | Type 1 DM | Slowed decline in GFR | No | ... |
| Peterson et al. *(63)* | Nondiabetic | Slowed decline in GFR | No | ... |
| Lewis et al. *(77)* | Type 1 DM | Decreased risk for ESRD, doubling SCr, and death | Yes, ACEI | Yes |
| Bakris et al. *(83)* | Type 2 DM | Slowed decline in GFR | Yes, ACEI | Yes |
| UK Prospective Diabetes Study group *(84)* | Type 2 DM | Decreased risk of proteinuria | Yes, ACEI | No |
| Zucchelli et al. *(80)* | NDRD | Slowed decline in GFR | Yes, ACEI | No |
| Hannedouche et al. *(81)* | NDRD | Slowed decline in GFR | Yes, ACEI | No |
| Kamper et al. *(78)* | NDRD | Slowed decline in GFR | Yes, ACEI | Yes |
| Toto et al. *(74)* | Hypertensive nephrosclerosis | Slowed decline in GFR | Yes, ACEI | No |
| Ihle et al. *(82)* | NDRD | Slowed decline in GFR | Yes, ACEI | Yes |
| Maschio et al. *(75)* | NDRD | Decreased risk for ESRD | Yes, ACEI | Yes |
| Gisen Group *(76)* | Glomerulonephritis | Decreased risk for ESRD | Yes, ACEI | Yes |
| AASK Group *(97)* | NDRD | Decreased risk for ESRD, 50% GFR loss, and death | Yes, ACEI | Yes |
| Parving et al. *(88)* | Type 2 DM | Decreased risk of proteinuria | Yes, ARB | Yes |
| Lewis et al. *(89)* | Type 2 DM | Decreased risk for ESRD, doubling Scr | Yes, ARB | Yes |
| RENAAL Group *(90)* | Type 2 DM | Decreased risk for ESRD, doubling Scr | Yes, ARB | Yes |

ACEI indicates angiotensin-converting enzyme inhibitor; ARB, angiotensin Type I receptor blocker; AHT, antihypertensive agents; DM, diabetes mellitus; GFR, glomerular filtration rate; ESRD, end-stage renal disease; SCr, serum creatinine; Nondiabetic renal disease (NDRD) includes patients with hypertensive nephrosclerosis, glomerular disease, tubulointerstitial diseases and autosomal dominant polycystic disease. Adapted from Toto *(104)*.

radation. Their renal effects may be counteracted in the long-term by compensatory upregulation of ACE-independent angiotensin production by as yet incompletely characterized alternative tissue-converting enzymes (e.g., chymase and ACE-II) *(86)*. ARBs effectively block angiotensin type I receptor actions but permit, and even stimulate, signaling via the type II receptor. All major angiotensin effects, including vasoconstriction, salt and water retention, aldosterone release, and subsequent hyperkalemia, glomerular hypertrophy, and augmentation of sympathetic activity are controlled via the ANG II type I receptor. Animal studies, however, have suggested vasodilatory and antiproliferative effects of the ANG II type II receptor *(87)*. The clinical relevance of these differences is yet unclear. The available evidence from studies in adults with imminent *(88)* or established diabetic nephropathy *(89,90)* indicates that ARBs are as effective as ACE inhibitors in preventing or slowing the course of renal disease, with a slightly better side effect profile. Long-term comparative studies are needed to define a potential therapeutic advantage of ARBs over ACE inhibitors.

In several animal models of progressive renal failure, the administration of aldosterone receptor blockers at sub-antihypertensive doses can mimic most of the antiproteinuric and antifibrotic effects of RAS antagonists, and add to their effects upon co-administration. Conversely, aldosterone reverses the renoprotective effects of ACE inhibitors and ARBs *(91)*. In patients with essential HTN treated with ACE inhibitors, plasma aldosterone levels increased over time, despite continued suppression of plasma ACE activity (aldosterone "escape" phenomenon) *(92)*. In a recent prospective trial in patients with severe heart failure, the addition of spironolactone to an ACE inhibitor markedly reduced patient morbidity and mortality, with a clinically insignificant increase in plasma potassium levels (93). The recent advent of a selective mineralocorticoid receptor blocker with reduced antiandrogenic side effects has given us hope that combined angiotensin and aldosterone antagonism may provide an acceptable treatment option in patients with chronic kidney disease resistant to RAS antagonist monotherapy. Of course, hyperkalemia may become a limiting factor with this therapeutic approach, and potassium levels must be monitored.

### *Pharmacological Renoprotection in Children*

The clinical evidence for the renoprotective efficacy of RAS blockade has been established exclusively in adults, mainly those with acquired glomerulopathies. In children with CRF, glomerulopathies account for fewer than 15% of cases, the vast majority being caused by hypo/dysplastic renal malformations and other congenital or hereditary disorders. Given that it is yet unproven whether RAS inhibition is equally renoprotective in pediatric kidney disorders as it is in typical adult nephropathies, the hyperfiltering nephrons in renal hypoplasia may be considered an experiment of nature to assess the validity of the Brenner hypothesis. Hypertension and proteinuria are also proven predictors of renal failure progression in children *(64)*, and extensive tubulointerstitial fibrosis is commonly found in progressive pediatric nephropathies, such as obstructive uropathy, reflux nephropathy, cystinosis, etc. These features provide a rationale for pharmacological renoprotection by ACE inhibition in children with CRF. However, individual subsets of pediatric kidney disease may remain unresponsive to ACE inhibition. It is important to note that polycystic kidney disease is the only disease entity identified to date in which ACE inhibition has not proven renoprotective *(94)*. In order to clarify the efficacy of ACE inhibition and BP control in children with CRF, a consortium of 33 European pediatric nephrologists has launched a prospective randomized trial in 400 pediatric CRF patients (ESCAPE Study). Following a baseline observation period, all patients receive a fixed dose of the ACE inhibitor ramipril, and are randomized to conventional or intensified BP control (target <50th ambulatory blood pressure monitoring [ABPM] percentile for height). The children will be monitored for CRF progression for a total of 5 yr; the first results are expected in 2005.

### *Clinical Strategies in Renoprotective Pharmacotherapy*

The growing experience with RAS antagonists as renoprotective agents has stimulated the development of diversified strategies aimed at optimizing the long-term preservation of renal function. At the current state of knowledge, there is broad consensus that renoprotective pharmacotherapy, using an ACE inhibitor or an ARB, should be initiated as early as possible, ideally upon diagnosis of chronic renal disease. RAS antagonists should be applied whenever a trend or potential for progressive renal damage exists, even in patients with low-grade proteinuria and mildly elevated or high-normal BP. The drug dose should be titrated to the level that provides maximal suppression of proteinuria. The maximally effective antiproteinuric dose may exceed by several times the dose that provides a maximal antihypertensive effect. While the dose should be increased gradually, an early rise in serum creatinine of up to 35% should be tolerated. The initial drop in GFR, which is mediated by the desired change in glomerular hemodynamics, quantitatively predicts the long-term renoprotective efficacy of RAS antagonism *(95)*. If the antihypertensive and/or antiproteinuric efficacy of a single RAS antagonist is unsatisfactory, addition of a thiazide (or a loop diuretic if GFR is <30 mL/min/ 1.73 $m^2$) is the next therapeutic option. The currently recommended target BP in adults with chronic kidney disease is <130/80 mmHg *(96)*. In children, we propose that BP should be lowered to below the 90th percentile for height. These strict target criteria mandate the use of 2–3 additional antihypertensive agents in many patients. If add-on antihypertensive agents are chosen, dihydropyridine calcium channel antagonists (e.g., nifedipine or amlodipine) should probably be avoided, since they increase glomerular HTN and proteinuria and, when used as monothererapy, are associated with poorer renal survival than β-blockers or ACE inhibitors *(97)*. In contrast, non-dihydropyridine-type calcium channel blockers (e.g., verapamil) reduce proteinuria in diabetic nephropathy, in part by increasing glomerular size permselectivity *(98)*. Their antiproteinuric effect is independent of, and an additive to, that of ACE inhibition *(99)*.

There is preliminary evidence that the combination of an ACE inhibitor with an ARB may enhance the antiproteinuric efficacy *(100–102)* and provide superior renoprotection compared to monotherapy with either agent alone *(102)*. At least in the short term (5 wk of observation), hyperkalemia or rapidly worsening renal function were not observed more frequently with combined treatment than with ARB monotherapy, despite superior antihypertensive and antiproteinuric efficacy of the combination therapy *(103)*. Although it is yet unclear whether the observed effects were truly synergistic, or merely additive with either drug administered at a submaximally effective dose, combination therapy appears to be a safe and effective way to provide maximal renoprotective efficacy without exceeding the legally approved doses (established for antihypertensive use) of each agent alone.

## ACKNOWLEDGMENTS

This work was supported by grants from the 5th Framework Program of the European Union (QLG1-2002-00908), the Boehringer Ingelheim Foundation and the Baxter Extramural Grant program.

## REFERENCES

1. Schärer K. Hypertension in children and adolescents. In: Malluche HH, Sawaya BP, Hakim RM, Sayegh MH, eds. Clinical Nephrology, Dialysis and Transplantation: A Continuously Updated Textbook. Deisenhofen: Dustri-Verlag, 1999;1–28.
2. Wühl E, Schaefer F, Mehls O. Prevalence and current treatment policies of hypertension and proteinuria in children with chronic renal failure in Europe. In: Timio M, Wizemann V, Venanzi S, eds. Cardionephrology. Cosenza: Editoriale Bios, 1999;85–88.
3. Brun P. Hypertension artérielle rénovasculaire. In: Loirat C, Niaudet P, eds. Néphrologie pédiatrique. Paris: Doin, 1993;203–211.
4. Hiner L, Falkner B. Renovascular hypertension in children. Pediatr Clin North Am 1993;40:123–140.
5. Deal JE, Snell MF, Barratt TM, Dillon MJ. Renovascular disease in childhood. J Pediatr 1992;121:378–384.

6. Rushton AR. The genetics of fibromuscular dysplasia. Arch Intern Med 1980;140:233–236.
7. Pilmore HL, Na Nagara MP, Walker RI. Neurofibromatosis and renovascular hypertension in early pregnancy. Nephrol Dial Transplant 1997;12:187–189.
8. Pober BR, Lacro RV, Rice C, Mandell V, Teele RL. Renal findings in 40 individuals with Williams syndrome. Am J Med Gene 1993;46:271–274.
9. Sumboonanouda A, Robinson BL, Gedroye WMW, Saxton HM, Reidy JF, Haycock GB. Middle aortic syndrome. Arch Dis Child 1992;67:501–505.
10. Wiggelinkhuizen J, Cremin BJ. Takayasu arteritis and renovascular hypertention in childhood. Pediatrics 1978;62:209–217.
11. Coleman TG, Guyton AM. Hypertension caused by salt loading in the dog. 3. Onset transients of cardic output and other circulatory variables. Circ Res 1969;25:153–160.
12. Charra B, Calemard E, Ruffet M, et al. Survival as an index of adequacy of dialysis. Kidney Int 1992;41: 1286–1291.
13. Ozkahya M, Toz H, Unsal A, et al. Treatment of hypertension in dialysis patients by ultrafiltration: role of cardiac dilatation and time factor (see comments). Am J Kid Dis 1999;34:218–222.
14. Sorof JM, Brewer ED, Portmann RJ. Ambulatory blood pressure monitoring and interdialytic weight gain in children receiving chronic hemodialysis. Am J Kidney Dis 1999;33:667–674.
15. Rahman M, Fu P, Sehgal AR, Smith MC. Interdialytic weight gain, compliance with dialysis regime, and agere are independent predictors of blood pressure in hemodialysis patients. Am J Kidney Dis 2000;35: 257–265.
16. Rahman M, Dixit A, Donley V, et al. Factors associated with inadequate blood pressure control in hypertensive hemodialysis patients. Am J Kidney Dis 1999;33:498–506.
17. Lingens N, Soergel M, Loirat C, Busch C, Lemmer B, Schärer K. Ambulatory blood pressure monitoring in paediatric patients treated by regular hemodialysis and peritoneal dialysis. Pediatr Nephrol 1995;9:167–172.
18. Chazot C, Charra B, Laurent G, et al. Interdialysis blood pressure control by long hemodialysis sessions. Nephrol Dial Transplant 1995;10:831–837.
19. Savage T, Fabbian F, Giles M, Tomson CRV, Raine AEG. Interdialytic weight gain and 48-hr blood pressure in haemodialysis patients. Nephrol Dial Transplant 1997;12:2308–2311.
20. Blumberg A, Nelp WB, Hegström RM, Scribner BH. Extracellular volume in patients with chronic renal disease treated for hypertension by sodium restriction. Lancet 1967;2:69–73.
21. Fine LG, Bourgoignie JJ, Weber H, Bricker NS. Enhanced end-organ responsiveness of the uremic kidney to the natriuretic factor. Kidney Int 1976;10:364–372.
22. Muniz P, Fortuno A, Zalba G, Fortuno MA, Diez J. Effects of loop diuretics on angiotensin II-stimulated vascular smooth muscle cells growth. Nephrol Dial Transplant 2001;16(Suppl 1):14–17.
23. Fortuno A, Muniz P, Zalba G, Fortuno MA, Diez J. The loop diuretic torasemide interferes with endothelin-1 actions in the aorta of hypertensive rats. Nephrol Dial Transplant 2001;16(Suppl I):18–21.
24. Brass H, Ochs HG, Armbruster H, Heintz R. Plasma renin activity (PRA) and aldosteroone (PA) in patients with chronic glomerulonephritis (GN) and hypertension. Clin Nephrol 1976;5:57–60.
25. Warren DJ, Ferris TF. Renin secretion in renal hypertension. Lancet 1970;1:159–162.
26. Campese VM. The kidney and the neurogenic control of blood pressure in renal disease. J Nephrol 2003;13: 221–224.
27. Ligtenberg G, Blankenstijn PJ, Oey PL, et al. Reduction of sympathetic hyperactivity by enalapril in patients with chronic renal failure. N Engl J Med 1999;340:1321–1328.
28. Converse RL, Jacobsen TN, Toto RD, et al. Sympathetic overactivity in patients with chronic renal failure. N Engl J Med 1992;327:1912–1918.
29. Baylis C, Vallance P. Effects of NO deficiency. Curr Opin Nephrol Hypertens 1996;5:80–88.
30. Morris STW, McMurray JJV, Rodger RSC, Jardine AG. Impaired endothelium-dependent vasodilatation in uremia. Nephrol Dial Transplant 2000;15:1194–2000.
31. Schmidt RJ, Domico J, Samsell LS, et al. Indices of activity of the nitric oxide system in hemodialysis patients. Am J Kidney Dis 1999;34:228–234.
32. Schmitt CP, Yokota S, Tracy C, Sorkin MI, Baylis C. Nitric oxide production is low in end-stage renal disease patients on peritoneal dialysis. Am J Physiol 1999;276:794–797.
33. Vallance P, Leone A, Calver A, Collier J, Moncada S. Accumulation of an endogenous inhibitor of nitric oxide synthesis in chronic renal failure. Lancet 1992;339:572–575.

34. Kielstein JT, Böger RH, Bode-Böger SM, et al. Asymmetric dimethylarginine plasma concentrations differ in patients with end-stage renal disease: relationship to treatment method and atherosclerotic disease. J Am Soc Nephrol 1999;10:594–600.
35. Anderstam B, Katzarski K, Bergström J. Serum levels of NO, NG-dimethyl-L-Arginine, a potential endogenous nitric oxide inhibitor in dialysis patients. J Am Soc Nephrol 1997;8:1437–1442.
36. Sumino H, Sato K, Sakamaki T, Kanda T, Nakamura T, Takahashi T, Sakamoto H, Kabayashi I, Nagai R. Reduced production of nitric oxide during hemodialysis. J Hum Hypertens 1999;13:437–442.
37. Vaziri ND, Ni X, Wang Q, Oveisi F, Zhou XJ. Downregulation of nitric oxide synthase in chronic renal insufficiency: role of excess PTH. Am J Physiol Renal Physiol 1998;274:F642–F649.
38. Agapitov AV, Haynes WG. Role of endothelin in cardiovascular disease. J Renin Angiotensin Aldosterone Syst 2002;3(1):1–15.
39. Shindo T, Kurihara H, Maemura K, et al. Renal damage and salt-dependent hypertension in aged transgenic mice overexpressing endothelin-1. J Mol Med 2002;80(2):69–70.
40. Lariviere R, Lebel M. Endothelin-1 in chronic renal failure and hypertension. Can J Physiol Pharmacol 2003;81(6):607–621.
41. Largo R, GomezGarre D, Liu XH, Alonso J, Blanco J, Plaza JJ, Egido J. Endothelin-1 upregulation in the kidney of uninephrectomized spontaneously hypertensive rats and its modification by the angiotensin-converting enzyme inhibitor quinapril. Hypertension 1997;29(5):1178–1185.
42. Elmarakby AA, Morsing P, Pollock DM. Enalapril attenuates endothelin-1-induced hypertension via increased kinin survival. Am J Physiol Heart Circ Physiol 2003;284(6):1899–1903.
43. McCarron DA, Ellison DH, Anderson S. Vasodilatation mediated by human PTH 1.34 in the spontaneously hypertensive rats. Am J Physiol 1984;246:96–100.
44. Raine AE, Bedford L, Simpson AW, et al. Hyperparathyroidism, platelet intracellular free calcium and hypertension in chronic renal failure. Kidney Int 1993;43:700–705.
45. Iseki K, Massry SG, Campese VM. Effects of hypercalcemia and parathyroid hormone on blood pressure in normal and renal failure rats. Am J Physiol 1986;250:924–929.
46. Schiffl H, Fricke H, Sitter T. Hypertension secondary to early-stage kidney disease: the pathogenetic role of altered cytosolic calcium ($Ca2^+$) homeostasis of vascular smooth muscle cells. Am J Kidney Dis 1993;21(2): 51–57.
47. Barker DJ, Eriksson JG, Forsen T, Osmond C. Fetal origins of adult disease: strength of effects and biological basis. Int J Epidemiol 2002;31:1235–1239.
48. Baum M, Ortiz L, Quan A. Fetal origins of cardiovascular disease. Curr Opin Pediatr 2003;12(2):166–170.
49. Silver LE, Decamps PJ, Kost LM, Platt LD, Castro LC. Intrauterine growth restriction is accompanied by decreased renal volume in the human fetus. Am J Obstet Gynecol 2003;188:1320–1325.
50. Manalich R, Reyes L, Herera M, Melendi C, Fundora I. Relationship between weight at birth and the number and size of renal glomeruli in humans: a histomorphometric study. Kidney Int 2000;58:770–773.
51. Keller G, Zimmer G, Mall G, Ritz E, Amann K. Nephron number in patients with primary hypertension. N Engl J Med 2003;348:101–108.
52. Brenner BM. Nephron adaptation to renal injury or ablation. Am J Physiol 1985;249:F324–F327.
53. Woods LL. Fetal origins of adult hypertension; a renal mechanism? Curr Opin Nephrol Hypertens 2000;9: 419–425.
54. Moritz KM, Wintour EM, Dodic M. Fetal uninephrectomy leads to postnatal hypertension and compromised renal function. Hypertension 2002;39:1071–1076.
55. Mei-Zahav M, Korzets Z, Cohen I, et al. Ambulatory blood pressure monitoring in children with a solitary kidney—a comparison between unilateral renal agensis and uninephrectomy. Blood Press Monit 2001;6(5):263–267.
56. Moritz KM, Johnson K, Douglas-Denton R, Wintour EM, Dodic M. Maternal glucocorticoid treatment programs alterations in the renin-angiotensin system of the ovine fetal kidney. Endocrinology 2002;143: 4455–4463.
57. Manning J, Beutler K, Knepper MA, Vehaskari VM. Upregulation of renal BSC1 and TSC in prenatally programmed hypertension. Am J Physiol Renal Physiol 2002;283:F202–F206.
58. Langley-Evans S, Langley-Evans A, Marchand M. Nutritional programming of blood pressure and renal morphology. Arch Physiol Biochem 2003;111(1):8–16.
59. Ingelfinger JR. Is microanatomy destiny? N Engl J Med 2003;348:99–100.
60. Klag MJ, Whelton PK, Randall BL, et al. Blood pressure and end-stage renal disease in men. Hypertension 1996;13:180–193.

61. Bakris GL. Progression of diabetic nephropathy: a focus on arterial pressure level and methods of reduction. Diabetes Res Clin Pract 1998;39:35–42.
62. Remuzzi G, Ruggenenti P, Benigni A. Understanding the nature of renal disease progression. Kidney Int 1997;51:2–15.
63. Peterson JC, Adler S, Burkart JM, et al. Blood pressure control, proteinuria, and the progression of renal disease: the modification of diet in renal disease study. Ann Intern Med 1995;123:754–762.
64. Wingen AM, Fabian Bach C, Schaefer F, Mehls O, European Study Group for Nutritional Treatment of Chronic Renal Failure in Childhood. Randomised multicentre study of a low-protein diet on the progression of chronic renal failure in children. Lancet 1997;349(9059):1117–1123.
65. Christensen PK, Hommel EE, Clausen P, Feldt-Rasmussen B, Parving HH. Impaired autoregulation of the glomerular filtration rate in patients with nondiabetic nephropathies. Kidney Int 1999;56:1517–1521.
66. Largo R, Gomez-Garre D, Soto K, et al. Angiotensin-converting enzyme is upregulated in the proximal tubules of rats with intense proteinuria. Hypertension 1999;33:732–739.
67. Benigni A, Remuzzi G. How renal cytokines and growth factors contribute to renal disease progression. Am J Kidney Dis 2001;37(2):21–24.
68. Gomez-Garre D, Largo R, Tejera N, Fortes J, Manzabeitia F, Egidio J. Activation of NF-Kappa B in tubular epithelial cells of rats with intense proteinuria: role of angiotensin II and endothelin-1. Hypertension 2001;37:1171–1178.
69. Nangaku M, Pippin J, Couser W. Complement membrane attack complex (C5b-9) mediates interstitial disease in experimental nephrotic syndrome. J Am Soc Nephrol 1999;10:2323–2331.
70. Nangaku M, Pippin J, Couser W. C6 mediates chronic progression of tubulointerstitial damage in rat with remnant kidneys. J Am Soc Nephrol 2002;13:928–936.
71. Tang S, Lai KN, Chan TM, Lan HY, Ho SK, Sacks SH. Transferrin but not albumin mediates stimulation of complement C3 biosynthesis in human proximal tubular epithelial cells. Am J Kidney Dis 2001;37:94–103.
72. Chen L, Zhang BH, Harris DC. Evidence suggesting that nitric oxide mediates iron-induced toxicity in cultured proximal tubule cells. Am J Physiol 1998;274:18–25.
73. Kriz W, Hartmann I, Hosser H, et al. Tracer studies in the rat demonstrate misdirected filtration and pertubular filtrate spreading in nephrons with segmental glomerulosclerosis. J Am Soc Nephrol 2001;12:496–506.
74. Toto RD, Mitchell HC, Smith RD, Lee HC, McIntire D, Pettinger WA. “Strict” blood pressure control and progression of renal disease in hypertensive nephrosclerosis. Kidney Int 1995;48:851–859.
75. Maschio G, Alberti D, Janin G, et al. Effect of angiotensin-converting-enzme inhibitor benazepril on the progression of chronic renal insufficiency. N Engl J Med 1996;334:939–945.
76. The GISEN Group (Gruppo Italiano di Studi Epidemiologici in Nefrologia). Randomised placebo-controlled trial of effect of ramipril on decline in glomerular filtration rate and risk of terminal renal failure in proteinuric, non-diabetic nephropathy. Lancet 1997;349:1857–1863.
77. Lewis EJ, Hunsicker LG, Raymond PB, Rohde RD, for the Collaborative Study Group. The effect of angiotensin-converting-enzyme inhibition on diabetic nephropathy. N Engl J Med 1993;329:1456–1462.
78. Kamper AL, Strandgaard S, Leyssac P. Effect of enalapril on the progression of chronic renal failure: a randomized controlled trial. Am J Hypertens 1992;5:423–430.
79. Parving HH, Andersen AR, Smidt UM, Svendsen PA. Early aggressive antihypertensive treatment reduces rate of decline in kidney function in diabetic nephropathy. Lancet 1983;1:1175–1179.
80. Zucchelli P, Zuccalà A, Borghi M, et al. Long-term comparison between captopril and nifidepin in the progression of renal insufficiency. Kidney Int 1992;42:452–458.
81. Hannedouche T, Landais P, Goldfarb B, et al. Randomised controlled trial of enalapril and beta blockers in non-diabetic chronic renal failure. Brit Med J 1994;309:833–837.
82. Ihle BU, Whitworth JA, Shahinfar S, Cnaan A, Kincaid-Smith PS, Becker GJ. Angiotensin-converting-enzyme inhibition in non-diabetic progressive renal insufficiency: a controlled double-blind trial. Am J Kidney Dis 1996;27:489–495.
83. Bakris GL, Copley JB, Vicknair N, Sadler R, Leurgans S. Calcium channel blockers vs. other antihypertensive therapies on progression of NIDDM associated nephropathy. Kidney Int 1996;50:1641–1650.
84. UK Prospective Diabetes Study Group. Efficacy of atenolol and captopril in reducing risk of macrovascular and microvascular complications in type-II diabetes. Brit Med J 1998;317:713–720.
85. Jafar TH, Schmid CH, Landa M, et al., for the ACE Inhibition in Progressive Renal Disease Study Group. Angiotensin-converting enzyme inhibitors and progression of nondiabetic renal disease. Ann Intern Med 2001;135:73–87.

86. Huang XR, Chen WY, Truong LD, Lan HY. Chymase is upregulated in diabetic nephropathy: implications for an alternative pathway of angiotensin II-mediated diabetic renal and vascular disease. J Am Soc Nephrol 2003;14:1738–1747.
87. Ma J, Nishimura H, Fogo A, Kon V, Inagami T, Ichikawa I. Accelerated fibrosis and collagen deposition develop in the renal interstitium of angiotensin type 2 receptor null mutant mice during ureteral obstruction. Kidney Int 1998;53:937–944.
88. Parving H, Lehnert H, Brochner-Mortensen J, Gomis R, Andersen S, Arner P, Irbesartan in Patients with Type 2 Diabetes and Microalbuminuria Study Group. The effect of irbesartan on the development of diabetic nephropathy in patients with type 2 diabetes. N Engl J Med 2001;345:870–878.
89. Lewis EJ, Hunsicker LG, et al., Collaborative Study Group. Renoprotective effect of the angiotensin-receptor antagonist irbesartan in patients with nephropathy due to type 2 diabetes. N Engl J Med 2001;345:851–860.
90. Brenner BM, Cooper ME, DeZeeuw D, et al., RENAAL Study Investigators. Effects of losartan on renal and cardiovascular outcomes in patients with type 2 diabetes and nephropathy. N Engl J Med 2001;345:861–869.
91. Epstein M. Aldosterone and the hypertensive kidney: its emerging role as a mediator of progressive renal dysfunction: a paradigm shift. J Hypertens 2001;19:829–842.
92. Sato A, Suzuki Y, Shibata H, Saruta T. Plasma aldosterone concentrations are not related to the degree of angiotensin-converting enzyme inhibition in essential hypertensive patients. Hypertens Res 2000;23:25–31.
93. Pitt B, Zannad F, Remme WJ, et al. The effect of spironolactone on morbidity and mortality in patients with severe heart failure. N Engl J Med 1999;341:709–717.
94. Ruggenenti P, Perna A, Gherardi G, Benigni A, Remuzzi G. Chronic proteinuric nephropathies: outcomes and response to treatment in a prospective cohort of 352 patients with different patterns of renal injury. Am J Kidney Dis 2000;35:1155–1165.
95. Bakris GL, Weir MR. Angiotensin-converting enzyme inhibitor-associated elevation in serum creatinine: is this a cause for concern? Arch Int Med 2000;160:685–693.
96. Joint National Committee on Prevention Detection, Evaluation, and Treatment of High Blood Pressure. The Seventh Report of the Joint National Committee on Prevention, Detection, Evaluation, and Treatment of High Blood Pressure. 2003. National Institutes of Health, National Heart, Lung, and Blood Institute, National High Blood Pressure Education Program, NIH Publication No. 03-5233.
97. Wright JTJ, Bakris G, Greene T, et al. Effect of blood pressure lowering and antihypertensive drug class on progression of hypertensive kidney disease. JAMA 2002;288:2421–2431.
98. Smith AC, Toto R, Bakris GL. Differential effects of calcium channel blockers on size selectivity of proteinuria in diabetic nephropathy. Kidney Int 1998;54:889–896.
99. Bakris GL, Weir MR, De Quattro V, McMahon FG. Effects of an ACE inhibitor/calcium antagonists combination on proteinuria in diabetic nephropathy. Kidney Int 1998;54:1283–1289.
100. Russo D, Pisani A, Balletta MM, DeNicola.L, Savino FA, Andreucci M, Minutolo R. Additive antiproteinuric effect of converting enzyme inhibitor and losartan in normotensive patients with IgA nephropathy. Am J Kidney Dis 1999;33:851–856.
101. Campbell R, Sangalli F, Perticucci E, et al. Effects of combined ACE inhibitor and angiotensin II antagonist treatment in human chronic nephropathies. Kidney Int 2003;63:1094–1103.
102. Nakao N, Yoshimura A, Morita H, Takada M, Kayano T, Ideura T. Combination treatment of angiotensin-II receptor blocker and angiotensin-converting-enzyme inhibitor in non-diabetic renal disease (COOPERATE): a randomised controlled trial. Lancet 2003;361:117–124.
103. Ruilope LM, Aldigier JC, Ponticelli C, Oddou-Stock P, Botteri F, Mann JF. Safety of the combination of valsartan and benazepril in patients with chronic renal disease. European Group for the Investigation of Valsartan in Chronic Renal Disease. J Hypertens 2000;18:89–95.
104. Toto R. Angiotensin II subtype 1 receptor blockers and renal function. Arch Intern Med 2001;161:1492–1499.
105. de Man SA, André JL, Bachmann HJ, Grobbee DE, Ibsen KK, Laaser U, Lippert P, Hofmann A. Blood pressure in childhood: pooled findings of six European studies. J Hypertens 1991;9:109–114.

# 22 Hypertension in End-Stage Renal Disease

*Karl Schärer,* MD

***Contents***



## INTRODUCTION

The preceding chapter demonstrated that blood pressure (BP) generally rises with progression of chronic renal failure (CRF), now known as chronic kidney disease (CKD). By the time end-stage renal disease (ESRD) occurs, the majority of affected children (approx 95%) have hypertension (HTN). The degree of BP elevation depends primarily on cardiovascular status, sodium balance, and the antihypertensive strategies prescribed. In many cases, drug-resistant HTN is the signal to start renal replacement therapy.

## MEASUREMENT OF BLOOD PRESSURE

### *Casual Blood Pressure*

The same guidelines for measuring BP used for normal children (*see* Chapter 5) apply to children on peritoneal dialysis (PD) and after transplantation. However, in measuring BP in children on hemodialysis (HD) treatment, the general rule to use the nondominant upper extremity must often be disregarded because the compression of an arteriovenous fistula or a vascular graft (usually on the nondominant arm) may cause access failure *(1)*. Sometimes the presence of an arteriovenous anastomosis leads to a diastolic runoff and to increased pulse pressure.

From: *Clinical Hypertension and Vascular Disease: Pediatric Hypertension*
Edited by: R. J. Portman, J. M. Sorof, and J. R. Ingelfinger © Humana Press Inc., Totowa, NJ

In order to avoid difficulties in measuring BP in the upper extremities, some authors proposed to use the legs to measure BP. However, systolic BP readings from the dorsalis pedis artery have yielded values 15 mmHg higher than arm pressures *(2)* and therefore not comparable. Automated oscillometric BP monitors should be avoided for casual measurements because they give significantly higher values than manual auscultatory readings, at least in adult HD patients *(3)*.

Some controversy exists surrounding the *timing* of BP measurements in HD patients. Casual readings are traditionally taken immediately after the start of HD sessions, but this so-called predialysis BP overestimates the mean systolic interdialytic systolic BP by 10 mmHg, whereas the postdialysis BP may underestimate it by 7 mmHg in adult patients *(4)*. Some authors believe that postdialysis readings reflect the interdialytic BP better *(5)*, whereas others prefer predialysis BP as a guide for treatment *(6)*. A variety of influences account for these differences before, during, and after HD changes in volume, neural signaling, local and systemic hormonal release, and vascular tone. Similarly, volume-related differences might be present between morning and evening BP in patients undergoing automated overnight PD with significant ultrafiltration, although such effects have not been studied in detail.

### *Continuous Blood Pressure Monitoring by Automated Oscillometric Methods*

Ambulatory BP monitoring (ABPM) improves the evaluation of the BP status in HD as well as in PD and transplanted patients. The advantages of ABPM (*see* Chapter 6) are particularly evident in ESRD patients. The white coat effect might play a more minor role than in other patient groups *(7)*, but this issue deserves further investigation in pediatric patients. Studies in adult HD patients have shown that ABPM is relatively reproducible and less variable than casual pre- or postdialysis BP; however, the reproducibility of the BP decrease during sleep (nocturnal dip) is poor, because up to 43% of patients change their nocturnal dip category after repeated measurements *(8)*.

The main advantage of ABPM, the possibility to evaluate circadian changes of BP, is particularly important in ESRD patients, in view of the prognostic significance of nocturnal dipping *(9)*. ABPM also allows the measurement of the BP load, defined as the amount of time that the systolic BP exceeds normal values, as an indicator of the degree of HTN, although this variable has not yet been satisfactorily evaluated in children. Finally, ABPM is helpful for adjusting the dosage of antihypertensive drugs.

In dialysed children, casual BP measurements and ABPM results are poorly correlated. A third of children appearing normotensive by casual readings have to be reclassified to hypertensive when examined by ABPM or the converse *(10)*. Sorof et al. *(11)* found a wide range of error for casual BP relative to ABPM, confirming the unreliable character of casual readings. Similar discrepancies were observed in allografted patients.

## DEFINITION OF HYPERTENSION IN END-STAGE RENAL DISEASE

Since children with ESRD are often growth-retarded, problems with the definition of HTN may occur, because no normative data for casual BP and ABPM are available for children with heights below the 5th or 3rd height percentile. It has been suggested that looking at norms for the age at which the child's height would fall in the 50th percentile should suffice. However, this maneuver may result in an underestimate of the normal BP range for such children *(1)*. Transplanted children often suffer from obesity which, by itself, may lead to HTN. Given the lack of BP standards for overweight children, it is often difficult to correctly categorize such patients.

In general, casual BP readings in dialyzed patients are subject to sampling errors, mainly because of the great influence of the rapidly changing volume status (as previously noted). Even repeated casual measurements are not able to reflect circadian changes. It appears that in all ESRD patients, HTN can be better defined by applying ABPM than by casual recordings, provided that well defined normative standards are available *(12)*. The best expression of the degree of HTN may occur after correction of the skewed distribution of normal BP data assessed by ABPM, using a new statistical tool (the LMS method) to calculate accurate standard deviation (SD) scores *(13)*.

## CLINICAL ASPECTS OF BLOOD PRESSURE MONITORING ASSESSMENT IN END-STAGE RENAL DISEASE

### *Dialysis Treatment*

In the first weeks or months after the start of dialysis therapy, BP tends to decrease, and often allows reduction in antihypertensive medication *(14)*. However, HTN persists in a high proportion in chronically dialysed children. This observation was confirmed in large pediatric dialysis populations followed in registry studies. In Europe, 55% of patients under 15 yr of age on maintenance dialysis received antihypertensive drugs. Despite receiving antihypertensive therapy, 45% of HD patients, and 31% of PD patients, maintained BP levels of 10 mmHg or more above the 95th percentile *(15)*. More recently, an American multicenter study reported that 53% of HD and 40% of PD patients (including adolescents) received antihypertensive drugs 2 yr after dialysis initiation *(16)*. Similar observations were reported by the Mid-European Pediatric Peritoneal Dialysis Study Group *(17)*. These multicenter studies, as well as most recent single center studies *(18)*, were based on casual BP measurements.

Using ABPM, which provides a more detailed analysis, Lingens et al. *(10)* found that 33% of children and adolescents on long-term HD, and 70% on PD, were hypertensive, as defined by standard reference data obtained from casual readings. Although no correlation was found between mean daytime BP and interdialytic weight gain, the predialysis plasma levels of atrial natriuretic peptide (ANP), as an indicator of the volume status, correlated highly with daytime BP in both HD and PD patients.

These observations were recently confirmed in PD children *(19)*. In a controlled ABPM study of 12 HD children, Sorof et al. *(11)* reported increased BP loads, and a linear relationship between the interdialytic weight gain and the corresponding increase in systolic BP.

An attenuated nocturnal dip in BP has been observed in many adult patients receiving dialysis treatment. This reduced nocturnal dipping may lead to nocturnal HTN, which presents an unfavorable prognostic sign. In the study by Lingens et al. *(10)*, the median nocturnal decline of mean systolic and diastolic BP was reduced by 4 and 7% in children on HD, and by 9 and 12% in those on PD, respectively. However, the mean nighttime values did not exceed daytime values by more than 1 mmHg in any subject. Figure 1 demonstrates the variations of median systolic and diastolic BP levels obtained by ABPM in this study. In the Finnish investigation, a decreased nocturnal decline of BP was noted in 40% of children on PD *(19)*.

### *Transplantation*

After renal transplantation, HTN can occur in both acute and chronic forms, and is an important predictor of patient and graft survival *(20)*. Earlier studies found an overall prevalence of 85–93% in grafted children *(21,22)*. The European Dialysis and Transplant Association (EDTA) reported that 57% of all transplanted children in Europe were treated by antihypertensive drugs, similar to the percentage found in HD or PD patients *(15)*. According to an American multicenter study, 70% of young graft recipients required antihypertensive medication at 1 mo, and 59 % at 2 yr after transplant *(23)*. Recent reports from various single centers suggest that this high proportion of children and adolescents with posttransplant HTN has not decreased significantly.

It should be stressed, however, that the data for posttransplant HTN summarized above were obtained from casual BP recordings which are poorly reproducible by ABPM in transplanted patients *(26)*. In the Lingens et al. series *(24)*, 56% of transplanted children regarded as hypertensive by casual BP recordings had to be reclassified by ABPM as normotensive. In the Soergel et al. study, systolic and/or diastolic HTN was found either at daytime or at nighttime in 60% of patients when compared with a suitable healthy population examined by ABPM. A similar investigation using a different ABPM monitor revealed only 35% of hypertensive children with transplants *(25)*. In other pediatric studies applying ABPM in grafted children, the prevalence of HTN is difficult to evaluate because reference standards were taken from casual recordings *(26–28)*.

Most reports agree that posttransplant HTN is predominantly observed at night. The degree of nocturnal HTN may be evaluated by calculating the mean drop of BP from daytime to nighttime. In the studies cited above and additional pediatric reports, the mean nocturnal dipping after transplant ranged 3–9% for systolic BP and 5–14% for diastolic BP, compared to 13% and 23%, respectively, in normal children *(12)*. Applying strict criteria, the proportion of “nondippers” was 30% *(24)*. Sorof et al. *(27)* found that during sleep mean BP exceeded awake systolic and diastolic BP in 24% and 17% of pediatric transplant patients, respectively. Consequently, the normal circadian BP rhythm is severely distorted after renal transplant, as shown by more sophisticated forms of analysis *(24)*.

The BP load assessed by ABPM monitoring, as a measure of hemodynamic stress, is significantly increased in transplanted children. Even with normal mean daytime BP values, Sorof et al. *(11)* reported increased diastolic BP loads in 56% of patients. In a similar pediatric study by Morgan et al. *(28)*, 24-h BP loads were slightly lower. Serial studies of BP profiles in adult patients showed a significant drop of daytime and nocturnal systolic BP during the first posttransplant year, associated with a reduction of left ventricular hypertrophy *(29)*.

## ETIOLOGY AND PATHOGENESIS OF HYPERTENSION IN CHILDREN WITH END-STAGE RENAL DISEASE

### *Dialysis Therapy*

The two main pathogenic mechanisms contributing to HTN, before and after initiation of dialysis therapy, are hypervolemia and increased vasoconstriction. Volume overload seems to be the major pathogenic factor, first outlined by Guyton et al. *(30)*. Diminished glomerular filtration rate and sodium excretory capacity result in sodium and water retention in the body, thereby increasing venous return and cardiac output. In order to prevent hyperperfusion of tissues, vasoconstriction ensues via autoregulation. This mechanism operates, however, only after some time lag. For example, it may take several weeks until volume changes in dialyzed adult patients are translated into changes in BP *(31)*. After the disappearance of edema, HTN may persist until a strict control of hypervolemia, e.g., by extension of the dialysis time, may finally reduce BP *(32)*. However, hypervolemia may also occur in the absence of HTN.

Increased peripheral vascular resistance caused by humoral factors inappropriate to the volume state is another explanation of HTN in dialyzed patients. Activation of the renin-angiotensin system (RAS) was demonstrated by high plasma renin activity in pediatric *(33)* as well as adult patients on HD treatment. In addition, the local RAS in the vessel walls appears to be activated in renal failure. Furthermore, increased sympathetic activity, correlating highly with systemic BP, was documented in dialyzed adults *(34)*. In children, a two- to fourfold increase of plasma noradrenalin and adrenalin levels was noted during an HD session *(33)*. Sympathetic overactivity appears to be mediated by an afferent signal arising in the failing kidney. The finding of structural abnormalities of coronary and great arteries in experimental CRF and dialyzed patients further support the role of elevated peripheral vascular resistance and impaired elasticity of great vessels in the pathogenesis of HTN in ESRD *(35,36)*.

Another concept used to explain HTN in ESRD relates to the abnormal endothelial release of hemodynamically active compounds. Elevated plasma levels of the vasoconstrictor endothelin-1 have been reported in hemodialyzed children *(39)*. Endothelium-dependent vasodilatation has been reported to be impaired in uremia, reflected by reduced release or action of nitric oxide *(37)*, possibly related to the accumulation of circulating inhibitors of nitric oxide synthetase (e.g., asymmetric dimethyl-L-arginine) in the plasma of adult ESRD patients *(38)*.

Finally, HTN in ESRD is related to the duration of HTN in the predialysis period and, therefore, to the original renal disease as well as to declining residual renal function during dialysis *(40)*. The same pathogenetic factors that contribute to HTN on dialysis may contribute to HTN in the predialysis period.

### *Transplantation*

Posttransplant HTN may be caused by a variety of etiological factors, which are summarized in Table 1 *(22,41,42)*. In the early posttransplant period, volume expansion, acute rejection with concomitant graft dysfunction, and high doses of glucocorticoids appear to play predominant roles. In the later posttransplant period, the most frequent cause of HTN is chronic allograft rejection and chronic allograft nephropathy, largely caused by toxicity from immunosuppressive agents such as calcineurin inhibitors. Calcineurin inhibitors are known to interfere with the action of endothelin and have other hypertensinogenic actions. Some authors reported that a high frequency (up to 20%) of children with renal allografts have renal artery stenosis *(21)*. Posttransplant renal artery stenosis appears to be caused primarily by vascular damage at the time of harvesting the organ, and by small vessel caliber in allografts from young donors.

## COMPLICATIONS FROM HYPERTENSION

Complications from HTN are mainly produced by vascular damage and may concern different organs. Before efficient antihypertensive therapy became available, involvement of the central nervous system was one of the most frightening manifestations of severe HTN in children with ESRD *(43)*.

The kidneys may be damaged further, even by mild elevation of BP in CRF. This was demonstrated in predialysis children in whom systolic HTN is an independent predictor of the progression of CRF *(44)*. Residual renal function may also be compromised by elevated BP during dialysis therapy. Likewise, HTN in renal transplant recipients with chronic rejection *(20)* may suffer additional renal damage from HTN. It should be noted, however, that the progression of CRF is also accelerated by vascular lesions not directly related to systemic or glomerular HTN.

In the long run, functional and structural abnormalities of the heart are the most important consequences of chronic HTN in pediatric ESRD patients. Systolic and diastolic cardiac function in CRF and ESRD have recently been reviewed *(45)*. Echocardiography and Doppler ultrasonography usually revealed normal systolic left ventricular (LV) function in the absence of severe HTN, anemia, or cardiac failure in children with ESRD, and LV contractility was regarded as normal *(46)*. However, LV diastolic dysfunction occurs in about half of adult dialysis patients and was also demonstrated in children *(47,48)*.

Four main structural abnormalities of the heart have been described in adult patients with CRF and ESRD with or without systemic HTN *(35)*: (1) LV hypertrophy (LVH); (2) expansion of the nonvascular cardiac interstitium leading to intracardial fibrosis; (3) changes of the vascular architecture (thickening of intramyocardial arterioles and reduction of capillary length density); and (4) myocardial calcifications. LVH is most relevant in children.

LVH is a strong and independent predictor of death and cardiac failure in adult dialysis patients *(49,50)*. Risk factors for the development of LVH are chiefly systolic HTN, anemia, hyperparathyroidism, coronary artery disease, hypervolemia, and prolonged dialysis therapy. Two forms of LVH may be distinguished *(51)*: pressure overload, leading to disproportionate overgrowth of cardiomyocytes and concentric (symmetric) LVH, with thickening of both ventricular septum and posterior wall, but normal cavity dimensions; and volume overload, resulting primarily in dilatation of the LV chamber and increased wall thickness sufficient to counterbalance the dilatation (eccentric or asymmetric LVH), with predominant thickening of the septum and a low LV mass to volume ratio. In ESRD, both forms of hypertrophy may be present and have also been described in dialyzed and grafted children *(18,52)*.

Although LVH is an adaptive response to chronic pressure or volume overload (allowing maintenance of systolic function), its persistence may become detrimental because it impairs diastolic compliance and reduces coronary perfusion reserve *(53,50)*. Reduced diastolic filling is closely associated with LVH and increased stiffness of the LV chamber owing to collagen accumulation.

Many reports have described LVH in children with CRF and ESRD (*see* ref. *45*). However, techniques such as electrocardiography used in earlier studies were often inappropriate for correct assessment of LV mass. Modern echocardiographic examination requires large experience and cooperative patients. In addition, there is controversy surrounding the optimal expression of LV mass data in children with renal disease.

LVH may be observed in children in the predialysis period *(48)*. In the largest echocardiographic study reported in children with ESRD (aged <l5 yr), 51% of patients on HD, 29% on PD, and 22% after transplant exhibited LVH. However, no methodological details were collected *(15)*. Since then, several single centers have published detailed data on LV mass in children and adolescents with ESRD determined by Doppler ultrasonography.

In children on dialysis, LV mass was increased up to twice that of mean control values *(45)*; recent investigators found LVH in 72% to 75% of pediatric patients *(18,28)*. In the Mitsnefes et al. study *(54)*, LV mass was increased by the start of dialysis therapy and did not change after a mean of 10 mo. After dialysis, a third of the subjects showed either a significant decrease or increase in LV mass, apparently related to the pressure load. However, the subjects in this study are atypical for current dialysis conditions in that the children had a high prevalence of HTN and anemia *(54)*.

The degree of LVH indexed to body size seems to be similar in pediatric and adult patients, although small children were rarely assessed. In adults on long-term HD, LVH may regress; this has been attributed to control of HTN, hypervolemia, or anemia *(55)*. Such regression of LV mass is associated with better survival *(56)*. In adults, LV mass may also decrease after conversion from conventional to daily nighttime HD, associated with a drop of BP *(57)*.

In children receiving continuous ambulatory or cycling PD, LVH is less frequent (45%), highly correlated with the severity of HTN and atrial natriuretic peptide, a marker of hypervolemia *(19)*. According to two studies, LVH also appears to be less severe in children receiving PD compared to those receiving HD treatment *(58,18)*. However, our own experience showed a similar LV mass index with both modes of treatment *(45)*.

After transplantation, LV mass and the overall prevalence of LVH remain about the same as in dialyzed children (56–82%) *(25,28,48)*, but the majority of pediatric patients who were dialyzed previously had a change in LV mass, either a significant (<20%) increase of LV mass with time, or a corresponding decrease *(52)*. In a study by Matteucci et al. *(25)*, LV mass and 24-h systolic BP were highly correlated, but there was poor correlation between LVH and the dose of immunosuppressive therapy by corticosteroids, cyclosporin, or antihypertensive medication.

LVH hypertrophy in ESRD is frequently associated with vascular lesions in the heart and great vessels, which have been extensively investigated in adult patients *(35,36)*. Two recent studies, which used new noninvasive imaging techniques, revealed a high prevalence of coronary calcifications and wall thickening of the carotid arteries in former pediatric patients evaluated as adults after long-standing dialysis treatment and transplantation *(59,60)*. A pathoanatomical study of the internal iliac arteries at the time of transplantation (after long-term dialysis) confirmed these clinical investigations *(61)*. Although no association was found with actual BP measurements, these findings demonstrate the early evolution of cardiovascular morbidity in pediatric ESRD patients, which seems to be more severe in those who received long-term dialysis treatment than in those who have had successful transplants.

It is well established that the high mortality of adult patients with ESRD is related to long-standing HTN. The mortality risk is increased by a large interdialytic weight gain, a high nocturnal BP, and an increased pulse pressure (difference systolic BP minus diastolic BP) *(62,63)*. Long-term studies have demonstrated that adequate BP control improves the survival of adult ESRD patients *(64)*.

Since the start of the dialysis era, there has been a remarkable decrease in early cardiovascular mortality in children and adolescents with ESRD *(65,66)*. However, late cardiovascular mortality has not been sufficiently explored in pediatric patients. It should be stressed that late fatal cardiovascular events, such as myocardial infarction and cerebrovascular accidents, are the result of both specific (uremic) and unspecific (traditional atherosclerotic) risk factors *(67)*. According to the US Renal Data System, 1.1 and 2.0 cardiac deaths per 100 patient years were recorded in dialyzed pediatric ESRD patients at the age of 0–15 yr in white and black subjects, respectively (normal about 0.1), rising to 2.3 for all patients reaching the age of 20–30 yr *(68)*. According to this study, cardiovascular mortality corresponds to approx 20–30% of all deaths encountered in dialyzed children and young adults up to 30 yr .

Another recent and somewhat more detailed study from the Netherlands analyzed the data from patients who had required the initiation of renal replacement therapy from birth to 15 yr of age between 1972 and 1992. Such children had an overall mortality of 1.6 per 100 patient years, a 31-fold increase in death rate compared to a normal population of same-aged children

*(66)*. Patients who had spent more time on dialysis than with a functioning renal allograft had a 7 times higher mortality rate. Altogether, 41% of deaths in children on both treatments were attributed to cardiovascular causes. Patients with long-standing HTN had a threefold higher risk of death. Cerebrovascular accidents on dialysis treatment were by far the most frequent cardiovascular cause encountered in this study.

## DIAGNOSTIC EVALUATION OF HYPERTENSION IN CHILDREN WITH END-STAGE RENAL DISEASE

Every pediatric patient with ESRD should be regarded as potentially hypertensive and should undergo a systematic evaluation. Casual BP recordings obtained by oscillometric devices should be checked by manual auscultatory methods and, preferably, by ABPM as well (*see* "Measurement of BP" and "Definition of HTN in ESRD"). ABPM is especially helpful in HD patients, because it allows a better recognition of intra- and postdialytic (particularly nocturnal) BP changes when continued over 24 or 48 h *(9)*. It is also recommended for the management of transplanted children, because it detects even minor degrees of HTN at daytime, and especially at nighttime. ABPM allows better monitoring of antihypertensive treatment and improves patient compliance in children on all forms of renal replacement therapy (RRT).

Given the known prognostic significance of cardiovascular lesions and hypertensive end-organ damage in pediatric ESRD patients, early and regularly repeated monitoring is required, even in the absence of any clinical signs. The investigations should include an assessment of cardiac structure and function by M-mode echocardiography, two-dimensional echocardiography, or Doppler ultrasonography *(45)*. There is no doubt that the collaboration of the nephrologist with an experienced (pediatric) cardiologist and/or radiologist considerably facilitates the cardiovascular care of ESRD children.

Volume changes should regularly and carefully be checked in hypertensive patients undergoing HD or PD. The absence of edema and normal pre- and postdialysis BP values are not reliable signs of normovolemia. Therefore, additional methods to recognize increased vascular volume should be applied as needed in children with severe HTN, marked lability of BP, or other instability. These methods include bioimpedance *(69)*, sonography of the inferior vena cava diameter *(70)*, and determination of the atrionatriuretic peptide in plasma *(19)*. Although these methods are not sufficiently validated in large series of ESRD children, their use may help in determining the individual "dry weight" at which the child must carefully be maintained. It should be noted that intravascular volume is reconstituted only a few hours after the end of an HD session *(5)*.

The diagnostic evaluation in transplanted children should consider the multiple etiologies of posttransplanted HTN (Table 1). Newer imaging techniques, such as magnetic resonance arteriography (MRA) and three-dimensional computed tomography, greatly aid the search for renal artery stenosis in the allograft.

## TREATMENT OF HTN IN THE PEDIATRIC END-STAGE RENAL DISEASE PATIENT

### *Treatment of Hypertension in the Dialysis Patient*

Control of volume status is the primary goal in the treatment of hypertensive children and adolescents undergoing long-term HD or PD *(71,72)*. In some patients, this may be obtained without antihypertensive medication. In every patient newly-admitted to dialysis therapy, one

Table 1
Factors Related to Posttransplant HTN

| |
|---|
| *Pretransplant factors* |
| Pre-existing HTN |
| Primary kidney disease |
| Recurrence of primary kidney disease (e.g., glomerulonephritis, HUS) |
| Atherosclerotic risk factors (e.g., obesity) |
| *Donor-related* |
| Very young donor (small vessels) |
| Hypertensive donor |
| *Transplantation-related* |
| Prolonged ischemia time |
| Delayed graft function |
| Volume expansion |
| *Immunologic/vascular factors* |
| Acute graft rejection |
| Chronic graft nephropathy (dysfunction) |
| Renal transplant artery stenosis or thrombosis |
| Remnant (hypoperfused) kidney |
| *Immunosuppressive therapy* |
| Corticosteroids |
| Calcineurin inhibitors (cyclosporin, tacrolimus) |
| *Other drugs* |
| Sympathicomimetic agents |
| *Lower urinary tract obstruction* |
| Ureteral stenosis |
| Lymphocele |
| *Hypercalcemia* |
| Hyperparathyroidism |

should try to gradually withdraw any antihypertensive medication within 1–2 mo in concert with a tolerable dietary salt and fluid restriction (which also helps to decrease thirst). During this period the true "dry weight" should become evident (*see* "Diagnostic Evaluation"), and the exact limits of pre- and postdialysis BP should be fixed. In general, the aim should be to attain casual BP readings below the 95th percentile. If possible, the therapeutic results should be checked regularly by ABPM, with the aim to obtain normal nocturnal, as well as daytime, BP values.

Since compliance with the strict procedures necessitated by ESRD and dialysis is often difficult, the dialysis prescription often has to be modified, e.g., switching to longer, more frequent (e.g., daily) or nocturnal HD sessions or by minimizing the sodium content of food and dialysate fluid. In a recent randomised crossover study performed in adult patients, daily HD sessions (6 times 2 h/wk over 6 mo) were able to reduce extracellular water, mean 24-h BP and LV mass significantly, compared with conventional HD (3 times 4 h/wk), and antihypertensive medication were able to be stopped or lowered in most subjects *(73)*. Similar results were obtained in a study in which patients switched from conventional to nocturnal dialysis *(57)*. In other studies, reduction of predialysis BP was obtained by gradually lowering the dialysate sodium content during HD sessions *(74)*. However, fluid removal is sometimes limited by hypotensive episodes occurring during the HD procedure, related either to exaggerated ultrafiltration or to concurrent use of high doses of diuretics or antihypertensive drugs.

Whether conversion from HD to PD (which allows a smoother fluid removal) has any persistent favorable effect on the BP status is controversial. On the other hand, a prolonged conservation of residual urine volume during HD or PD treatment generally allows for dialysis with a less stringent dialytic volume control. Above all, application of all criteria for adequate dialysis is important in both hypertensive and normotensive pediatric dialysis patients.

It is generally agreed that antihypertensive drugs should be used in dialysed children only if BP remains elevated, despite seemingly adequate volume control. Since no controlled studies have been performed in this group of patients, the optimal drug therapy remains empirical, based on investigations performed in other hypertensive populations. Angiotensin-converting enzyme (ACE) inhibitors and calcium channel blockers (CCBs) (usually as long-acting compounds) appear to be the most frequently used antihypertensive agents used in dialysed children. In the EDTA study, they were given to 62% and 56% of children on HD and PD, respectively, followed by β-blocking agents (35% and 44%, respectively), alone or in combination with other drugs *(15)*. The antihypertensive drugs mentioned are usually well tolerated, but the prescribing physician must note their multiple side effects, contraindications, and dose modifications required in renal failure most carefully (*see* Chapter 27).

ACE inhibitors have a favorable effect not only on BP but also on LVH *(75)*. Experience with ANG II receptor antagonists is still limited, even in adult patients receiving dialysis. CCBs have also been shown to reduce LV mass and may be used, even in the presence of volume overload. Nifedipine, as a rapidly acting compound, is widely used for treating hypertensive crises, despite the concern its use has raised in adults. The less frequent application of β-blocking agents in children with RRT may be related to their side effects (bradycardia, CNS symptoms, etc.), but according to a recent study in adults, they contribute to improved survival *(63)*. In many cases, the hypotensive agents already mentioned, as well as additional agents (including loop diuretics), have to be combined in order to obtain adequate BP control. In general, it is sufficient to apply these oral drugs once daily, preferably in the evening. Drug-resistant HTN is rare and usually the result of inadequate ultrafiltration, but may also be due to a paradoxical (heightened) response of the RAS to ultrafiltration.

### *Treatment of Posttransplant Hypertension*

The close association between interval changes in BP and LV mass in transplanted children *(52)* points to the importance of treating high BP early and aggressively before chronic rejection occurs. As in dialysed patients, the regular application of ABPM may help to detect minor degrees of HTN (especially when occurring at night), and to adjust antihypertensive strategies accordingly.

Before the introduction of or any change in the practice of antihypertensive medication is considered, one should consider modifying the immunosuppressive regimen by reducing the dose of corticosteroids or cyclosporine without compromising graft function. A number of new immunosuppressive drugs have been recently introduced. These drugs are less nephrotoxic and are not associated with HTN *(76)*.

All classes of antihypertensive drugs have been used in transplanted children; according to a NAPRTCS study, combination therapy was employed in two-thirds of cases *(23)*. According to a recent study in adult renal transplant patients, calcium channel antagonists (nifedipine) seemed to be superior to an ACE inhibitor (lisinopril) because the calcium channel antagonist appeared to improve renal function (by 20% after 2 yr) *(41)*. When using ACE inhibitors, graft function must be watched carefully, especially in the presence of a suspected renal artery stenosis. β-blocking agents are not regarded as first-line therapy because of their dyslipidemic and diabetogenic potential. Atherosclerotic risk factors should be avoided, but it is controversial if the presence of hyperlipidemia lipid-lowering drugs (e.g., statins) are indicated. In rare cases of renovascular HTN, transluminal angioplasty or surgery may be considered.

## REFERENCES


1. Samuels JA, Sorof JM. Blood pressure management in the dialysis patient. In: Warady BA, Schaefer FS, Fine RN, Alexander SR eds. Pediatric Dialysis. Boston: Kluwer Academic, 2004, in press.
2. Frauman AC, LansingLM, Fennell RS. Indirect blood pressure measurement in children undergoing hemodialysis: a comparison of brachial and dorsalis pedis auscultatory sites. AANNT J 1984;11:19–21.
3. Rahman M, Griffin V, Kumar A, Manzoor F, Wright JT Jr, Smith MC. A comparison of standardized versus "usual" blood pressure measurements in hemodialysis patients. Am J Kidney Dis 2002;39:1226–1230.
4. Coomer RW, Schulman G, Breyer JA, Shyr Y. Ambulatory blood pressure monitoring in dialysis patients and estimation of mean interdialytic blood pressure. Am J Kidney Dis 1997;29:678.
5. Luik AJ, Kooman P, Leuwissen KML. Hypertension in haemodialysis patients: is it only hypervolemia? Nephrol Dial Transplant 1997;12:1557–1560.
6. Conion PJ, Walshe JJ, Heinle S. Predialysis systolic blood pressure correlates strongly with mean 24-hour systolic blood pressure and left ventricular mass in stable hemodialysis patients. J Am Soc Nephrol 1996;7:2658–2663.
7. Ritz E, SchwengerV, Zeier M, Rychlik I. Ambulatory blood pressure monitoring: fancy gadgetry or clinically useful exercise? Nephrol Dial Transplant 2001;16:1550–1554.
8. Peixoto AJ, Santos SF, Mendes, RB, et al. Reproducibility of ambulatory blood pressure monitoring in hemodialysis patients. Am J Kidney Dis 2000;36:983–990.
9. Covic A, Goldsmith D. Ambulatory blood pressure monitoring: an essential tool for blood pressure assessment in uraemic patients.Nephrol Dial Transplant 2002;17:1737–1741.
10. Lingens N, Soergel M, Loirat C, Busch D, Lemmer B, Schärer K. Ambulatory blood pressure monitoring in pediatric patients treated by regular haemodialysis and peritoneal dialysis. Pediatr Nephrol 1995;9:167–172.
11. Sorof JM, Brewer ED, Portman RJ. Ambulatory blood pressure monitoring and interdialytic weight gain in children receiving chronic hemodialysis. Am J Kidney Dis 1999;33:667–674.
12. Soergel M, Kirschstein M, Busch C, et al. Oscillometric twenty-four hour ambulatory blood pressure values in healthy children and adolescents. A multicenter trial including 1141 subjects. J Pediatr 1997;129:178–184.
13. Wühl E, Witte K, Soergel M, et al. Distribution of 24-h ambulatory blood pressure in children: normalized reference values and role of body dimensions. J Hypertension 2002;20:1995–2007.
14. Schärer K, Rauh W, Ulmer HE. The management of hypertension in children with chronic renal failure. In: Giovannelli G, New MI, Gorini S, eds. Hypertension in children and adolescents. New York: Raven, 1981; 239–250.
15. Loirat C, Ehrich JMH, Geerlings W, et al. Report on management of renal failure in Europe XXII, 1992. Nephrol Dial Transplant 1994;9(Suppl 1):26–40.
16. Lerner GR, Warady BA, Sullivan EK, Alexander SR. Chronic dialysis in children and adolescents. The 1996 report of the North American Pediatric Renal Transplant Cooperative Study. Pediatr Nephrol 1999;13: 404–417.
17. Schaefer F, Klaus G, Müller-Wiefel D, Mehls O. Mid-European Pediatric Peritoneal Dialysis Study Group. Current practice of peritoneal dialysis in children: results of a longitudinal survey. Perit Dial Int 1999;19:S445–S449.
18. Mitsnefes MM, Daniels SR, Schwartz SM, Meyer RA, Khoury P, Strife CF. Severe left ventricular hypertrophy in pediatric dialysis: prevalence and predictors. Pediatr Nephrol 2000;14:898–902.
19. Holttä T, Happonen JM, Rönnholm K, Fyhrquist F, Holmberg C. Hypertension, cardiac state, and the role of volume overload during peritoneal dialysis. Pediatr Nephrol 2001;16:324–331.
20. Opelz G, Wuciak T, Ritz E. Association of chronic kidney graft failure with recipient blood pressure. Collaborative Transplant study. Kidney Int 1998;53:217–222.
21. Broyer M, Guest G, Gagnadoux MF, Beurton D. Hypertension following renal transplantation in children. Pediatr Nephrol 1987;1:16–21.
22. Ingelfinger JA, Brewer ED. Pediatric post-transplant hypertension. Child Nephrol Urol 1992;12:139–146.

23. Baluarte HI, Gruskin AB, Ingelfinger IR, Stablein D, Tejani A. Analysis of hypertension in children posttransplantation. A report of the North American Pediatric Renal Transplant Cooperative Study. Pediatr Nephrol 1994;8:570–573.
24. Lingens N, Dobos E, Witte K, et al. Twenty-four hour ambulatory blood pressure profiles in pediatric patients after renal transplantation. Pediatr Nephrol 1997;11:23–26.
25. Matteucci MC, Giordano U, Calzolari A, Turchetta A, Santilli A, Rizzoni G. Left ventricular hypertrophy, treadmill tests, and 24-hour blood pressure in pediatric transplant patients. Kidney Int 1999;56:1566–1570.
26. Soergel M, Maisin A, Azancot-Benisty A, Loirat C. Ambulante Blutdruckmessung bei nierentransplantierten Kindern und Jugendlichen. Z Kardiol 1992;81(Suppl 2):67–70.
27. Sorof JM, Poffenbarger T, Portman R. Abnormal 24-hour blood pressure pattern in children after renal transplantation. Am J Kidney Dis 2000;35:681–686.
28. Morgan H, Khan I, Hashmi A, Hebert D, Mc Crindle BW, Balfe W. Ambulatory blood pressure monitoring after renal transplantation in children. Pediatr Nephrol 2001;16:843–847.
29. Ferreira SR, Morisco VA, Taveres A, Pachero-Silva A. Cardiovascular effects of successful transplantation: a 1year sequential study of left ventricular morphology and function, and 24-hour blood pressure profile. Transplantation 2002;74:1580–1587.
30. GuytonAC, Granger HJ, Coleman TG. Autoregulation of the total systemic circulation and its relation to control of cardiac output and arterial pressure. Circ Res 1971;28(Suppl 1):93–97.
31. Charra B, Bergstrom J, Scribner BH. Blood pressure control in dialysis patients: importance of the lag phenomenon. Am J Kidney Dis 1998;32:720–724.
32. Katzarski KS, Charra B, Luik AJ, et al. Fluid state and blood pressure control in patients treated with long and short hemodialysis Nephrol Dial Transplant 1999;14:369–375.
33. Rauh W, Hund E, Sohl G, Rascher W, Mehls O, Schärer K. Vasoactive hormones in children with chronic renal failure. Kidney Int 24(Suppl 15):16–21.
34. Orth SR, Amann K, Strojek K, Ritz E. Sympathetic overactivity and arterial hypertension in renal failure. Nephrol Dial Transplant 2001;16(Suppl 1):67–69.
35. Ritz E, Amann K, Törnig J, Schwartz U, Stein G. Some cardiac abnormalities in renal failure. Adv Nephrol 1997;27:85–103.
36. Schwartz U, Buzello M, Ritz E, et al. Morphology of coronary atherosclerotic lesions in patients with end-stage renal failure. Nephrol Dial Transplant 2000;15:218–223.
37. Passauer J, Bussemaker E, Range U, Plug M, Gross P. Evidence in vivo showing increase of nitric oxide generation and impairment of endothelium dependent vasodilatation in normotensive patients on chronic hemodialysis. J Am Soc Nephrol 2000;11:1726–1734.
38. Xiao S, Wagner L, Schmidt RJ, Baylis C. Circulating endothelial nitric oxide synthase inhibitory factor in some patients with chronic renal disease. Kidney Int 2001;59:1466–1472.
39. Erkan E, Devarajan P, Kaskel F. Role of nitric oxide, endothelin-1, and inflammatory cytokines in blood pressure regulation in hemodialysis patients. Am J Kidney Dis 2002;40:76–81.
40. Menon MK, Naimark DM, Bargman JM, Vas SI, Oreopoulos DG. Long-term blood pressure control in a cohort of periteoneal dialysis patients and its association with residual renal function. Nephrol Dial Transplant 2001;16:2207–2213.
41. Midtvedt K, Hartmann A. Hypertension after kidney transplantation: are treatment guidelines emerging? Nephrol Dial Transplant 2002;17:1166–1169.
42. Gruskin AB, Darbagh S, Fleischmann LF, Apostol EM, Mattoo TK. Mechanisms of hypertension in childhood diseases. In: Barratt TM, Avner ED, Harmon WE, eds. Pediatric Nephrology. 4th edition. Baltimore: Lippincott Williams and Wilkins, 1999;987–1005.
43. Schärer K, Benninger C, Heimann A, Rascher W. Involvement of the central nervous system in renal hypertension. Eur J Pediatr 1993;152:59–63.
44. Wingen AM, Fabian-Bach C, Schaefer F, Mehls O. Randomised multicenter study of a low-protein diet on the progression of chronic renal failure in children. Lancet 1997;349:1117–1123.
45. Schärer K, Schmidt KG, Soergel M. Cardiac function and structure in patients with chronic renal failure. Pediatr Nephrol 1999;13:951–965.
46. Colan SD, Sanders SP, Ingelfinger JR, Harmon W. Left ventricular mechanics and contractile state in children and young adults with end-stage renal disease: effect of dialysis and transplantation. J Am Coll Cardiol 1987;10:1085–1094.

47. Goren A, Glaser I, Drukker A. Diastolic function in children and adolescents on dialysis and after kidney transplantation: an echocardiographic assessment. Pediatr Nephrol 1993;7:725–728.
48. Johnstone LM, Jones CL, Grigg LE, Wikinson JL, Walker RG, Powell HR. Left ventricular abnormalities in children, adolescents and young adults with renal disease. Kidney Int 1996;50:998–1006.
49. Parfrey PS, Foley RN, Harnett JD, Kent GM, Murray DC, Barre PE. Outcome and risk factors for left ventricular disorders in chronic uraemia. Nephrol Dial Transplant 1996;11:1277–1285.
50. Middleton RJ, Parfrey PS, Foley RN. Left ventricular hypertrophy in the renal patient. J Am Soc Nephrol 2001;12:1079–1084.
51. London GM. The concept of ventricular vascular coupling: functional and structural alterations of the heart and arterial vessels of the heart go in parallel. Nephrol Dial Transplant 1998;13:250–253.
52. Mitsnefes MM, Schwartz SM, Daniels SR, Kimball TR, Khoury P, Strife CF. Changes in left ventricular mass index in children and adolescents after renal transplantation,. Pediatr Transplant 2001a;5:279–284.
53. Raine AEG, Schwarz U, Ritz E. Hypertension and cardiac problems. In: Davison AM, Cameron JS, Grunfeld J-P, Kerr DNS, Ritz E, Winearls CG, eds. Oxford Textbook of Clinical Nephrology. 2nd ed. Oxford: Oxford University Press, 1998;1885–1918.
54. Mitsnefes MM, Daniels SR, Schwartz SM, Khoury P, Strife CF. Changes in left ventricular mass in children and adolescents during chronic dialysis. Pediatr Nephrol 2001b;16:318–325.
55. Washio M, Okuda S, Mizou CT, et al. Risk factors for left ventricular hypertrophy in chronic hemodialysis patients. Clin Nephrol 1997;47:362–366
56. London GM, Pannier B, Guerin AP, et al. Alterations of left ventricular hypertrophy and survival of patients receiving hemodialysis: follow-up of an interventional study. J Am Soc Nephrol 2001;12:2759–2767.
57. Chan CF, Floras JS, Miller JA, Richardson RM, Pierratos A. Regression of left ventricular hypertrophy after conversion to nocturnal hemodialysis. Kidney Int 2002;61:2235–2239.
58. Litwin M, Kawalec W, Grenda R. Left ventricular changes in the course of chronic renal failure and during dialysis therapy. In: Timio M, Wizemann V, Venanzi S, eds. 6th European Meeting on Cardionephrology. Cosenza: Editoriale Bios, 1997;93–96.
59. Goodman WG, Goldin J, Kuizon BD, et al. Coronary artery calcification in young adults with end-stage renal disease who are undergoing dialysis. New Engl J Med 2000;342:1478–1483.
60. Oh J, Wunsch R, Turzer M, et al. Advanced coronary and carotid arteriopathy in young adults with childhood-onset chronic renal failare. Circulation 2002;106:100–105.
61. Nayir A, Bilge L, Kilicaslan I, Ander H, Emre S, Sirin A. Arterial changes in paediatric haemodialysis patients undergoing renal transplantation. Nephrol Dial Transplant 2001;16:2041–2047.
62. Amar J, Vernier I, Rossignol E. Nocturnal blood pressure and 24-hour pulse pressure are potent indicators of mortality in hemodialysis patients. Kidney Int 2000;57:2485–2491.
63. Foley RN, Herzog CA, Collins AJ. Blood pressure and long-term mortality in United States hemodialysis patients: USRDS waves 3 and 4 study. Kidney Int 2002;62:1784–1790.
64. Mailloux LU, Haley WE. Hypertension in the ESRD patient: pathophysiology, therapy, outcomes, and future directions. Am J Kidney Dis 1998;32:705–719.
65. Reiss U, Wingen AM, Schärer K. Mortality trends in pediatric patients with chronic renal failure. Pediatr Nephrol 1996;10:602–605.
66. Groothof JW, Gruppen MP, Offringa M, et al. Mortality and causes of death of end-stage renal disease in children: a Dutch cohort study. Kidney Int 2002;61:621–629.
67. Locatelli F, Bommer JK, London GM. Cardiovascular disease determinant in chronic renal failure: clinical approach and treatment. Nephrol Dial Transplant 2001;16:459–468.
68. Parekh RS, Carroll CE, Wolfe RA, Port FK. Cardiovascular mortality in children and young adults with end-stage kidney disease. J Pediatr 2002;141:191–197.
69. Wühl E, Frisch C, Schärer K, Mehls O. Assessment of total body water in pediatric patients on dialysis. Nephrol Dial Transplant 1996;11:75–80.
70. Dietel T, Filler G, Grenda R, Wolfish N. Bioimpedance and inferior vena cava diameter for assessment of dialysis dry weight. Pediatr Nephrol 2000;14:903–907.
71. D Amico M, Locatelli F. Hypertension in dialysis: pathophysioligy and treatment. J Nephrol 2002;25:438–445.
72. Horl MP, Horl WH. Hemodialysis associated hypertension: pathophysiology and therapy. Am J Kidney Dis 2002;39:227–244.
73. Fagugli RM, Reboldi G, Quintaliani G, et al. Short daily hemodialysis: blood pressure control and left ventricular mass reduction in hypertensive hemodialysis patients. Am J Kidney Dis 2001;38:371–376.

74. Krautzig S, Janssen U, Koch KM, Granolleeras C, Shaldon S. Dietary salt restriction and reduction of dialysate sodium to control HTN in maintenance hemodialysis patients. Nephrol Dial Transplant 1998;13:552–553.
75. Cannella G, Paoletti E, Barocci S, et al. Angiotensin converting enzyme gene polymorphism and reversibility of uremic left ventricular hypertrophy following long-term antihypertensive therapy. Kidney Int 1998;54:618–626.
76. Morales JM. Influence of the new immunosuppressive combinations on arterial hypertension after renal transplantation. Kidney Int 2002;62(Suppl 82):81–87.

# IV Evaluation and Management of Pediatric Hypertension

# 23 Diagnostic Evaluation of Pediatric Hypertension

*Rita D. Swinford*, MD,
*and Ronald J. Portman*, MD

*CONTENTS*



## INTRODUCTION

A clinical challenge to the successful treatment of children with hypertension (HTN) is in the identification and evaluation of those children who will benefit from antihypertensive therapy *(1)*. Additionally, consideration must be given to the causative spectrum of HTN in pediatric patients, as it is broad and changes with age. Most infants, toddlers, and school-aged children must be presumed to have secondary HTN. Essential HTN is most prevalent in adolescence and not dissimilar from that found in adults. For children with severe HTN—those above the 99th percentile—careful, comprehensive and immediate evaluation is required. A general rule for the identification of children at higher risk for secondary HTN is: the younger the child and the more severe the HTN, the more likely it is that a secondary cause will be found. Nontheless, older pediatric patients are still at risk and evaluation is important. The cause(s) of the child's HTN may be remediable and may benefit from pharmacologic therapy. Also important to consider are children with diabetes and/or chronic kidney disease (CKD). Recent recommendations for these children include beginning therapy with antihypertensive medications, although the patient may be normotensive. Another recommendation for kidney and cardiovascular protection is that blood pressure (BP) be lowered to below the 90th percentile in children and <130/80 mmHg in older adolescents and adults *(2)*. This chapter has been organized as a guideline for the clinician evaluating a new pediatric patient with HTN, with references to other chapters in this book for more detailed information of secondary HTN in children.

Despite numerous guidelines, the diagnosis of pediatric HTN is not evidence-based, but is still based on statistical data *(3)* (as delineated in other chapters in this book). For example, Rocchini and colleagues *(4)* reported poor BP measurement standardization, and surveys indicate that approx 40% of British pediatricians did not routinely measure BPs. Nurses and

From: *Clinical Hypertension and Vascular Disease: Pediatric Hypertension*
Edited by: R. J. Portman, J. M. Sorof, and J. R. Ingelfinger © Humana Press Inc., Totowa, NJ

Table 1
Staging of HTN in Children by ABPM

| *Classification* | *Clinic BP* | *Mean systolic ambulatory BP* | *SBP load* |
|---|---|---|---|
| Normal BP | <95th percentile | <95th percentile | <25% |
| WCH | >95th percentile | <95th percentile | <25% |
| Stage 1 HTN | >95th percentile | <95th percentile | 25–50% |
| Stage 2 HTN | >95th percentile | >95th percentile | 25–50% |
| Stage 3 HTN | >95–99th percentile | >95th percentile | >50% |

In the future, the addition of the BP index will be included in this table for improved staging *(8)*.

doctors who did take BP measurements were found to use a variety of definitions and techniques for the diagnosis of HTN. As a further example of the conundrum, elevation of systolic BP, not diastolic BP, is now recognized to be most closely related to cardiovascular events in adults. Data to support this pediatric guideline have only recently become available *(5)*. For example, in 2002, Sorof and colleagues demonstrated in children that mild to moderate increases in systolic BP were more closely linked to left ventricular hypertrophy (LVH) than diastolic BP, and that treatment should be aimed at normalization of systolic BP *(6)*.

Technologic advances have seen the widespread introduction of oscillometric devices, which have the advantage of ease of use and little interobserver variability. These devices determine BP by measuring the mean arterial pressure from the point of maximum oscillations in the artery and calculating the systolic BP and diastolic BP using proprietary and unpublished algorithms. Unfortunately, the studies that compare these devices to auscultatory sphygmomanometry give highly variable results, most frequently showing poor correlation (*see* Chapter 4). Because BP is a continuous variable, assuming that a casual BP measurement is representative of the patient's true BP pattern may not be reasonable. Ambulatory BP monitoring (ABPM), on the other hand, is now commonly used in pediatric settings and effectively captures a child's BP pattern. ABPM provides evidence for defining a patient as having HTN by showing persistent BP elevation in a nonmedical setting by an elevated mean BP *(7)*, by calculation of the BP load (the percentage of BP exceeding the 95th percentile for age and height), or by calculation of the BP index (the patient's BP divided by their age, gender- and height-specific 95th percentile). As outlined elsewhere in this book, ABPM can be most useful in diagnosing white coat HTN (WCH), a condition felt not to require immediate pharmacologic therapy (*see* Chapter 8). Children with WCH have an elevated BP in the presence of a health care professional but normal in their own environment. The definition includes normal 24-h mean BP and BP load (Table 1) *(8)*. Mild HTN is found more frequently in patients with WCH than in those with severe HTN.

In adults, self-measurement of BP (SMBP) is becoming an important technique for BP monitoring. SMBP can be effective in suggesting the diagnosis of WCH and in monitoring antihypertensive therapy. However, there are two major considerations that make the use of this technology for children less attractive at this time. First, as in adults, patients and their parents do not truthfully record the data. This has also been observed with the use of glucometers in diabetic patients. The lack of reliability can be overcome by the use of monitors that objectively record the data for subsequent download. Secondly, and more importantly, BP monitors and cuffs have not been validated in children in a rigorous manner *(2)*.

Table 2
Phases of HTN Evaluation

*Phase 1: Is the patient truly hypertensive in the nonmedical setting?*
- Ambulatory BP monitoring
- Self-monitoring of BP
- School-based BP measurements

*Phase 2: Screening*
- CBC
- Urinalysis
- Urine culture
- Serum chemistries
  - electrolytes (potassium, sodium, chloride, bicarbonate, glucose)
  - creatinine, BUN
- Lipoprotein profiling (serum total cholesterol, with high density lipoprotein, low-density lipoprotein, and triglycerides)
- Renal ultrasound with Doppler
- Echocardiogram/EKG

*Phase 3: Definition of abnormalities*
- Renal imaging
  - renal ultrasound with Doppler plus/minus
  - radionuclide scan
  - Voiding cystourethrogram
- Renovascular imaging (noninvasive), computed tomography (CT) or magnetic resonance imaging
- Angiography
- Captopril challenge
- Renin profiling (plasma renin activity or direct renin assay)
- Aldosterone, catecholamine profiling
- Abdominal imaging; CT or ultrasound

*Phase 4: Determination of significance and remediability of abnormalities*
- Arteriography (conventional or digital subtraction angiography)
- Renal vein renin collection
- Renal biopsy
- MIBG scans (pheochromocytoma)

That said, the traditional pattern of a higher prevalence of secondary HTN compared to essential HTN in adolescence is changing. Essential HTN is becoming increasingly evident during late childhood and early adolescence. Indeed, with the exception of childhood asthma, HTN may now be the most common chronic disease of childhood. The causal factor responsible for the apparent dramatic increase in the prevalence of essential HTN is *obesity*, now considered a global phenomenon associated with an increased risk for the development of cardiovascular and renal disease *(9)*. Once it has been determined that a child has an elevated BP, and that this BP is persistently elevated, the following guide will serve to aid in the diagnostic evaluation (Tables 2 and 3). We use the term "phase" of evaluation in an attempt to avoid confusion with "stages" of HTN used in Table 1.

Phase 1: *Is the patient truly hypertensive in the nonmedical setting?*
(Confirmation of hypertension with ABPM or objective SMBP)

Phase 2: *Screening for HTN*

Table 3
**Questions to be Addressed in Phase 2 Evaluation After the HTN Has Been Confirmed**

| *Test* | *Design* |
|---|---|
| *What has HTN done to the patient?* | |
| Examination of history | |
| Measurement of growth | |
| Urinalysis | Renal disease (microalbuminuria, proteinuria, hematuria) |
| Chest radiogram and electrocardiogram or echocardiogram | Left ventricular hypertrophy |
| Poor growth | Chronic kidney disease |
| Fundoscopic exam | Chronic hypertension |
| Hemoglobin/hematocrit | Renal dysfunction/anemia of CRF |
| Serum electrolytes, Ca and phosphate dysregulation | Renal dysfunction |
| *What other risk factors for cardiovascular/kidney disease are present?* | |
| Fasting blood sugar | Diabetes |
| Elevated HgA1c | Diabetes |
| Glucosuria | Diabetes |
| Weight | Obesity |
| Lipoprotein analysis | Hypercholesterolemia; hypertriglyceridemia |
| Family history | Cardiovascular, obesity |
| Personal history | Medications, smoking, inactivity |
| *Why does the patient have HTN?* | |
| Serum electrolytes | $1^0$ or $2^0$ aldosteronism |
| BUN and serum creatinine | Renal dysfunction |
| Uric acid | Primary hypertension marker (?) |
| Renal ultrasound | Anatomic or pathologic etiology |
| Urinalysis | Hematuria/proteinuria (nephritis, renal masses) |
| Weight | Obesity |

A. Why does the patient have HTN? (Etiology)
B. What has HTN already done to the patient's body? (End-organ damage)
C. What other risk factor(s) for cardiovascular/kidney disease does the patient have? (Co-morbidities)

Phase 3: *Definition of Abnormalities*
Phase 4: *Determination of Significance and Remediability of Abnormality*

## EVALUATION

*Phase 1: Is the patient truly hypertensive in the nonmedical setting?*

When a child is found to have an elevated BP, this should elicit, *before* a thorough evaluation is performed, further validation of the possible HTN. At least two, preferably three, measurements should be taken at least 2 min apart, and the average of these measurements compared to the Task Force normograms *(2)* at each measurement session. If the BP is confirmed to be elevated, BP measurement should be repeated on at least two separate occasions unless it is severe (>99th percentile) or the child is symptomatic. In the latter case, one should make immediate referral to a specialist in pediatric HTN or admission to a hospital or emergency room.

Self-monitoring of BP (SMBP) can also be performed, preferably with a recording monitor and with attention paid to the caveats previously mentioned. School nurses can be useful in collecting additional measurements, which can then be faxed to complete the record. While school BP equipment is often not well-calibrated and nurses' training varies, proper training of nurses and time spent monitoring validation at local schools is time well spent. Ideally, an ABPM should be used to confirm the diagnosis of HTN and to exclude the diagnosis of white coat HTN (WCH). A small percentage of patients, similar to those reported by Lurbe and colleagues *(10)*, may have normal casual BP measurements but elevated ambulatory BP measurement, i.e., masked HTN- organ damage for adults and children, normotensive subjects and those with WCH have the same prevalence of end-organ damage. Conversely, those with masked HTN have an end-organ damage prevalence similar to true hypertensives *(11)*. A paradigm for the evaluation of HTN using different BP measurement techniques can be found in Fig. 1.

*Phase 2: Screening for HTN*

*a. Why does the patient have HTN?*

The etiology of HTN by age group is listed in Table 4. The exact percentages for each age group are unknown. However, the younger the patient and the more severe the HTN, the more likely the HTN is secondary. Most adolescents have essential HTN. The percentage of secondary causes in this age group remains higher than in adults. Consequently, all pediatric patients must be screened for secondary causes. Renal or renovascular causes of HTN account for approx 90% of secondary causes, with 2% caused by abnormalities of the aorta and 0.5% from pheochromocytoma *(12)*.

The personal and family history of HTN (Table 5) is a key starting point for the assessment of childhood HTN. Symptoms related to HTN may be caused by the disease, related to the cause of the HTN, nonspecific, or absent. The newborn may appear to have sepsis, feeding disorders, or neurologic abnormalities, while older patients are frequently asymptomatic, but may complain of nonspecific symptoms such as abdominal pain, epistaxis, chest pain or headache. Children can have subtle abnormalities that are difficult to attribute to HTN, such as personality changes, irritability, or changes in school performance. The HTN-oriented history should be directed at eliciting evidence of systemic diseases, use of medications, including those which elevate BP (oral contraceptives, bronchodilators, cyclosporin, corticosteroids, decongestants), congenital disorders, symptoms related to HTN (headache, irritability), neonatal history (use of umbilical catheters, neonatal asphyxia), growth pattern, present and past history of kidney or urologic disorders including urinary tract infections, symptoms suggestive of an endocrine etiology (change in weight, sweating, flushing, fevers, palpitations, muscle cramps), and family history of HTN or other cardiovascular morbid or mortal events.

The physical examination should address direct attention to detecting causes of secondary HTN (Table 6). For a child in the first year of life, secondary causes of HTN are the rule. Secondary HTN is still suspect when no etiology is detected (Table 4). Secondary HTN has a different spectrum in older children (Table 4). The physical examination should focus on symptoms and signs of HTN (Table 7). For all age groups with HTN, kidney disease is a common etiology. Approximately 60–90% is secondary to renal parenchymal or renovascular disease. A physical examination may reveal cranial (infants), neck, back, or abdominal bruits, where stenotic lesions cause turbulent blood flow, or asymmetric lower vs upper extremity pulses, signifying a possible aortic coarctation. Evidence for secondary HTN can also be

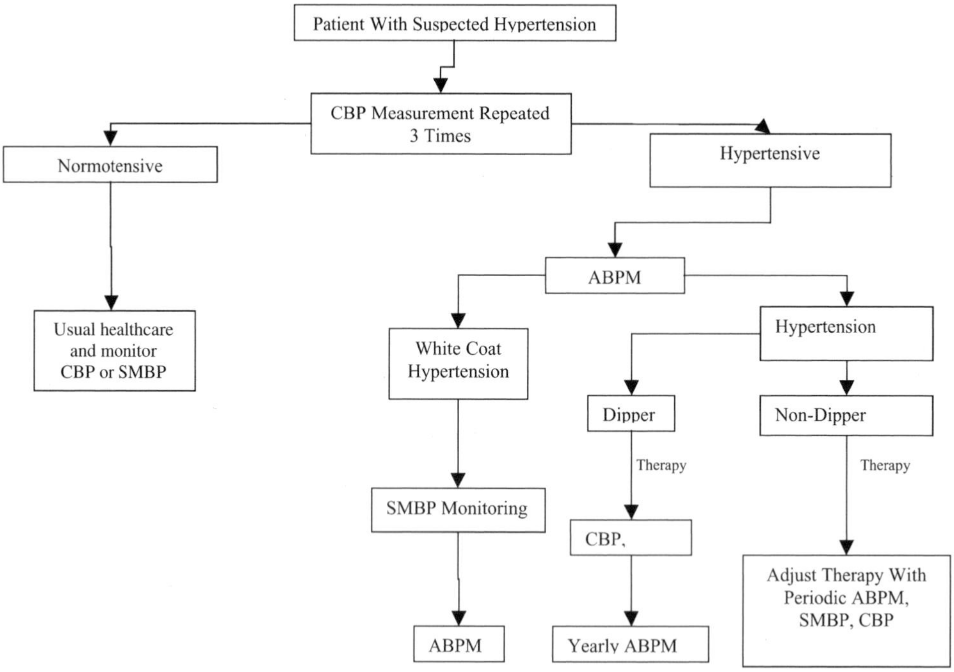


Fig. 1. When a patient is found to have an elevated blood pressure (BP) on initial evaluation or screening, BP should be repeated at two more sessions. If the patient is determined to be normotensive after repeated measures, follow-up BP measurements should be taken every 6 mo to 1 yr. One must be mindful that the patient may still have a nondipping pattern placing them in a higher risk category or masked hypertension (HTN). One should follow the patient's clinical course and if proceeds as expected, casual BP or self-measurement of BP (SMBP) can be used to follow the patient. However, if features are unexplained, such as proteinuria, or symptoms are present with elevation of BP, an ambulatory BP monitoring (ABPM) should be performed. CBP = Casual BP.

If the patient has HTN by casual measurement, ABPM may be performed to diagnose white coat HTN (WCH) as well as determine altered BP patterns. If WCH is found, SMBP can be effective in monitoring the WCH and ABPM can be repeated if clinical course varies from expected. If ABPM confirms the HTN, the patient can then be categorized by dipping status. A patient with a dipping pattern may be followed with casual BP or, ABPM with occasional ABPM monitoring as needed. However, a patient with a nondipping pattern can only be practically monitored by ABPM which should be used along with casual BP and SMBP as needed to maintain and assure adequate circadian BP control. The significance and chronicity of BP abnormalities should also be confirmed by assessment of end-organ damage.

supported by a finding of hypertensive retinopathy, neurofibromas, café-au-lait spots, lesions of tuberous sclerosis, or thyromegaly during the physical examination. Initial evaluation should also assess four extremity BP measurements to screen for coarctation of the aorta.

A serum creatinine and estimation (Schwartz formula) *(13)* of glomerular filtration rate (GFR), or actual GFR measurement, either by 24-h urine collection for creatinine or by using a radioisotope tagged study—e.g., iothalamate—is also fundamental *(14)*. The importance of a complete urinalysis with urinary protein or microalbumin and sterilely collected urine for culture cannot be overemphasized. Proteinuria or hematuria may be revealed, indicating possible glomerular disease or other nonglomerular conditions, such as pyelonephritis, obstructive uropathy, and interstitial nephritis. The proteinuria may be exacerbated with exercise or may change in quantity with the circadian pattern. The examination of a newly voided and cen-

Table 4
**Most Common Causes of Secondary Hypertension: By Age**

| *Age group* | *Etiology* |
|---|---|
| Newborn | Renal artery or venous thrombosis |
| | Renal artery stenosis |
| | Congenital renal abnormalities |
| | Coarctation of the aorta |
| | Bronchopulmonary dysplasia |
| First year | Coarctation of the aorta |
| | Renovascular disease |
| | Renal parenchymal disease |
| | Iatrogenic (medication, volume) |
| | Tumor |
| Infancy to 6 yr | Renal parenchymal disease |
| | Renovascular disease |
| | Coarctation of the aorta |
| | Tumor |
| | Endocrine causes[a] |
| | Iatrogenic |
| | Essential HTN |
| Age 6–10 yr | Renal parenchymal disease |
| | Essential HTN |
| | Renovascular disease |
| | Coarctation of the aorta |
| | Endocrine causes |
| | Tumor |
| | Iatrogenic |
| Adolescence, age 12–18 yr | Essential HTN |
| | Iatrogenic |
| | Renal parenchymal disease |
| | Endocrine causes |
| | Coarctation of the aorta |

[a]Shaded areas are uncommon for category.

trifuged urine specimen can reveal important information (e.g., red cells casts, white cells, red blood cells, bacteria, etc.), which may further illuminate the causal relationship to the HTN.

A renal ultrasound is a simple and informative noninvasive test and appropriate for the initial screening. The prevalence of abnormalities revealed by a renal ultrasound may be low. However, the importance of findings and noninvasive nature make it a valued screening test. The information provided can reveal asymmetrically sized kidneys, which would suggest vesicoureteral reflux, obstruction, unilateral infection, or possible kidney dysplasia; symmetrically enlarged kidneys indicate potential infective (pyelonephritis) or glomerular disease. Additionally, the renal ultrasound easily documents renal calculi, nephrocalcinosis, renal parenchymal cysts, polycystic kidney disease, or multicystic dysplastic disorder. Doppler waveform analysis of the renal hilum can also provide information about the patency of the vessels. However, its sensitivity is limited, particularly in infants and children, and in the detection of intrarenal lesions and incomplete stenoses in older children or adolescents *(15,16)*.

**Table 5**
**Relevant Questions for the Hypertensive Evaluation of Patient History**

- Family history
  - Essential HTN
    - medications/diet control
    - salt-sensitive
    - obesity
  - Systemic Disease
    - endocrine
      - hyperthyroidism, diabetes
    - obesity
    - cardiovascular disease
      - early myocardial infarction/stroke
    - hyperlipoproteinemia
    - kidney disease
      - kidney failure, dialysis or transplantation
- Medications
  - Antiinflammatory agents: steroidal and nonsteroidal
  - Decongestants
  - Stimulants: caffeine, ritalin, adderal
  - Antidepressants: tricyclics
  - Immunosuppression: Cyclosporin, FK506
- Weight change
  - Weight loss or gain?
  - Time frame for interval change in weight
    - Weight loss as with pheochromocytoma
    - Weight gain as with exogenous or endogenous steroids
- Neonatal history: umbilical arterial catheter; neonatal asphysia, bronchopulmonary dysplasia
- Trauma
- Systemic disease
  - Systemic lupus erythematosus
  - Polyarteritis
  - Flushing, sweating, headaches, palpitations as in pheochromocytoma or neuroblastoma
  - Neurofibromatosis
  - Scleroderma
  - Urinary tract infections or history of unexplained or explained fevers
- Substance abuse
  - Amphetamines
  - Other (e.g., cocaine, PCPs)

Serum electrolytes will most commonly be normal. However, alterations of potassium concentrations can indicate primary or secondary hyperaldosteronism, particularly when the potassium is low and there is a concomitant metabolic alkalosis. Liddle's syndrome, the syndrome of apparent mineralocorticoid excess, Gordon's Syndrome, glucocorticoid remediable aldosteronism, and other forms of monogenic HTN are often associated with this electrolyte pattern and altered renin and aldosterone levels (Fig. 2) *(17)*. By contrast, an elevated potassium level in conjunction with a metabolic acidosis may suggest kidney disease. Indeed, this diagnosis may be supported by an elevation in serum creatinine, or one may find nephrocal-

Table 6
Physical Examination: Clues to the Etiology of HTN

| | |
|---|---|
| Body habitus | Thinness—pheochromocytoma, hyperthyroidism, renal disease (growth failure) |
| | Obesity—metabolic syndrome |
| | Central obesity—Cushing's syndrome |
| | Virilized—congenital adrenal hyperplasia |
| | Rickets—chronic renal disease |
| Skin | Neurofibromas—neurofibromatosis |
| | Café-au-lait spots—pheochromocytoma |
| | Tubers, ash-leaf spots—tuberous sclerosis |
| | Bruising—Cushing's disease, trauma |
| | Rashes: vasculitis—collagen vascular disease or nephritic |
| | impetigo—acute nephritis |
| | striae—Cushing's disease |
| | Needle tracks—iatrogenic HTN |
| Head and face | Unusual shape—mass lesion |
| | Round facies (moon)—Cushing's syndrome |
| | Elfin facies—William's syndrome |
| | Seventh nerve palsy—severe HTN |
| Eyes | EOM palsy—nonspecific |
| | Fundal changes—nonspecific |
| | Proptosis—hyperthyroidism |
| Neck | Goiter— ? hyperthyroid goiter |
| | Bruit |
| Lungs | Rales, rhonchi—nonspecific ? cardiac decompensation |
| Heart | Failure—same as for enlarged heart |
| | Rub— ? chronic renal disease with HTN |
| | Enlargement |
| Abdomen | Masses—Wilms tumor, neuroblastoma, hydronephrosis, polycystic kidney disease |
| | Hepatomegaly—heart failure |
| | Hepatosplenomegaly—infantile polycystic disease |
| | Scars—GU surgery |
| | Bruit—renovascular disease |
| | Edema—renal/renovascular disease |
| Back/flank | Bruit—renovascular disease |
| | Flank tenderness—pyelonephritic, obstruction, acute nephritis |
| | Scoliosis—? HTN secondary to procedures |
| Pelvis | Mass—obstructive neurophathy, neuroblastoma |
| Genitalia | Ambiguous, virilized—congenital adrenal hyperplasia |
| Extremities | Disparity in BP, pulse, delayed refill—coarctation |
| | Edema |
| Neurologic | Bell's palsy—nonspecific |
| | Encephalopathy—nonspecific |
| | Personality changes—nonspecific |
| | Changes in school performance—nonspecific |

**Table 7**
**Physical Signs or Symptoms Suggestive of Secondary HTN**

| *Sign or symptom* | *Comment* |
|---|---|
| *CNS* | |
| Hypertensive crisis | Severe HTN with underlying encephalopathy |
| Bell's palsy | Often associated with severe HTN |
| Hypertensive retinopathy | In children, rarely found in essential HTN but good staging unavailable |
| *Skin* | |
| Neurofibromas | Pheochromocytoma/renovascular lesions |
| Café-au-lait spots | Pheochromocytoma/renovascular lesions |
| Lesions of tuberous sclerosis | Renal cysts, vascular lesions |
| Rash | |
| of systemic lupus erythematosus | Lupus nephritis |
| or Henoch–Schonlein purpura | Henoch-Schonlein nephritis/vasculitis |
| Needle tracks | Drug abuse, iatrogenous hypertension |
| *Goiter* | |
| | Hyperthyroidism |
| *Lungs* | |
| Picture of bronchopulmonary dysplasia | Associated HTN |
| Pulmonary edema | Volume overload associated hypertension: acute glomerulo-nephritis or chronic renal insufficiency |
| *Heart* | |
| Failure | Volume overload associated HTN: acute glomerulonephritis or chronic renal insufficiency |
| *Endocrine/genetic* | |
| Multiple endocrinopathy | Pheochromocytoma |
| Turner's syndrome | Coarctation of the aorta |
| William's syndrome | Renovascular hypertension |
| Van Hippel–Lindau | Pheochromocytoma |
| *Abdominal* | |
| Bruits | Renovascular HTN |
| Enlarged kidneys | Polycystic disease, obstructive uropathy, renal inflammatory disorders (pyelonephritis, nephritis) |

cinosis on renal ultrasound, indicating a renal tubular defect. Importantly, values of serum creatinine for pediatric patients differ with increasing age and often can be misinterpreted as "normal" when, in fact, a significant loss of kidney mass/function has occurred, despite the use of the Schwartz formula *(13)*.

An echocardiogram performed for the assessment of end-organ damage can also diagnose the presence of coarctation of the aorta. Further studies to assess the presence of endocrine abnormalities, such as pheochromocytoma or Cushing's disease, should depend on signs or symptoms consistent with the diagnosis.

*b. What are the consequences of the HTN: end-organ damage?*

The relationship of HTN to end-organ damage is critical to the true definition of HTN and discussed in detail by Sorof (*see* Chapter 8). The evaluation of HTN is not solely to determine

| | Laboratory Results | | | | | | |
|---|---|---|---|---|---|---|---|
| Syndrome | $K^+$ | pH | Renin | Aldo | Specific Treatment | Gene Loci | Gene |
| GRA | ↓ | ↑ | ↓ | ↑ | Spironolactone (Amiloride, triamterene) | 8q | Chimeric gene (CYP11B1/ CYP11B2) |
| Liddle's syndrome | ↓ | ↑ | ↓ | ↓ | Amiloride, triamterene | 16p | $\beta$ and $\gamma$ subunit of ENaC |
| AME | ↓ | ↑ | ↓ | ↓ | Spironolactone (Amiloride, triamterene) | 16q | 11-$\beta$-HSD |
| MR | ↓ | ↑ | ↓ | ↓ | None, multiple drug therapy | 4q | MR |
| Gordon's syndrome | ↑ | ↓ | ↓ | ↓ | Hydrochlorothiazide | 1q<br>12p13<br>17p | WNK1<br>WNK4 |
| HBS | N | N | N (↓) | N | None, multiple drug therapy | 12p11 | Unknown |

NOTE. Contrary to the rest, the HBS is not salt sensitive and features normal values for the shown parameters. Abbreviations: $K^+$, potassium; Aldo, aldosterone.

Fig. 2. Monogenic forms of hypertension (HTN). Abbreviations: GRA, glucocorticoid-remediable aldosteronism; AME, apparent mineralocorticord excess; MR, mineralocorticoid receptor mutation; HBS, HTN brachydactyly syndrome

where the measured level of BP exceeds some epidemiologically derived number, but rather to ascertain the level of this endothelial disease marker associated with end-organ damage. The evaluation of end-organ damage should include a complete assessment of the eyes, cardiovascular system (including blood vessels), kidneys, and nervous system. This assessment can assist in determining the chronicity and severity of the HTN. Fundoscopy rarely discloses hemorrhages or exudates, but may reveal arteriolar narrowing and arteriovenous nicking. Unfortunately, there has been no development of a standardized grading system for hypertensive retinopathy in children.

LVH is a clear and independent risk factor for cardiovascular morbidity and mortality in adult patients, but its significance is less clear for children unless it is severe and compromising cardiac function. The echocardiogram is more sensitive than the electrocardiogram for the determination of left ventricular hypertrophy/index *(18)*. ABPM has been shown to have a high correlation with LV mass index where casual BP (CBP) measurements do not.

Specifically the best predictors include the 24 h, wake or sleep mean BP, BP load or BP index *(19)*. Additionally, further evidence for HTN's role in causing end-organ damage in pediatrics emanates from the correlation of the carotid intimal-medial thickness and LV mass index with hypertension and obesity *(20)*. There is a growing body of evidence that demonstrates an association with nondipping status and an increased risk of adverse events *(21–22)*. Additional markers of end-organ damage include elevated microalbumin excretion, which is especially important in diabetics, patients with CKD, obesity. The presence of end-organ damage in a child is an absolute indication for pharmacologic treatment of HTN.

The majority of pediatric hypertensive patients with a secondary cause have CKD, which is commonly associated with alterations in the circadian patterns of BP. The most frequent of these rhythmic abnormalities is nocturnal (sleep) period HTN and a nondipping BP pattern *(23,24)*. As stated in The Seventh Report of the Joint National Committee on the Prevention, Detection, Evaluation, and Treatment of High Blood Pressure (JNC 7) *(25)*, "The level of mean ABP or BP load correlates better than office measurements with target organ injury." Abnormal ambulatory BP patterns have been shown to be related to varying degrees of abnormal protein excretion (Fig. 3) *(26)*, more rapid progression of kidney disease *(27–29)*, and to cardiovascular damage and events *(30)*. In this regard, the correlation between CBP and ABP is poor, as is the relationship of CBP to end-organ damage *(31,32)*.

*c. What other risk factors for cardiovascular disease may be present?*

The major modifiable cardiovascular risk factors are HTN, diabetes, smoking, hyperlipidemia, and proteinuria (CKD), and should be evaluated during the initial screening process. A reasonable list of tests for screening includes a fasting lipoprotein analysis, including cholesterol, triglycerides, high-density lipoprotein (HDL), low-density lipoprotein (LDL), and very low-density lipoprotein (VLDL), a fasting glucose and insulin for assessment of insulin resistance, microalbumin excretion, echocardiography, and kidney function.

*Phase 3: Definition of Abnormalities*

Phase 3 evaluation is designed to further clarify and define abnormalities identified during Phase 1 in any of the three categories of etiology, risk factors, and end-organ damage determination. Concerning etiology, performance of stage 3 evaluation should be done for the very young hypertensive patient or for those with severe HTN, even if Phase 1 is unremarkable (Table 1). At this point, we aim to find the abnormality, but specifically limit the diagnostic tests to match the patient. For instance, if it is revealed, through the patient history and/or physical examination that the patient has stigmata of hyperthyroidism, e.g., weight loss,

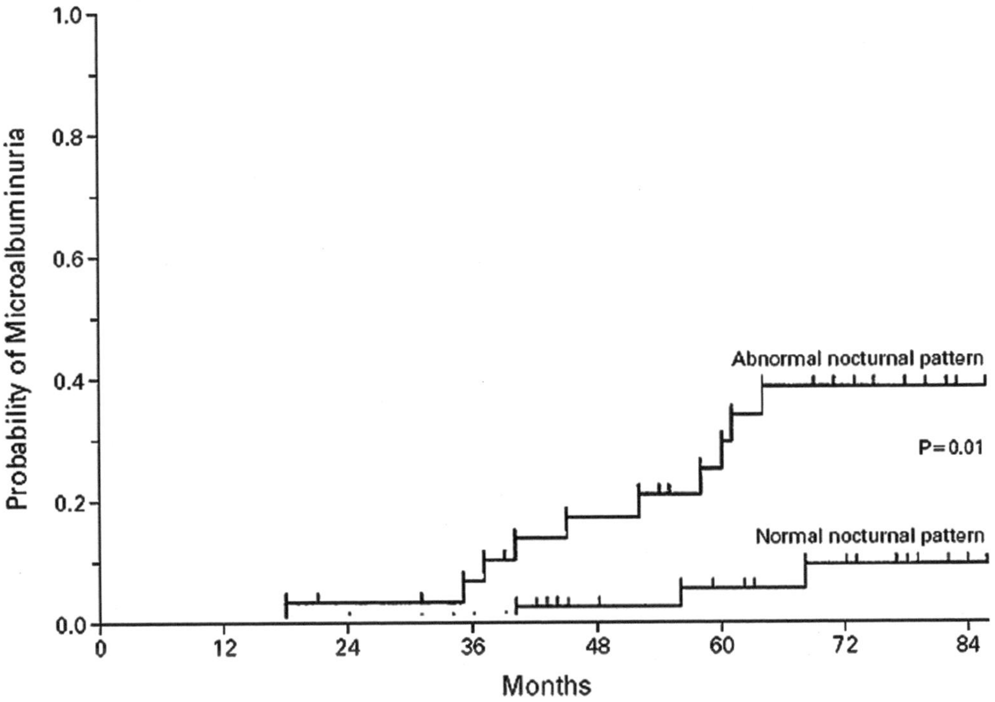


Fig. 3. Kaplan-Meier curves showing the probability of microalbuminuria according to the pattern of daytime and nighttime systolic pressure. The probability of microalbuminuria differed significantly between the two groups ($p = 0.01$ by the log-rank test; $\chi^2 = 6.217$ with 1 df). The risk of microalbuminuria was 70% lower in the subjects with a normal nocturnal pattern than in those with an abnormal nocturnal pattern *(27)*. Reproduced from ref. *26*, with permission.

enlargement of thyroid, or proptosis, we might perform a thyroid panel, but not necessarily on all patients fitting this profile. Individual consideration should be given to the measurement of plasma levels of various endocrine or vasoactive hormones, as well as 24-h excretion rates of various hormones based on prior findings. Imaging studies provide information on the condition of the renal parenchyma and renovascular dysfunction. Renal ultrasound with Doppler flow analysis, in conjunction with other studies, can reveal the etiology for diagnosis of certain kidney lesions. Radionuclide renal scanning can be very helpful, since it can assess both renal function, perfusion, obstruction, and presence of renal scarring. Radionuclide scintigraphy, used to to assess scarring, may use either $^{99m}$Tc dimercaptosuccinic acid (DMSA), $^{99m}$Tc glucoheptonate (DTPA), or $^{99m}$Tc mercaptoacetyltriglycine ($Mag_3$), and can be done with diuretics to help assess if the presence of hydronephrosis presents an obstruction. A voiding cystourethrogaphy should also be performed in children with a history of urinary tract infections and for whom the diagnosis of vesicoureteral reflux or bladder abnormalities is considered. Detection of proteinuria requires either quantitation of protein excretion with the first morning urine using a urinary protein to creatinine ratio, or a 24-h urine collection for protein and creatinine (split into supine and upright fractions to assess for orthostatic proteinuria).

Abnormalities of the mesenteric, splenic, and hepatic vessels often accompany renovascular disease in children. A certain percentage of these children may have neurofibromatosis type 1 (NF-1) *(33,34)*, abdominal coarctation *(35–37)* or intracranial disease *(38)*. In our experience, Doppler ultrasound is a very specific but insensitive test for renovascular HTN. Screening for renal artery stenosis in children with captopril scans has also been unrewarding. Magnetic resonance angiography may become a valuable tool for detection of renal artery stenosis in children, but no large studies have yet validated the technology. It may be used as a screening test but if there is a high index of suspicion, arteriography, the gold standard, should still be performed.

If other risk factors are identified, testing and/or appropriate referral should be performed. For example, glucose intolerance should be further evaluated with an assessment of glycosylated hemoglobin or proteins, a glucose tolerance test, and a referral to endocrinology. Elevated serum lipoproteins in the obese could suggest dietary causes or, rarely, hypothyroidism. Familial forms of hyperlipidemia, such as abnormalities in the number or function of LDL receptors, should also be assessed.

*Phase 4: Determination of the Significance and Remediability of Abnormality*

At this point, having found an abnormality, we now look for a test, or series of tests, that will provide information regarding the medical or surgical correctablity of the problem. If a renal artery stenosis is detected by renovascular imaging, renal vein renins may provide further evidence for surgical correction. If either an elevated serum metanephrine or urinary catecholamines is found, suggesting a pheochromocytoma, then an octreotide or metaiodobenzylguanidine (MIBG) scan would aid in localization for surgical correction. A finding of significant proteinuria or hematuria with red blood cell casts would suggest the need for a renal biopsy. This information is also helpful in determining the type of antihypertensive therapy to be used. If abnormalities in serum renin or aldosterone consistent with the genetic syndromes outlined in Fig. 2 are found, specific therapies, such as amiloride or spironolactone, are suggested (*see* Chapter 12). A finding of CKD or diabetes can suggest the use of drugs affecting the renin-angiotensin system, such as ACE inhibitors or angiotension receptor blockade.

## SUMMARY

An end-organ damage assessment should be the basis for the definition of pediatric HTN. However, the current definition is not based on this. Primary HTN, defined by BP measurements exceeding the 95th percentile for height, is increasing in prevalence, particularly in older children and adolescents with HTN risk factors, e.g., obesity. We recommend the evaluation of the pediatric hypertensive patient in phases, beginning with the confirmation of HTN beyond the office measurement (Phase 1). This confirmation is followed by the screening phase, Phase 2, which further defines: (a) the etiology of the HTN, with the knowledge that younger patients are more likely to have a secondary etiology and older essential HTN; (b) other risk factors for cardiovascular/kidney disease; (c) hypertensive end-organ damage. Phase 3 defines the abnormalities in either a, b, or c, and the fourth and final phase is the determination of the significance of observed findings.

We believe that pharmacological treatment of all children and adolescents with persistent HTN is needed because of the risk of end-organ damage and the lack of long-term efficacy of nonpharmacologic therapy as a sole therapy. Evidence-based definitions of pediatric HTN, and the indication for treatment, are currently evolving. Also evolving is the introduction of new information for areas of pre- and postnatal causes of HTN; genetics of HTN; the relationship of obesity, diabetes, and CKD to HTN; the use of ABPM in the evaluation of childhood HTN; and the introduction of new pharmacologic therapy. Clearly, the information presented in this text has improved our understanding of the pathogenesis, diagnosis and treatment of childhood HTN. However, there remains a need for significant advancements. The most efficient tests and evaluation pathways for determining which children have secondary forms of HTN, or who is at risk for end-organ damage, have yet to be determined.

## REFERENCES


1. Falkner BE. Treatment of hypertensive children and adolescents. In: Isso JL, Black HR, eds. Hypertension Primer, 3rd Edition. Philadelphia: American Heart Association, 2003;494–497.
2. Portman RJ. Guideline 3, Measurement of Blood Pressure. Kidney Disease Quality Outcome Initiative, in press.
3. Update on the 1987 Task Force Report on High Blood Pressure in Children and Adolescents: A Working Group Report from the National High Blood Pressure Education Program Pediatrics 1996;98:649–658.
4. Rocchini, AP. Pediatric hypertension 2001. Curr Opin Cardiol 2002;17:385–389.
5. Rucki S, Feber J. Repeated ambulatory blood pressure monitoring in adolescents with mild hypertension. Pediatr Nephrol 2001;16:911–915.
6. Sorof JM, Cardwell G, Franco K, Portman RJ. Ambulatory blood pressure and left ventricular mass index in hypertensive children. Hypertension 2002;39:903–908.
7. Soergel M, Kirschstein M, Busch C, et al. Oscillometric twenty-four hour ambulatory blood pressure values in health children and adolescents: a multicenter trial including 1141 subjects. J Pediatr 1997;130:178–184.
8. Lurbe E, Sorof JM, Daniels SR. Clinical and research aspects of ambulatory blood pressure monitoring in children. J Pediatr 2004;144(7):7–16.
9. Lurbe E, Alvarez V, Redon J. Obesity, body fat distribution, and ambulatory blood pressure in children and adolescents. J Clin Hypertens 2001;3:362–367.
10. Lurbe E, Toor I, Paya R, Alvarez V, Redon J. Masked hypertension in adolescents. Am J Hypertens 2003;16:237A.
11. Clement DL, De Buyzere ML, De Bacquer DA, et al. (Office versus Ambulatory Pressure Study Investigators). Prognostic value of ambulatory blood-pressure recordings in patients with treated hypertension New Engl J Med 2002;348:2407–2415
12. Londe S. Causes of hypertension in the young. Pediatr Clin North Am 1978;25(1):55–65.
13. Schwartz GJ, Brion LP, Spitzer A. The use of plasma creatinine concentration for estimating glomerular filtration rate in infants, children, and adolescents. Pediatr Clin North Am 1987;34(3):571–590.
14. Hall PM, Rolin H. Iothalmate clearance and its use in large-scale clinical trials. Current Opin Nephrol Hypertens 1995;3:510–513.
15. Olin JW, Piedmonte MA, Young JR. The utility of duplex ultrasound scanning of the renal arteries for diagnosing significant renal artery stenosis. Ann Intern Med 1995;122:833–838.
16. Brun P, Kchouk H, Mouchet B. Value of Doppler ultrasound for the diagnosis of renal artery stenosis in children. Pediatr Nephrol 1997;11:27–30.
17. Toka HR, Luft FC. Monogenic forms of human hypertension. Semin Nephrol 2002;22(2):81–88.
18. Daniels SR, Loggie JM, Khoury P, Kimball TR. Left ventricular geometry and severe left ventricular hypertrophy in children and adolescents with essential hypertension. Circulation 1998;97:1907–1911.
19. Sorof JM, Poffenbarger T, Franco K, Portman R. Evaluation of white coat hypertension in children: importance of the definitions of normal ambulatory blood pressure and the severity of casual hypertension. Am J Hypertens 2001;14:855–860.
20. Sorof JM, Alexandrov AV, Cardwell G, Portman RJ. Carotid artery intimal-medial thickness and left ventricular hypertrophy in children with elevated blood pressure. Pediatrics 2003;111:61–66.
21. Covic A, Goldsmith DJA, Georgescu GC, Ackrill P. Relationships between blood pressure variability and left ventricular parameters in hemodialysis and renal transplant patients. Nephrology 1998;4:87–94.
22. Appel LJ, Robinson KA, Guallar E, et al. Utility of Blood Pressure Monitoring Outside of the Clinic Setting. Summary, Evidence Report/Technology Assessment: Number 63. AHRQ Publication No. 03-E003, March 2002. Agency for Healthcare Research and Quality, Rockville, MD. Retrieved from http://www.ahrq.gov/clinic/epcsums/utilbpsum.htm.
23. Baumgert P, Walger P, Gemen S, von Eiff M, Raidt H, Rahn, KH. Blood pressure elevation during the night in chronic renal failure, hemodialysis and after renal transplantation. Nephron 1991;57:293–298.
24. Middeke M, Schrader J. Nocturnal blood pressure in normotensive subjects and those with white coat, primary, and secondary hypertension. Brit Med J 1994;308:630–632.

25. Chobanian AV, Bakris GL, Black HR, et al. and the National High Blood Pressure Education Program Coordinating Committee. The Seventh Report of the Joint National Committee on the Prevention, Detection, Evaluation and Treatment or High Blood Pressure. JAMA 2003;289:2560–2572.
26. Lurbe E, Redon J, Kesani A, et al. Increase in nocturnal blood pressure and progression to microalbuminuria in type I diabetes. N Engl J Med 2002;347:797–805.
27. Csiky B, Kovacs T, Wagner L, Vass T, Nagy J. Ambulatory blood pressure and progression in patients with IgA nephropathy. Nephrol Dial Transplant 1999;14:86–90.
28. Timio M, Venanzi S, Lolli S, et al. "Non-dipper" hypertensive patients and progressive renal insufficiency: a 3-year longitudinal study. Clin Nephrol 1995;43(6):382–387.
29. Farmer KT, Goldsmith DJA, Quin JD, et al. Progression of diabetic nephropathy—is diurnal blood pressure rhythm as important as absolute blood pressure level. Nephrol Dial Transplant 1998;13:635–639.
30. Nakano S, Fukuda M, Hotta F, et al. Reversed circadian blood pressure rhythm is associated with occurrences of both fatal and nonfatal vascular events in NIDDM subjects. Diabetes 1998;47:1501–1506.
31. Mcgregor DO, Olsson C, Lynn, Kevin L. Autonomic dysfunction and ambulatory blood pressure in renal transplant recipients. Transplantation 2001;71:1277–1281.
32. Tucker B, Fabbian F, Giles M, Thurasingham RC, Raine AEG, Baker LRI. Left ventricular hypertrophy and ambulatory blood pressure monitoring in chronic renal failure. Nephrol Dial Transplant 1997;12:724–728.
33. Loughridge LW. Renal abnormalities in the Marfan syndrome. Q J Med 1959;28:531–544.
34. Glushien AS, Mansuy MM, Littman DS. Pheaechromocytoma: its relationship to neurocutaneous syndromes. Am J Med 1953;14:318–327.
35. Alpert BS, Bain HH, Balfe JW. Role of the renin-angiotensin-aldosterone system in hypertensive children with coarctation of the aorta. Am J Cardiol 1979;43:828–831.
36. Becker AE, Becker MJ, Edward JE. Anomalies associated with coarctation of aorta. Circulation 1979;41:1067–1069.
37. Morriss M, McNamara D. Coarctation of the aorta. In: Garson A, Bricker J, McNamara D, eds. Science and Practice of Pediatric Cardiology. Philadelphia: Lea & Febiger, 1990;1353–1365.
38. Wiggelinkhuizen J, Cremin BJ. Takayasu arateritis and renovascular hypertension in childhood. Pediatrics 1978;62:209–217.

# 24 Nonpharmacologic Treatment of Pediatric Hypertension

*Bruce S. Alpert*, MD, *Michael Hasselle*, BS, *and Sidney Orndu*ff, PhD

*Contents*



## INTRODUCTION

During childhood, elevated systolic and/or diastolic blood pressure (BP) is commonly secondary to diseases of the kidneys, endocrine system, and/or cardiovascular system. When diagnostic evaluation does not reveal a cause for the elevation in BP, we call that condition essential, or idiopathic, hypertension (HTN). Over 90% of HTN in adults is essential HTN; there are well over 60 million Americans with essential HTN. Much has been written about research to control essential HTN in adults; relatively less work has been done concerning children. Many pharmacologic approaches, such as β-blockade, angiotensin-converting enzyme (ACE) inhibition, afterload reduction, α-blockade, etc., have been successful in lowering BP. When essential HTN occurs in childhood, a nonpharmacologic approach to lowering BP is preferable so that the patient may not require life-long medication. Long-term use of medications may be associated with significant side-effects and produce associated morbidity and/or mortality.

Several nonpharmacologic approaches have been successful in lowering BP in adults and children. These include weight loss, exercise, stress reduction, and alterations in electrolyte intake, in particular $Na^+$, $K^+$, and $Cl^-$. Chapter 18, by Dr. Wilson, discusses the effects of dietary electrolytes on BP. Chapter 20, by Dr. Rocchini, provides evidence that weight loss may control essential HTN. These findings will not be repeated in this chapter. The specific areas covered herein are exercise and stress reduction. More research is needed in both areas.

## EXERCISE

Several years ago, Alpert and Wilmore *(1)* published a review of data relating to the effects of activity/exercise on BP in healthy children and adolescents, as well as in those with elevated

From: *Clinical Hypertension and Vascular Disease: Pediatric Hypertension*
Edited by: R. J. Portman, J. M. Sorof, and J. R. Ingelfinger © Humana Press Inc., Totowa, NJ

BP. If BP was normal prior to the exercise intervention, there was no measurable change in systolic BP or diastolic BP after the program. At the time of that review, there were seven studies that reported data relating to changes in BP in children and adolescents with essential HTN in response to an exercise/activity intervention. An extensive literature review by one author (MH) failed to find additional, recent studies addressing this issue.

The first documented research concerning exercise was an abstract in 1979 by Laird, Fixler, and Swanborn *(2)*. They studied seven boys, aged 15–16 yrs. The intervention was a 2-mo program of weight lifting, presumably both an aerobic and an isometric activity. They measured systolic BP, diastolic BP, and left ventricular (LV) mass. The change in systolic BP was small, from a mean of 134 mmHg–131 mmHg. The inclusion criteria of essential HTN identified in these subjects, whose systolic BP prior to the intervention was only 134 mmHg, weakens the value of the study somewhat. The diastolic BP change pre- to postexercise was from a mean of 78 mmHg–80 mmHg. A similar, insignificant change in LV mass occurred, from 198–202 g. The important conclusion from this abstract was that resistance training did not lead to an increase in BP, which had been thought of as a possibility. The authors concluded that "hypertensive" youth did not need to be restricted from resistance training.

Shortly thereafter, Frank and co-workers *(3)* reported data from the Bogalusa Heart Study on 48 children (gender unspecified) from 8 to18 yr of age whose BPs were in the top decile of a group of 1604 youth followed in that study. The subjects were receiving antihypertensive medications. The intervention included both dietary and exercise components; the exercise component was not rigorously described. The intervention was successful, lowering both systolic BP and diastolic BP by 9 mmHg each. Because the patients had dietary, exercise, and pharmacologic treatments simultaneously, no conclusions may be drawn as to the effectiveness of exercise alone in this group of Caucasians and African-Americans.

In 1983 and 1984, Hagberg and colleagues *(4,5)* published two articles from studies in 25 children, 19 of whom were boys. The mean age was 15.6 yr, and all attended public schools. There were 6 African-Americans and 19 Caucasians. A control group was included, rendering these findings statistically more robust. The subjects underwent a 3 d/wk, 30–40 min/d aerobic program supervised by school physical education faculty. The subjects were identified as hypertensive by a carefully done set of screenings. The variables measured prior to the 6-mo training period and after 9 mo of detraining included systolic BP, diastolic BP, and $VO_2$ max. The study results are summarized in Table 1. The effects of the program were more pronounced in boys compared to girls; the mixed-gender control group experienced no training-induced changes. There were no racial differences. The positive changes were all reversed with detraining. This small controlled trial supports the hypothesis that aerobic exercise lowers BP in adolescents with essential HTN. The expected drops in BP should be approximately 8 mmHg for systolic BP and 5 mmHg for diastolic BP.

In the following year, the Hagberg team *(6)* expanded their studies by utilizing an aerobic program followed by weight training. There were 6 children in the treatment group and 17 controls. The aerobic program consisted of 5 mo of endurance training (running) at 60–75% of $VO_2$ max. Each session lasted 30–50 min and occurred 3 d/wk. After the aerobic training phase, the youths switched to a weight training program consisting of 12–15 repetitions of 14 exercises. That phase also lasted 5 mo. The subjects then detrained for 12 mo. The systolic BP fell from 143 mmHg to 130 mmHg following the aerobic sessions, and to 126 mmHg at the end of the endurance training. After detraining it rose to 142 mmHg. The changes with exercise were of statistical significance. The parallel changes of diastolic BP were from 80 mmHg to

Table 1
Hagberg et al. *(4,5)* Study Results

| | *Systolic BP (mmHg)* | *Diastolic BP (mmHg)* | *$VO_2$ max (ml/kg/min)* |
|---|---|---|---|
| Pretraining | 137 | 80 | 43 |
| End of training | 129[a] | 75[a] | 48 |
| Detraining | 139 | 78 | 43 |

[a] $p < 0.01$.

77 mmHg, 73 mmHg, and 74 mmHg, none of which were statistically significant. There were decreases in measured systemic vascular resistance in response to both the endurance and weight training. These studies continue to support the concept that both endurance and weight training have beneficial effects on systolic BP and, to a lesser degree, diastolic BP in youth with essential HTN. The group of six children was too small to draw conclusions with respect to either gender or ethnicity.

More recently, Danforth et al. *(7)* used a simple cycle ergometer or jogging/walking program in a group of 12 African-American children (mean age 11.5 yr, low socio-economic status). The sessions were 30 min/d, 3 d/wk, for 12 wk. The target intensity was 60–80% of maximal heart rate (HR). The results are shown in Table 2. The intervention led to a 9 mmHg reduction in systolic BP and a 9 mmHg decrease in diastolic BP, both of which were statistically significant. The diastolic BP returned to baseline after detraining; however, there was a lasting effect of the reduction after detraining for systolic BP. The compliance (attendance) was an outstanding 96%. The decrease in BP was not related to a change in weight. This study shows that inexpensive programs may yield results similar to those involving more expensive equipment or which last more than 3 mo.

The final study on which we comment comes from a very productive research team in Denmark *(8)*. The Odense Schoolchild Study has produced numerous significant results. In this particular publication, results from 137 children were reported, 68 normotensives and 69 hypertensives. The children were 9–11 yr of age. The 8 mo intervention involved three additional 50-min sessions of school physical education per week. The variables reported were systolic BP, diastolic BP, and $VO_2$ max. The systolic BP in the "hypertensive" boys decreased 113 mmHg–107 ($p < 0.05$). No significant change occurred in the diastolic BP values. There was a slight but significant increase in $VO_2$, 52–54 mL/min/kg. No statistically significant changes in systolic BP or diastolic BP occurred in the hypertensive girls. During the 8-mo study, data were collected at 3 mo to assess interval changes; none occurred. The significant results all occurred at the end of the 8 mo. This is the largest series published to date, and concludes that boys appear to benefit more than girls from an intensive exercise intervention.

In summary, endurance (aerobic) exercise led to reductions of systolic BP and diastolic BP, but seldom to completely normal levels. The "hypertensives" generally did not have BP elevations much greater than the normotensive/hypertensive cut-offs. The one study that used only resistance training *(2)* did not show a reduction in BP, but when resistance training was performed following an aerobic program, the reductions in BP were maintained. There has been a concern that children with essential HTN should not participate in resistance training. No study showed a deleterious effect. Accordingly, we do not believe that children with essential HTN who do not show evidence of end-organ damage such as stroke, renal failure, or increased LV mass need to be excluded from resistance training.

Table 2
Danforth et al. *(7)* Study Results

| | *Systolic BP (mmHg)* | *Diastolic BP (mmHg)* |
|---|---|---|
| Initial | 130 | 84 |
| Posttraining | 121[a] | 75[a] |
| Detraining | 123[a] | 85 |

[a] $p < 0.01$ vs initial.

From available data, it is not possible to state what is the minimal frequency, intensity, or duration of exercise that will lead to reductions of systolic BP or diastolic BP. From a public health standpoint, exercise should be life-long in duration. Recent recommendations *(1)* have been for three or more sessions per week, 30 or more minutes per day, and at least at 60% $VO_2$ max.

Future studies should enroll children with more severe elevations of BP. Children of all ethnicities should be included. The reason for the apparently better results in male, compared to female, children needs to be investigated. For optimal efficiency these studies should be multicenter. An organization such as the North American Society for Pediatric Exercise Medicine could be a valuable resource for such a study. We hope that the readers of this chapter will appreciate the paucity of rigorous data and will seek to provide future studies to define the much-needed data.

## STRESS REDUCTION

The relevance of stress reduction for the treatment of essential HTN dates back to early theories regarding the pathogenesis of the disorder. Clinical and empirical data implicate stress as an important factor for the development and maintenance of HTN in certain persons, and provide a rationale for the use of stress management techniques in at-risk persons. With respect to children and adolescents, such nonpharmacologic approaches are especially important, since elevated BP in childhood often relates to essential HTN in early adulthood, and clinical trials have not conclusively determined the long-term risk-benefit ratio of antihypertensive drug therapy for youth *(9)*. Consequently, current guidelines for treating childhood HTN are conservative; when essential HTN is the likely diagnosis in the context of mild BP elevations, interventions that emphasize lifestyle or health-promoting behavioral changes are recommended.

In general, nonpharmacologic therapies for essential HTN encompass strategies aimed at weight reduction, dietary modification, and physical activity. Considerably less attention has been devoted to stress reduction, *per se*; this disparity is even more apparent for pediatric HTN patients. This is surprising given the effectiveness of stress reduction techniques such as biofeedback and relaxation training for a variety of medical conditions affecting children, including fecal *(10)* and urinary *(11)* incontinence, headache *(12,13)*, and asthma *(14)*. One possible explanation for the lack of carry-over may be the relatively recent incorporation of BP measurement in the routine pediatric examination *(9)*. Reluctance on the part of some physicians to inquire about recreational behaviors (e.g., drinking, smoking) that may have negative overall effects on young patients *(15)* also may contribute to a lack of perceived need for more formal treatment recommendations that emphasize stress-reduction in children and adolescents with essential HTN.

Research has demonstrated that stress elicits significant increases in BP and other hemodynamic parameters in children. Furthermore, a number of studies have shown that these BP responses to stress predict future elevations in resting BP in children and adolescents over periods of several months to years *(16–22)*. Consequently, the utilization of techniques to reduce reactivity to stress during childhood may prevent the development of essential HTN across the lifespan.

Two studies provide some support for the use stress reduction in children at risk for developing essential HTN *(23,24)*. Utilizing nonsomatic therapies, these studies reported substantial changes in BP, or behaviors associated with elevated BP, in disparate samples of children. Although the lasting effects of these interventions are not known, these studies underscore the importance of stress and stress reduction in childhood HTN.

The first investigation examined the effects of Medical Resonance Therapy Music (MRT-Music) in a sample of children with transient HTN following the nuclear accident in Chernobyl *(23)*. Sixty children with varying degrees of BP elevation were exposed to twice-daily MRT-Music treatments for three weeks while in the hospital. Treatment sessions lasted 20–30 min and occurred under conditions designed to maximize relaxation. Pre- and posttreatment comparisons of basic hemodynamic parameters revealed a strong treatment effect for both systolic BP and diastolic BP, with a normalization of overall BP to age-appropriate levels. This effect was particularly pronounced for those children with higher, compared to lower, levels of HTN at the onset of treatment.

The second study examined the relationship between religion and various parameters of cardiovascular (CV) health in a sample of 137 immigrants between 18 and 71 yr of age *(24)*. Regression analyses indicated strong associations among demographic, social support, and physical health measures for this group of individuals deemed to be at risk for BP elevations secondary to immigration-related stress. After ruling out a number of competing explanations for the observed relationships, the author concluded that religious commitment had a beneficial effect on CV health, as indicated by significantly lower rates of HTN, as well as significantly lower systolic BP and diastolic BP levels among those high on both quantitative and qualitative indices of religious commitment. This association was particularly robust for younger persons in the sample. The author discussed this relationship in terms of social support, and noted that religious participation appeared to remove a source of stress among immigrants by facilitating feelings of social cohesion and a sense of belonging. Although over one-third of the sample was classified as hypertensive, it is unclear how many participants were adolescents, as opposed to adults. Nevertheless, the study provided support for the positive effects of church attendance and religious commitment on CV health in general and BP elevations in particular, among both youthful and older immigrants.

Four studies of nonpharmacologic, stress reduction treatments for normotensive children have implications for the management of childhood HTN. One study evaluated the effects of gender and family support on dietary compliance and BP in a sample of 184 African-American adolescents who participated in a 5-d low Na+ diet as part of a HTN prevention program *(16)*. Compliance was defined as urine Na+ excretion ≤50 mEq/24 h at the completion of the dietary intervention. A trend toward lower systolic BP was observed among compliant participants, but the effect diminished after controlling for body mass index. Moreover, dietary compliance was moderated by social support and gender. These findings suggest that social support may play a role in improving dietary compliance, and, subsequently, BP control, among adolescents at risk for developing essential HTN.

Another study evaluated the impact of Transcendental Meditation (TM) at rest and during acute psychological stress in high school students *(26)*. Adolescents with high normal BP were randomly assigned to either a TM or health education control group. Pre- and postintervention comparisons revealed significant group differences, with TM participants exhibiting greater decreases in resting systolic BP and greater declines in systolic BP during a car driving simulation task compared to control group peers.

In contrast, generally unfavorable results have been reported for the use of progressive muscle relaxation (PMR) in the treatment of adolescents with high BP *(27,28)*. Compared to wait-list controls, significant declines in systolic BP were observed in teenagers upon completion of a 3-mo school-based PMR program. At follow-up 4 mo later, however, group differences in BP were no longer significant *(27)*. Similarly, 4 mo of relaxation training, combined with increased physical activity, failed to yield BP differences in comparisons of community boys with nontreated peers *(28)*.

## SUMMARY

Given the link between elevated BP during childhood and the development of adult HTN, the need for interventions aimed at reducing disease development in at-risk youth is apparent. Stress has been identified as an important contributor to the progression and maintenance of HTN in certain individuals. Nonpharmacologic techniques that minimize stress to achieve and maintain normal BP are particularly relevant for children because clinical trials have not conclusively determined the long-term risk–benefit ratio of antihypertensive drug therapy for young patients. When essential HTN is the likely diagnosis in the context of mild BP elevations in children and adolescents, interventions that emphasize lifestyle or health-promoting behavioral changes are recommended *(9)*. Stress reduction is an example of such an approach. In addition to using stress reduction techniques to treat children with essential HTN, these methods may be useful for children with high-normal BP, and may provide adjunctive benefit to more intensive therapies for young patients with severe disease.

## REFERENCES

1. Alpert BS, Wilmore JH. Physical activity and blood pressure in adolescents. Ped Exerc Sci 1994;6:361–380.
2. Laird WP, Fixler DE, Swanborn CD. Cardiovascular effects of weight training in hypertensive adolescents. Med Sci Sports Exerc 1979;11:78 (abstract).
3. Frank GC, Farris RP, Ditmarsen P, Voors AW, Berenson GS. An approach to primary preventive treatment for children with high blood pressure in a total community. J Am College Nutr 1982;1:357–374.
4. Hagberg JM, Goldring D, Ehsani AA, et al. Effect of exercise training on the blood pressure and hemodynamic features of hypertensive adolescents. Am J Cardiol 1983;52:763–768.
5. Hagberg JM, Goldring D, Heath GW, et al. Effect of exercise training on plasma catecholamines and haemodynamics of adolescent hypertensives during rest, submaximal exercise and orthostatic stress. Clin Physiol 1984;4:117–124.
6. Hagberg JM, Ehsani AA, Goldring D, Hernandez A, Sinacore DR, Holloszy JO. Effect of weight training on blood pressure and hemodynamics in hypertensive adolescents. J Pediatrics 1984;104:147–151.
7. Danforth JS, Allen KD, Fitterling JM, et al. Exercise as a treatment of hypertension in low-socioeconomic-status Black children. J Consulting Clin Psych 1990;58:237–239.
8. Hansen HS, Froberg K, Hyldebrandt N, Nielsen JR. A controlled study of eight months of physical training and reduction of blood pressure in children: the Odense schoolchild study. Brit Med J 1991;303:682–685.
9. Update on the Task Force (1987) on High Blood Pressure in Children and Adolescents: a working group report from the National High Blood Pressure Education Program. Pediatrics 1996;98:649–658.

10. Borowitz SM, Cox DJ, Sutphen JL, Kovatchev B. Treatment of childhood encopresis: a randomized trial comparing three treatment protocols. J Pediatr Gastroenterol Nutr 2002;34:378–384.
11. Rhodes C. Effective management of daytime wetting. Paediatr Nurs 2000;12:14–17.
12. Arndorfer RE, Allen KD. Extending the efficacy of a thermal biofeedback treatment package to the management of tension-type headaches in children. Headache 2001;41:183–192.
13. Grazzi L, Andrasik F, D'Amico D, Leone M, Moschiano F, Bussone G. Electrohyographic biofeedback-assisted relaxation training in juvenile episodic tension-type headache: clinical outcome at three-year follow-up. Cephalalgia 2001;21:798–803.
14. Malhi P. Psychosocial issues in the management and treatment of children and adolescents with asthma. Indian J Pediatr 2001;68 (Suppl 4):S48–S52.
15. Ellen JM, Franzgrote M, Irwin CE, Millstein SG. Primary care physicians' screening of adolescent patients: a survey of California physicians. J Ado Health 1998;22:433–38.
16. Murphy JK, Alpert BS, Walker SS, Wilkey ES. Children's cardiovascular reactivity: stability of racial differences and relation to subsequent blood pressure over a one-year period. Psychophysiology 1991;28:447–457.
17. Murphy JK, Alpert BS, Walker SS. Ethnicity, pressor reactivity, and children's blood pressure: five years of observations. Hypertension 1992;20: 327–332.
18. Malpass D, Treiber FA, Turner JR, et al. Relationships between children's cardiovascular stress responses and resting cardiovascular functioning 1 year later. Int J Psychophysiol 1997;25:139–144.
19. Treiber FA, Turner JR, Davis H, Thompson W, Levy M, Strong WB. Young children's cardiovascular stress responses predict resting cardiovascular functioning 2 1/2 years later. J Cardiovasc Risk 1996;3:95–100.
20. Kelsey RM, Barnard M, Alpert BS. Race, SES, and cardiovascular reactivity to cold stress as longitudinal predictors of blood pressure in adolescents. Am J Hypertens 2001;14:250A.
21. Borghi C, Costa FV, Boschi S, Mussi A, Ambrosioni E. Predictors of stable hypertension in young borderline subjects: a five-year follow-up study. J Cardiovasc Pharmacol 1986;S138–S141.
22. Falkner B, Kushner H, Onesti G, Angelakos ET. Cardiovascular characteristics in adolescents who develop essential hypertention. Hypertension 1981;3:521–527.
23. Sidorenko VN. Effects of the medical resonance therapy music on haemodynamic parameter in children with autonomic nervous system disturbances. Integrative Physiological and Behavioral Science 2000;35: 208–211.
24. Walsh A. Religion and hypertension: testing alternative explanations among immigrants. Beh Med 1998;24: 122–130.
25. Wilson D, Ampey-Thornbill G. The role of gender and family support on dietary compliance in an African American adolescent hypertension prevention study. Ann Behav Med 2001;23:59–67.
26. Barnes VA, Treiber FA, Davis, H. Impact of Transcendental Meditation on cardiovascular function at rest and during acute stress in adolescents with high normal blood pressure. J Psychosom Res 2001;51:597–605.
27. Ewart CK, Harris WL, Iwata MM, Coates TJ, Bullock R, Simon B. Feasibility and effectiveness of school-based relaxation in lowering blood pressure. Health Psychol 1987;65:399–416.
28. Rauhala E, Alho H, Hanninen O, Helin P. Relaxation training combined with increased physical activity lowers the psychophysiological activation in community-home boys. Int J Psychophysiol 1990;101:63–68.

# 25 Approach to the Pharmacologic Treatment of Pediatric Hypertension

*Douglas L. Blowey,* MD

*CONTENTS*



## INTRODUCTION

Hypertension (HTN) is present in 50 million adult Americans and is clearly associated with an increased risk of cardiovascular disease (CVD), stroke, and kidney failure *(1)*. Untreated or inadequately treated HTN is an enormous financial burden for society, with an estimated annual cost in the United States of $329 billion *(2)*. The risk for cardiovascular morbidity and mortality is related to the severity of HTN and other independent risk factors, such as the presence or absence of target organ damage, dyslipidemia, smoking, diabetes mellitus, male sex, and a family history of CVD. Lowering of BP by lifestyle modifications or antihypertensive drug therapy reduces the risk for cardiovascular-, stroke-, and kidney-related complications. Certain antihypertensive drugs improve the cardiovascular or kidney outcome independent of their BP-lowering effect, such as the improved renal and cardiac survival observed in patients receiving angiotensin-converting enzyme (ACE) inhibitors *(3,4)*. Antihypertensive drug therapy in adults is guided by large, randomized trials that have demonstrated a treatment-related decline in cardiovascular morbidity and mortality, dose-BP lowering-response relationships, and a comprehensive characterization of the drug's adverse effect profile.

In contrast, the risk of future CVD, stroke, and kidney failure in the 1–4% of children with HTN *(5,6)* is unclear, although there is accumulating evidence that the antecedents of CVD are

From: *Clinical Hypertension and Vascular Disease: Pediatric Hypertension*
Edited by: R. J. Portman, J. M. Sorof, and J. R. Ingelfinger © Humana Press Inc., Totowa, NJ

in childhood. Longitudinal epidemiological studies have shown that elevated BP in childhood and the acquisition of obesity are important predictors of adult high BP *(7)*. Left ventricular hypertrophy (LVH), an independent risk factor for adult CVD, is common in children with HTN, and highly correlates with obesity *(8,9)*, an emerging epidemic in pediatrics.

Coronary artery fatty streaks, in autopsy specimens taken from deceased young people that participated as youths in the Bogalusa Heart Study, were more common in those with high BP readings as a youth *(10)*. Taken together, these studies suggest that the pathological processes responsible for CVD begins in childhood, and that treatment of high BP during childhood may delay or modify future morbidity and mortality.

Prior to initiating antihypertensive treatment in a child with high BP, the high BP readings are confirmed with repeated measurements or ambulatory BP monitoring (ABPM), an investigation is completed for secondary causes of HTN and target organ damage, and the history is reviewed for coexisting conditions and current medications, both prescribed and over the counter. Although BP measurements tend to track over time in children, not all children with mild BP elevations remain hypertensive with repeated measurements and time. The strongest correlation for adult HTN is in the adolescent with persistently high BP measurements *(7)*. The potential for normalization of BP with time was noted in a recent study where 17% of hypertensive children enrolled in an antihypertensive drug trial had normalization of their BP during the 2-wk placebo screening period, and 34% of children randomized to placebo had normalization of BP during the 12-wk study *(11)*. Secondary HTN, when identified, is potentially correctable, and can avoid the need for long-term drug therapy or helps guide the initial antihypertensive drug regimen. Concurrent disease states and concomitant medications may modify the cardiovascular risk associated with HTN, or modify the antihypertensive drug's pharmacokinetic/pharmacodynamic profile, and are important to consider when designing an antihypertensive regimen.

Any child who consistently has BP measurements exceeding the 95th percentile for age, sex, and height when measured with the appropriate techniques *(12)* warrants some form of intervention directed at lowering BP and modifying other cardiovascular risk factors, whether it be lifestyle modifications or pharmacologic therapy. Intervention at lower BPs (e.g., 90–95th percentile) should be strongly considered in children with evidence of target organ damage or children at risk for progressive kidney disease, such as those with diabetes mellitus, proteinuric kidney disease, chronic kidney disease, and polycystic kidney disease.

All children with HTN should be encouraged to adopt lifestyle changes and become educated about other risk factors for CVD. Lifestyle modifications include weight loss for overweight children, enhanced physical activity, and reduction of sodium intake. The adolescent should be counseled on the adverse effects of smoking, alcohol, and illicit drugs (*see* Chapter 24).

The decision to begin antihypertensive drug therapy is based on the degree of BP elevation, the presence of cardiovascular risk factors, and the presence of target organ damage or a potentially progressive kidney disease. Figure 1 follows the risk stratification schema adopted by Joint National Committee VI *(1)*, and attempts to incorporate the current treatment trend among experts in the field of pediatric HTN. The BP cut-off values for the initiation of antihypertensive drug therapy are clearly arbitrary, as there are no studies in children that correlate the degree of BP elevation with long-term outcome. A 10 mmHg rise above the 95th percentile for age, sex, and height is approx 3 standard deviations (SD) above the mean. The treatment of pediatric hypertensive emergencies is covered in Chapter 27 and neonatal HTN in Chapter 20.

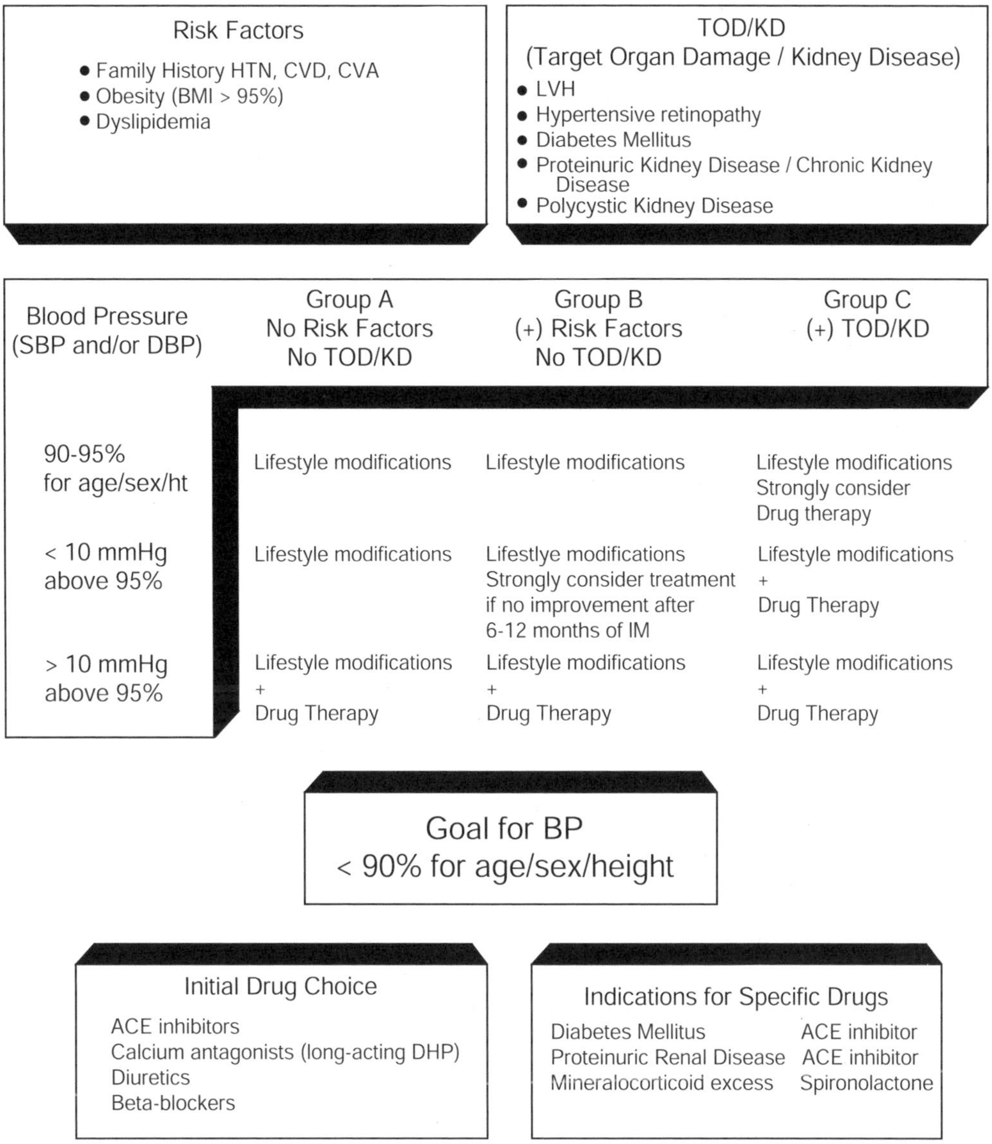


Fig. 1. Treatment recommendations for pediatric hypertension. TOD, target organ disease; LVH, left ventricular hypertrophy.

Owing to the heterogeneous nature of childhood HTN with a high rate of secondary causes, especially in the young child, most pediatricians have abandoned the indiscriminant stepped-care approach recommended for adults for an individualized approach to antihypertensive drug therapy *(13)*. With an individualized approach, the initial antihypertensive drug is chosen based on the presumed mechanism and severity of HTN, concomitant diseases and therapies, availability of appropriate formulations (e.g., suspension and dosage choices), and, when available, pediatric safety and efficacy data. Encouragingly, after implementation of the 1997 US Food and Drug Administration (FDA) Modernization Act, several pharmacokinetic and efficacy studies of antihypertensive agents in children have been completed or are in progress (*see* Chapter 26). In general, individualized therapy begins with a low dose of the initial drug (Table 1) and is slowly titrated upward, based on the BP response or side effects. Unless

Table 1
Antihyptertensive Agents in Children

| *Drug* | *Pediatric dosing* | *Adult dosing* | *Formulation* |
|---|---|---|---|
| *ACE inhibitors* | | | |
| Benazepril[a,b] | Initial: 0.2 mg/kg/d<br>Max: 10 mg QD | Initial: 10 mg/d<br>Max: 80 mg/d | T: 5 mg/10/20/40 |
| Captopril[a] | Initial: 0.2–0.5 mg/kg ÷ BID/TID<br>Max: 5 mg/kg/d | Initial: 25 mg BID/TID<br>Max: 450 mg/d | T:12.5 mg/25/50/100<br>Extemp: 1 mg/mL |
| Enalapril[a] | Initial: 0.08 mg/kg QD<br>Max: 0.6 mg/kg/d | Initial: 2.5–5 mg QD<br>Max: 40 mg/d | T: 2.5 mg/5/10/20<br>Extemp: 1 mg/ml |
| Fosinopril[b] | Initial: 0.1 mg/kg/d<br>Max: 10 mg QD | Initial: 10 mg QD<br>Max: 80 mg/d | T: 10 mg/20/40 |
| Lisinopril[a] | Initial: 0.08 mg/kg QD<br>Max: 0.6 mg/kg/d | Initial: 10 mg QD<br>Max: 80 mg/d | T: 2.5 mg/5/10/20/30/40 |
| Moexipril[a] | No data | Initial: 7.5 mg QD<br>Max: 60 mg/d | T: 7.5 mg/15 |
| Perindopril[a] | No data | Initial: 4 mg QD<br>Max: 16 mg/d | T: 2 mg/4/8 |
| Quinapril[a] | 5–10 mg QD | Initial: 10 mg QD<br>Max: 80 mg/d | T: 5 mg/10/20/40 |
| Ramipril[a] | No data | Initial: 2.5 mg QD<br>Max: 20 mg/d | C: 1.25 mg/2.5/5/10<br>Extemp: capsule with H2O |
| Trandolapril[a] | No data | Initial: 1 mg QD<br>Max: 8 mg/d | T: 1 mg/2/4 |
| *ANG II receptor antagonists* | | | |
| Candesartan | No data | Initial: 16 mg QD<br>Max: 32 mg/d | T: 4 mg/8/16/32 |
| Eprosartan | No data | Initial: 600 mg QD<br>Max: 800 mg/d | T: 400 mg/600 |
| Irbesartan | Initial: > 6 yr 75 mg QD<br>Max: 150 mg/d | Initial: 150 mg QD<br>Max: 300 mg/d | T: 75 mg/150/300 |
| Losartan[b] | Initial: 0.75 mg/kg/d<br>Max: 50 mg QD | Initial: 50 mg QD<br>Max: 100 mg/d | T: 25 mg/50/100 |
| Telmisartan | No data | Initial: 40 mg QD<br>Max: 80 mg/d | T: 20 mg/40/80 |
| Valsartan | No data | Initial: 80 mg QD<br>Max: 320 mg/d | C: 80 mg/160 |
| *CCBs* | | | |
| Amlodipine | Initial: 0.1–0.2 mg/kg QD<br>Max: 0.6 mg/kg | Initial: 5 mg QD<br>Max: 10 mg/d | T: 2.5 mg/5/10<br>Extemp: 1 mg/mL |
| Felodipine ER | No data[b] | Initial: 5 mg QD<br>Max: 10 mg/d | T: 2.5 mg/5/10 |
| Isradipine | Initial: 0.1 mg/kg Q 6-8 hr<br>Max: 1.2 mg/kg/d | Initial: 2.5 mg BID<br>CR: 5 mg QD<br>Max: 20 mg/d | C: 2.5 mg/5<br>CR: 5 mg/10<br>Extemp: 1 mg/mL |
| Nifedipine | 0.25 mg/kg/dose Q 4–6 hr | | C: 10 mg/20 |
| Nifedipine SR/XL | Initial: 0.25 mg/kg ÷ QD/BID<br>Max: not established | Initial: 30 mg QD<br>Max: 180 mg/d | T: 30 mg/60/90 |
| Nisoldipine | No data | Initial: 20 mg QD<br>Max: 60 mg/d | T: 10 mg/20/30/40 |

(continued)

Table 1 (continued)

| *Drug* | *Pediatric dosing* | *Adult dosing* | *Formulation* |
|---|---|---|---|
| *Diuretics* | | | |
| Chlorothiazide | Initial: 10–20 mg/kg ÷ QD/BID<br>Max: <2 yr 375 mg/d<br>>2 yr 1 gm/d | Initial: 500 mg QD/BID<br>Max: 2 g/d | T: 250 mg/500<br>Susp: 250 mg/5mL |
| Chlorthalidone[a] | Initial: 1–2 mg/kg QD/QOD<br>Max: not established | Initial: 15 mg QD<br>Max: 50 mg QD | T: 25 mg/50 |
| Hydrochloro-thiazide | Initial: 1–2 mg/kg ÷ QD/BID<br>Max: <2 yr 37.5 mg/d<br>> 2 yr 100 mg/d | Initial: 25 mg QD/BID<br>Max: 100 mg/d | C: 12.5 mg<br>T: 25 mg/50<br>Soln: 50 mg/5 mL |
| Spironolactone[a] | Initial: 1 mg/kg ÷ QD/BID<br>Max: 3 mg/kg/d (may need higher doses with mineralocorticoid excess) | Initial: 25 mg QD/BID<br>Max: 200 mg/d | T: 25 mg/50/100<br>Extemp: 5 mg/mL; 1 mg/mL |
| *Vasodilators* | | | |
| Hydralazine[a] | Initial: 1 mg/kg ÷ BID/QID<br>Max: 7 mg/kg/d | Initial: 10 mg QID<br>Max: 300 mg/d | T: 10 mg/25/50/100<br>Extemp: 20 mg/5 mL |
| Minoxidil[a] | Initial: 0.1–0.2 mg/kg ÷ QD/BID<br>Max: not established | Initial: 5 mg QD<br>Max: 100 mg/d | T: 2.5 mg/10<br>Extemp: 2 mg/mL |
| *β-Adrenergic antagonists* | | | |
| Acebutolol[a] | No data | Initial: 400 mg QD<br>Max: 1200 mg/d | C: 200 mg/400 |
| Atenolol[a] | Initial: 0.8–1 mg/kg QD<br>Max: 2 mg/kg/d | Initial: 50 mg QD<br>Max: 100 mg/d | T: 25 mg/50/100<br>Extemp: 2 mg/mL |
| Bisoprolol[a] | No data[c] | Initial: 5 mg QD<br>Max: 20 mg/d | T: 5 mg/10 |
| Metoprolol XL | No data | Initial: 50–100 mg QD<br>Max: 400 mg/d | T(XL): 25 mg/50/100/200<br>Extemp: 10 mg/mL |
| Nadolol[a] | No data | Initial: 40 mg QD<br>Max: 320 mg/d | T: 20 mg/40/80/120/160 |
| Propranolol | Initial: 0.5–1 mg/kg ÷ BID/TID<br>Max: 8 mg/kg/d | Initial: 40 mg BID<br>LA: 80 mg QD<br>Max: 640 mg/d | T: 10 mg/20/40/60/80<br>LA: 60 mg/80/120/160<br>Extemp: 1 mg/mL |
| Timolol | No data | Initial: 10 mg BID<br>Max: 60 mg/d | T: 5 mg/10/20 |
| Labetalol (α- and β-) | Initial: 4 mg/kg ÷ BID<br>Max: not established | Initial: 100 mg BID<br>Max: 2.4 g/d | T: 100 mg/200/300<br>Extemp: 10 mg/mL |
| Carvedilol (α- and β-) | No data | Initial: 6.25 mg BID<br>Max: 50 mg/d | T: 3.125 mg/6.25/12.5/25 |
| *Central α-adrenergic agonists* | | | |
| Clonidine | Initial: 5–10 μg/kg ÷ BID/TID<br>Max: 0.9 mg/d | Initial: 0.1 mg BID<br>Max: 2.4 mg/d | T: 0.1 mg/0.2/0.3<br>Transdermal: 0.1 mg/0.2/0.3 |
| Guanfacine[a] | No data | Initial: 1 mg QD<br>Max: 2 mg/d | T: 1 mg/2 |
| *α-Adrenergic antagonists* | | | |
| Doxazosin | No data | Initial: 1 mg QD<br>Max: 16 mg/d | T: 1 mg/2/4/8 |
| Prazosin | Initial: 5–25 μg/kg BID/TID<br>Max: 400 μg/kg/d | Initial: 1 mg BID<br>Max: 40 mg/d | C: 1 mg/2/5 |
| Terazosin | No data | Initial: 1 mg QD<br>Max: 20 mg/d | C: 1 mg/2/5/10 |

[a]Dosage adjustment required for renal failure. T, tablet; C, capsule; ER, extended release.
[b]Being studied.
[c]Data available for Ziac (bisoprolol/HCTC)

Table 2
Clinical Problems with Antihypertensive Drugs

| |
|---|
| *ACE inhibitors / ANG II receptor antagonist* |
| Use with caution in patients with bilateral renal artery stenosis or renal artery stenosis in a solitary kidney |
| Use during 2nd–3rd trimester of pregnancy associated with fetal and neonatal toxicity |
| Cough, hypotension, angioedema, renal failure, hyperkalemia, neutropenia |
| *CCBs* |
| Profound and unexpected drops in BP seen with short-acting nifedipine |
| Flushing, headache, fatigue, palpitations, edema |
| *Vasodilators* |
| Fluid retention, edema, palpitations |
| Minoxidil—Hypertrichosis |
| Hydralazine—Lupus-like syndrome (greater in slow acetylators) |
| *β-Adrenergic antagonists* |
| Use with caution in patients with bronchial asthma, heart failure, diabetes mellitus |
| Fatigue, cold extremities, sedation, bradycardia, abnormalities of lipid and glucose metabolism |
| *Peripheral α-adrenergic antagonist* |
| Orthostatic hypotension with first dose "First Dose Effect" |
| *Centrally acting α-adrenergic agonist* |
| Rebound HTN with abrupt withdrawal |
| Sedation, dry mouth, headache |
| *Diuretics* |
| Potassium loss, volume depletion |
| Hearing loss (loop diuretics), hyperkalemia (potassium-sparing diuretics) |

clinically warranted, dose titration should proceed slowly, especially with antihypertensive drugs that have a long biological half-life (e.g., amlodipine), so that the BP response at each dose level can be fully evaluated. An alternative antihypertensive agent can be substituted if no response or significant side effects are observed (Table 2). A second drug is added to the current regimen if the response to the first drug is inadequate, but well tolerated, and correctable causes of an inadequate response are addressed (Table 4). If BP is controlled with a second drug, a fixed combination preparation can be substituted if the appropriate dosing formulation is available (Table 3). Once BP is controlled for 6–12 mo, and target organ damage has regressed or resolved, an effort to decrease the dosage or the number of antihypertensive medications should be considered. Lifestyle modifications are maintained during step-down therapy and drug reductions should be made methodically and slowly in order to fully assess the BP response with each change.

There are clinical situations where a specific class of drug has proven more effective or beneficial for reasons independent of BP lowering *(14,15)* (Fig. 1). In the child with diabetes mellitus and microabluminuria or proteinuria, an angiotensin-converting enzyme (ACE) inhibitor is recommended. ACE inhibitors have been shown to slow the loss of renal function in adults with diabetic proteinuric renal disease *(3)*. Although outcome studies have not been performed with angiotensin II (ANG II) receptor antagonists, these agents may also be beneficial for patients in whom ACE inhibitors are indicated but who are unable to tolerate ACE inhibitors. ACE inhibitors are also recommended for children with proteinuric kidney disease

Table 3
Fixed-Drug Combinations

| | |
|---|---|
| *ACE inhibitors (+) diuretics* | |
| Benazepril (+) Hydrochlorothiazide | 5 mg/6.25 mg; 10/12.5; 20/12.5; 20/25 |
| Captopril (+) Hydrochlorothiazide | 25 mg/15 mg; 50/15; 25/25; 50/25 |
| Enalapril (+) Hydrochlorothiazide | 5 mg/12.5 mg; 10/25 |
| Fosinopril (+) Hydrochlorothiazide | 10 mg/12.5 mg; 20/12.5 |
| Lisinopril (+) Hydrochlorothiazide | 10 mg/12.5 mg; 20/12.5; 20/25 |
| Moexipril (+) Hydrochlorothiazide | 7.5 mg/12.5 mg; 15/25 |
| Quinapril (+) Hydrochlorothiazide | 10 mg/12.5 mg; 20/12.5; 20/25 |
| *ANG II receptor antagonists (+) diuretics* | |
| Candesartan (+) Hydrochlorothiazide | 16 mg/12.5 mg; 32/12.5 |
| Irbesartan (+) Hydrochlorothiazide | 150 mg/12.5 mg; 300/12.5 |
| Losartan (+) Hydrochlorothiazide | 50 mg/12.5 mg; 100/25 |
| Telmisartan (+) Hydrochlorothiazide | 40 mg/12.5 mg; 80/12.5 |
| Valsartan (+) Hydrochlorothiazide | 80 mg/12.5 mg; 160/12.5 |
| *ACE inhibitors (+) CCBs* | |
| Benazepril (+) Amlodipine | 10 mg/2.5 mg; 10/5; 20/5 |
| Enalapril (+) Felodipine ER | 5 mg/2.5 mg; 5/5 |
| *β-adrenergic antagonist (+) diuretics* | |
| Atenolol (+) Chlorthalidone | 50 mg/25 mg; 100/25 |
| Bisoprolol (+) Hydrochlorothiazide | 2.5 mg/6.25 mg; 5/6.25; 10/6.25 |
| Nadolol (+) Bendroflumethiazide | 40 mg/5 mg; 80/5 |
| Propranolol (+) Hydrochlorothiazide | 40 mg/25 mg; 80/25 |
| Propranolol LA (+) Hydrochlorothiazide | 80 mg/50 mg; 120/50; 160/50 |
| Timolol (+) Hydrochlorothiazide | 10 mg/25 mg |
| *Vasodilators (+) diuretics* | |
| Hydralazine (+) Hydrochlorothiazide | 25 mg/25 mg; 50/50; 100/50 |
| *Sympatholytics (+) diuretics* | |
| Clonidine (+) Chlorthalidone | 0.1 mg/15 mg; 0.2/15; 0.3/15 |
| Prazosin (+) Polythiazide | 1 mg/0.5 mg; 2/0.5; 5/0.5 |

or chronic kidney disease. The loss of kidney function in adults with proteinuric kidney disease is slowed in those receiving ACE inhibitors *(16,17)*.

In the absence of an absolute indication for a specific antihypertensive drug, the trend in the treatment of HTN in children has been the use of ACE inhibitors, long-acting dihydropyridine calcium channel blockers (CCBs), and, most recently, ANG II receptor antagonists. These agents have gained favor owing to the low side-effect profile, long duration of action requiring once- or twice-daily dosing, and the availability of formulations that allow for pediatric dosing. For many of the newer antihypertensive drugs, pharmacokinetic and efficacy studies providing for the rational use of these agents in children have been completed or are in progress (*see* Chapter 26). Although many of the traditional agents are still available for use in children with HTN, it is unlikely that efficacy and pharmacokinetic studies will be performed. Therefore, the pediatric dosing information will continue to be based on the reported experience in a few patients. Other antihypertensive agents that may be reasonably used as first line agents include thiazide-type diuretics, β-adrenergic antagonists, and peripheral α-adrenergic antagonists. The α-adrenergic antagonists, such a doxazosin, prazosin, and terazosin may be useful in the

Table 4
Causes of Inadequate Response to Antihypertensive Therapy

| |
|---|
| Inappropriate measurement technique |
| Damaged/Improperly calibrated equipment |
| Noncompliance with prescribed therapy |
| Medication noncompliance |
| Dietary noncompliance (e.g., low salt, fluid restriction) |
| Lifestyle modification noncompliance (failure to lose weight, exercise, etc.) |
| Progression of underlying disease |
| Worsening renal failure |
| Arteritis/vasculitis |
| Inappropriate drug for underlying mechanism of HTN |
| Dose of antihypertensive medications too low |
| Drug interactions |
| Sympathomimetics, illicit drugs |
| Caffeine |
| Oral contraceptives, corticosteroids, cyclosporine, tacrolimus |
| NSAIDs |
| Drug metabolism |
| Rapid inactivation (e.g., rapid acetlylator with hydralazine) |
| Slow bioactivation of prodrug (e.g., losartan, irbesartan) |

obese adolescent with "insulin resistant syndrome" owing to the minimal effect of the drug on lipid and carbohydrate metabolism and the reported enhanced sympathetic activity in such patients *(18,19)*. Vasodilators (e.g., hydralazine, minoxidil) and central α-adrenergic agonists (e.g., clonidine, guanfacine) are to be considered second line agents. See Table 1 for dosing recommendations.

## ANGIOTENSIN-CONVERTING ENZYME INHIBITORS

ACE catalyzes the conversion of ANG I to ANG II, which in turn influences BP by direct vasoconstriction of the arterial vasculature, increased sympathetic nervous system activity, direct cardiovascular inotropic effect, and aldosterone-enhanced salt and water retention. ACE inhibitors, such as benazepril, captopril, enalapril, fosinopril, lisinopril, moexipril, perindopril, quinapril, ramipril, and trandolapril reversibly inhibit the enzyme and block the formation of ANG II and the degradation of the vasodilatory peptide bradykinin.

Because renal and renovascular disease are frequent causes of childhood HTN, ACE inhibitors are commonly prescribed. ACE inhibitors are well tolerated by children, and they lower BP in hypertensive children in a dose-dependent manner *(20–28)*. Neonates appear to be extremely sensitive to the BP-lowering effects of ACE inhibitors. The dosage should be significantly lower than the dosage recommended for older children *(29,30)* (*see* Chapter 20).

Captopril has a beneficial BP-lowering effect in children with renal parenchymal and renovascular disease *(20,22–25)*. However, the increased incidence of cough and need for more frequent dosing has led to greater use of the newer, longer-acting ACE inhibitors (e.g., enalapril, lisinopril). Once-daily dosing with enalapril or lisinopril lowers trough BP in a dose-dependent manner in children with HTN *(26,27)*. In these prospective studies, the lowest dosage group

(0.02 mg/kg) did not have a consistent BP-lowering response, and the initial recommended dosage for both agents is 0.08 mg/kg given once daily. If a child is receiving a moderate dose of an ACE inhibitor and the BP-lowering effect diminishes towards the end of the dosing interval (e.g., trough BP), twice-daily dosing should be considered prior to adding a second antihypertensive drug. The pharmacokinetic parameters of enalapril in hypertensive children aged 2–16 yr were similar to those reported for adults *(31)*.

The most common adverse effects reported in children receiving ACE inhibitors include cough, hypotension, and deterioration of renal function *(32,33)*. The decline in renal function and hypotension is noted most in neonates or in children with preexisting renal disease or volume depletion, and is uncommon in the well hydrated child with normal renal function. Less common adverse effects include angioedema, hyperkalemia, rash, anemia, and leucopenia *(34)*.

The use of ACE inhibitors during the second and third trimester of pregnancy has been associated with fetal and neonatal toxicity. ACE inhibitor fetopathy is characterized by fetal hypotension, anuria-oliogohydramnios, growth restriction, pulmonary hypoplasia, renal tubular dysplasia, and hypocalvaria *(35)*. Adolescents of childbearing potential are to be informed of these potential risks and counseled on proper birth control measures. ACE inhibitors are contraindicated in children with a history of angioedema and should be used with great caution in children with bilateral renal artery stenosis, or renal artery stenosis in a solitary kidney.

## CALCIUM CHANNEL BLOCKERS

The contraction of cardiac and vascular smooth muscle is dependent on the inward flux of calcium. Dihydropyridine CCBs, such as amlodipine, felodipine, isradipine, nicardipine, nifedipine, and nitrendipine, inhibit the inward movement of calcium and cause relaxation of the arterial vasculature and decreased peripheral vascular resistance. In contrast to nondihydropyridine CCBs, such as verapamil and diltiazem, dihydropyridine CCBs have a negligible effect on cardiac conduction and contractility.

CCBs effectively lower BP in hypertensive children and are well tolerated *(36,37)*. Amlodipine lowered the systolic and diastolic BP of hypertensive children in a dose-dependent manner when administered once-daily *(38)*. Amlodipine is ideally suited for the treatment of childhood HTN because the prolonged elimination half-life (e.g., >30 h) permits once-daily dosing. Also, the physicochemical properties allow the drug to be compounded as a liquid suspension (extemporaneous formulation) that permits treatment of children unable to swallow tablets or capsules. These same physiochemical properties allow dose titration in small increments. In children able to swallow a tablet or capsule formulation, sustained release nifedipine appears to be well tolerated.

The most common adverse effects reported in children receiving CCBs include flushing, headache, peripheral edema, and fatigue *(32,39–41)*. Other reported adverse effects include gingival hyperplasia, chest pain, and nausea and vomiting *(34)*.

The use of short-acting nifedipine or other short-acting CCBs in children with HTN is not recommended for long-term therapy while their use to control acute elevations of BP is controversial *(42–45)*. Short-acting nifedipine in adult patients is associated with an increased risk of adverse cardiac and neurologic events *(15,46)*. In general, short-acting nifedipine appears to be effective in children with acute BP elevation *(42)*, however, profound and unpredictable drops in BP have been observed in children receiving short-acting nifedipine, occasionally with catastrophic central nervous systems (CNS) events *(47)*. When used, the initial nifedipine dosage should be 0.1–0.25 mg/kg and should be avoided in children with an underlying acute CNS injury*(42,48)*.

## ANGIOTENSIN II RECEPTOR ANTAGONISTS

ANG II receptor antagonists block the binding of ANG II to the angiotensin receptor (type 1) located in vascular smooth muscle and the adrenal gland. ANG II receptor antagonists prevent the pressor effect of ANG II and inhibit ANG II-stimulated aldosterone secretion from the adrenal gland.

Results from the ongoing pediatric trials investigating the efficacy of ANG II receptor antagonist have not been published. In adults with HTN, ANG II receptor antagonists effectively lower BP and are extremely well tolerated with an adverse effect profile similar to placebo.

Owing to the fetal and neonatal toxicity noted with drugs that act on the RAS *(35)*, ANG II receptor antagonist should not be given during the second and third trimester of pregnancy. Adolescents of childbearing potential are to be informed of these potential risks and counseled on proper birth control measures.

## DIURETICS

Thiazide diuretics are the most common and effective diuretics prescribed for HTN in adults. Loop diuretics are not useful as long-term antihypertensive agents because of the adaptive processes that limit their effectiveness *(49)*. Loop diuretics may be effective, however, as adjuvant therapy in volume-overloaded patients who are resistant to the effects of thiazide diuretics, such as those with chronic renal failure. The potassium-sparing diuretics (e.g., spironolactone and amiloride) are specifically indicated for HTN caused by mineralocorticoid excess, and thiazide and loop diuretic-induced hypokalemia.

The initial BP-lowering effect of thiazide diuretics results from an increased urinary loss of sodium and extracellular fluid volume contraction. With chronic dosing, sodium balance and extracellular fluid volume return towards normal. However, the lower BP is maintained by a decline in peripheral vascular resistance. The mechanism(s) responsible for the changes in vascular resistance are unclear. The antihypertensive response to thiazide diuretics is dependent on sodium intake, and a high sodium intake will attenuate the antihypertensive effect and is a common cause of apparent resistance to therapy (Table 4).

Thiazide diuretics, alone or in combination with β-adrenergic antagonists, lowers BP in children with HTN *(11,50)*. In a recently published placebo-controlled trial examining the BP-lowering effect of the combination drug bisoprolol/hydrochlorothiazide, systolic and diastolic BP were significantly reduced compared to a group of children randomized to placebo *(11)*.

The thiazide dose-antihypertensive response relationship in adults is relatively flat; there is little further BP lowering, but increased incidence of adverse effects, with larger doses. Common adverse effects with diuretics are hypokalemia, hyponatremia, alkalosis, and extracellular fluid volume depletion. Caution is suggested when adding an ACE inhibitor to a child receiving diuretics as the diuretic-induced volume depletion may increase the risk of hypotension and renal dysfunction. Ototoxicity is a reported side effect of loop diuretics, and the risk increases with high doses, kidney failure, and concomitant use of other ototoxic drugs such as aminoglycosides.

## β-ADRENERGIC RECEPTOR ANTAGONISTS

β-adrenergic receptor antagonists decrease BP through several mechanisms including decreased cardiac output, decreased secretion of renin and aldosterone, altered CNS sympathetic activity, and potentiation of natriuretic peptides.

Cardioselective β-adrenergic receptor antagonists such as acebutolol, atenolol, bisoprolol, and metoprolol have a greater affinity for the $\beta_1$-adrenergic receptor, whereas nonselective drugs such as carvedilol, labetalol, nadolol, propranolol, and timolol interact with both $\beta_1$- and $\beta_2$-adrenergic receptors. The preferential effect of cardioselective drugs for $\beta_1$-adrenergic receptors is relative, and at higher doses, cardioselective drugs will inhibit the $\beta_2$-adrenergic receptors that are located in bronchial musculature. The clinical importance of intrinsic sympathetic activity is not well defined. Carvedilol and labetalol are nonselective β-adrenergic receptor antagonists that also have peripheral $\alpha_1$-adrenergic blocking activity.

β-adrenergic receptor antagonists lower BP in hypertensive children when used alone or in combination with other antihypertensive agents *(11,50–52)*. Great interindividual variation exists in the amount of propranolol needed to lower BP; propranolol is metabolized by the liver prior to entering the systemic circulation (e.g., first pass effect). This results in unpredictable plasma concentrations following oral administration and a wide range of effective dosages. The combination drug bisoprolol and hydrochlorothiazide lowered systolic and diastolic BP in children with HTN *(11)*. Metoprolol, a cardioselective agent, effectively lowered BP in a group of hypertensive adolescents *(53)*.

The most common adverse effects from β-adrenergic receptor antagonists are related to the CNS and include dizziness, light-headedness, fatigue, depression, and hallucinations. Other adverse effects are bradycardia, postural hypotension, cold extremities, and nausea. β-adrenergic receptor antagonists can mask the premonitory signs associated with hypoglycemia in diabetic patients and should not be used in patients with bronchospastic disease.

## CENTRALLY ACTING SYMPATHOLYTIC AGENTS

Stimulation of the $\alpha_2$-adrenergic receptors in the CNS decreases sympathetic outflow. Centrally acting agents, such as clonidine and guanabenz, are commonly reserved for HTN recalcitrant to multiple antihypertensive drugs. Clonidine may be the preferred antihypertensive agent in children receiving pharmacologic treatment of a hyperactivity disorder. The reported experience with centrally acting agents is limited to adolescents with essential HTN *(54–56)*.

Side effects are common with the use of centrally acting agents. Dry mouth, sedation, fatigue, dizziness, weakness, and constipation are typically dose-related and tend to decrease with continued dosing. Discontinuation of centrally acting agents should be gradual because abrupt withdrawal can result in symptoms such as agitation, headache, tremor, and HTN.

## PERIPHERAL ADRENERGIC ANTAGONIST

$\alpha_1$-adrenergic receptor antagonists, such as doxazosin, prazosin, and terazosin, block the pressor effect of adrenergic stimulation on the vasculature, resulting in reduced arteriolar resistance and venous capacitance. $\alpha_1$-adrenergic receptor antagonists are usually reserved for severe or drug-resistant HTN and are infrequently prescribed in children. The $\alpha_1$-adrenergic receptor antagonists can be considered for initial therapy in children with the insulin-resistant syndrome, a syndrome characterized by obesity, insulin resistance, lipid abnormalities, and

HTN; the syndrome is associated with sympathetic overactivity *(5)* and $\alpha_1$-adrenergic receptor antagonists have a positive effect on the lipid profile.

The first dose phenomenon, a marked postural hypotensive response that occurs shortly after the initial dose or with a dosage increase, is common and more likely to occur in patients receiving diuretics or β-adrenergic receptor antagonists. The most common adverse effects associated with $\alpha_1$-adrenergic receptor antagonists are dizziness, headache, fatigue, palpitations, and nausea.

## VASODILATORS

Vasodilators, such as hydralazine and minoxidil, produce arteriolar vasodilation through a direct action on vascular smooth muscle. Minoxidil successfully lowers BP in children *(57,58)* but is best reserved for severe and drug-resistant forms of HTN.

The predominant side effects of vasodilators are fluid and salt retention and cardiac stimulation. Cardiac output is increased by enhanced venous return and sympathetic activity. Patients with poorly compliant ventricles, such as those with severe LVH and diastolic dysfunction, may develop heart failure when they take prescribed vasodilators. Subsequent treatment with diuretics, or β-adrenergic receptor antagonist, may modify the fluid retention and cardiac stimulation. Flushing, headache, palpitations, hypotension, and palpitation are commonly observed with vasodilators. Growth of hair on the face, back, arms, and legs occurs in all patients receiving minoxidil and can be very distressing for young girls. Hydralazine can cause a drug-induced lupus syndrome, particularly in slow acetylators.

## REFERENCES

1. National Institutes of Health, National Heart, Lung, and Blood Institute, National High Blood Pressure Program. The sixth report of the joint national committee on prevention, detection, evaluation, and treatment of high blood pressure. Report No. 98-4080. 1997.
2. National Heart, Lung and Blood Institute (NHLBI). Fact Book Fiscal Year 2001. US Department of Health and Human Services, Bethesda, MD: National Institute of Health. 2002.
3. Lewis EJ, Hunsicker LG, Bain RP, Rohde RD. The effect of angiotensin-converting-enzyme inhibition on diabetic nephropathy. The Collaborative Study Group. N Engl J Med 1993;329:1456–1462.
4. Pfeffer MA, Braunwald E, Moye LA, et al. Effect of captopril on mortality and morbidity in patients with left ventricular dysfunction after myocardial infarction. Results of the survival and ventricular enlargement trial. The SAVE Investigators. N Engl J Med 1992;327:669–677.
5. Sorof JM. Systolic hypertension in children: benign or beware? Pediatr Nephrol 2001;16:517–525.
6. Sinaiko AR, Gomez-Marin O, Prineas RJ. Prevalence of "significant" hypertension in junior high school-aged children: the children and adolescent blood pressure program. J Pediatr 1989;114:664–669.
7. Lauer RM, Clarke WR. Childhood risk factors for high adult blood pressure: the Muscatine study. Pediatrics 1984;84:633–641.
8. Sorof JM, Cardwell G, Franco K, Portman RJ. Ambulatory blood pressure and left ventricular mass index in hypertensive children. Hypertension 2002;39(4):903–908.
9. Sorof J, Hanevold C, Portman R, Daniels S. Left ventricular hypertrophy in hypertensive children: a report from the international pediatric hypertension association. Am J Hypertens 2002;15[4 (part 2 of 2)]:31A. Abstract
10. Tracy RE, Newman WP, III, Wattigney WA, Berenson GS. Risk factors and atherosclerosis in youth autopsy findings of the Bogalusa Heart Study. Am J Med Sci 1995;310 (Suppl 1):S37–S41.
11. Sorof JM, Cargo P, Graepel J, et al. beta-Blocker/thiazide combination for treatment of hypertensive children: a randomized double-blind, placebo-controlled trial. Pediatr Nephrol 2002;17:345–350.
12. National High Blood Pressure Education Program Working Group on Hypertension Control in Children and Adolescents. Update on the 1987 Task Force Report on High Blood Pressure in Children and Adolescents: A

Working Group Report from the National High Blood Pressure Education Program. Pediatrics 1999;98:649–658.
13. Wells T, Stowe C. An approach to the use of antihypertensive drugs in children and adolescents. Curr Ther Res Clin Exp 2001;62:329–350.
14. Agodoa LY, Appel L, Bakris GL, et al. Effect of ramipril vs amlodipine on renal outcomes in hypertensive nephrosclerosis: a randomized controlled trial. JAMA 2001;285:2719–2728.
15. Pahor M, Psaty BM, Alderman MH, et al. Health outcomes associated with calcium antagonists compared with other first-line antihypertensive therapies: a meta-analysis of randomized controlled trials. Lancet 2000;356:1949–1954.
16. Ruggenenti P, Perna A, Gherardi G, Benini R, Remuzzi G. Chronic proteinuric nephropathies: outcomes and response to treatment in a prospective cohort of 352 patients with different patterns of renal injury. Am J Kidney Dis 2000;35:1155–1165.
17. Gansevoort RT, de Zeeuw D, de Jong PE. Long-term benefits of the antiproteinuric effect of angiotensin-converting enzyme inhibition in nondiabetic renal disease. Am J Kidney Dis 1993;22:202–206.
18. Sorof JM, Poffenbarger T, Franco K, Bernard L, Portman RJ. Isolated systolic hypertension, obesity, and hyperkinetic hemodynamic states in children. J Pediatr 2002;140:660–666.
19. Rocchini AP. Adolescent obesity and hypertension. Pediatr Clin N Am 1993;40:81–92.
20. Leckman JF, Detlor J, Harcherik DF, et al. Acute and chronic clonidine treatment in Tourette's syndrome: a preliminary report on clinical response and effect on plasma and urinary catecholamine metabolites, growth hormone, and blood pressure. J Child Psychiatry 1983;22:433–440.
21. Miller K, Atkin B, Rodel Jr PV, Walker JF. Enalapril: a well-tolerated and efficacious agent for the pediatric hypertensive patient. J Cardiovasc Pharmacol 1987;10(Suppl 7):S154–S156.
22. Morsi MR, Madina EH, Anglo AA, Soliman AT. Evaluation of captopril versus reserpine and furosemide in treating hypertensive children with acute post-streptococcal glomerulonephritis. Acta Paediatr 1992;81: 145–149.
23. Bendig L, Temesvari A. Indications and effects of captopril therapy in childhood. Acta Physiologica Hungarica 1988;72:121–129.
24. Sagat T, Sasinka M, Furkova K, Milovsky V, Riedel R, Tordova E. Treatment of renal hypertension in children by captopril. Clin Exp Hypertens A 1986;8:853–857.
25. Callis L, Vila A, Catala J, Gras X. Long-term treatment with captopril in pediatric patients with severe hypertension and chronic renal failure. Clin Exp Hypertens A 1986;8:847–851.
26. Soffer BA, Shahinfar S, Shaw WC, et al. Effects of the Ace inhibitor, enalapril, in children age 6–16 years with hypertension. Pediatr Res 2000;47. Abstract.
27. Herrera P, Soffer B, Zhang Z, et al. Effects of the ACE inhibitor, lisinopril (L), in children age 6–16 years with hypertension. Am J Hypertens 2002;14(4 part 2):32A. Abstract.
28. Seeman T, Dusek J, Feber J, Vondrak K, Janda J. Treatment of hypertension with ramipril in children with renal diseases. Am J Hypertens 2002;15(4 par 2):204A–205A. Abstract.
29. Tack ED, Perlman JN. Renal failure in sick hypertensive premature infants receiving captopril therapy. J Pediatr 1988;112:805–810.
30. Sinaiko AR, Mirkin BL, Hendrick DA, Green TP, O'Dea RF. Antihypertensive effect and elimination kinetics of captopril in hypertensive children with renal disease. J Pediatr 1983;103:799–805.
31. Wells T, Rippley R, Hogg R, et al. The pharmacokinetics of enalapril in children and infants with hypertension. J Clin Pharmacol 2001;41:1064–1074.
32. von Vigier RO, Mozzettini S, Truttmann AC, Meregalli P, Ramelli GP, Bianchetti MG. Cough is common in children prescribed converting enzyme inhibitors. Nephron 2000;84:98.
33. Bianchetti MG, Caflisch M, Oetliker OH. Cough and converting enzyme inhibitors. Eur J Pediatr 1992;151: 225–226.
34. Blowey DL. Safety of the newer antihypertensive agents in children. Expert Opin Drug Saf 2002;1:39–43.
35. Sedman AB, Kershaw DB, Bunchman TE. Recognition and management of angiotensin converting enzyme inhibitor fetopathy. Pediatr Nephrol 1995;9:382–385.
36 Flynn JT, Pasko D. Calcium channel blockers: pharmacology and place in therapy of pediatric hypertension. Pediatr Nephrol 2000;15:302–316.
37. Sinaiko AR. Clinical pharmacology of converting enzyme inhibitors, calcium channel blockers and diuretics. J Hum Hypertens 1994;8:389–394.

38. Flynn JT, Hogg RJ, Portman RJ, et al. A randomized, placebo-controlled trial of amlodipine in the treatment of children with hypertension. Am J Hypertens 2002;15(4 part 2):31A–32A. Abstract.
39. Flynn JT, Smoyer WE, Bunchman TE. Treatment of hypertensive children with amlodipine. Am J Hypertens 2000;13:1061–1066.
40. Silverstein DM, Palmer J, Baluarte HJ, Brass C, Conley SB, Polinsky MS. Use of calcium-channel blockers in pediatric renal transplant recipients. Pediatr Transplant 1999;3:288–292.
41. Tallian KB, Nahata MC, Turman MA, Mahan JD, Hayes JR, Mentser MI. Efficacy of amlodipine in pediatric patients with hypertension. Pediatr Nephrol 1999;13:304–310.
42. Egger DW, Deming DD, Hamada N, Perkin RM, Sahney S. Evaluation of the safety of short-acting nifedipine in children with hypertension. Pediatr Nephrol 2002;17:35–40.
43. Truttmann AC, Zehnder-Schlapbach S, Bianchetti MG. A moratorium should be placed on the use of short acting nifedipine for hypertensive crises (letter). Pediatr Nephrol 1998;12:259–261.
44. Sinaiko AR, Daniels S. The use of short-acting nifedipine in children with HTN: another example of the need for comprehensive drug testing in children. J Pediatr 2001;139:7–9.
45. Flynn JT. Nifedipine in the treatment of hypertension in children. J Pediatr 2002;140:787–788.
46. Psaty BM, Heckbert SR, Koepsell TD, et al. The risk of myocardial infarction associated with antihypertensive drug therapies. JAMA 1995;274:620–625.
47. Gauthier B, Trachtman H. Short-acting nifedipine (letter). Pediatr Nephrol 1997;11:786–787.
48. Levene MI, Gibson NA, Fenton AC, Papathoma E, Barnett D. The use of a calcium-channel blocker, nicardipine, for severely asphyxiated newborn infants. Dev Med Child Neurol 1990;32:567–574.
49. Ellison D. Adaptation to diuretic drugs. In: Seldin D, Giebisch G, eds. Diuretic agents: clinical physiology and pharmacology. San Diego: Academic, 1997;209–232.
50. Bachmann H. Propranolol versus chlorthalidone—a prospective therapeutic trial in children with chronic hypertension. Helv Paediat Acta 1984;39:55–61.
51. Potter DE, Schambelan M, Salvatierra Jr O, Orloff S, Holliday MA. Treatment of high-renin hypertension with propranolol in children after renal transplantation. J Pediatr 1977;90:307–311.
52. Griswold WR, McNeal R, Mendoza SA, Sellers BB, Higgins S. Propranolol as an antihypertensive agent in children. Arch Dis Child 1978;53:594–596.
53. Falkner B, Lowenthal DT, Affrime MB. The pharmacodynamic effectiveness of metoprolol in adolescent hypertension. Pediatr Pharmacol 1982;2:49–55.
54. Falkner B, Onesti G, Lowenthal DT, Affrime MB. Effectiveness of centrally acting drugs and diuretics in adolescent hypertension. Clin Pharmacol Ther 1982;32:577–583.
55. Walson PD, Rath A, Kilbourne K, Deitch MW. Guanabenz for adolescent hypertension. Pediatr Pharmacol 1984;4:1–6.
56. Falkner B, Lowenthal DT, Onesti G. Dynamic exercise response in hypertensive adolescent on clonidine therapy: clonidine therapy in adolescent hypertension. Pediatr Pharmacol 1980;1:121–128.
57. Sinaiko AR, Mirkin BL. Management of severe childhood hypertension with minoxidil: a controlled clinical study. J Pediatr 1977;91:138–142.
58. Pennisi AJ, Takahashi M, Bernstein BH, et al. Minoxidil therapy in children with severe hypertension. J Pediatr 1977;90:813–819.

# 26 Pediatric Antihypertensive Trials

*Thomas G. Wells,* MD

*Contents*



## INTRODUCTION

Because hypertension (HTN) is prevalent in the adult population and is often a chronic, nonremitting condition associated with morbidity and mortality, pharmaceutical firms have committed significant resources to the development of effective antihypertensive medications. Under the regulatory guidance of the US Food and Drug Administration (FDA) and similar agencies in other countries, these new drugs were evaluated for safety and effectiveness in adults before marketing approval was granted. Until recently, antihypertensives were rarely studied adequately in children, but were still prescribed for patients less than 18 yr of age. Off-label use, with all of its implied risks, was often the only option available to physicians who treated children with HTN *(1)*.

Recognizing the need to address this potentially dangerous inequity, several federal initiatives designed to include children in the drug development process were proposed. In 1994, the FDA promulgated the Pediatric Rule, which was expanded in 1998 and required manufacturers to perform limited studies in children if a new drug offered any potential health benefits in the pediatric population *(2,3)*. With the passage of the FDA Modernization Act (FDAMA) in 1997 and later the Best Pharmaceuticals for Children Act (BPCA) in 2002, pharmaceutical firms were granted meaningful financial incentives in exchange for conducting appropriate pediatric studies *(4,5)*.

Since 1998, many antihypertensive drugs have been successfully studied in children and more studies are currently underway or planned *(6–13)*. An ideal clinical trial would yield useful information and at the same time minimize the risks to the children participating in the

From: *Clinical Hypertension and Vascular Disease: Pediatric Hypertension*
Edited by: R. J. Portman, J. M. Sorof, and J. R. Ingelfinger © Humana Press Inc., Totowa, NJ

study. Traditional methods used to determine the safety and effectiveness of antihypertensive agents in adults must be modified to meet the challenges presented by pediatric patients.

## THE DRUG DEVELOPMENT PROCESS

The traditional drug development process is divided into several phases, beginning with the discovery phase during which a new chemical entity is developed (Fig. 1). Extensive preclinical testing determines key safety factors. The results of the preclinical studies are used to develop early phase clinical trials, which yield information that is used to design subsequent studies. When the clinical trials are complete, a New Drug Application (NDA) is filed with the FDA. Postmarketing studies are conducted after the NDA has been approved and the drug reaches the market. This traditional process is not strictly sequential and development phases may overlap.

Clinical trials may be defined as studies conducted using human subjects and designed to determine the pharmacological properties of a drug in a biological system, characterize its effectiveness in treating or ameliorating a disease, condition, or symptom, and define its safety. Pharmacokinetic studies determine the absorption, distribution, metabolism, and elimination of the drug, define the appropriate dose and dosing interval for a given formulation, and assess the effects of inherited or acquired alterations in metabolism, impaired clearance, or other relevant factors on drug disposition. Clinical trials are typically conducted in four phases, although these phases should not be viewed as absolutes and in some cases are not clearly separable.

The clinical phases of the drug development process commence with the filing of the Investigational New Drug (IND) Application. In this application, the sponsor formally requests permission to study a drug for a specific indication. If a drug is found to be safe and effective during clinical trials, a New Drug Application (NDA) is filed with the FDA. In the NDA, the sponsor requests approval to market the drug for a specific indication or set of indications. Drug development may be halted for lack of safety and effectiveness, or for other reasons at any stage in the process.

Phase I studies are typically safety studies involving relatively few subjects. These early trials are "first exposure" studies and are usually performed in healthy subjects unless the expected toxicity of the drug is significant (e.g., chemotherapeutic agents used to treat cancer). Extensive sampling of blood, urine, and other body fluids to determine drug disposition is usually accomplished during Phase I.

Phase II studies are typically conducted in patients who have the target disease or condition that the drug has been designed to treat. These studies usually involve up to several hundred subjects. The primary purpose of most Phase II studies is safety, but efficacy data that will be used to design Phase III studies are generally collected. Trials conducted early in Phase II may be designated as Phase IIA studies and those conducted later may be designated as Phase IIB.

Phase III studies are typically large, multicenter trials designed to collect data to support the effectiveness claims that will be part of the NDA. Several Phase III studies may be ongoing at the same time. Although Phase III trials are designed primarily to demonstrate that the study drug provides effective treatment for the condition or disease under study (i.e. the indication), additional safety data are collected. As with Phase II studies, Phase III trials may be designated Phase IIIA or IIIB. Phase IIIB trials are usually conducted after the NDA has been submitted but before marketing approval is granted.

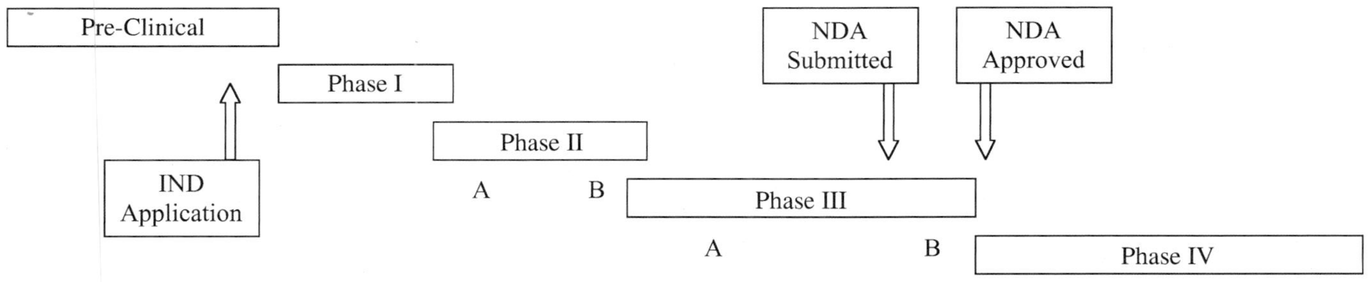


Fig. 1. The traditional drug development process.

Phase IV studies, also known as postmarketing studies, are conducted for many reasons. The FDA may request additional safety data. Occasionally, rare adverse effects that were not apparent in earlier trials are uncovered after a drug is brought to market during Phase IV "surveillance" studies. Phase IV trials may also be conducted to study a new formulation or evaluate additional indications. However, many Phase IV studies are designed to increase physician awareness and use of a new product.

The antihypertensive studies conducted in children under FDAMA after 1997 have followed a special set of laws and regulations determined by Congress and the FDA *(2–5,14–16)*. The original FDAMA legislation had two specific provisions that were important to pediatric drug development *(17)*. First, the law required the FDA to compile a list of drugs for which additional pediatric information may be beneficial. Second, for drugs that were already on the market and were determined to have potentially beneficial effects in children, a Written Request for additional pediatric studies was issued for specified clinical studies. An additional six months of market exclusivity were granted to sponsors that submitted data judged by the FDA to be responsive to the terms of the Written Request.

The market exclusivity provision of FDAMA was extended in the BPCA legislation passed by Congress in 2002 *(5)*. In addition, the BPCA created a new mechanism to study off-patent drugs. In this alternate mechanism, a prioritized list of off-patent drugs that may produce health benefits in children, or that may require reformulation for pediatric use, was developed with input from a wide variety of experts. The sponsor will be offered the chance to conduct appropriate studies, but it is anticipated that almost all will decline. If the sponsor refuses to conduct the studies, a Request for Proposals (RFP) mechanism, similar to other requests issued by the National Institutes of Health (NIH), will be developed for each specific compound and indication. Applicants are given guidelines and are asked to design studies that address specific points in the RFP. A request to study nitroprusside for induction of controlled hypotension during surgical or medical procedures in children was recently released *(18)*.

Studies of drugs that are already off-patent, as well as trials conducted for those drugs with remaining patent protection, will address very similar clinical questions. The FDA released a sample Written Request to provide sponsors with recommended study designs for antihypertensive trials in children *(19)*. However, after several studies conducted in response to early Written Requests failed to yield interpretable data, the guidance was withdrawn and is under revision.

## CURRENT STUDY DESIGN ELEMENTS

While many factors surrounding the design of antihypertensive trials in children are non-controversial, other issues are still intensely debated. Guidance documents from the FDA are subject to change. However, such changes reflect an ongoing commitment by all interested parties to improve the quality and interpretability of the data collected in pediatric antihypertensive trials.

Presently, the Written Requests issued by the FDA contain several important elements. Key elements of a standard Written Request are presented in Table 1. The three key elements of studies conducted under a Written Request are: (1) a pharmacokinetic study; (2) a dose-ranging study to determine effectiveness; and (3) safety data from the controlled trials and an extended open label treatment period. The dose-ranging study must be interpretable or the study will not be considered responsive to the Written Request, and exclusivity will not be granted.

Table 1
Key Features of a Standard Written Request

*Study aims*
- Pharmacokinetic data
- Dose-ranging trial to determine effectiveness
- Safety data

*Age groups*
- Infants and toddlers (aged 1 to <2 yr)
- Preschool children (aged 2 to <6 yr)
- School-aged children (aged 6 to Tanner stage <3 or aged <12 yr)
- Adolescents (Tanner stage 3 or aged 12 to <17 yr)

*Racial groups*
- 40–60% black subjects (ACE inhibitor and ANG II receptor antagonist drugs)

*Formulation issues*
- Potentially marketable formulation or if not possible, documented efforts to do so

*Dose-ranging trial design*
- Double blind
- Minimum of 3 dose levels
- Primary endpoint: absolute or percentage change in systolic or diastolic BP
- Trial A: Randomized to placebo or one of three doses
- Trial B: Randomized to one of three doses (no placebo)
- Trial C: Two study periods: (1) Same as trial B<br>(2) Randomized withdrawal to drug or placebo
- Trial D: Randomized withdrawal to drug or placebo

*Pharmacokinetic trial design*
- Same dose range as doses studied for effectiveness
- Same ages as studied for effectiveness

Antihypertensive trials conducted in the United States, European Union, and Japan in adult subjects typically adhere to the International Conference on Harmonisation (ICH) guidelines, first signed in 2000 *(20)*. There are many similarities between accepted methodologies in pediatric and adult antihypertensive trials *(20)*. The ICH Consensus Principle recognizes that the primary endpoint may be the change in either systolic or diastolic BP. Assessment of therapeutic and adverse effects in the short- and long-term is a critical element of preferred study designs in both the adult and pediatric populations. Finally, inclusion of a wide range of doses is encouraged.

Several significant differences exist between the ICH Consensus Principle and the Pediatric Written Requests. Apart from considerations related to the age and the number of subjects, the ICH guidelines encourage the use of ambulatory blood pressure monitoring (ABPM) to determine effectiveness, require more strict criteria for assessing the time course of the response to therapy and any possible adverse effects using trough/peak ratios, provide more liberal criteria for including a placebo arm, encourage the use of active control drugs as a comparison to standard therapy, provide specific suggested safety assessments, and recommend assessment of withdrawal effects *(20)*.

Table 2
Antihypertensive Agents Studied Under a Written Request and Granted Pediatric Exclusivity

| *Drug* | *Manufacturer* | *Pediatric labeling approved* |
|---|---|---|
| Amlodipine | Pfizer | |
| Benazepril | Novartis | |
| Bisoprolol | Wyeth Ayerst | |
| Enalapril | Merck | Feb. 13, 2001 |
| Felodipine | Astra Zeneca | |
| Fosinopril | Bristol-Myers Squibb | May 27, 2003 |
| Lisinopril | Merck, Astra Zeneca | May 29, 2003 |
| Losartan | Merck | |
| Quinapril | Parke-Davis | |

Source: http://www.fda.gov/cder/pediatric/exgrant.htm.

## ANTIHYPERTENSIVE TRIALS IN CHILDREN

Between 1980 and 1998, none of the new antihypertensive agents granted marketing approval in the US were formally evaluated in children and, consequently, none were labeled for use in the pediatric population. From June of 1998 to August of 2003, the FDA issued formal Written Requests for 25 marketed drugs that are used to lower BP *(6)*. As of August 2003, studies have been completed and exclusivity granted for nine antihypertensive agents (Table 2). Additional studies are underway or planned.

More importantly, inclusion of pediatric information in the product label has been approved for several of the drugs that received exclusivity *(7)*. Enalapril was the first antihypertensive agent to receive approval for pediatric labeling in more than 20 yr *(7)*. Included in the new label is specific information concerning dose, pharmacokinetics, and instructions for the preparation of an extemporaneous suspension useful in children unable to swallow tablets *(21)*. In 2003, fosinopril and lisinopril also received approval for inclusion of pediatric data in the product label. These changes should appear in reference manuals, such as the Physicians' Desk Reference, in 2004.

## DILEMMAS IN THE DESIGN OF PEDIATRIC TRIALS

The intent of the Pediatric Rule, and elements of the FDAMA, was to develop and disseminate important information concerning drug use in children and, in doing so, improve pediatric therapeutics. The early studies conducted under the provisions of FDAMA highlighted some of the peculiarities of pediatric HTN that created unique challenges for study design and implementation. First and foremost, the goals of the parties involved in studying antihypertensives in children must be understood because these goals directly affect the quantity and type of information that is collected. The sponsor may desire to use accepted methods to meet the minimum requirements for exclusivity in the Written Request. For example, if the primary outcome measure for the dose ranging study is measurable reduction in systolic or diastolic BP, additional testing beyond required safety monitoring may not receive support. Academicians may desire to address valid scientific questions not directly pertinent to the primary endpoint in the Written Request. However, this goal may conflict with the sponsor's desire to conduct a cost-effective study and to minimize the collection of information unrelated to the primary outcome measure that, if adverse in nature, could prompt additional questions from the FDA. Ultimately, the sponsors and the FDA must agree to a rational study design and data analysis plan that are likely to yield information that is interpretable and clinically useful.

## SPECIFIC ISSUES RELATED TO THE DESIGN OF PEDIATRIC ANTIHYPERTENSIVE TRIALS

### *Measurement of Blood Pressure*

Under the current guidelines, the difference between end-of-study and baseline systolic or diastolic BPs is the primary endpoint for antihypertensive trials conducted in children. Typically, the 24-h trough BP is used to determine response to therapy. Comparisons are made between the changes in BP from baseline to the end of the study across dosing groups.

The importance of measuring BP accurately cannot be overstated. Casual BP measurements are subject both to bias, which can be reduced using a randomized, double-blind design and/or placebo, and measurement error. Strict adherence to accepted measurement techniques *(22)* and observer training are essential.

Casual BP may be measured using a variety of instruments. The mercury manometer, once considered the standard device, has been removed from many locations because of environmental concerns. Aneroid manometers or oscillometric devices have replaced the mercury manometers. Each device has unique strengths and limitations that have been previously described *(22–25)*. It is important to understand how each device determines BP and the appropriate maintenance schedules for any instruments used to measure BP during a trial. If possible, each subject should have BPs measured, using the same type of device at each visit.

ABPM is frequently used in antihypertensive trials in adult subjects *(26)*. ABPM offers several advantages, including removal of observer bias and error, detection of subjects who have white coat hypertension (WCH), assessment of duration of action and correlation of adverse effects with dosing, and calculation of trough/peak ratios that can be used to demonstrate adequate BP control throughout the dosing interval *(26)*. In long-term effectiveness and safety studies, ABPM may correlate better than casual measurements with important clinical outcome measures *(27)*. However, younger children often have difficulty complying with the requirements of ABPM. Furthermore, there are no uniform standards for measurement protocols.

Finally, the use of home monitoring in pediatric trials has been limited to safety monitoring *(11)*. In adults, there is some evidence to suggest that home monitoring may be superior to office measurement for long-term clinical care *(28)*.

Accurate BP measurement is critical to the success of pediatric trials. In designing pediatric trials, consideration should be given to the age of the subjects, measurement techniques, observer training, the number and timing of critical measurements, the white coat effect, and device selection and maintenance. No standard approach exists, but one should be defined for each study to minimize the effect of measurement error on the outcome of the study.

### *Defining the Study Population*

Several issues must be considered in selecting the target population for any trial. The definition of HTN that is most widely accepted comes from the 1996 Update to the 1987 Task Force Report on High BP in Children and Adolescents *(22)*. It is generally accepted that systolic and/or diastolic BP greater than or equal to the 95th percentile for age, gender, and height constitutes HTN in children *(22)*. The Task Force recommends that the average of multiple measurements be taken over weeks to months to avoid the accommodation effect and regression to the mean *(22)*. The Task Force guidelines represent a balanced approach that attempts to distinguish between children with truly elevated BP and those who may have elevated readings, either temporarily or inconsistently.

Less-strict standards have generally been employed to identify potential subjects for inclusion in antihypertensive trials. The number of elevated readings prior to inclusion, the conditions under which the qualifying measurements were obtained, and the timing of the measurements varied among studies. Few, if any, studies encouraged the use of ABPM to exclude subjects with WCH. To increase the pool of potentially eligible subjects, patients with BP at or above the 90th percentile, who also have diabetes or a strong family history of HTN, are included. In some trials, there was no concordance between the BP used to determine eligibility and that used as the primary endpoint. For example, entry criteria allowed children with systolic, diastolic, or systolic and diastolic HTN to be included in the study, but the primary endpoint was defined as either systolic or diastolic BP. In most trials, inclusion criteria allowed a mix of treatment-naïve subjects with established patients who were receiving drug therapy and agreed to a withdrawal phase that often included a brief placebo run-in period. All of these issues create tradeoffs between the homogeneity of the study population and the size of the pool of potential study subjects.

## *Dose-Ranging Studies*

Several possible designs can be employed to determine the minimum effective dose, the maximum useful dose, and the therapeutic dosing range. In adult trials, the simplest design employs a single fixed dose compared with placebo. This design yields little information about dose–response relationships and has not been included in the options for studies conducted under a Written Request. Other schemes employ an optional titration in which the dose of study drug is increased only if subjects fail to reach predetermined BP criteria, or a forced titration scheme in which the dose is increased whether or not subjects have achieved the target BP. Also, children may be randomly assigned to one of at least three groups that employ different (i.e., high, medium, low) fixed doses of the study medication. In adults, a placebo arm is generally included in all of these schemes. In children, concerns over the use of placebo, even for brief periods of time, lead to dosing regimens that permitted randomization and double-blinding, but in some cases lacked a placebo control group.

Many studies conducted under FDAMA Written Requests employ a two-phased approach, in which dose–response relationships are explored during the first phase, and withdrawal to active drug or placebo occurs during the second phase. For safety reasons, BP is monitored closely, either by frequent visits to the research center or monitoring home BPs during all phases of the study. Subjects who manifest severe, symptomatic HTN at any point during the study are generally dropped from the study or allowed rescue therapy. There are often no set criteria to determine when consideration should be given to withdrawing the subject from the study, but in some cases severe HTN, defined as BP above the 99th percentile, has been used as a criterion for withdrawal *(10)*. Instead, the decision to discontinue a subject has often been left to the discretion of the investigator with input from the treating physician, subject, and parents.

Two other issues critical to defining the study population are whether to include patients with primary and/or secondary HTN, and whether to allow concomitant therapy during the study. Secondary HTN is more prevalent in young children and in children aged less than 6 yr; very few children less than 6 yr of age have essential HTN. In contrast, adolescents frequently have primary HTN, raising the question of whether the study population needs to be restricted, or simply subjected to a *post hoc* analysis based on known diagnoses at the time of enrollment. The latter approach does not restrict the pool of potential subjects. However, because Written Requests now mandate inclusion of children 1–16 yr of age, it is no longer feasible to restrict the study population to those children with primary HTN.

Because children with treated HTN receive a variety of antihypertensive therapies, most studies have chosen to withdraw subjects from current therapy prior to enrollment. The decision as to whether withdrawal of therapy is safe or advisable should be left to the treating physician. In situations where withdrawal of therapy is not permitted, an "add-on" treatment design has been used. The obvious drawback of this approach is the difficulty in distinguishing the effect of the study drug alone from any synergistic effects. For this reason, the "add-on" design has not been used in recent trials conducted under Written Requests but should be considered in children aged >6 yr. If a combination product is being evaluated, a factorial design may permit determination of the optimal ratio of the two individual drugs *(20)*.

One significant issue related to pediatric trials is dosing of study medications. Most children under 6 yr of age have difficulty swallowing a tablet or capsule. Significant effort and expense is needed to develop and test liquid formulations that are stable and palatable. In children who are able to swallow tablets or capsules, a fixed-dose scheme may not be appropriate for children of all ages. Strict dosing schemes based on body weight or body surface area are not possible using fixed doses. Development and testing of tablets or capsules using doses that have not been evaluated previously is costly and time consuming. For this reason, the tablets or capsules used in the trials are often the same fixed doses as marketed drugs. Furthermore, children ages 6–16 yr may vary more than sixfold in body weight and, as a result, weight-based stratification schemes have often been used to maintain reasonably similar drug exposure. The dilemma of how to stratify based on the body weight of the subjects is a critical decision and becomes significantly more challenging if optional or forced titration schemes are used in a randomized, double-blind, placebo-controlled trial.

Development and testing of age-appropriate formulations are critical elements of pediatric antihypertensive studies. Although several stable extemporaneous preparations have been developed, there are no commercially available liquid preparations for any of the angiotensin-converting enzyme (ACE) inhibitors, angiotensin II (ANG II) receptor antagonists, or calcium channel antagonists. In an attempt to rectify this situation, the FDA now mandates that sponsors undertake a good faith attempt to develop a marketable liquid formulation as part of the response to the Written Request.

Outcome measures are clearly important to the dose-ranging study. Systolic HTN is more common in children *(29)*, but may be more labile as well. Some trials have used diastolic BP as the primary endpoint *(11,13)*, whereas others have used both systolic and diastolic BP *(10)*. Because the standard deviation for systolic BP is larger, more subjects may be required to achieve statistical significance. Whichever measure is chosen as the primary endpoint, the other should be used as a secondary endpoint.

ABPM offers some significant advantages in antihypertensive trials that have been previously discussed. At present, trough casual measurements are used to define outcomes. If ABPM is to become more widely used in pediatric antihypertensive trials, validation of the instruments, selection of a primary endpoint, and the use of standard methods will become important considerations. Ultimately, the advantages of ABPM may lead to increased use in pediatric trials, similar to what has already occurred in the adult population.

### *Data Analysis in Dose-Ranging Studies*

Response to therapy can be defined in absolute terms or as a percentage change in BP. Because the absolute values used to define normal and high BPs change significantly over the pediatric age range, some believe that examining the percentage change in BP may be more appropriate than using the absolute change. For example, an absolute difference of 5 mmHg represents a greater percentage change in BP for a toddler than for an adolescent. Either method is acceptable in pediatric studies.

Determination of sample size is often difficult but critically important. Recently, the FDA mandated that dose–response studies must be powered to detect a 3 mmHg difference between high and low doses in a dose-ranging study, or between placebo and active drug in a placebo-controlled withdrawal study. Previously, some studies had used a 5 mmHg difference to determine sample size *(11)*. Selection of appropriate standard deviations for systolic and diastolic BPs is also critical. Published data provide some guidance *(24,30)*.

The type of data analysis will depend on protocol design. Both intention to treat and per protocol analyses have been used *(10,11,13)*. Secondary subgroup analyses should be included in the analysis plan. Important considerations include age, gender, race, primary vs secondary HTN, and sexual maturation.

Some studies have examined response defined as the percentage of subjects whose BP returns to normal while taking the study drug. It is important to compare the response to the study drug to that of the placebo when this measure is used. This measure is useful in that it allows clinicians to estimate the likelihood of response in an unselected population of children with HTN.

While short-term endpoints are generally accepted in pediatric trials, the effect of maintaining a normal BP over the long term requires consideration of additional outcome measures. Surrogate endpoints, such as microalbuminuria, renal function, vascular wall thickness, left ventricular mass index, BP load, and other outcome measures are feasible, but it remains uncertain whether or not these will be studied routinely in industry-sponsored clinical trials in the absence of any regulatory requirement.

### *Pharmacokinetic Studies*

Basic pharmacokinetic and pharmacodynamic principles, as applied to pediatric antihypertensive studies, have been previously considered *(31)*. The FDA has mandated that pharmacokinetic studies should be conducted in children who are the same ages as subjects enrolled in the dose ranging study. There are compelling reasons to conduct these studies in children. Developmental changes in body composition, gastrointestinal transit time, the activity of drug metabolizing enzymes, the efficiency of drug elimination mechanisms, and concentration-response relationships for some substrates have been well described *(31–33)*. Formulations appropriate for younger children should be studied in the pediatric population.

The FDA presently requires relatively few pharmacokinetic parameters to define the disposition of antihypertensive agents in children. Typically, requested data include the area under the concentration vs time curve (AUC), the maximum plasma or serum concentration ($C_{max}$), and the time at which the maximal concentration is observed ($T_{max}$). Often, the elimination half-life ($t_{1/2}$) is reported. However, the elimination half-life is a derived parameter that changes as both clearance and the volume of distribution change.

Additional information that may be collected for selected drugs includes disposition of metabolites, renal clearance of parent drug and any metabolites, drug accumulation, and the effect of food on absorption. Occasionally, the effects of gender, sexual maturation, or race may be relevant to drug metabolism. Also, patients taking medications that may induce or inhibit relevant drug-metabolizing enzymes are typically prohibited from participating in the study.

In designing pharmacokinetic studies, consideration must be given to the unique pharmacokinetic properties of the study drug. If accumulation is expected, it may be necessary to perform the study at steady state rather than after administration of a single dose. Separating the pharmacokinetic and dose-ranging studies permits use of a substitution scheme in which a single dose of the study drug is substituted for a single dose of the subjects' usual antihypertensive therapy. If a pharmacokinetic arm is included in the dose-ranging study, then it is possible to perform the pharmacokinetic study after the first dose, after multiple doses, or both. If the dose-ranging and pharmacokinetic studies are combined, it is advisable to make the pharmacokinetic study optional, or enrollment in the study may be compromised. Furthermore, in a combined design, the anxiety concerning phlebotomy that many children experience may raise BP and compromise the validity of BP measurements done to measure the effectiveness of the study drug.

The number, timing, and volume of blood samples needed to define the pharmacokinetics of antihypertensives in children are critical considerations, particularly in infants and toddlers. Frequent samples are best collected through an indwelling intravenous catheter placed with the aid of a topical anesthetic preparation. The estimated volume of blood discarded must be added to the total volume withdrawn for pharmacokinetic samples and other laboratory studies. The Institutional Review Board at each site will determine the maximum volume of blood that can be safely withdrawn for research purposes. For studies involving young children, it is imperative to develop microassays that detect drug and metabolites using a small sample volume. Otherwise, the sampling scheme will be severely restricted. Alternatively, a population pharmacokinetic approach may be possible.

## FUTURE DIRECTIONS

As important to children as the past five years have been, the future of pediatric antihypertensive trials promises to be even more exciting. Several key developments may contribute to better study designs that will yield more information.

As ABPM becomes more readily available and more widely accepted, it is likely that routine use of ABPM in pediatric clinical trials will occur. Widespread use awaits validation of one or more instruments in children and the results of several ongoing projects to define normative data. ABPM could be used to exclude children with WCH whenever feasible. In designing these studies, it is important to identify subjects who are truly hypertensive because the drug effect may be smaller or inconsistent in subjects with white coat or labile HTN. A standard ABPM protocol for clinical trials would permit comparisons between drugs. Also, ABPM could be used as it is in the adult population to define peak and trough reductions in BP which, in turn, will permit improved assessment of the duration of action and the relationship of clinically apparent adverse effects to the dosing schedule.

The information collected from ongoing trials must be disseminated. Sponsors must be encouraged to publish study data and to apply not just for exclusivity, but labeling changes that publicize pediatric dosing. Ultimately, placing dosing and safety information into the hands of practitioners may reduce errors and associated morbidity.

Finally, the environment for conducting pediatric antihypertensive trials is rapidly improving. As more studies are conducted, study sites become more adept. There are many relevant and interesting questions of a scientific nature that could be added to ongoing clinical trials. However, industry cannot be expected to shoulder the burden for all of these needed studies. With the passage of the BPCA, the NIH and the FDA are engaged in an historic cooperative effort to study off-patent drugs. Many antihypertensive agents commonly used in children are off-patent, and without the mechanisms established by the BPCA to support these studies, it is likely that many useful drugs will not be studied. Beyond this effort, there are many comparative studies examining the long-term effectiveness and safety of antihypertensives in children that need to be conducted. These studies are of a generic nature and address issues that have been addressed in adults, such as the effect of race on response to different classes of drugs, and how best to measure therapeutic success. It is these questions that the NIH, working with clinical investigators, is best suited to answer.

## REFERENCES

1. Wells TG. Underserved therapeutic classes: examples which should not be ignored in infants and children. Drug Inf J 1996;30:1179–1186.
2. Specific requirements on content and format of labeling for human prescription drugs; revision of "Pediatric Use" subsection in the labeling; final rule. Food and Drug Administration, Department of Health and Human Services. Federal Register 1994;59:64240–64250, December 13, 1994.
3. Food and Drug Administration, Department of Health and Human Services. Regulations requiring manufacturers to assess the safety and effectiveness of new drugs and biologic products in pediatric patients; final rule. Federal Register 1998;63:66631–66672, December 2, 1998.
4. Food and Drug Administration Modernization Act of 1997. Public Law 105-115, 1997.
5. Best Pharmaceuticals for Children Act. Public Law 107-001, 2002.
6. United States Food and Drug Administration Center for Drug Evaluation and Research (n.d.). Approved active moieties to which the FDA has issued a Written Request for pediatric studies under section 505A of the Federal Food, Drug, and Cosmetic Act. Retrieved August 29, 2003, from http://www.fda.gov/cder/pediatric/wrlist/htm.
7. United States Food and Drug Administration Center for Drug Evaluation and Research. (n.d.) Pediatric exclusivity labeling changes. Retrieved August 29, 2003, from http://www.fda.gov/cder/pediatric/labelchange/htm.
8. Sakarcan A, Tenney F, Wilson JT, et al. The pharmacokinetics of irbesartan in hypertensive children and adolescents. J Clin Pharmacol 2001;41:742–749.
9. Wells TG, Rippley R, Hogg R, et al. The pharmacokinetics of enalapril in children and infants with hypertension. J Clin Pharmacol 2001;41:1064–1074.
10. Sorof JM, Cargo P, Graepel J, et al. β-blocker/thiazide combination for treatment of hypertensive children: a randomized double-blind, placebo-controlled trial. Pediatr Nephrol 2002;17:345–350.
11. Wells TG, Frame V, Soffer B, et al. A double-blind, placebo-controlled, dose-response study of the effectiveness and safety of enalapril for children with hypertension. J Clin Pharmacol 2002;42:870–880.
12. Blumer JL, Daniels SR, Dreyer WJ, et al. Pharmacokinetics of quinapril in children: assessment during substitution for chronic angiotensin-converting enzyme inhibitor treatment. J Clin Pharmacol 2003;43:128–132.
13. Trachtman H, Frank R, Mahan JD, et al. Clinical trial of extended-release felodipine in pediatric essential hypertension. Pediatr Nephrol 2003;18:548–553.
14. Center for Drug Evaluation and Research, Food and Drug Administration, United States Department of Health and Human Services. General considerations for the clinical evaluation of drugs in infants and children. HEW (FDA) 77-3041, 1977.
15. Center for Drug Evaluation and Research and Center for Biologics Evaluation and Research, Food and Drug Administration, United States Department of Health and Human Services. Guidance for industry: qualifying for pediatric exclusivity under section 505A of the Federal Food, Drug and Cosmetic Act. Docket No. 98D-0265, June 30, 1998.

16. Food and Drug Administration, United States Department of Health and Human Services. Additional safeguards for children in clinical investigations of FDA-regulated products. Federal Register 2001;66:20589–20598.
17. Center for Drug Evaluation and Research, Food and Drug Administration, United States Department of Health and Human Services. List of drugs for which additional pediatric information may produce health benefits in the pediatric population. Docket No. 98N-0056, 1998.
18. National Institute of Child Health and Human Development, National Institutes of Health, United States Department of Health and Human Services. Pediatric Off-Patent Drug Study (PODS) - Sodium Nitroprusside NICHD-2003-09. Retrieved August 29, 2003, from: http://www2.eps.gov/spg/HHS/NIH/NICHD/NICHD-2003-09/Attachments.html.
19. Center for Drug Evaluation and Research, Food and Drug Administration, United States Department of Health and Human Services. Sample written request for oral antihypertensives. Retrieved April 1999 from: http://www.fda.gov/cder/pediatric/htnwr.htm.
20. ICH Steering Committee. International Conference on Harmonisation of Technical Requirements for Registration of Pharmaceuticals for Human Use. Principles for clinical evaluation of new antihypertensive drugs. March 2, 2000.
21. Physicians' Desk Reference (57th Edition), Montvale, NJ: Thomson PDR, 2003.
22. National High Blood Pressure Education Program Working Group on Hypertension Control in Children and Adolescents. Update on the 1987 Task Force Report on High Blood Pressure in Children and Adolescents: a working group report from the National High Blood Pressure Education Program. Pediatrics 1996;98:649–658.
23. Morgenstern B. Blood pressure, hypertension, and ambulatory blood pressure monitoring in children. Am J Hypertens 2002;15:64S–66S.
24. Task Force on Blood Pressure Control in Children. Report of the Second Task Force on Blood Pressure Control in Children–1987. Pediatrics 1987;79:1–25.
25. Wells TG, Neaville WA, Arnold JR, Belsha CW. Evaluation of manual and semi-automated home blood pressure monitors in children and adolescents. Amer J Med Sci 1998;315:110–117.
26. Myers MG. Ambulatory blood pressure monitoring in the assessment of antihypertensive therapy. Blood Pressure Monitoring 1999;4:185–188.
27. Sorof JM. Ambulatory blood pressure monitoring in pediatric end-stage renal disease: chronic dialysis and transplantation. Blood Pressure Monitoring 1999;4:171–174.
28. Calvo-Vargas C, Padilla-Rios V, Troyo-Sanroman R. Loaned self-measurement equipment model compared with ambulatory blood pressure monitoring. Blood Press Monit 2003;8:63–70.
29. Sorof JM. Prevalence and consequences of systolic hypertension in children. Am J Hypertens 2002;15:57S–60S.
30. Wells TG, Zhang Z, Soffer BA, Shaw WC, Herrera PL, Shahinfar S. Antihypertensive trial design in children: blood pressure variability among the hypertensive children enrolled in the enalapril pediatric study (Abstract). Am J Hypertens 2001;14:109A.
31. Wells TG. Antihypertensive therapy: basic pharmacokinetic and pharmacodynamic principles as applied to infants and children. Am J Hypertens 2002;15:34S–37S.
32. Kearns GL, Reed MD. Clinical pharmacokinetics in infants and children: a reappraisal. Clin Pharmacokinet 1989;17(Suppl I):29–67.
33. Blumer JL, Reed MD. Principles of neonatal pharmacology. In: Yaffe SJ, Aranda JV, eds. Pediatric Pharmacology: Therapeutic Principles in Practice. Philadelphia: W.B. Saunders, 1992;164–177.

# 27 Management of Hypertensive Emergencies

*Raymond D. Adelman*, MD

*CONTENTS*



## INTRODUCTION

Severe hypertension (HTN) in childhood is uncommon but may have life-threatening consequences when it occurs. The concern of the clinician is the immediate and effective reduction of blood pressure (BP) to safer levels in order to mitigate the development or exacerbation of target organ injury. Equally important, the physician must avoid overly aggressive therapy that may in itself cause injury equal to or exceeding that of the presenting HTN *(1–4)*. A large and varied number of medications is currently available to lower blood pressure safely. This chapter will discuss etiology, clinical presentation, evaluation, pathophysiology, and treatment of severe HTN.

## DEFINITIONS OF HYPERTENSIVE EMERGENCIES AND URGENCIES

Hypertensive emergency *(2,5–9)*, the focus of this chapter, is defined as HTN that represents a threat to life or involves vital organs such as the brain, kidney, and heart. It may manifest with retinal hemorrhages, papilledema, encephalopathy, cardiac failure, pulmonary edema, renal insufficiency, or proteinuriua. In older terminology, hypertensive emergency would be termed malignant or accelerated hypertension *(2,5,6,10,11)*. While organ involvement is felt by some experts to be necessary to define hypertensive emergency, it would seem prudent to broaden the definition; it should also include any patient who, at the time of presentation, or in the very

From: *Clinical Hypertension and Vascular Disease: Pediatric Hypertension*
Edited by: R. J. Portman, J. M. Sorof, and J. R. Ingelfinger © Humana Press Inc., Totowa, NJ

near future, manifests, or will likely manifest, serious clinical signs, symptoms, or organ involvement. While this may necessitate management of some patients who do not ever progress to significant organ involvement, it is a clinically sensible approach, given the rapidity with which acute and significant deterioration may occur in a patient.

There is no absolute level of BP elevation that defines severe HTN. There are widely divergent opinions in this area. While the Second Task Force *(12)* defined severe HTN as exceeding the 99th percentile for age, others have suggested a diastolic BP in excess of 110 mmHg. Patients with BP above the 99th percentile frequently go unrecognized as having severe or even moderate HTN. This is especially true in the neonatal population, despite the availability of BP norms for gestational age, birthweight, and conceptual age *(13)*. Other patients with sustained chronic HTN may have levels well in excess of the 99th percentile and not have a hypertensive emergency. The preexisting BP, the chronicity of the HTN, and the acuteness and degree of elevation of BP at presentation are as important as the absolute BP value *(4)*. A 10-yr-old with acute glomerulonephritis, for example, and with acute HTN of 160/90 mmHg, may present with a seizure, whereas another 10-yr-old, with chronic HTN and a BP of 180/110 mmHg, may be relatively asymptomatic *(2)*.

## THE IMPORTANCE OF DEFINING SEVERE HYPERTENSION

A hypertensive emergency, as opposed to a hypertensive urgency, refers to how imminent serious clinical sequelae are, and the rapidity with which drug pressure must be lowered. The definition often dictates both the kinds of medications and the intensity of clinical surveillance. A hypertensive emergency requires immediate intervention within minutes to hours *(2,5–9)*, whereas a hypertensive urgency may be gradually managed over a period of a few days *(2)*. An emergency will require intravenous therapy and inpatient monitoring; an urgency is often treated with oral medications and, when deemed safe, in an outpatient setting.

## ETIOLOGIES OF SEVERE HYPERTENSION

Most patients with severe HTN have some underlying disease, usually renal in nature *(1,5,14)*. While essential HTN can present as a hypertensive emergency, it is uncommon in the pediatric population, especially in prepubertal children. Renal scarring, caused by reflux nephropathy or obstructive uropathy, various glomerulopathies, and renovascular disease are the most common etiologies *(1)*. Other causes include end stage renal disease in patients on dialysis, renal transplants (especially early in the posttransplant period), hemolytic uremic syndrome, cystic diseases of the kidneys, coarctation of the aorta, increased intracranial pressure and, less commonly, endocrine causes such as pheochromocytoma. In adolescents, one must also consider oral contraceptives, illicit drugs such as cocaine *(15)* and amphetamines, diet pills, and chewing tobacco *(16)*. The acute cessation of prescribed antihypertensives such as clonidine or β-blockers has also been associated with hypertensive crisis.

In the neonate, common etiologies include umbilical artery catheter-associated renal artery thrombosis and aortic thrombosis *(17)*, chronic pulmonary disease, and coarctation of the aorta. HTN is also seen with fluid and electrolyte excess related to undiagnosed renal insufficiency, or with administration of excessive sodium or calcium in parenteral nutrition. Frequently, severe HTN in the neonate goes unrecognized because BPs in vulnerable patients may not be routinely measured, levels in excess of the 99th percentile aren't recognized, or acute increments over baseline BP are not clinically appreciated *(17)*.

Table 1
Symptoms and Signs of Hypertensive Emergency

| | |
|---|---|
| Hypertensive retinopathy | 27% |
| Hypertensive encephalopathy | 25% |
| Convulsions | 25% |
| Left ventricular hypertrophy | 13% |
| Facial palsy | 12% |
| Visual symptoms | 9% |
| Hemiplegia | 8% |
| Cranial bruits | 5% |
| BP >99% without organ damage | 29% |

Modified from ref. *1*. Abbreviations: BP, blood pressure.

While a hypertensive emergency may occur with an acute illness such as poststreptococcal glomerulonephritis, patients have often had sustained HTN prior to presentation owing to chronic underlying renal disease or an undiagnosed coarctation.

## CLINICAL MANIFESTATIONS

Children with a hypertensive emergency usually present with signs and symptoms involving the central nervous system (CNS), heart, and kidneys. In a series of patients presenting at Great Ormond Street Hospital *(1)*, hypertensive retinopathy occurred in 27%, hypertensive encephalopathy in 25%, convulsions in 25%, left ventricular (LV) hypertrophy in 13%, facial palsy in 12%, visual symptoms in 9%, and hemiplegia in 8%. Interestingly, 29% of patients with BP greater than the 99th percentile had no end-organ damage (Table 1) *(1)*.

Visual symptoms included blurred vision, double vision, or loss of visual acuity and were caused by retinopathy, cortical damage, vitreous hemorrhage, or anterior ischemic optic neuropathy *(1)*. Optic neuropathy may lead to infarction of the optic nerve caused by ciliary arterial hypertensive damage, especially if BP is reduced too quickly *(18–20)*. In some cases, visual symptoms remitted with antihypertensive therapy, but patients subsequently developed blindness *(21)*. Encephalopathy may present with seizures, severe headaches (often described as splitting), altered sensorium, visual changes, dysarthria, and coma *(22,23)*. The diagnosis of severe HTN must always be considered in a patient presenting with an isolated Bell's palsy or a recurrent Bell's palsy *(24)*. Interestingly, the association between Bell's palsy and HTN was recognized by Moxon *(25)* in 1869.

The electroencephelogram (EEG) may be normal or display focal or diffuse delta slowing, especially in parietal or occipital areas. Head computed tomography (CT) may show diffuse, symmetric, well demarcated areas of hypodense white matter. Magnetic resonance imaging (MRI) often shows widespread lesions with focal increased T2 weight signals in the white matter and cortex, especially in the occipital area. Head CT and MRI studies may be completely normal in hypertensive encephalopathy *(26)*. The prognosis for children with hypertensive encephalopathy is unclear. Uhari *(22)* reported that 6 of 11 patients had long-term stigmata and that one child died in hypertensive crisis. Trompeter *(23)* reported no permanent neurological deficits among 45 patients, each of whom had each suffered a single episode of hypertensive encephalopathy.

Cardiac symptoms may include frank congestive failure associated with severe pulmonary edema *(27)*. LV hypertrophy is common *(2)*. Renal involvement may include a significant elevation in serum creatinine and/or proteinuria and hematuria. Proteinuria is usually in the nonnephrotic range *(2)*. Renal impairment may be the result of both a sustained hypertensive insult to the kidneys and/or an underlying renal condition that may have worsened with HTN. Some patients may have gastrointestinal symptoms, such as abdominal pain with hemorrhage secondary to microvascular damage. Patients with severe HTN may have a microangiopathic hemolytic anemia.

In neonates, common clinical manifestations of severe HTN include tachypnea, cardiomegaly, congestive heart failure, lethargy, seizures, retinopathy, and failure to thrive. Many severely hypertensive neonates are asymptomatic *(17)*.

## EVALUATION OF CHILDREN WITH HYPERTENSIVE CRISIS

The initial evaluation should include a complete history and physical examination focused towards identifying and treating underlying secondary causes of HTN. The clinician should inquire about inherited conditions, such as polycystic kidney disease, neurofibromatosis, or early onset HTN in family members. The neonatal course may provide clues such as prematurity, prolonged mechanical ventilation, or umbilical artery catheterization.

A history of urinary tract infections, vesicoureteral reflux, hospitalizations, and previous surgery should be explored. The clinician should ask about any current prescribed medications, over-the-counter medications such as decongestants, and, in adolescent, use of contraceptives and street drugs. In patients with known preexisting renal disease, the possibility that there has been worsening of the underlying condition, or failure to take prescribed medications with subsequent poor BP control or rebound HTN, should be considered *(28)*.

The physical examination should evaluate growth parameters, presence of dysmorphic features, unusual secondary sexual characteristics, and cutaneous abnormalities that might be associated with acute HTN. A careful fundoscopic exam may reveal retinal hemorrhages, papilledema, or exudates *(14,26,29)*. A thorough cardiovascular and neurological examination should be performed, including assessment for heart failure and abnormal mental status. BPs should be measured with the appropriate arm/leg-sized cuffs in upper and lower extremities to rule out coarctation or middle aortic syndrome *(30)*.

Initial laboratory studies should include a urinalysis, a complete blood count with a peripheral smear, electrolytes, calcium blood urea nitrogen, serum creatinine, a chest x-ray, and an electrocardiogram. A renal ultrasound with Doppler flow determination may be useful *(2)*. A cranial CT scan or MRI may be considered in order to evaluate for hypertensive encephalopathy, cerebral vascular ischemia, or hemorrhage, and also to evaluate a patient who is comatose *(31)*. If the CT scan or MRI is unrevealing in a patient with severe neurological dysfunction, especially an adolescent, a toxicology screen should be considered *(27)*.

## PATHOPHYSIOLOGY

The pathologic findings in severe HTN have been well documented, especially with regard to the kidneys *(32)*. Grossly, kidneys have subcapsular petechial hemorrhages that involve the cortex as well. Microscopically, glomeruli show fibrinoid necrosis, tubules have marked atrophy, and the interstitium displays fibrosis, hemorrhage, and patchy inflammation. The most dramatic changes are usually within the vasculature. Arterioles may display fibrinoid necrosis *(6,33)* with subendothelial plasma insudation. Intravascular hyaline thrombi may be present. The interlobular arteries may show marked intimal hyperplasia and proliferative endarteritis. The proliferation of intimal cells is described as "onion skin" changes and may be seen in larger vessels as well. There may also be medial hypertrophy and perivascular fibrosis. These changes can lead to virtually complete vascular occlusion and renal ischemia *(4)*, eliciting release of renin and resulting in the generation of Angiotensin II (ANG II) *(27)*. High peripheral renin levels may be primary or secondary to renal ischemia. Increased ANG II leads to further renal vasoconstriction and ischemia *(2)*.

CNS abnormalities *(29)* involve chronic changes in the vasculature, with fibrinoid necrosis of arterioles and recent changes caused by acute encephalopathy *(26)*. In the latter, there is breakdown of the blood brain barrier, and transudation of fluid into the brain resulting in localized or widespread edema *(27)*. Microinfarctions and petechial hemorrhages may occur *(2)*. Changes seen on CT include white matter hypodensity and generalized or focal edema. The MRI may show focal cortical and white matter increased T2 signal *(26,34)*. A condition called occipital parietal encephalopathy (PRES) *(35)*, with headaches, seizures, altered mental status, and cortical blindness has been described involving the parietal occipital region, with characteristic CT and MRI findings. PRES is reversible upon lowering BP.

The primary pathophysiological concern with severe HTN is the adverse impact on vascular autoregulation—that is, on the ability of renal and cerebral vasculature to maintain adequate blood flow to these organs across a wide range of arterial pressures *(36,37)*. This is especially of concern relative to the renal and cerebral circulations. Normally, with a decline in BP, the myogenic reflex in the afferent arteriole causes it to dilate *(38)*, which will maintain organ perfusion; a decline beyond a certain level is associated with a fall in renal blood flow and glomerular filtration rate. With increases in BP, arteriolar vasoconstriction diminishes the impact of high pressure on vulnerable organs. Above the upper end of the autoregulatory curve, preglomerular vasoconstriction is overcome by high pressure directly transmitted to the glomeruli *(38)*. The anatomic changes seen with severe HTN shift vascular responsiveness. In this setting, rigid vessels function more as pipes than as vasoreactive tissue, allowing the high pressures to be transmitted directly to viscera. Also in this setting, decreases in high BP cause exaggerated decreases in organ perfusion. Individual patients may no longer compensate for sudden falls in BP, which affects "watershed" areas and can lead to cerebral infarction, transverse ischemic myelopathy, or blindness *(6,18–20)*. Although most studies regarding the consequences of impaired autoregulation have concerned adult subjects, several reports in the pediatric population testify to the fact that children with sustained severe HTN are highly vulnerable to sudden drops in BP, usually as a result of overly-aggressive antihypertensive therapy (Table 2) *(3)*. Neonates are at particular risk for intracranial hemorrhage and other CNS sequelae related to both acute rises and declines in BP. Not only is there poor cerebral autoregulation in this age group, but neonates have highly vulnerable blood vessels in the subependymal germinal matrix *(17,39,40)*. The absence of clinically recognizable sequelae to dramatic changes in BP in some neonates shouldn't lull the clinician into minimizing the potential for injury.

## TREATMENT

The goal of treatment of a hypertensive emergency is the safe, well controlled lowering of BP, with preservation of target organ function and avoidance of therapeutic complications such as ischemic neuropathy of the optic nerve, transverse ischemic myelopathy, and renal impair-

Table 2
Signs and Symptoms Developed During Treatment of Hypertensive Emergency

| | *Bolus* *(n = 13)* | *Infusion* *(n = 2)* |
|---|---|---|
| Transient visual loss | 6 | 0 |
| Transient acute renal failure | 5 | 2 |
| Permanent visual loss | 4 | 0 |
| Transverse ischemic myelopathy | 1 | 0 |
| % complications | 23 | 4 |
| % permanent complications | 7 | 0 |

Modified from ref. *1*.

ment *(3,6,18–20)*. These complications largely occur when BP is lowered too quickly in the face of a loss of autoregulatory function caused by chronic HTN. Deal et al. *(1)* evaluated 110 severely hypertensive pediatric patients presenting over a 10-yr period. 57 patients were treated with intravenous boluses of diazoxide or hydralazine with intent to normalize BP in 12–24 h. 13 patients developed significant complications (Table 2) including 4 who suffered irreversible neurological damage. Subsequently, in a later era, 53 patients were treated with a controlled, gradual BP reduction over 96 h using labetolol and/or nitroprusside. Only 2 patients among these 53 developed transient hypotensive complications.

Similar experiences of complications caused by abrupt and profound changes in BP have been reported in neonates *(41)* and adults *(42)*. It is recommended *(3)* that patients with hypertensive emergency be placed in an intensive care setting with careful monitoring and experienced nursing and physician support. BP should be reduced by 25–30% of the desired amount in the first 6 h, another 25–30% in the next 24–36 h, and then to the final desired level over 48–72 h *(2,3)*. The desired level in the acute setting should be a safe BP, for example, near the 95th percentile, and not necessarily at a normal BP. The patient should have BP monitored carefully, as well as frequent clinical evaluations for pupillary reactivity, visual acuity, level of consciousness, and other neurological findings. Fluid balance and renal function should be carefully monitored *(2)*. An intravenous line for volume expansion with normal saline should be available in the event that hypotension occurs.

Because of changes in renal vascular autoregulation caused by chronic HTN, it is not uncommon for renal function to decline initially*(38)*. However, the renal function in most patients will improve over time. In some patients, long-term control of BP has allowed patients to be removed from dialysis *(43,44)*.

There is a variety of medications available to treat hypertensive emergencies. Ideally, medicines should be given intravenously, be easily titratable to effect, have short half lives, and produce minimal side effects. Among the preferred medications are sodium nitroprusside *(1,5,9,28,45–48)*, labetalol *(1,5,9,28,45,46,49–51)*, nicardipine *(52–60)*, and, recently, fenoldopam. While each agent has distinct pharmacologic actions, most can be used in most cases of severe HTN, regardless of the underlying etiology. Occasionally, a specific agent may be more tailored to a specific clinical condition, such as the use of labetelol in high catecholamine-induced HTN. It is important for the clinician to gain familiarity and comfort with one or more of these agents. Other agents that have been used in acute HTN include intravenous diazoxide, hydralazine, esmolol, and enalaprilat. Diazoxide, a direct arteriolar vasodilator, may be given in pulse dosages or by slow intravenous infusion *(61–66)*. Pediatric experience with intravenous infusion of diazoxide is limited; hypotensive complications may occur, as well as significant hyperglycemia *(28)*. Hydralazine *(5,28,46)*, a direct arteriolar vasodilator, causes significant reflex tachycardia and headaches, and has an unacceptably long half-life. Experience with esmolol *(9,46,67,68)*, a cardio-selective β-blocker, is limited in the pediatric population. Because esmolol is short-acting, titratable, cardioselective, and parenterally administered, it may be particularly useful in catecholamine-mediated HTN such as post-coarctation repair *(68)*, or in theophylline and caffeine overdosages. Esmolol has no direct vascular action; its hypotensive effect is owing to decreased cardiac output associated with reduced heart rate and cardiac index *(67)*. Enalaprilat *(69,70)*, an angiotensin converting enzyme (ACE) inhibitor, has a slower onset of action and an unacceptably long half-life. It should not be administered to patients with bilateral renal artery stenosis or single kidneys, or to children with renal transplants in whom posttransplant renal artery stenosis is a consideration *(28)*. If use of an ACE inhibitor increases initial serum creatinine by more than 30%, or causes a progressive rise in serum creatinine, it should be discontinued and the patient investigated for renal artery stenosis *(38)*. ACE inhibitors may also be associated with hyperkalemia.

A number of oral drugs have been used to treat hypertensive emergencies, the most popular of which is nifedipine *(71–81)*, a calcium channel blocker (CCB) with a fairly rapid onset. Although nifedipine has been widely used, this agent and other oral or sublingual agents are not recommended in the treatment of a hypertensive emergency *(3,81)*. Sublingual absorption of nifedipine is unpredictable, as is the extent and duration of its hypotensive action. The risk of overshooting a desired level, as well as a prolonged duration of effect of several hours, makes this drug particularly inappropriate. Although a recent survey of pediatric nephrologists suggests continued use of this drug, especially for asymptomatic patients with severe HTN *(78)*, 10% of respondents identified serious adverse consequences. The adult literature also carries reports of serious consequences owing to profound falls in BP *(79)*. Other oral agents such as captopril *(41,82–86)* and minoxidil *(28,45,46)* carry similar risks.

Table 3 lists the commonly used antihypertensive drugs for severe HTN, noting those favored by the author. Sodium nitroprusside *(1,5,9,28,45–48)* is a potent dilator of arteriolar and venous beds, acts within seconds, has a very short half-life of seconds to minutes, and is quite easy to titrate. Exposure to light must be avoided, since it is inactivated by light. Sodium nitroprusside can cause hypotension and reflex tachycardia. Though it is metabolized to thiocyanate, high thiocyanate levels *(88,89)* are uncommon and mainly seen with high drug dosages, prolonged administration, or renal insufficiency. The risk of cyanide toxicity is substantially reduced by the addition of sodium thiosulfate to sodium nitroprusside. The necessity to monitor plasma cyanide/thiocyanate levels, and the need to cover the medication and infusion lines, make use of this drug cumbersome.

Labetolol *(1,5,9,28,45,46,49–51)*, a combined α- and β-blocker, has an onset of action within 5–10 min, a relative moderate duration of action of 2–3 h, and is especially useful in HTN associated with increased circulating catecholamines and CNS-mediated HTN. Since vasodilators such as sodium nitroprusside and hydralazine increase intracranial pressure *(28,57)*, labetolol has a role in such patients. It should be avoided in patients with heart failure or asthma. It has also been associated with significant hyperkalemia in patients with end stage renal disease *(90,91)*.

Nicardipine *(52-60)*, a CCB with an onset of action within minutes and a half-life of 10 min, acts primarily as a peripheral vasodilator. Baseline blood pressure is reached in about 30–60

Table 3
Recommended Drugs for Treatment of a Hypertensive Emergency

| *Drug* | *Route* | *Dose* | *Action* | *Onset of action* | *Duration* | *Comment* |
|---|---|---|---|---|---|---|
| Labetalol | IV | 0.5–3 mg/kg per h | α and β sympathetic blocker | 5–10 min | 2–3 h | Contraindicated in patients with asthma. May cause bradycardia and worsen heart failure |
| Sodium nitroprusside[a] | IV | 0.5–8 μg/kg per min | Vasodilator of arteriolar and venous beds. Acts as endogenous NO | Within s | Short half-life—s to min. | Inactivated by light. May cause hypotension, reflex tachycardia, cyanide and thiocyanate toxicity. May cause increased cerebral blood flow and intra cranial pressure |
| Nicardipine[a] | IV | 0.5–3 μg/kg per min | CCB | Within min | 15–30 min | Reflex tachycardia. May increase cyclosporin A levels. Thrombophlebits |
| Fenoldopam[a] | IV | 0.5–2 μg/kg per min | Dopamine 1 receptor agonist | 15 min | 15-30 min | May cause headaches, tachycardia. Contraindicated with glaucoma |
| Hydralazine | IV | 0.1–0.5 mg/kg | Direct arteriolar vasodilator | 10–30 min | 4–12 h | Causes reflex tachycardia, headaches, flushing, fluid retention |
| Clonidine | IV | 2–6 μg/kg | Central α adrenergic stimulation | 10 min | 3–7 h | Rebound HTN reported after use |
| Esmolol | IV | 50–300 μg/kg per min | Cardio-selective β adrenoceptive antagonist | Within s | 10–20 min | Not compatible with $NaHCO_3$ Avoid if history of asthma May cause bradycardia |
| Enalaprilat | IV | 0.005–0.01 mg/kg 8–24 hourly | Angiotensin converting enzyme inhibitor | Within 15 min | 12–24 h | Should not be used if severe renal artery stenosis present or suspected, especially if bilateral |

[a] Preferred by author
Abbreviations: CCB, calcium channel blocker; HTN, hypertension.

min *(56,58)*. There is now much more pediatric experience with nicardipine, which has proven safe, effective, easy to use, and responsible for minimal side effects in patients with hypertensive emergencies of a variety of etiologies. It has been used in all age ranges, including neonates, is usually effective as a single agent, and appears safe and effective when given for prolonged periods *(60,87)* (Fig. 1). For many, nicardipine is the preferred drug for treatment of a hypertensive emergency.

Fenoldopam *(92–99)* is a selective dopamine-1-receptor agonist that has been tested extensively in adults and, to a limited extent, in children. It is a short-acting, parenteral arteriolar vasodilator that acts on dopamine 1 receptors present in mesenteric, renal, coronary, and

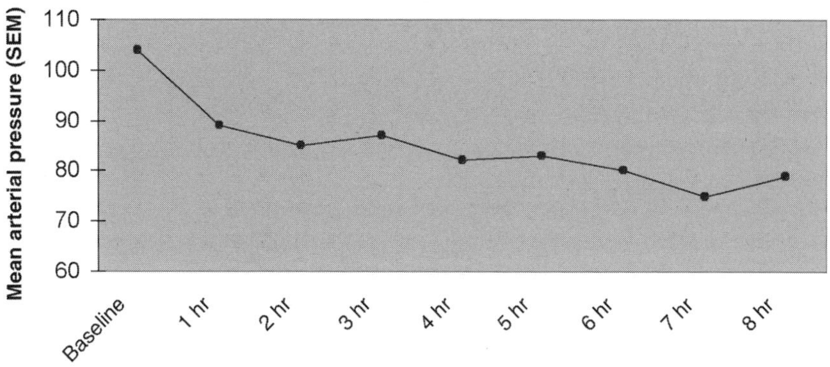


Fig. 1. Antihypertensive effect of nicardipine in 15 pediatric patients (modified from ref. *55*).

cerebral arterioles. It is also a direct inhibitor of proximal and distal tubular sodium transport. In a number of studies, fenoldopam has shown hypotensive effectiveness comparable to nitroprusside in patients with severe HTN. Furthermore, there have been impressive improvements in creatinine clearance, urine flow, and urinary sodium excretion *(92,93,96)* when this agent is used. Accordingly, it would seem that this drug might be especially useful in patients with compromised renal function because of its salutory effects on renal function. Furthermore, since fenoldopam is cleared via hepatic conjugation, dosages need not be adjusted for renal insufficiency *(97)*. The recommended dosage in children is 0.5 μg/kg/min to 2.0 μg/kg/min—somewhat higher than in adults; some patients have required as much as 5 μg/kg/min *(97)*. Hemodynamic studies show dramatic decreases in peripheral vascular resistance, modest decreases in pulmonary vascular resistance, and increased cardiac ejection fraction. Target BPs have been reached quickly. Side effects include headaches and cutaneous flushing. Because fenoldopam increases intraocular pressure, it is contraindicated in patients with glaucoma *(94)*. Fenoldopam is considerably more expensive than other drugs used for hypertensive emergencies, but may have a role in selected patients, such as those with significant renal compromise.

Whereas α adrenergic blockade with phenoxybenzamine given preoperatively is the ideal approach to the patient with a diagnosed pheochromocytoma, phentolamine is the recommended drug for patients with pheochromocytoma presenting with an acute hypertensive emergency, developing hypertensive crisis during radiographic evaluation, or in the perioperative period. Phentolamine is a potent adrenergic inhibitor with an onset of 1–2 min and a duration of 10–30 min. The recommended dose is 0.05–0.10 mg/kg/dose intravenously.

In summary, a hypertensive emergency, though uncommon, may have life-threatening consequences, as well as serious CNS, cardiac, and renal sequelae. After a careful history and physical examination, attention must be directed toward the immediate reduction of BP to a safe, though not necessarily normal, level. The appropriate medications should be intravenous, have short half-lives, be easily titratable, and have few side effects. Patients should be monitored in an intensive care setting with appropriately trained medical staff. Sodium nitroprusside, nicardipine, labetolol, and, in certain cases, fenoldopam and esmolol, are drugs of choice. Gradual, controlled, and moderate reduction in BP reduces the risk of serious complications that occur when BP is lowered too quickly. The aggressive use of intravenous medications, or the use of oral medications, should be avoided.

## REFERENCES


1. Deal JE, Barratt TM, Dillon MJ. Management of hypertensive emergencies. Arch Dis Child 1992;67:1089–1092.
2. Kitiyakara C, Guzman NJ. Malignant hypertension and hypertensive emergencies. J Am Soc Nephrol 1998;9:133–142.
3. Adelman RD, Coppo R, Dillon MJ. The emergency management of severe hypertension. Pediatr Nephrol 2000;14:422–427.
4. Elliott WJ. Hypertensive emergencies. Crit Care Clin 2001;17:435–451.
5. Arbus GS, Farine M. Management of hypertensive emergencies in children. In: Loggie JMH, ed. Pediatric and Adolescent Hypertension. Oxford: Blackwell Scientific, 1992;369–377.
6. Isles CG. Hypertensive emergencies: malignant hypertension and hypertensive encephalopathy. In: Swales JD, ed. Textbook of Hypertension. Oxford: Blackwell Scientific, 1994;1233–1248.
7. Abdelwahab W, Frishmen W, Landau A. Management of hypertensive urgencies and emergencies. J Clin Pharmacol 1995;35:747–762.
8. Zampaglion B, Pascale C, Marchisio M, Cavallo Perin P. Hypertensive urgencies and emergencies. Prevalence and clinical presentation. Hypertension 1995;27:144–147.
9. Fivush B, Neu A, Furth S. Acute hypertensive crisis in children: emergencies and urgencies. Curr Opin Pediatr 1996;9:233–236.
10. World Health Organization. Arterial hypertension. World Health Organ Tech Rep Ser 1978;628–657.
11. Cetta F, Hurley RM, Hatch D, Castelli M. Malignant hypertension. J Pediatr 1991;118:981–986.
12. National Heart, Lung and Blood Institute. Report of the second task force on blood pressure control in children 1987. Pediatrics 1987;79:1–25.
13. Zubrow AB, Hulman S, Kushner H, Falkner B. Determinants of blood pressure in infants admitted to neonatal intensive care units: a prospective multicenter study. J Perinatol 1995;15:479.
14. Sadowski RH, Falkner B. Hypertension in pediatric patients. Am J Kidney Dis 1996;27:305–315.
15. Thakur V, Godley C, Weed S, Cook ME, Hoffman E. Case reports: cocaine-associated accelerated hypertension and renal failure. Am J Med Sci 1996;312:295–298.
16. Adelman RD. Smokeless tobacco and hypertension in an adolescent. Pediatrics 1987;79:837–838.
17. Adelman RD. The hypertensive neonate. Clin Perinatol 1988;15:567–585.
18. Ledingham JG, Rajagopalan B. Cerebral complications in the treatment of accelerated hypertension. Q J Med 1997;48:25–41.
19. Hulse JA, Taylor DS, Dillon MJ. Blindness and paraplegia in severe childhood hypertension. Lancet 1979;II:553–556.
20. Taylor D, Ramsay J, Day S, Dillon M. Infarction of the optic nerve head in children with accelerated hypertension. Br J Opthalmol 1981;65:153–160.
21. Browning AC, Mengher LS, Gregson RM, Amoaku WM. Visual outcome of malignant hypertension in young people. Arch Dis Child 2001;85:401–403.
22. Uhari M, Saukkonen AL, Koskimies O. Central nervous system involvement in severe arterial hypertension of childhood. Eur J Pediatr 1979;132:141–146.
23. Trompeter RS, Smith RL, Hoare RD, Neville BG, Chantler C. Neurological complications of arterial hypertension. Arch Dis Child 1982;57:913–917.
24. Harms MM, Rotteveel JJ, Kar NC, Gabreels FJ. Recurrent alternating facial paralysis and malignant hypertension. Neuropediatrics 2001;31:318–320.
25. Moxon W. Apoplexy into canal of fallopius in a case of Bright's disease, causing facial paralysis. Trans Pathol Soc Lond 1869;20:420–422.
26. Wright RR, Mathews KD. Hypertensive encephalopathy in childhood. J Child Neurol 1996;11:193–196.
27. Phillips RA, Greenblatt J, Krakoff LR. Hypertensive emergencies: diagnosis and management. Prog Cardiovasc Dis 2002;45:33–48.
28. Dillon MJ, Inglefinger JR. Pharmacological treatment of hypertension. In: Holiday MA, Barratt TM, Avner ED, eds. Pediatric Nephrology, 3rd ed. Baltimore: Williams Wilkins, 1994;1165–1174.
29. Menkes JH, Fink BW, Hurvitz CGH, Hyman CB, Jordan SC, Watanabe F. Neurological manifestations of systemic disease. In: Menkes JH, Sarnat HB. eds. Child Neurology, 6th ed. Philidelphia: Williams Wilkins, 2000;1120–1121.
30. Panayiotopoulos YP, Tyrrell MR, Koffman G, Reidy JF, Haycock GB, Taylor PR. Mid-aortic syndrome presenting in childhood. Br J Surg 1996;83:235–240.

31. Vidt DG. Emergency room management of hypertensive urgencies and emergencies. J Clin Hypertens 2001;3:158–164.
32. Goldblatt PJ, Gohara AF, Khan NH, Hampton JA. Benign and malignant nephrosclerosis and renovascular hypertension. In: Tisher CC, Brenner BM, eds. Renal Pathology with Clinical and Functional Correlations. Philidelphia: Lippincott, 1989;II:1131–1159.
33. Kincaid Smith P. Malignant hypertension. J Hypertens 1991;9:893–899.
34. Jones BV, Egelhoff JC, Patterson RJ. Hypertensive encephalopathy in children. Am J Neuroradiol 1997;18: 101–106.
35. Hinchey J, Chaves C, Appignani B, et al. A reversible posterior leukoencephalopathy syndrome. N Engl J Med 1996;334:494–500.
36. Strandgaard S, Paulson OB. Cerebral autoregulation. Stroke 1984;15:413–416.
37. Strandgaard S, Olesen J, Skinhoj E, Lassen NA. Autoregulation of brain circulation in severe arterial hypertension. BMJ 1973;1:507–510.
38. Palmer BF. Renal dysfunction complicating the treatment of hypertension. N Eng J Med 2002;347:1256–1261.
39. Goddard J, Lewis RM, Armstrong DL, et al. Moderate rapidly induced hypertension as a cause of intraventricular hemorrhage in the newborn beagle model. J Pediatr 1980;96:1057–1060.
40. Perlman J. Intrapartum hypoxic-ischemic cerebral injury and cerebral palsy. Pediatrics 1997;99:851–859.
41. Perlman JM, Volpe JJ. Neurologic complications of captopril treatment of neonatal hypertension. Pediatrics 1989;83:47–52.
42. Hoshide S, Kario K, Fujikawa H, Ikeda U, Shimada K. Hemodynamic cerebral infarction triggered by excessive blood pressure reduction in hypertensive emergencies. J Am Geriatr Soc 1998;46:1179–1180.
43. Mroczek WJ, Davidov M, Gavrilovich L, Finnerty FA. The value of aggressive therapy in the hypertensive patient with azotemia. Circulation 1969;40:893.
44. Adelman RD, Russo J. Malignant hypertension: recovery of renal function after treatment with antihypertensive medications and hemodialysis. J Pediatr 1981;98:766–768.
45. Houtman PN, Dillon MJ. Medical management of hypertension in childhood. Child Nephrol Urol 1992;12: 154–161.
46. Sinaiko AR. Treatment of hypertension in children. Pediatr Nephrol 1994;8:603–609.
47. Gordillo Paniagua G, Velasquez Jones L, Martini R, Valdez Bolanos E. Sodium nitroprusside treatment of severe arterial hypertension in children. J Pediatr 1975;87:799–802.
48. Luderer JR, Hayes AH Jr, Dubnsky O, Cerlin CM. Long-term administration of sodium nitroprusside in childhood. J Pediatr 1977;91:490–491.
49. Cumming AM, Davies DL. Intravenous labetalol in hypertensive emergency. Lancet 1979;I:929–930.
50. Cressman MD, Vidt DG, Gifford RW, Moore WS, Wilson DJ. Intravenous labetalol in the management of severe hypertension and hypertensive emergencies. Am Heart J 1984;107:980–985.
51. Bunchman TE, Lynch RE, Wood EG. Intravenously administered labetalol for treatment of hypertension in children. J Pediatr 1992;120:140–144.
52. Wallin JD, Fletcher, Ran CVS, et al. Intravenous nicardipine for the treatment of severe hypertension. Arch Intern Med 1989;149:2662–2669.
53. Tjoa HI, Ram CVS. Immediate control of severe hypertension with intravenous nicardipine or sodium nitroprusside. Am J Hypertens 1990;3:104A.
54. Treluyer JM, Hubert P, Jouvet P, Couderc S, Cloup M. Intravenous nicardipine in hypertensive children. Eur J Pediatr 1993;152:712–714.
55. Sartori SC, Nakagawa TA, Solhaug MJ, Morris A, Adelman RD. Intravenous nicardipine for treatment of systemic hypertension in children. Pediatr Res 1999;45:A258.
56. Hersey SL, O'Dell NE, Lowe S, et al. Nicardipine versus nitroprusside for controlled hypotension during spinal surgery in adolescents. Anesth Analg 1997;84:1239–1244.
57. Micheal J, Groshong T, Tobias JD. Nicardipine for hypertensive emergencies in children with renal disease. Pediatr Nephrol 1998;12:40–42.
58. Tenney F, Sakarcan A. Nicardipine is a safe and effective agent in pediatric hypertensive emergencies. Am J Kidney Dis. 2000;35:E20.
59. Tobias JD. Nicardipine to control mean arterial pressure after cardiothoracic surgery in infants and children. Am J Ther 2001;8:3–6.
60. Flynn JT, Mottes TA, Brophy PD, Kershaw DB, Smoyer WE, Bunchman TE. Intravenous necardipine for treatment of severe hypertension in children. J Pediatr 2001;139:38–43.

61. McLaine PN, Drummond KN. Intravenous diazoxide for severe hypertension in childhood. J Pediatr 1971;79:829–832.
62. Henrich WL, Cronin R, Miller PD, Anderson RJ. Hypotensive sequelae of diazoxide and hydralazine therapy. JAMA 1977;237:264–265.
63. McCrory WW, Kohaut EC, Lewy JE, Lieberman E, Travis LB. Safety of intravenous diazoxide in children with severe hypertension. Clin Pediatr (Phila) 1979;18:661–663, 666–667, 671.
64. Wilson DJ, Lewis RC, Vidt DG. Control of severe hypertension with pulse diazoxide. Cardiovasc Clin 1981;12:79–91.
65. Thien TA, Huysmans FT, Gerlag PG, Koene RA, Wijdeveld PG. Diazoxide infusion in severe hypertension and hypertensive crisis. Clin Pharmacol Ther 1979;25:795–799.
66. Ram CV, Kaplan NM. Individual titration of diazoxide dosage in treatment of severe hypertension. Am J Cardiol 1979;43:627–630.
67. Cuneo BF, Zales VR, Blahunka PC, Benson DW Jr. Pharmacodynamics and pharmacokinetics of esmolol, a short-acting beta-blocking agent, in children. Pediatr Cardiol 1994;15:296–301.
68. Wiest DB, Garner SS, Uber WE, Sade RM. Esmolol for the management of pediatric hypertension after cardiac operations. J Thorac Cardiovasc Surg 1998;115:890–897.
69. Hirschl MM, Binder M, Bur A, et al. Clinical evaluation of different doses of intravenous enalaprilat in patients with hypertensive crisis. Arch Intern Med 1995;155:2217–2223.
70. Strauss R, Gavras I, Vlahakos D, Gavras H. Enalaprilat in hypertensive emergencies. J Clin Pharmacol 1986;26:39–43.
71. Bertel O, Conen D, Radu EW, Muller J, Lang C, Dubach UC. Nifedipine in hypertensive emergencies. Brit Med J 1983;286:19–21.
72. Dilmen U, Caglar MK, Senses DA, Kinik E. Nifedipine in hypertensive emergencies of children. Am J Dis Child 1983;137:1162–1165.
73. Rascher W, Bonzel KE, Ruder H, Muller Wiefel DE, Scharer K. Blood pressure and hormonal responses to sublingual nifedipine in acute childhood hypertension. Clin Exp Hypertens A 1986;8:859–869.
74. Roth B, Herkenrath P, Krebber J, Abu Chaaban M. Nifedipine in hypertensive crisis of infants and children. Clin Exp Hypertens A 1986;8:871–877.
75. Wachter RM. Symptomatic hypotension induced by nifedipine in the acute treatment of severe hypertension. Arch Intern Med 1987;147:556–558.
76. Lopez Herce J, Albajara L, Cagigas P, Garcia S, Ruza R. Treatment of hypertensive crisis in children with nifedipine. Intensive Care Med 1988;14:519–521.
77. van Harten J, Burrraaf K, Danhof M, van Brummelen P, Breimer DD. Negligible sublingual absorption of nifedipine. Lancet 1987;II:1363–1365.
78. Gauthier B, Trachtman H. Short acting nifedipine. Pediatr Nephrol 1997;11:786–787.
79. Grossman E, Messerli FH, Grodzicki T, Kowey P. Should a moratorium be placed on sublingual nifedipine capsules given for hypertensive emergencies and pseudoemergencies? JAMA 1996;276:1328–1231.
80. Blaszak RT, Savage JA, Ellis EN. The use of short-acting nifedipine in pediatric patients with hypertension. J Pediatr 2001;139:34–37.
81. Calvetta A, Martino S, von Vigier RO, Schmidtko J, Fossali E, Bianchetti MG. "What goes up must immediately come down!" Which indication for short-acting nifedipine in children with arterial hypertension? Pediatr Nephrol 2003;18:1–2.
82. Griswold W, McNeal R, O'Connor D, Reznik V, Mendoza D. Oral converting enzyme inhibitor in malignant hypertension. Arch Dis Child 1982;57:235–237.
83. Biollaz J, Waeber B, Brunner HR. Hypertensive crisis treated with orally administered captopril. Eur J Clin Pharmacol 1983;25:145–149.
84. Hauger Klevene JH. Captopril in hypertensive crisis. Lancet 1985;II:732–733.
85. Angeli P, Chiesa M, Caregaro L, et al. Comparison of sublingual captopril and nifedipine in immediate treatment of hypertensive emergencies. A randomized, single-blind clinical trial. Arch Intern Med 1991;151:678–682.
86. O'Dea RF, Mirkin BL, Alward CT, Sinaiko AR. Treatment of neonatal hypertension with captopril. J Pediatr 1988;113:403–406.
87. Gouyon JB, Geneste B, Semama DS, Francoise M, Germain JF. Intravenous nacardipine in hypertensive preterm infants. Arch Dis Child 1997;76:F126–F127.

88. Kunathai S, Sholler GF, Celermajer J, O'Halloran M, Cartmill TB, Nunn GR. Nitroprusside in children after cardio-pulmonary bypass: a study of thiocyanate toxicity. Pediatr Cardiol 1989;10:121–124.
89. Linakis JG, Lacouture PG, Woolf A. Monitoring cyanide and thiocyanate concentrations during infusion of sodium nitroprusside in children. Pediatr Cardiol 1991;12:214–218.
90. Hamad A, Salameh M, Zihlif M, Feinfeld DA, Carvounis CP. Life-threatening hyperkalemia after intravenous labetolol injection for hypertensive emergency in a hemodialysis patient. Am J Nephrol 2001;21:241–244.
91. Arthur S, Greenburg A. Hyperkalemia associated with intravenous labetalol therapy for acute hypertension in renal transplant recipients. Clin Nephrol 1990;33:269–271.
92. Elliott WJ, Weber RR, Nelson KS, et al. Renal and hemodynamic effects of intravenous fenoldopam versus nitroprusside in severe hypertension. Circulation 1990;81:970–977.
93. Shusterman NH, Elliott WJ, White WB. Fendoldopam, but not nitroprusside, improves renal function in severly hypertensive patients with impared renal function. Am J Med 1993;95:161–168.
94. Post JB 4$^{th}$, Frishman WH. Fenoldopam: a new dopamine agonist for the treatment of hypertensive urgencies and emergencies. J Clin Pharmacol 1998;38:2–13.
95. Tumlin JA, Dunbar LM, Oparil S, et al. Fenoldopam, a dopamine agonist, for hypertensive emergency: a multicenter randomized trial. Fenoldopam Study Group. Acad Emerg Med 2000;7:653–662.
96. Murphy MB, Murray C, Shorten GD. Fenoldopam: a selective peripheral dopamine-receptor agonist for the treatment of severe hypertension. N Engl J Med 2001;345:1548–1557.
97. Strauser LM, Pruitt RD, Tobias JD. Initial experience with fenoldopam in children. Am J Ther 1999;6: 283–288.
98. Tobias JD. Fenoldopam for controlled hypotension during spinal fusion in children and adolescents. Paediatr Anaesth 2000;10:261–266.
99. Tobias JD. Controlled hypotension in children: a critical review of available agents. Pediatr Drugs 2002;4: 439–453.

# Appendix

## *Blood Pressure Tables From the Fourth Report on the Diagnosis, Evaluation, and Treatment of High Blood Pressure in Children and Adolescents*

This appendix contains the recently published blood pressure (BP) normative tables, definitions of hypertension, and techniques to calculate a child's exact BP percentile. This appendix is published with the permission of the NHLBI Working Group Report of the Fourth Report on the Diagnosis, Evaluation and Treatment of High Blood Pressure in Children and Adolescents and the American Academy of Pediatrics, who will publish the entire report in *Pediatrics*.

### DEFINITIONS OF HYPERTENSION

In children and adolescents, the normal range of BP is determined by body size and age. BP standards that are based on sex, age, and height provide a more precise classification of BP according to body size. This approach avoids misclassifying children who are very tall or very short.

The BP tables are revised to include the new height percentile data (http://www.cdc.gov/growthcharts/) (Centers for Disease Control and Prevention and National Center for Health Statistics, 2000) as well as the addition of BP data from the NHANES 1999–2000. The 50th, 90th, 95th, and 99th percentiles of systolic blood pressure (SBP) and diastolic blood pressure (DBP) (using K5) for height by sex and age are given for boys and girls in Tables 3 and 4. Although new data have been added, the sex, age, and height BP levels for the 90th and 95th percentiles have changed minimally from the last report. The 50th percentile has been added to the tables to provide the clinician with the BP level at the midpoint of the normal range. Although the 95th percentile provides a BP level that defines hypertension, management decisions in children with hypertension should be determined by the degree or severity of hypertension. Therefore, the 99th percentile has been added to facilitate clinical decision making in the plan for evaluation. Standards for SBP and DBP for infants aged younger than 1 yr are available (Task Force on Blood Pressure Control in Children, 1987).

To use the tables in a clinical setting, the height percentile is determined by using the newly revised CDC Growth Charts (http://www.cdc.gov/growthcharts). The child's measured SBP and DBP are compared with the numbers provided in the table (boys or girls) according to the child's age and height percentile. The child is normotensive if the BP is below the 90th percentile. If the BP is equal to or above the 90th percentile, the BP measurement should be repeated at that visit to verify an elevated BP. BP measurements between the 90th and 95th percentiles indicate prehypertension and warrant reassessment and consideration of other risk

From: *Clinical Hypertension and Vascular Disease: Pediatric Hypertension*
Edited by: R. J. Portman, J. M. Sorof, and J. R. Ingelfinger © Humana Press Inc., Totowa, NJ

factors (*see* Table 5). In addition, if an adolescent's BP is greater than 120/80 mmHg, the patient should be considered to be prehypertensive even if this value is less than the 90th percentile. This BP level typically occurs for SBP at age 12 yr and for DBP at age 16 yr. If the child's BP (systolic or diastolic) is at or above the 95th percentile, the child may be hypertensive, and the measurement must be repeated on at least two additional occasions to confirm the diagnosis. Staging of BP, according to the extent to which a child's BP exceeds the 95th percentile, is helpful in developing a management plan for evaluation and treatment that is most appropriate for an individual patient. On repeated measurement, hypertensive children may have BP levels that are only a few mmHg above the 95th percentile; these children would be managed differently from hypertensive children who have BP levels that are 15–20 mmHg above the 95th percentile. An important clinical decision is to determine which hypertensive children require more immediate attention for elevated BP. The difference between the 95th and 99th percentiles is only 7–10 mmHg and is not large enough, particularly in view of the variability in BP measurements, to adequately distinguish mild hypertension—where limited evaluation is most appropriate—from more severe hypertension where more immediate and extensive intervention is indicated. Therefore, Stage 1 hypertension is the designation for BP levels that range from the 95th percentile to 5 mmHg above the 99th percentile. Stage 2 hypertension is the designation for BP levels that are higher than the 99th percentile plus 5 mmHg. Once confirmed on repeated measures, Stage 1 hypertension allows time for evaluation before initiating treatment unless the patient is symptomatic. Patients with Stage 2 hypertension may need more prompt evaluation and pharmacologic therapy. Symptomatic patients with Stage 2 hypertension require immediate treatment and consultation with experts in pediatric hypertension. These categories are parallel to the staging of hypertension in adults, as noted in JNC 7 (Chobanian et al., 2003).

## *Using the BP Tables*

1. Use the standard height charts to determine the height percentile.
2. Measure and record the child's SBP and DBP.
3. Use the correct gender table for SBP and DBP.
4. Find the child's age on the left side of the table. Follow the age row horizontally across the table to the intersection of the line for the height percentile (vertical line).
5. There, find the 50th, 90th, 95th, and 99th percentiles for SBP in the left columns and for DBP in the right columns.

   - BP less than the 90th percentile is normal.
   - BP between the 90th and 95th percentile is prehypertension. BP equal to or exceeding 120/80 but remains less than the 95th percentile is prehypertension, even if this figure is less than the 90th percentile.
   - BP greater than the 95th percentile may be hypertension.

6. If the BP is greater than the 90th percentile, the BP should be repeated twice at the same office visit, and an average SBP and DBP should be used.
7. If the BP is greater than the 95th percentile, BP should be staged. If Stage 1 (95th percentile to the 99th percentile plus 5 mmHg), BP measurements should be repeated on two more occasions. If hypertension is confirmed, evaluation should proceed as noted in the Working Group Report. If BP is Stage 2 (>99th percentile plus 5 mmHg), prompt referral should be made for evaluation and therapy. If the patient is symptomatic, immediate referral and treatment are indicated. Those patients with a compelling indication, as noted in Table 6 would be treated as the next higher category of hypertension.

## *Computation of Blood Pressure Percentiles*

To compute the SBP percentile of a boy who is aged *y* years and height *h* inches with SBP = *x* mmHg:

1. Refer to the most recent CDC growth charts, which are available online, and convert the height of *h* inches to a height Z-score relative to boys of the same age; this is denoted by Zht.
2. Compute the expected SBP ($\mu$) for boys of age *y* years and height *h* inches given by

$$\mu = \alpha + \sum_{j=1}^{4} \beta_j (y-10)^j + \sum_{k=1}^{4} \gamma_k (Zht)^k$$

   where $\alpha$, $\beta_1 \ldots$, $\beta_4$ and $\gamma_1 \ldots$, $\gamma_4$ are given in the third column of Table 2.

3. Then convert the boy's observed SBP to a Z-score (Zbp) given by Zbp = $(x - \mu)/\sigma$ where $\sigma$ is given in the third column of Table 2.
4. To convert the BP Z-score to a percentile (P) compute P = $\Phi$ (Zbp) × 100% where $\Phi$ (Z) = area under a standard normal distribution to the left of Z. Thus, if Zbp = 1.28, then $\Phi$ (Zbp) = .90 and the BP percetnile = .90 × 100% = 90%.
5. To compute percentiles for SBP for girls, DBP (K5) for boys, and DBP (K5) for girls, use the regression coefficients from the fourth, fifth, and sixth columns of Table 2.

   For example, a 12-yr-old boy, with height at the 90th percentile for his age-sex group, has a height Z-score = 1.28, and his expected SBP ($\mu$) is

   $\mu = 102.19768 + 1.82416(2) + 0.12776(2^2) + 0.00249(2^3) - 0.00135(2^4) + 2.73157(1.28) - 0.19618(1.28)^2 - 0.04659(1.28)^3 + 0.00947(1.28)^4 = 109.46$ mmHg

**Table 1**
**Oscillometric Mean Ambulatory BP Values in Healthy Children: Summary for Clinical Use**

| | | *24-h Percentile* | | *Daytime percentile*[c] | | *Nighttime percentile*[b] | |
|---|---|---|---|---|---|---|---|
| | *Height (cm) (n)* | *50th* | *95th* | *50th* | *95th* | *50th* | *95th* |
| *Boys* | | | | | | | |
| | 115–124.9 (33) | 105/65 | 113/72 | 112/73 | 123/85 | 95/55 | 104/63 |
| | 125–134.9 (62) | 105/65 | 117/75 | 113/73 | 125/85 | 96/55 | 107/65 |
| | 135–144.9 (102) | 107/65 | 121/77 | 114/73 | 127/85 | 97/55 | 110/67 |
| | 145–154.9 (108) | 109/66 | 124/78 | 115/73 | 129/85 | 99/56 | 113/67 |
| | 155–164.9 (115) | 112/66 | 126/78 | 118/73 | 132/85 | 102/56 | 116/67 |
| | 165–174.9 (83) | 115/67 | 128/77 | 121/73 | 135/85 | 104/56 | 119/67 |
| | 175–184.9 (69) | 120/67 | 130/77 | 124/73 | 137/85 | 107/56 | 122/67 |
| *Girls* | | | | | | | |
| | 115–124.9 (40) | 103/65 | 113/73 | 111/72 | 120/84 | 96/55 | 107/66 |
| | 125–134.9 (58) | 105/66 | 117/75 | 112/72 | 124/84 | 97/55 | 109/66 |
| | 135–144.9 (70) | 108/66 | 120/76 | 114/72 | 127/84 | 98/55 | 111/66 |
| | 145–154.9 (111) | 110/66 | 122/76 | 115/73 | 129/84 | 99/55 | 112/66 |
| | 155–164.9 (156) | 111/66 | 124/76 | 116/73 | 131/84 | 100/55 | 113/66 |
| | 165–174.9 (109) | 112/66 | 124/76 | 118/74 | 131/84 | 101/55 | 113/66 |
| | 175–184.9 (25) | 113/66 | 124/76 | 120/74 | 131/84 | 103/55 | 114/66 |

[a]Daytime: 8 AM to 8 PM
[b]Nighttime: midnight to 6 AM

Suppose his actual SBP is 120 mmHg (x); his SBP Z-score is then:

SBP Z-score = $(x - \mu)/\sigma = (120 - 109.46)/10.7128 = 0.984$

The corresponding SBP percentile = $\phi$ (0.984) × 100% = 83.7th percentile.

**Table 2**
**Regression Coefficients From Blood Pressure Regression Models[a]**

| *Variable name* | *Symbol* | *Systolic BP* | | *Diastolic BP5* | |
|---|---|---|---|---|---|
| | | *Male* | *Female* | *Male* | *Female* |
| Intercept | $\alpha$ | 102.19768 | 102.01027 | 61.01217 | 60.50510 |
| Age | | | | | |
| Age –10 | $\beta_1$ | 1.82416 | 1.94397 | 0.68314 | 1.01301 |
| $(Age -10)^2$ | $\beta_2$ | 0.12776 | 0.00598 | –0.09835 | 0.01157 |
| $(Age -10)^3$ | $\beta_3$ | 0.00249 | –0.00789 | 0.01711 | 0.00424 |
| $(Age -10)^4$ | $\beta_4$ | –0.00135 | –0.00059 | 0.00045 | –0.00137 |
| Normalized height | | | | | |
| Zht | $\gamma_1$ | 2.73157 | 2.03526 | 1.46993 | 1.16641 |
| $Zht^2$ | $\gamma_2$ | –0.19618 | 0.02534 | –0.07849 | 0.12795 |
| $Zht^3$ | $\gamma_3$ | –0.04659 | –0.01884 | –0.03144 | –0.03869 |
| $Zht^4$ | $\gamma_4$ | 0.00947 | 0.00121 | 0.00967 | -0.00079 |
| Standard deviation | $\sigma$ | 10.7128 | 10.4855 | 11.6032 | 10.9573 |
| $\rho$[b] | | 0.4100 | 0.3824 | 0.2436 | 0.2598 |
| n (persons) | | 32,161 | 31,066 | 24,057 | 23,443 |
| n (*visits*) | | *42,074* | *41,017* | *29,182* | *28,794* |

BP, blood pressure; Diastolic BP5, diastolic measurement at Korotkoff 5.

[a]Obtained from mixed effects linear regression models.

[b]The value of $\rho$ represents the correlation between BP measurements at different ages for the same child after correcting for age and Zht. This computation was necessary because some studies contributing to the childhood BP database provided BP at more than one age.

**Table 3**
**Blood Pressure Levels for Boys by Age and Height Percentile**

| *Age (yr)* | *BP percentile* | *Systolic BP (mmHg)* *Percentile of height* 5th | 10th | 25th | 50th | 75th | 90th | 95th | *Diastolic BP (mmHg)* *Percentile of height* 5th | 10th | 25th | 50th | 75th | 90th | 95th |
|---|---|---|---|---|---|---|---|---|---|---|---|---|---|---|---|
| 1 | 50th | 80 | 81 | 83 | 85 | 87 | 88 | 89 | 34 | 35 | 36 | 37 | 38 | 39 | 39 |
| | 90th | 94 | 95 | 97 | 99 | 100 | 102 | 103 | 49 | 50 | 51 | 52 | 53 | 53 | 54 |
| | 95th | 98 | 99 | 101 | 103 | 104 | 106 | 106 | 54 | 54 | 55 | 56 | 57 | 58 | 58 |
| | 99th | 105 | 106 | 108 | 110 | 112 | 113 | 114 | 61 | 62 | 63 | 64 | 65 | 66 | 66 |
| 2 | 50th | 84 | 85 | 87 | 88 | 90 | 92 | 92 | 39 | 40 | 41 | 42 | 43 | 44 | 44 |
| | 90th | 97 | 99 | 100 | 102 | 104 | 105 | 106 | 54 | 55 | 56 | 57 | 58 | 58 | 59 |
| | 95th | 101 | 102 | 104 | 106 | 108 | 109 | 110 | 59 | 59 | 60 | 61 | 62 | 63 | 63 |
| | 99th | 109 | 110 | 111 | 113 | 115 | 117 | 117 | 66 | 67 | 68 | 69 | 70 | 71 | 71 |
| 3 | 50th | 86 | 87 | 89 | 91 | 93 | 94 | 95 | 44 | 44 | 45 | 46 | 47 | 48 | 48 |
| | 90th | 100 | 101 | 103 | 105 | 107 | 108 | 109 | 59 | 59 | 60 | 61 | 62 | 63 | 63 |
| | 95th | 104 | 105 | 107 | 109 | 110 | 112 | 113 | 63 | 63 | 64 | 65 | 66 | 67 | 67 |

Table 3 (*continued*)

| Age (yr) | BP percentile | Systolic BP (mmHg) Percentile of height 5th | 10th | 25th | 50th | 75th | 90th | 95th | Diastolic BP (mmHg) Percentile of height 5th | 10th | 25th | 50th | 75th | 90th | 95th |
|---|---|---|---|---|---|---|---|---|---|---|---|---|---|---|---|
| | 99th | 111 | 112 | 114 | 116 | 118 | 119 | 120 | 71 | 71 | 72 | 73 | 74 | 75 | 75 |
| 4 | 50th | 88 | 89 | 91 | 93 | 95 | 96 | 97 | 47 | 48 | 49 | 50 | 51 | 51 | 52 |
| | 90th | 102 | 103 | 105 | 107 | 109 | 110 | 111 | 62 | 63 | 64 | 65 | 66 | 66 | 67 |
| | 95th | 106 | 107 | 109 | 111 | 1012 | 114 | 115 | 66 | 67 | 68 | 69 | 70 | 71 | 71 |
| | 99th | 113 | 114 | 116 | 118 | 120 | 121 | 122 | 74 | 75 | 76 | 77 | 78 | 78 | 79 |
| 5 | 50th | 90 | 91 | 93 | 95 | 96 | 98 | 98 | 50 | 51 | 52 | 53 | 54 | 55 | 55 |
| | 90th | 104 | 105 | 106 | 108 | 110 | 111 | 112 | 65 | 66 | 67 | 68 | 69 | 69 | 70 |
| | 95th | 108 | 109 | 110 | 112 | 114 | 115 | 116 | 69 | 70 | 71 | 72 | 73 | 74 | 74 |
| | 99th | 115 | 116 | 118 | 120 | 121 | 123 | 123 | 77 | 78 | 79 | 80 | 81 | 81 | 82 |
| 6 | 50th | 91 | 92 | 94 | 96 | 98 | 99 | 100 | 53 | 53 | 54 | 55 | 56 | 57 | 57 |
| | 90th | 105 | 106 | 108 | 110 | 111 | 113 | 113 | 68 | 68 | 69 | 70 | 71 | 72 | 72 |
| | 95th | 109 | 110 | 112 | 114 | 115 | 117 | 117 | 72 | 72 | 73 | 74 | 75 | 76 | 76 |
| | 99th | 116 | 117 | 119 | 121 | 123 | 124 | 125 | 80 | 80 | 81 | 82 | 83 | 84 | 84 |
| 7 | 50th | 92 | 94 | 95 | 97 | 99 | 100 | 101 | 55 | 55 | 56 | 57 | 58 | 59 | 59 |
| | 90th | 106 | 107 | 109 | 111 | 113 | 114 | 115 | 70 | 70 | 71 | 72 | 73 | 74 | 74 |
| | 95th | 110 | 111 | 113 | 115 | 117 | 118 | 119 | 74 | 74 | 75 | 76 | 77 | 78 | 78 |
| | 99th | 117 | 118 | 120 | 122 | 124 | 125 | 126 | 82 | 82 | 83 | 84 | 85 | 86 | 86 |
| 8 | 50th | 94 | 95 | 97 | 99 | 100 | 102 | 102 | 56 | 57 | 58 | 59 | 60 | 60 | 61 |
| | 90th | 107 | 109 | 110 | 112 | 114 | 115 | 116 | 71 | 72 | 72 | 73 | 74 | 75 | 76 |
| | 95th | 111 | 112 | 114 | 116 | 118 | 119 | 120 | 75 | 76 | 77 | 78 | 79 | 79 | 80 |
| | 99th | 119 | 120 | 122 | 123 | 125 | 127 | 127 | 83 | 84 | 85 | 86 | 87 | 87 | 88 |
| 9 | 50th | 95 | 96 | 98 | 100 | 102 | 103 | 104 | 57 | 58 | 59 | 60 | 61 | 61 | 62 |
| | 90th | 109 | 110 | 112 | 114 | 115 | 117 | 118 | 72 | 73 | 74 | 75 | 76 | 76 | 77 |
| | 95th | 113 | 114 | 116 | 118 | 119 | 121 | 121 | 76 | 77 | 78 | 79 | 80 | 81 | 81 |
| | 99th | 120 | 121 | 123 | 125 | 127 | 128 | 129 | 84 | 85 | 86 | 87 | 88 | 88 | 89 |
| 10 | 50th | 97 | 98 | 100 | 102 | 103 | 105 | 106 | 58 | 59 | 60 | 61 | 61 | 62 | 63 |
| | 90th | 111 | 112 | 114 | 115 | 117 | 119 | 119 | 73 | 73 | 74 | 75 | 76 | 77 | 78 |
| | 95th | 115 | 116 | 117 | 119 | 121 | 122 | 123 | 77 | 78 | 79 | 80 | 81 | 81 | 82 |
| | 99th | 122 | 123 | 125 | 127 | 128 | 130 | 130 | 85 | 86 | 86 | 88 | 88 | 89 | 90 |
| 11 | 50th | 99 | 100 | 102 | 104 | 105 | 107 | 107 | 59 | 59 | 60 | 61 | 62 | 63 | 63 |
| | 90th | 113 | 114 | 115 | 117 | 119 | 120 | 121 | 74 | 74 | 75 | 76 | 77 | 78 | 78 |
| | 95th | 117 | 118 | 119 | 121 | 123 | 124 | 125 | 78 | 78 | 79 | 80 | 81 | 82 | 82 |
| | 99th | 124 | 125 | 127 | 129 | 130 | 132 | 132 | 86 | 86 | 87 | 88 | 89 | 90 | 90 |
| 12 | 50th | 101 | 102 | 104 | 106 | 108 | 109 | 110 | 59 | 60 | 61 | 62 | 63 | 63 | 64 |
| | 90th | 115 | 116 | 118 | 120 | 121 | 123 | 123 | 74 | 75 | 75 | 76 | 77 | 78 | 79 |
| | 95th | 119 | 120 | 122 | 123 | 125 | 127 | 127 | 78 | 79 | 80 | 81 | 82 | 82 | 83 |
| | 99th | 126 | 127 | 129 | 131 | 133 | 134 | 135 | 86 | 87 | 88 | 89 | 90 | 90 | 91 |
| 13 | 50th | 104 | 105 | 106 | 108 | 110 | 111 | 112 | 60 | 60 | 61 | 62 | 63 | 64 | 64 |
| | 90th | 117 | 118 | 120 | 122 | 124 | 125 | 126 | 75 | 75 | 76 | 77 | 78 | 79 | 79 |
| | 95th | 121 | 122 | 124 | 126 | 128 | 129 | 130 | 79 | 79 | 80 | 81 | 82 | 83 | 83 |
| | 99th | 128 | 130 | 131 | 133 | 135 | 136 | 137 | 87 | 87 | 88 | 89 | 90 | 91 | 91 |
| 14 | 50th | 106 | 107 | 109 | 111 | 113 | 114 | 115 | 60 | 61 | 62 | 63 | 64 | 65 | 65 |
| | 90th | 120 | 121 | 123 | 125 | 126 | 128 | 128 | 75 | 76 | 77 | 78 | 79 | 79 | 80 |
| | 95th | 124 | 125 | 127 | 128 | 130 | 132 | 132 | 80 | 80 | 81 | 82 | 83 | 84 | 84 |

(*continued*)

Table 3 (*continued*)

| Age (yr) | BP percentile | Systolic BP (mmHg) Percentile of height 5th | 10th | 25th | 50th | 75th | 90th | 95th | Diastolic BP (mmHg) Percentile of height 5th | 10th | 25th | 50th | 75th | 90th | 95th |
|---|---|---|---|---|---|---|---|---|---|---|---|---|---|---|---|
| | 99th | 131 | 132 | 134 | 136 | 138 | 139 | 140 | 87 | 88 | 89 | 90 | 91 | 92 | 92 |
| 15 | 50th | 109 | 110 | 112 | 113 | 115 | 117 | 117 | 61 | 62 | 63 | 64 | 65 | 66 | 66 |
| | 90th | 122 | 124 | 125 | 127 | 129 | 130 | 131 | 76 | 77 | 78 | 79 | 80 | 80 | 81 |
| | 95th | 126 | 127 | 129 | 131 | 133 | 134 | 135 | 81 | 81 | 82 | 83 | 84 | 85 | 85 |
| | 99th | 134 | 135 | 136 | 138 | 140 | 142 | 142 | 88 | 89 | 90 | 91 | 92 | 93 | 93 |
| 16 | 50th | 111 | 112 | 114 | 116 | 118 | 119 | 120 | 63 | 63 | 64 | 65 | 66 | 67 | 67 |
| | 90th | 125 | 126 | 128 | 130 | 131 | 133 | 134 | 78 | 78 | 79 | 80 | 81 | 82 | 82 |
| | 95th | 129 | 130 | 132 | 134 | 135 | 137 | 137 | 82 | 83 | 83 | 84 | 85 | 86 | 87 |
| | 99th | 136 | 137 | 139 | 141 | 143 | 144 | 145 | 90 | 90 | 91 | 92 | 93 | 94 | 94 |
| 17 | 50th | 114 | 115 | 116 | 118 | 120 | 121 | 122 | 65 | 66 | 66 | 67 | 68 | 69 | 70 |
| | 90th | 127 | 128 | 130 | 132 | 134 | 135 | 136 | 80 | 80 | 81 | 82 | 83 | 84 | 84 |
| | 95th | 131 | 132 | 134 | 136 | 138 | 139 | 140 | 84 | 85 | 86 | 87 | 87 | 88 | 89 |
| | 99th | 139 | 140 | 141 | 143 | 145 | 146 | 147 | 92 | 93 | 93 | 94 | 95 | 96 | 97 |

BP, blood pressure.

The 90th percentile is 1.28 standard deviation (SD), 95th percentile is 1.645 SD, and the 99th percentile is 2.326 SD over the mean.

For research purposes, the standard deviations in Table 2 allow one to compute BP Z-scores and percentiles for boys with height percentiles given in Table 3 (i.e., the 5th,10th, 25th, 50th, 75th, 90th, and 95th percentiles). These height percentiles must be converted to height Z-scores given by (5% = –1.645; 10% = –1.28; 25% = –0.68; 50% = 0; 75% = 0.68; 90% = 1.28%; 95% = 1.645) and then computed according to the methodology in steps 2–4 as previously described in "Computation of Blood Pressure Percentiles." For children with height percentiles other than these, follow steps 1–4.

Table 4
Blood Pressure Levels for Girls by Age and Height Percentile

| Age (yr) | BP percentile | Systolic BP (mmHg) Percentile of height 5th | 10th | 25th | 50th | 75th | 90th | 95th | Diastolic BP (mmHg) Percentile of height 5th | 10th | 25th | 50th | 75th | 90th | 95th |
|---|---|---|---|---|---|---|---|---|---|---|---|---|---|---|---|
| 1 | 50th | 83 | 84 | 85 | 86 | 88 | 89 | 90 | 38 | 39 | 39 | 40 | 41 | 41 | 42 |
| | 90th | 97 | 97 | 98 | 100 | 101 | 102 | 103 | 52 | 53 | 53 | 54 | 55 | 55 | 56 |
| | 95th | 100 | 101 | 102 | 104 | 105 | 106 | 107 | 56 | 57 | 57 | 58 | 59 | 59 | 60 |
| | 99th | 108 | 108 | 109 | 111 | 112 | 113 | 114 | 64 | 64 | 65 | 65 | 66 | 67 | 67 |
| 2 | 50th | 85 | 85 | 87 | 88 | 89 | 91 | 91 | 43 | 44 | 44 | 45 | 46 | 46 | 47 |
| | 90th | 98 | 99 | 100 | 101 | 103 | 104 | 105 | 57 | 58 | 58 | 59 | 60 | 61 | 61 |
| | 95th | 102 | 103 | 104 | 105 | 107 | 108 | 109 | 61 | 62 | 62 | 63 | 64 | 65 | 65 |
| | 99th | 109 | 110 | 111 | 112 | 114 | 115 | 116 | 69 | 69 | 70 | 70 | 71 | 72 | 72 |
| 3 | 50th | 86 | 87 | 88 | 89 | 91 | 92 | 93 | 47 | 48 | 48 | 49 | 50 | 50 | 51 |
| | 90th | 100 | 100 | 102 | 103 | 104 | 106 | 106 | 61 | 62 | 62 | 63 | 64 | 64 | 65 |
| | 95th | 104 | 104 | 105 | 107 | 108 | 109 | 110 | 65 | 66 | 66 | 67 | 68 | 68 | 69 |
| | 99th | 111 | 111 | 113 | 114 | 115 | 116 | 117 | 73 | 73 | 74 | 74 | 75 | 76 | 76 |

Table 4 (*continued*)

| | | *Systolic BP (mmHg)* | | | | | | | *Diastolic BP (mmHg)* | | | | | | |
|---|---|---|---|---|---|---|---|---|---|---|---|---|---|---|---|
| | | *Percentile of height* | | | | | | | *Percentile of height* | | | | | | |
| *Age (yr)* | *BP percentile* | *5th* | *10th* | *25th* | *50th* | *75th* | *90th* | *95th* | *5th* | *10th* | *25th* | *50th* | *75th* | *90th* | *95th* |
| 4 | 50th | 88 | 88 | 90 | 91 | 92 | 94 | 94 | 50 | 50 | 51 | 52 | 52 | 53 | 54 |
| | 90th | 101 | 102 | 103 | 104 | 106 | 107 | 108 | 64 | 64 | 65 | 66 | 67 | 67 | 68 |
| | 95th | 105 | 106 | 107 | 108 | 110 | 111 | 112 | 68 | 68 | 69 | 70 | 71 | 71 | 72 |
| | 99th | 112 | 113 | 114 | 115 | 117 | 118 | 119 | 76 | 76 | 76 | 77 | 78 | 79 | 79 |
| 5 | 50th | 89 | 90 | 91 | 93 | 94 | 95 | 96 | 52 | 53 | 53 | 54 | 55 | 55 | 56 |
| | 90th | 103 | 103 | 105 | 106 | 107 | 109 | 109 | 66 | 67 | 67 | 68 | 69 | 69 | 70 |
| | 95th | 107 | 107 | 108 | 110 | 111 | 112 | 113 | 70 | 71 | 71 | 72 | 73 | 73 | 74 |
| | 99th | 114 | 114 | 116 | 117 | 118 | 120 | 120 | 78 | 78 | 79 | 79 | 80 | 81 | 81 |
| 6 | 50th | 91 | 92 | 93 | 94 | 96 | 97 | 98 | 54 | 54 | 55 | 56 | 56 | 57 | 58 |
| | 90th | 104 | 105 | 106 | 108 | 109 | 110 | 111 | 68 | 68 | 69 | 70 | 70 | 71 | 72 |
| | 95th | 108 | 109 | 110 | 111 | 113 | 114 | 115 | 72 | 72 | 73 | 74 | 74 | 75 | 76 |
| | 99th | 115 | 116 | 117 | 119 | 120 | 121 | 122 | 80 | 80 | 80 | 81 | 82 | 83 | 83 |
| 7 | 50th | 93 | 93 | 95 | 96 | 97 | 99 | 99 | 55 | 56 | 56 | 57 | 58 | 58 | 59 |
| | 90th | 106 | 107 | 108 | 109 | 111 | 112 | 113 | 69 | 70 | 70 | 71 | 72 | 72 | 73 |
| | 95th | 110 | 111 | 112 | 113 | 115 | 116 | 116 | 73 | 74 | 74 | 75 | 76 | 76 | 77 |
| | 99th | 117 | 118 | 119 | 120 | 122 | 123 | 124 | 81 | 81 | 82 | 82 | 83 | 84 | 84 |
| 8 | 50th | 95 | 95 | 96 | 98 | 99 | 100 | 101 | 57 | 57 | 57 | 58 | 59 | 60 | 60 |
| | 90th | 108 | 109 | 110 | 111 | 113 | 114 | 114 | 71 | 71 | 71 | 72 | 73 | 74 | 74 |
| | 95th | 112 | 112 | 114 | 115 | 116 | 118 | 118 | 75 | 75 | 75 | 76 | 77 | 78 | 78 |
| | 99th | 119 | 120 | 121 | 122 | 123 | 125 | 125 | 82 | 82 | 83 | 83 | 84 | 85 | 86 |
| 9 | 50th | 96 | 97 | 98 | 100 | 101 | 102 | 103 | 58 | 58 | 58 | 59 | 60 | 61 | 61 |
| | 90th | 110 | 110 | 112 | 113 | 114 | 116 | 116 | 72 | 72 | 72 | 73 | 74 | 75 | 75 |
| | 95th | 114 | 114 | 115 | 117 | 118 | 119 | 120 | 76 | 76 | 76 | 77 | 78 | 79 | 79 |
| | 99th | 121 | 121 | 123 | 124 | 125 | 127 | 127 | 83 | 83 | 84 | 84 | 85 | 86 | 87 |
| 10 | 50th | 98 | 99 | 100 | 102 | 103 | 104 | 105 | 59 | 59 | 59 | 60 | 61 | 62 | 62 |
| | 90th | 112 | 112 | 114 | 115 | 116 | 118 | 118 | 73 | 73 | 73 | 74 | 75 | 76 | 76 |
| | 95th | 116 | 116 | 117 | 119 | 120 | 121 | 122 | 77 | 77 | 77 | 78 | 79 | 80 | 80 |
| | 99th | 123 | 123 | 125 | 126 | 127 | 129 | 129 | 84 | 84 | 85 | 86 | 86 | 87 | 88 |
| 11 | 50th | 100 | 101 | 102 | 103 | 105 | 106 | 107 | 60 | 60 | 60 | 61 | 62 | 63 | 63 |
| | 90th | 114 | 114 | 116 | 117 | 118 | 119 | 120 | 74 | 74 | 74 | 75 | 76 | 77 | 77 |
| | 95th | 118 | 118 | 119 | 121 | 122 | 123 | 124 | 78 | 78 | 78 | 79 | 80 | 81 | 81 |
| | 99th | 125 | 125 | 126 | 128 | 129 | 130 | 131 | 85 | 85 | 86 | 87 | 87 | 88 | 89 |
| 12 | 50th | 102 | 103 | 104 | 105 | 107 | 108 | 109 | 61 | 61 | 61 | 62 | 63 | 64 | 64 |
| | 90th | 116 | 116 | 117 | 119 | 120 | 121 | 122 | 75 | 75 | 75 | 76 | 77 | 78 | 78 |
| | 95th | 119 | 120 | 121 | 123 | 124 | 125 | 126 | 79 | 79 | 79 | 80 | 81 | 82 | 82 |
| | 99th | 127 | 127 | 128 | 130 | 131 | 132 | 133 | 86 | 86 | 87 | 88 | 88 | 89 | 90 |
| 13 | 50th | 104 | 105 | 106 | 107 | 109 | 110 | 110 | 62 | 62 | 62 | 63 | 64 | 65 | 65 |
| | 90th | 117 | 118 | 119 | 121 | 122 | 123 | 124 | 76 | 76 | 76 | 77 | 78 | 79 | 79 |
| | 95th | 121 | 122 | 123 | 124 | 126 | 127 | 128 | 80 | 80 | 80 | 81 | 82 | 83 | 83 |
| | 99th | 128 | 129 | 130 | 132 | 133 | 134 | 135 | 87 | 87 | 88 | 89 | 89 | 90 | 91 |
| 14 | 50th | 106 | 106 | 107 | 109 | 110 | 111 | 112 | 63 | 63 | 63 | 64 | 65 | 66 | 66 |
| | 90th | 119 | 120 | 121 | 122 | 124 | 125 | 125 | 77 | 77 | 77 | 78 | 79 | 80 | 80 |
| | 95th | 123 | 123 | 125 | 126 | 127 | 129 | 129 | 81 | 81 | 81 | 82 | 83 | 84 | 84 |

(*continued*)

Table 4 (*continued*)

| Age (yr) | BP percentile | Systolic BP (mmHg) Percentile of height 5th | 10th | 25th | 50th | 75th | 90th | 95th | Diastolic BP (mmHg) Percentile of height 5th | 10th | 25th | 50th | 75th | 90th | 95th |
|---|---|---|---|---|---|---|---|---|---|---|---|---|---|---|---|
| | 99th | 130 | 131 | 132 | 133 | 135 | 136 | 136 | 88 | 88 | 89 | 90 | 90 | 91 | 92 |
| 15 | 50th | 107 | 108 | 109 | 110 | 111 | 113 | 113 | 64 | 64 | 64 | 65 | 66 | 67 | 67 |
| | 90th | 120 | 121 | 122 | 123 | 125 | 126 | 127 | 78 | 78 | 78 | 79 | 80 | 81 | 81 |
| | 95th | 124 | 125 | 126 | 127 | 129 | 130 | 131 | 82 | 82 | 82 | 83 | 84 | 85 | 85 |
| | 99th | 131 | 132 | 133 | 134 | 136 | 137 | 138 | 89 | 89 | 90 | 91 | 91 | 92 | 93 |
| 16 | 50th | 108 | 108 | 110 | 111 | 112 | 114 | 114 | 64 | 64 | 65 | 66 | 66 | 67 | 68 |
| | 90th | 121 | 122 | 123 | 124 | 126 | 127 | 128 | 78 | 78 | 79 | 80 | 81 | 81 | 82 |
| | 95th | 125 | 126 | 127 | 128 | 130 | 131 | 132 | 82 | 82 | 83 | 84 | 85 | 85 | 86 |
| | 99th | 132 | 133 | 134 | 135 | 137 | 138 | 139 | 90 | 90 | 90 | 91 | 92 | 93 | 93 |
| 17 | 50th | 108 | 109 | 110 | 111 | 113 | 114 | 115 | 64 | 65 | 65 | 66 | 67 | 67 | 68 |
| | 90th | 122 | 122 | 123 | 125 | 126 | 127 | 128 | 78 | 79 | 79 | 80 | 81 | 81 | 82 |
| | 95th | 125 | 126 | 127 | 129 | 130 | 131 | 132 | 82 | 83 | 83 | 84 | 85 | 85 | 86 |
| | 99th | 133 | 133 | 134 | 136 | 137 | 138 | 139 | 90 | 90 | 91 | 91 | 92 | 93 | 93 |

BP, blood pressure.

The 90th percentile is 1.28 standard deviation (SD), 95th percentile is 1.645 SD, and the 99th percentile is 2.326 SD over the mean.

For research purposes, the standard deviations in Table 2 allow one to compute BP Z-scores and percentiles for girls with height percentiles given in Table 4 (i.e., the 5th,10th, 25th, 50th, 75th, 90th, and 95th percentiles). These height percentiles ust be converted to height Z-scores given by (5% = –1.645; 10% = –1.28; 25% = –0.68; 50% = 0; 75% = 0.68; 90% = 1.28%; 95% = 1.645) and then computed according to the methodology in steps 2–4 as previously described in "Computation of Blood Pressure Percentiles." For children with height percentiles other than these, follow steps 1–4.

**Table 5**
**Classification of Hypertension in Children and Adolescents, With Measurement Frequency and Therapy Recommendations**

| | *SBP or DBP percentile*[a] | *Frequency of BP measurement* | *Therapeutic lifestyle changes* | *Pharmacologic therapy* |
|---|---|---|---|---|
| Normal | <90th | Recheck at next scheduled physical examination | Encourage healthy diet, sleep, and exercise | — |
| Prehypertension | 90th to <95th or if BP exceeds 120/80 even if below 90th percentile up to <95th percentile[b] | Recheck in 6 mo | Weight management counseling if overweight, introduce exercise and diet management | None unless compelling indications such as CKD, diabetes mellitus, heart failure, LVH |
| Stage 1 hypertension | 95th percentile to the 99th | Recheck in 1–2 wk; if persistently elevated | Weight management counseling if | Initiate therapy based on |

Table 5 (*continued*)

| | *SBP or DBP percentile*[a] | *Frequency of BP measurement* | *Therapeutic lifestyle changes* | *Pharmacologic therapy* |
|---|---|---|---|---|
| | percentile plus 5 mmHg | on two additional occasions, evaluate or refer to source of care within 1 mo or sooner if the patient is symptomatic | overweight, introduce exercise and diet management | indications in Table 6 or if compelling indications as above |
| Stage 2 hypertension | >99th percentile plus 5 mmHg | Evaluate or refer to source of care within 1 wk or immediately if the patient is symptomatic | Weight management counseling if overweight, introduce exercise and diet management | Initiate therapy[c] |

BP, blood pressure; CKD, chronic kidney disease; DBP, diastolic blood pressure; LVH, left ventricular hypertrophy; SBP, systolic blood pressure.

[a]For sex, age, and height measured on at least three separate occasions; if systolic and diastolic categories are different, categorize by the higher value.

[b]This occurs typically at 12 yr old for SBP and at 16 yr old for DBP.

[c]Frequently, more than one medication is required.

Table 6
**Indications for Antihypertensive Drug Therapy in Children**

| |
|---|
| Symptomatic hypertension |
| Secondary hypertension |
| Hypertensive target-organ damage |
| Diabetes (Types I and II) |
| Persistent hypertension despite nonpharmacologic measures |

# Index

**D**